INTERVENTIONS FOR STUDENTS WITH LEARNING DISABILITIES

Interventions for Students with Learning Disabilities

A Meta-Analysis of Treatment Outcomes

H. LEE SWANSON

with Maureen Hoskyn and Carole Lee

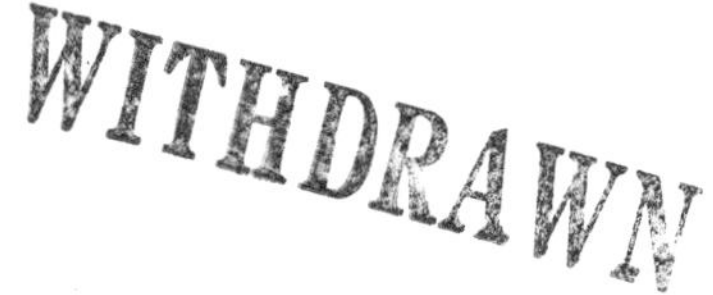

THE GUILFORD PRESS
New York London

A Division of Guilford Publications, Inc.
72 Spring Street, New York, NY 10012
http://www.guilford.com

Printed in the United States of America

This book is printed on acid-free paper.

Last digit is print number: 9 8 7 6 5 4 3 2 1

Library of Congress Cataloging-in-Publication Data
available from the Publisher.

ISBN 1-57230-449-9

About the Authors

H. Lee Swanson, PhD, is professor of educational psychology at the University of California at Riverside. His research interests focus on learning disabilities and memory. He served as editor of the *Learning Disabilities Quarterly* from 1989 to 1997.

Maureen Hoskyn, MA, is completing her doctorate in educational psychology, focusing on working memory and writing. She has served as a special education classroom teacher and school psychologist in Vancouver and Victoria, British Columbia.

Carole Lee, PhD, is currently the director of evaluation in the Fontana, California, school district. Her research expertise includes learning disabilities, working memory, and mathematical problem solving.

Acknowledgments

This book had its origins in a discussion with Drs. Karen Harris and Steve Graham, of the University of Maryland, and Chris Jennison, editor at The Guilford Press. I appreciate their encouragement through the various stages of this project. I am indebted to our research consultant, Dr. Harris Cooper, of the University of Missouri, who provided critical technical assistance throughout this project. The comprehensive meta-analysis of intervention research for students with learning disabilities reported in this volume was supported by a U.S. Department of Education Grant (No. H023E40014), the Chesapeake Institute, and Peloy Endowment Funds. I am deeply indebted to the assistance of two superb research associates, Carole Lee and Maureen Hoskyn, who invested over two years in the project. They labored on all aspects of data entry, coding, and recoding. Maureen played a major role in analyzing the subgroups in Chapter 3 and Carole played a major role in developing Appendix E. I would also like to thank Dr. Tam O'Shaugnessy, Georgia State University, who had a major part in the descriptive analysis of reading for studies that used single-subject designs (Chapter 4). I am also deeply indebted to Kathy Mattson, who transcribed tapes and all my hieroglyphics into coherent prose. Special appreciation is also given to Colleen M. McMahon for establishing the reliability of the coding scheme and participating in the early stages of this project. I am appreciative of additional coding assistance from graduate students Albert Restori, Jan Ruffner, Elissa McLaughlin-Cheng, Christi Carson, Bonnie Kraemer, Tam O'Shaughnessy, and Brian Murray from the University of California—Riverside. I am particularly appreciative of extensive comments made by Drs. Ellen Schiller, U.S. Department of Education; Bernice Wong, Simon Fraser University; Phil Winne, Simon Frasier University; Steve Forness, UCLA; Sharon Vaughn, University of Texas; Ed Kameenui, University of Oregon; and Reid Lyon, National Institute of Child Health and Human Development, on an earlier draft of this synthesis. The views reflected in this volume are my own, and do not necessarily reflect those of the U.S. Department of Education, the Chesapeake Institute, or the reviewers noted above.

H. LEE SWANSON

Contents

INTERVENTIONS FOR STUDENTS WITH LEARNING DISABILITIES

Introduction and Overview

The book provides a technical comprehensive report on approximately 30 years of intervention research for students with learning disabilities. The text follows a typical research organizational format that provides a justification for the synthesis (Chapter 1), describes the methods of analysis (Chapter 2), details the results (Chapters 3 and 4), and then concludes with a discussion of the most important findings (Chapter 5) and another on their implications (Chapter 6). The intended audience for this book is researchers and graduate students interested in learning disabled (LD) students. The text assumes graduate-level training in research design, as well as some familiarity with the field of learning disabilities.

The text details the procedures of analysis, summarizes the studies reviewed, and discusses the effect size for each study, coding formats, and so on for interested researchers. The procedure used throughout this text is meta-analysis. Simply stated, meta-analysis is a statistical reviewing technique that provides a quantitative summary of findings across an entire body of research. The results of individual studies are converted to a standardized metric or effect size (to be discussed in the text). Before I provide an overview of the text, I want to provide a little personal background for the reader regarding this project.

This work was originally motivated by a need to share with parents and teachers instructional programs that have been experimentally shown to work for LD students. Many a time I have shared the results of standardized and informal testing information on children suspected of having learning disabilities in school meetings with their teachers and/or parents. Parents have often asked me, "What would you recommend as an approach to help my child experience some academic success?" or said something like "We have tried several tutoring programs, but my child continues to get further behind and . . . I don't know what teaching approach works for a child like mine, do you?" Likewise, I have been asked by teachers, "What does research say about the reading or math approaches that work best for children with learning disabilities?" Questions such as these from professionals who work with students with learning disabilities require research-based answers. Thus, it seems very important at the practical level to dissect what the available research tells us about teaching LD children.

Although several practical questions directed my interest toward summarizing the intervention literature, the project was "hatched" from a preliminary synthesis carried out in collaboration with Cristi Carson, one of my doctoral students. Two things happened thanks to this earlier work with Cristi. One, Cristi never did an independent study with me again. I sensed some negative opinion on her part about the quality of research in the field of learning disabilities, as well as an aversion to meta-analysis research (to be discussed in Chapter 1) because it is labor-intensive work that may not yield results of theoretical import (i.e., the findings are only as good as the primary studies). Two, I discovered that we had only begun to scratch the surface in terms of uncovering what intervention research tells us. My work with Cristi left several questions unanswered. For example, Why is it that every intervention discussed in the literature seems to work? Or, What role does experimental intervention research have, if any, for policymakers and teachers? In my quest to answer these and other nagging questions, I was able to solicit, thanks to grant money, help from another doctoral student, Carole Lee, who summarized the various treatment studies for me. This preliminary work with Cristi and Carole was reported in *School Psychology Review* in 1996.

Based on this preliminary work, I submitted an application for a grant to the U.S. Department of Education. In my application I proposed to synthesize all the intervention literature published since the field's official inception (1963). I soon received proverbial "good news and bad news." The good news, much to my surprise, was that the U.S. Department of Education was willing to fund my grandiose scheme. The bad news was that all the work had to be completed within 2 years. During the first year of the project, four doctoral student assistants burned out while working for me. They were exhausted and frustrated by complex coding demands, interrater checks on the accuracy of their coding, long hours, and, frankly, the evaluation of methodological issues within studies not necessarily reflected in their current course work. I held weekly meetings with my assistants to address these issues, provide instruction, and keep up morale. To compound these problems, the U.S. Department of Education insisted that I submit a preliminary report within 14 months of starting this huge project. Dr. Ellen Schiller at the U.S. Department of Education was tremendously encouraging through all stages of the project. However, she demanded several external reviews of our preliminary report. Although I was allowed to select the reviewers, the reviewers I chose reflected a continuum of theoretical orientations and perspectives that no single report could satisfy. Based on their extensive feedback, however, I was left with the task of completely rewriting the final report. I say *I* for several reasons. First, I "lost" my two major research assistants. Maureen

Hoskyn's visa expired, so she had to return home to Canada and her teaching position there. Carole Lee had to shift her attention to finishing her dissertation within the time frame imposed by the university. Although both Maureen and Carole were deeply committed to my project, they couldn't afford to work for nothing after my grant funds ran out. Fortunately, thanks to Ellen Schiller and Mike Kane from the Chesapeake Institute, I received additional funds for Maureen and Carole to finish the coding of studies, which they did. Second, my co-principal investigator went on sick leave, and then on sabbatical. Thus, I was left with the task of analyzing all the coded data and writing the final report. I don't think I completed one other writing project during the 8 months it took me to write the final report, which is published here. Although I use the word "we" in the universal sense throughout the text, all errors of analysis are my own and do not reflect those of my research staff.

I will now provide an "advanced organizer" of what we did and what we found as the reader proceeds through the text. The text is divided into six chapters. The first chapter provides a justification for the review and formulates three general questions that directed the synthesis. These questions focused on (1) determining the best interventions, (2) determining the role of instructional domain (reading, mathematics, spelling) on treatment outcome, and (3) determining the role of sample variations, that is, aptitude, on treatment outcome.

Chapter 2 discusses in detail the methodology for synthesizing the literature. The project started as a search of all relevant literature identified from four online databases: (1) ERIC, a database of educational reports, evaluations, and research maintained by the Educational Research Information Center; (2) PsycLIT, a review of psychological journals; (3) MEDline, a review of all medical literature; and (4) comprehensive dissertation abstracts. Descriptors for the online search included "learning disabilities," "reading disabilities," "dyslexia," and related categories (e.g., "educationally handicapped") paired with the terms "instruction," "intervention," "remediation," "materials," and other related descriptors (e.g., "training"). In addition, all state departments and selected authors were sent letters requesting published or unpublished documents on intervention studies that utilized LD participants.

Studies in the synthesis had to meet four criteria. First, each study had to include LD students of (1) average intelligence who received intervention over a period of time (a minimum of three sessions) and (2) who were assigned to experimental and/or (depending on methodology) control instructional conditions. Second, each study had to include information on selection criteria for students with learning disabilities. Third, each study had to measure treatment outcomes quantitatively. Finally, the studies had to show no severe methodological flaw (e.g., results of control group were not reported, incorrect degrees of freedom).

Chapters 3 and 4 detail the search for relationships between study characteristics and study outcomes. Chapter 3 focuses on those relationships for group designs, and Chapter 4 focuses on those studies that rely on single-subject or time-series designs. The chapters indicate that the meta-analytic review include 272 intervention studies. Approximately 930 studies were identified as reporting

data, but only a third of these studies could be analyzed for effect sizes. Effect sizes for 180 group design and 85 single-subject design intervention studies were analyzed across instructional domains (e.g., reading, mathematics), sample characteristics (e.g., age, intelligence), intervention parameters (e.g., number of instructional sessions, instructional components), methodological procedures (e.g., internal validity, treatment integrity, random assignment), and article characteristics (e.g., funding source, number of coauthors, frequency of citations).

Chapter 5 provides a detailed analysis of the findings. The reader less interested in methodology, may want to read this chapter first. Some of the important findings highlighted in this chapter include the following:

1. *The magnitude of change is greater in some academic domains than others.* Based on Cohen's criteria of .80 effect size as a substantive finding, and when controlling for variations in methodology, only studies in the domains of reading comprehension, vocabulary, and creativity approached Cohen's .80 threshold for a large effect. For single-subject design studies (to be discussed), all domain areas except handwriting yield effect sizes at or above the .80 threshold.

2. *Not all treatments are equally effective.* A Combined Model that includes components of direct instruction and strategy instruction is an effective procedure for remediating learning disabilities when compared to other models. The instructional components that make up this treatment include attention to sequencing, drill–repetition–practice, segmentation and then synthesis of information, directed response and questioning, control of task difficulty, technology, the teacher systematically modeling problem-solving steps, making use of small interactive groups, and strategy cuing.

3. *Treatment effects are specific to the academic problems being addressed.* The Combined Model was more effective than competing models across academic domains. However, effect sizes were higher across measures of reading. Within the domain of reading, however, the effectiveness of the Combined Model is most pronounced on reading comprehension measures when compared to word recognition measures.

4. *LD children were closer in performance to non-learning-disabled (NLD) children when the treatment conditions included strategy instructions.* The results indicated that effect size differences between LD and NLD children were significantly smaller when LD children were exposed to treatments that included strategy conditions than when compared to competing treatment conditions (e.g., direct instruction).

5. *Variations in the definitions of learning disabilities influence treatment outcome.* The results suggest that studies that meet cutoff score criteria (IQ at or above 84 and reading scores below the 25th percentile) qualify treatment effects. For both group and single-subject design studies, the Combined Model yields higher effect sizes when cutoff scores can be computed than when cutoff scores cannot be computed.

6. *Variations in methodology have a significant impact on treatment outcomes.* Interventions that vary from the control condition in terms of setting, teacher, and number of instructional steps yield larger effect sizes than studies that fail to control

for such variations. A serious threat to interpreting treatment effects across group design and single-subject design studies occurred when studies "stacked" the treatment condition with substantially more steps and procedures than the control condition.

Chapter 6 discusses the implications of the findings. One of the most important implications relates to instruction. The results are supportive of the pervasive influence of strategy instruction and direct instruction models for remediating learning disabilities. However, the results also suggest that a Combined Model (which includes the instructional components related to controlling task difficulty, small group instruction, and structured verbal interaction) is a viable heuristic for positively influencing treatment outcomes. Chapter 6 also provides suggestions for developing principles of instruction and making applications to policy issues.

Chapter 1

Purpose and Perspective

In this chapter we will review the issues that justify the need for a comprehensive synthesis of intervention literature for children and adults with learning disabilities. We review the historical and contemporary context of intervention research and then lay a foundation for the research questions that direct this synthesis. The chapter addresses (1) historical and contemporary intervention research issues, (2) problems with previous meta-analyses, (3) procedures of direct and strategy instruction, and (4) major questions directing the current synthesis.

WHY DO A SYNTHESIS?

The number of children classified as learning disabled has increased substantially over the last 20 years. For example, 783,000 children were identified with learning disabilities in 1976, but by 1992–1993, the LD population exceeded 2.3 million. These children currently comprise almost 50% of all placements into special education (U.S. Office of Education, 1994). Although students with learning disabilities is the largest category of students receiving special education, questions such as "Which intervention is best suited for LD students?" or, more appropriately, "Which intervention works best for the type of learning problem experienced by the LD student?" cannot be answered. This is unfortunate because policy issues (such as "where" or "how" educational intervention should occur) related to instruction for LD students will not be resolved without a clear understanding of intervention research (Martin, 1988; also see Bateman, 1992; Graham & Harris, 1996; Hallahan, 1992; and Scruggs & Mastropieri, 1993, for a review). Kameenui (1991) recently assessed progress in the LD field, stating that "although we have made progress in recognizing the complexity of learning disabilities as a psychological, historical, and theoretical construct, very little progress has been made in recognizing . . . important developments of intervention for students with learning disabilities" (p. 365). Furthermore, a review of the LD literature reveals few systematic, quantitative (or qualitative) analyses of instructional approaches for students who are learning disabled (Lessen, Dudzinski, Karsh, & Van Acker, 1989). For example, Lessen et al. (1989) wrote one of the few comprehensive reviews of intervention research published on LD samples since 1973 (see Chalfant & Scheffelin, 1969; Hallahan & Cruickshank, 1973; and Kass, 1970, for a review of intervention studies prior to 1970). Lessen et al. (1989) suggested that "academic intervention research is crucial so that systematic analysis of a student's performance . . . should dictate teaching procedures, methods, and materials" (p. 107). Unfortunately, we have no clear understanding of the intervention approaches that work with a particular type of LD child as a consequence of gender, age, intelligence, and/or level of achievement.

Clearly, students with learning disabilities are a heterogeneous sample and no general treatment approach can be recommended for all of them. However, as a partial response to the concerns noted above, our purpose in this text is to synthesize the empirical evidence derived from educational interventions for LD students. We assume that without an attempt to sort and choose studies on the basis of method, treatment variants, respondents, and the like, very few conclusions can be drawn about intervention procedures that yield positive outcomes unique to the learning disabled. Recent narrative reviews of instructional research on learning disabilities, although of practical import, have been limited by their reliance on a narrow sample of interventions, domains (e.g., perceptual processing, social skills), and/or techniques to analyze studies.

Besides practical issues related to instruction, there are also theoretical reasons why a comprehensive synthesis of intervention research in the field of learning disabilities is needed. Intervention studies can test conceptual models or frameworks for understanding learning disabilities. One conceptual model that has achieved some consensus in the field is that LD children are of normal intelligence, but suffer information-processing difficulties (e.g., Borkowski, Estrada, Milstead, & Hale, 1989; Deshler & Shumaker, 1988; Fletcher et al., 1994; Stanovich & Siegel, 1994; Swanson & Alexander, 1997). A popular assumption that has emerged in the last few years is that LD children have specific processing deficits that are localized to low-order processes, particularly phonological coding (e.g., Francis, Shaywitz, Stuebing, Shaywitz, & Fletcher, 1996; Siegel, 1992; Stanovich & Siegel, 1994). Phonological processing is "the association between sounds with letters, that is, the understanding of the grapheme–phoneme conversion rules and the exceptions to these rules" (Siegel, 1993, p. 38). This assumption finds some consensus in the field because reading problems are pervasive in LD populations, and there is a plethora of research that suggests phonological coding underlies most of these problems (see Siegel, 1993, for a review). Although this may be true, no synthesis of intervention studies has been carried out to determine if specific processes or skills related to reading are more resistant to change than other academic domains. Thus, the common assumption that processing deficits underlie the poor performance of LD students, and therefore that one would expect some resistance to change in specific domains (such as reading) as a function of treatment, when compared to other domains (e.g., social skills), has not been tested. This is interesting in light of the fact that information processing and reading are sometimes seen as interactive with several other processes, and therefore processes that contribute to reading are seen by some researchers as neither top-down nor bottom-up in nature (see Frederiksen, 1981, and Rumelhart, 1977; then see Adams, 1990, and Seidenberg & McClelland, 1989, for a review).

To date, the characteristics and unique aptitudes of children with learning disabilities as a function of instruction are almost entirely based on research conducted within single testing sessions. In any given session, such research could yield an ambiguous mix of results: LD children's performance as a function of instruction remains lower than the performance of non-learning-disabled (NLD) children, LD children catch up to NLD children, or treatment effects yield inconclusive results. Intervention research based on the manipulation of psychological and educational variables that are intended to induce changes in learning over an extended time period can clarify such findings. More specifically, if (1) the deficient processes attributed to learning disabilities are compensated for and/or directly changed via an instructional approach, (2) the outcomes are predicted, (3) the correlates of the study match or parallel theoretical models derived from replicated laboratory findings, and (4) the intervention study meets the assumptions of statistical power, internal validity, and controlled artifacts (e.g., sampling error, reliability of dependent measures), then additional (or lack of) support can be found for the theoretical model under investigation. Thus, the stability of the construct under investigation is better studied over time rather than in isolated sessions (see Eagly & Wood, 1994; Hedges, 1982a, 1982b, 1982c; and Schmidt, 1992, for discussion on linking research synthesis to theory). That is, changes in behavior can be interpreted within a theoretical framework in the "real world" domains of application.

HISTORICAL CONTEXT

Prior to outlining the primary questions addressed in this synthesis, we will first establish a necessary historical context. Part of the LD field's claim to a unique professional identity resulted from its focus on identifying and remediating specific psychological processing difficulties (e.g., see Wiederholt, 1974, for a review). Several tests were used to identify specific processing disorders (e.g., the Frostig Developmental Test of Visual Perception [Frostig, Lefever, & Whittlesey, 1964], the Illinois Test of Psycholinguistic Abilities [McCarthy & Kirk, 1961]) and various programs designed to remediate these specific processing deficits were published (Cruickshank, Bentzen, Ratzeburg, & Tannhauser, 1961; Kirk, 1963; Strauss & Kephart, 1955). Popular intervention approaches during the 1960s and 1970s included visual–motor, auditory sequencing, visual perception, and cross modality training exercises. The rationale for these interventions was that the remediation of deficits underlying the learning process would bolster children's performance in such domains as reading and math.

Several criticisms were directed at these particular interventions on theoretical grounds (e.g., see Hallahan & Cruickshank, 1973, for a review). In addition, a number of empirical investigations questioned the efficacy of these processing approaches (Wiederholt & Hammill, 1971). Criticism of process training for students with learning disabilities spread from perceptual to psycholinguistic processes (Newcomer & Hammill, 1975), with reviews generally indicating that process training did not generalize to improvements in academics (e.g., Arter & Jenkins, 1979). Because of these controversies, the intervention focus of the field shifted. Process training as a means for treating learning disabilities was deemphasized, and the new focus became direct instruction of academic skills. In the words of Myers and Hammill (1990), "learning disabilities needed an approach with a better base for its foundation. . . . The principles of direct instruction satisfied this purpose" (p. 42).

By 1977, dissatisfaction with a processing orientation to remediation of learning disabilities and the influence of federal regulations implemented under Public Law 94-142 combined to reduce emphasis on treatment of "psychological processes" as part of remediating academic problems in LD children in the public schools. Although learning disabilities were still assumed to be related to basic psychological processes, such as memory deficits, the focus of assessment and intervention was now directed toward minimizing the "discrepancy" between general ability and poor academic achievement. Possibly because of the focus on the discrepancy between general ability and performance in a particular academic domain, many intervention programs during this time period for LD children were not distinct from remedial education (Martin, 1988; Myers & Hammill, 1990). These remediation programs focused on improving basic skills, such as reading and mathematics, via individualized programing, direct continuous measurement (e.g., precision teaching [Lindsley, 1964]), and criterion-based instruction (Stephens, 1977), with the setting of interventions usually occurring in resource rooms (i.e., the LD student spends a majority of his or her day in a regular classroom and goes to the resource room to work on specific academic deficits) (Wiederholt, Hammill, & Brown, 1978; see Mercer & Mercer, 1981, for a review).

The mid-1980s witnessed a shift from the more remedial–academic approach of teaching to instruction that included both cognitive and direct instruction. Instruction was geared toward providing students with information and metacognitive skills necessary for academic success through the use of principles of self-reinforcement, especially self-management and self-talk (e.g., Deshler, Schumaker, & Lenz, 1984a; Deshler, Schumaker, Lenz, & Ellis, 1984b; Wong, 1986). Studies published within this time period suggested that LD children have trouble accessing and mentally coordinating a number of cognitive activities. The research in this area may be summarized as follows: LD children experience difficulty with such self-regulating mechanisms as checking, planning, monitoring, testing, revising, and evaluating during an attempt to learn or solve problems (e.g., Bos & Anders, 1990; Palincsar & Brown, 1988; Wong & Jones, 1982).

In addition, these children were viewed as suffering from deficits in such mental operations as logically organizing and coordinating incoming information that requires carrying out mental operations (e.g., Borkowski et al., 1989; Swanson, 1982). Such children perform poorly on a variety of tasks requiring the use of the general control processes involved in solution strategies (e.g., see Wong, 1991, for a review). Under some conditions, well-designed strategy training improves performance (e.g., Gelzheiser, 1984), while at other times some general cognitive constraints prevent the effective use of control processes (see Cooney & Swanson, 1987, for a review). However, when training of information-processing components includes instruction related to self-evaluation (e.g., predicting outcomes, organizing strategies, using various forms of trial and error), enhancing attributions (beliefs) related to effective strategy use (e.g., Borkowski et al., 1989; see Harris & Pressley, 1991, for a review), and certain subprocesses are relatively familiar or automatized (see Spear-Swerling & Sternberg, 1994), training attempts are generally successful (e.g., Borkowski et al., 1989). The implication from findings during the 1980s and early 1990s is that the previous research, which focused on low-order processing deficits (e.g., attention, short-term memory), incorporated findings that suggest that LD children suffer from higher-order processing problems (processes that monitor the whole cognitive system) (e.g., Swanson, 1987; also see Swanson & Alexander, 1997).

Parallel to the cognitive literature, however, the early 1990s witnessed a resurgence of direct instruction intervention studies, primarily influenced by reading research, which suggested that phonological processes should be the primary focus of intervention. The rationale is that because a large majority of children with learning disabilities suffer problems in reading, some of these children's reading problems are exacerbated because of lack of systematic instruction in processes related to phonological awareness (the ability to hear and manipulate sounds in words and understand the sound structure of language). This lower-order skill was viewed as a specific processing deficiency that underlies higher-order cognitive problems. This view has given rise to several interventions that focus heavily on phonics instruction and intensive individual one-to-one tutoring to improve children's phonological awareness of word structures and sequences (e.g., Torgesen, Wagner, Rashotte, Alexander, & Conway, 1997; Vellutino et al., 1996).

CONTEMPORARY CONTEXT

Recent trends in the intervention literature suggest that research advances linking processing problems of the learning disabled to instruction practice have been in the domain of reading. Evidence shows that LD readers have problems processing phonological information (see Olson, Kliegl, Davidson, & Foltz, 1985; Olson, Wise, Conners, & Rack, 1990; Rack, Snowling, & Olson, 1992; and

Snowling, 1981, for a review). There have been some studies that suggest, however, that LD children may suffer other processing problems besides those related to phonological processing. Semantic and orthographic processes have also played an important role in predicting reading performance (e.g., Chabot, Petros, & McCord, 1983; Lovegrove, Martin, & Slaghuis, 1986; Swanson, 1987; Vellutino, Scanlon, & Spearing, 1995; Zecker & Zinner, 1987).

In contrast to phonological processing, however, the direct impact of semantic processing (e.g., understanding the meaning of words) and orthographic processing (e.g., understanding the writing conventions of the language and correct and incorrect spellings) on reading deficits is less clear (see Siegel, 1993, p. 47, for a discussion). For example, some studies suggest differences between reading ability groups in terms of semantic coding (e.g., Swanson, 1987; Vellutino et al., 1995; Zecker & Zinner, 1987), while others suggest no differences (e.g., Jorm, 1979; Siegel, 1985).

In terms of orthographic processing, Olson et al. (1985) presented LD readers with real and pseudowords (e.g., rain–rane) and required them to select the correct spelling. The tasks were designed so that only visual memory for orthography was used (phonological processes were not helpful for sounding out the word pairs since sounding out would produce the same word sounds) to select the real word. They found that LD readers' performance was comparable to the control group on orthographic tasks. In contrast, McBride-Chang, Manis, Seidenberg, Custodio, and Doi (1993) found that orthographic abilities were deficient in LD readers across a broad age range (grades 5–9). Further, a 2-year follow-up study (Manis, Custodio, & Szeszulski, 1993) indicated that orthographic processing difficulties persist in LD readers.

Metacognition (see Wong, 1991, for a review) is another process implicated in LD children's poor reading performance in some studies (e.g., Wong & Jones, 1982), but not others (e.g., McBride-Chang et al., 1993). Metacognition refers to an individual's awareness of, and ability to monitor, adjust, and regulate his or her cognitive actions in regard to learning (e.g., Palincsar, 1986a, 1986b; Paris, Cross, & Lipson, 1984). There are two reasons why metacognition has played a major role in explaining LD children's reading difficulties. First, the research suggests that when attempting to comprehend text, LD readers inefficiently access metacognitive strategies, as compared to skilled readers (e.g., Johnson, Graham, & Harris, 1997; Wong & Jones, 1982; Wong & Wong, 1986). Second, several studies (e.g., Graves, 1986; Wong & Jones, 1982) suggest that procedures that enhance metacognition positively influence LD readers' text comprehension. Although metacognition has played a role in explaining LD readers' poor comprehension performance (see Palincsar, 1986; and Wong, 1991, for a review), they do possess metacognitive knowledge to some degree (e.g., Wong & Wong, 1986). For example, McBride-Chang et al. (1993) found no differences between LD and skilled readers on a metacognitive questionnaire. Thus, although metacognitive knowledge may be adequately represented in LD readers' long-term memory (e.g., see Wong, 1991, pp. 267–268, for discussion), they do not always access the metacognitive base they possess.

A final influence that has been implicated as a source of LD children's poor reading is working memory (Siegel & Linder, 1984; Siegel & Ryan, 1989; Swanson, 1993a). Working memory is a processing resource of limited capacity that has been shown to be relevant to reading (e.g., Daneman & Carpenter, 1980; Dixon, Lefevre, & Twilley, 1988; Herdman & LeFevre, 1992; Just & Carpenter, 1992; Perfetti, 1985; Turner & Engle, 1989). Several studies suggest that LD readers can be characterized by their inability to retain information in memory while simultaneously processing the same or other information (e.g., Siegel & Ryan, 1989; Swanson, 1993a). This skill is critical to a wide range of reading tasks because an important feature of many reading activities is that incoming information must be temporarily preserved while other information is being acquired or manipulated.

Thus, because of the diversity of processing difficulties experienced by LD children, there are numerous treatment orientations regarding how to handle the various processing deficits attributed to these students. For example, sharp divisions exist about the most effective method of teaching reading (see Adams, 1990; Chall, 1967; Palincsar & Brown, 1984; Vellutino et al., 1996; and Williams, 1979, for a review). On one side of the continuum, several studies trying to decipher some of the features of learning disabilities have traced aspects of the condition to a deficit in phonological awareness, the ability to code words into individual assigned units. Advocates of the phonological deficit theory want to replace current context-based reading instruction with highly structured explicit and intensive instruction in phonological rules and other applications to print. On the other side of the continuum, there are those who argue that reading has meaning only within the context of language. Advocates of this approach point out that, research showing generalization of isolated word intervention to text reading fluency and comprehension is limited (e.g., Aaron, Frantz, & Manges, 1990; Kendall & Hood, 1979; Lomax, 1983; Pflaum, 1980; then see Byrne, Freebody, & Gates, 1992; Coltheart, Avons, Masterson, & Laxon, 1991; and Waters, Caplan, & Leonard, 1992), and argue that the primary function of reading is extracting meaning from text (Chall, 1967). They reason that there are strong links between reading acquisition and oral language acquisition, and further reason that when reading is accented, its meaning and purpose should be emphasized. That is, they argue that the purpose of reading is for meaning and that it is counterproductive to focus primarily on individual letters and sounds.

The implications of this debate are manifested in areas of reading and writing. For example, in the area of reading comprehension, some approaches emphasize accurate word recognition, either through segmented phonetic analysis or whole-word contextual procedures (e.g., Lovett, Ransby, Hardwick, Johns, & Donaldson, 1989), while other approaches emphasize cognitive strategies focusing on student-generated sentences (generative learning) and teacher–student dialogue (reciprocal teaching related to getting the gist of a passage, summarization, and inference from text; e.g., Palincsar & Brown, 1984).

In summary, over the last 30 years there have been several conceptual shifts, as well as paradigm debates, as to what underlies learning disabilities, which in turn raise questions about the best instructional intervention. Although the shifts in intervention focus and procedures over the last 30 years reflect debates within a relatively new field, the fundamental issue for this field is to determine effective academic interventions. Thus, an analysis of academic intervention research is crucial to any systematic understanding of the academic needs of LD students. The purpose of this synthesis is to provide a comprehensive quantitative synthesis of data-based and methodologically sound intervention studies that focus on intervention to improve LD students' academic, social, and behavioral performance.

META-ANALYSIS OF INTERVENTION RESEARCH

Given both the theoretical and practical interest for synthesizing intervention research, this text evaluates the empirical evidence derived from educational interventions for students with learning disabilities. Recent narrative reviews of instructional research and learning disabilities (e.g., Lessen et al., 1989), although of theoretical and practical import, have been limited by their reliance on a narrow sample of interventions, domains (e.g., perceptual processing, social skills), and/or techniques to analyze studies. The present review uses meta-analytic techniques to aggregate the research literature on intervention. Meta-analysis is a statistical reviewing technique that provides a quantitative summary of findings across an entire body of research (Cooper & Hedges, 1994; Hedges & Olkin, 1985). Of interest in this report is the meta-analysis of research on the effects of treatments that are based on the manipulation of instructional variables that are intended to induce educational change, whether in academic (e.g., reading, mathematics), cognitive (e.g., problem solving), or behavioral domains (e.g., social skills).

Previous Syntheses

A few meta-analyses of research in the field of learning disabilities (e.g., see Forness, Kavale, Blum, & Lloyd, 1997, for a review) have been published, but none to our knowledge have considered intervention research across a broad array of academic domains. The only synthesis we are aware of that provides an overall estimate of treatment effectiveness is that of Swanson, Carson, and Sachse-Lee (1996). They assembled a collection of group design studies (78) published between 1967 to 1993, that focused on youths 6–18 years of age, and reported from a total of 324 effect sizes a mean effect size of .85 for treatment versus control conditions. Using Cohen's (1988) threshold of .80 for a "large" effect, their meta-analysis suggests that various instructional approaches have a significant beneficial effect for children and adolescents with learning disabilities.

There were two important findings from this earlier synthesis. First, Swanson et al. suggest that *not all* forms of intervention work equally well. In their synthesis, studies were classified into one of four instructional orientations: therapeutic (eclectic), remedial, direct instruction, and strategy intervention. The authors based their classification treatments on the hypothesis of the primary study, as well as on key words in the introduction, abstract, and title of each article related to the treatment of choice. Mean effect size scores were .59 for the eclectic approaches (approaches not directed specifically to academic skills), .91 for direct instruction, .68 for remedial instruction, and 1.07 for strategy instruction. Thus, a higher effect size emerged for direct instruction and for strategy instruction when compared to the other two approaches.

Second, Swanson et al. found that no particular academic or behavioral domain (e.g., reading, mathematics, spelling, language, social skills, memory, cognition) was resistant to change as a function of intervention. Although most of the research related to intervention was conducted in the reading domain (e.g., reading comprehension, word recognition), no significant differences in effect sizes were found across targeted domains (e.g., reading, social skills, mathematics, spelling). There were qualifications, however, to these findings. For example, sample sizes were smaller for the categories of language, memory, and cognition than for the categories of writing, mathematics, spelling, reading, and intelligence. Younger children were more likely than older children to participate in studies on word skills, general intellectual processing, and perceptual training. There was also a bias related to publication year: those studies that primarily focused on general language skills were more likely to be in earlier publications. Regardless, the authors concluded that effect sizes were statistically comparable across domains of study, and that no deficit area emerged that was not responsive to treatment effects.

There were several limitations to this earlier synthesis that the current synthesis addresses. First, Swanson et al.'s results on treatment approaches are equivocal. Most problematic in the earlier syntheses was an overreliance in coding the intervention approaches on how the primary author labeled the experimental condition rather than coding the actual procedures and components of instruction reported by the authors. This is problematic for several reasons. The most obvious is that the distinction between various treatments may be more artificial than real. For example, the advantage of strategy instruction over direct instruction may not reflect a contrast between interventions. This is because direct instruction uses some of the same instruction techniques as the strategy models (or vice versa): corrective feedback, active frequent participation of the learner, teaching skills in a cumulative manner, and providing a reinforcement system.

Second, the previous analyses did not analyze the relationship between domain categories (targeted behaviors) and treatment. Therefore, we do not know if the various intervention approaches have broad general effects or whether treatments are more effective in some domains than in others. There was much speculation on this issue by the authors. For example, the syntheses suggested that effective procedures for reading comprehension were direct instruction (e.g., Darch & Kameenui, 1987), strategy instruction (e.g., Palincsar & Brown, 1984), summarization (e.g., Gajria & Salvia, 1992 simultaneous–successive processing (e.g., Brailsford, Snart, & Das, 1984), and attribution–cognitive training (e.g., Wong & Jones, 1982), whereas word recognition skills and spelling were best influenced by phonetic/decoding training (e.g., Gettinger, Bryant, & Fayne, 1982; Gittelman & Feingold, 1983). In addition, the authors noted that the effects of strategy instruction were most pronounced in the reading comprehension and writing domains, but also suggested such procedures may be effective in the communication-language domain (Olsen, Wong, & Marx, 1983). They also argued that "it appears that phonetically regular materials seem to have a special benefit to students experiencing word recognition and spelling difficulty, whereas other students seem to learn this quite well with standard materials. Thus, the domains of reading recognition and spelling may be better served by remedial than cognitive approaches" (p. 387). Although they did not investigate them directly, Swanson et al. (1996) also suggested that several domains were influenced by various treatment effects, even though these domains were not the main focus of intervention. For example, although strategy instruction was seen as robust treatment for reading comprehension and writing performance, Swanson et al. argued that when instruction focuses on a general domain (e.g., writing, reading) measures of cognitive processing were directly influenced, such as metacognition about the domain (e.g., Englert, Raphael, & Anderson, 1992). None of these assumptions, however, were tested in their synthesis.

Third, the authors failed to operationalize the term "learning disabilities." Selection criteria for article inclusion were (1) primary authors stated that LD subjects were provided treatment and (2) subject description was given to the notion of discrepancy (i.e., children and adolescents with learning disabilities suffer a discrepancy between their actual achievement and their expected level of achievement based on IQ scores). Swanson et al. (1996) assumed that broadly defined samples provide greater external validity for intervention effectiveness, although the inclusion of such studies sacrificed precision in predicting performance outcomes. Unfortunately, the usefulness of discrepancy criteria as a means of separating LD children from those who are generally poor learners is equivocal (see Stanovich & Siegel, 1994, for a review). To remedy this situation, the authors of the synthesis needed to compare discrepancy definitions with other operational definitions on treatment outcome. For example, recent operational definitions for defining learning disabilities have abandoned the discrepancy notions and now identify LD children by using a cutoff score on standardized reading tests (LD children usually perform academically below the 25th percentile; see Morrison & Siegel, 1991, for a discussion) and intelligence tests (a score at or above 85 on a standardized intelligence measure; see Swanson, 1991, for a review).

Fourth, as an extension of the above criticism, no explicit attempts were made at matching the various treatments to variation in aptitude. Thus, the previous synthesis adds little information about whether aptitude × treatment outcomes emerge across studies. Although these interactions were possibly overlooked because of the meager psychometric and demographic data reported in the primary studies, the previous synthesis failed to investigate treatment effects related to sample description. Thus, we cannot determine if many of the strategies or interventions that appear helpful to broadly defined "students with learning disabilities" may be helpful to a narrowly defined group of LD students as well. For example, intervention approaches that include (1) having the teacher describe and model the use of a strategy, (2) provide ample opportunity for students to apply the strategy and to practice conditions (provide assistance and feedback when needed), (3) help students to develop a verbal repertoire about the use of strategies, (4) encourage students to set goals for the strategy, and so on, may be more appropriate for higher IQ LD students than for relatively low IQ students. Without investigating this possibility, however, the generality of the results is in question.

Fifth, the authors failed to partial out the methodological artifacts from the effect sizes. Thus comparisons between treatment approaches are suspect. In the earlier syntheses, sample procedures for each study were classified into (1) intact groups in classroom or school, nonrandom assignment; (2) intact groups, but with counterbalancing of subjects in treatments on variables of gender, IQ, and ethnicity (subject-to-subject matching procedures); and (3) randomly assigned groups. The mean effect sizes for studies with LD controls across domain measures were 1.55, 1.41, and .77, for intact, subject matching, and random or stratified sampling, respectively. Thus, there was a clear bias in effect sizes as a function of sampling procedures. Other methodological artifacts should also have been considered. For example, in addition to random assignment, striking design problems to consider are (1) exposing control students to different training materials and (2) not checking to determine if participants completed the treatment as directed. Most critically, less than 2% of the studies reported in the Swanson et al. synthesis provide any information related to treatment integrity (fidelity, or the degree to which the intervention program was carried out on a session-by-session basis as planned). Treatment integrity assumes that each and every component or procedure of the intervention is carried out as intended and recommended. This is necessary in order to validate the different instructional approaches (also see Graham & Harris, 1993, for a discussion of this issue).

Finally, several methodological problems with the previous analysis and others (e.g., see Weisz, Weiss, Han, Granger, & Morton, 1995, for a review) relate to the statistical analysis of the data. Previous meta-analyses have used an unweighted least squares general linear (ULS) approach outlined by Smith, Glass, and Miller (1980). To use this approach several assumptions must be met: (1) comparisons (e.g., an analysis of variance [ANOVA] for the dependent variables for different methods such as direct instruction vs. strategy instruction) among different studies must be of approximate or equivalent sample size, and (2) the variance of individual effect sizes must be comparable across observations. In meta-analysis, Hedges and Olkin (1985) have argued that the variance of an effect size (i.e., the reliability) is not interpretable because it reflects, in part, the sample size of the study on which the effect size is based.

Current Synthesis

Given the historical context of intervention research and the limitations of previous meta-analyses, the current research was conducted to provide a comprehensive synthesis of intervention studies that address the aforementioned issues. Because of the vastness of the topic, however, some boundaries were necessary in our analysis. The intervention literature that focuses on administrative decisions and *does not* reflect a manipulation of treatment conditions (e.g., educational placement in a resource room) falls outside the boundaries. Educational research based on intervention that occurs as an extension of the educational placement of children, adolescents, and adults with LD within various educational (e.g., classroom or college) placements is included. Moreover, attention is directed to only those instructional interventions that include students with learning disabilities. Excluded from the analysis, however, are interventions in which the effects of intervention on students with learning disabilities cannot be directly analyzed or partialed out in the analysis. Also, within the area of educational intervention, it was necessary to place parameters on the level or scope of intervention. At one end of a rough continuum, we distinguished between treatment techniques that include separable elements, but that do not, by themselves, reflect a freestanding treatment (e.g., teacher presents advance organizers). At the other end of this continuum are broad approaches that reflect policies and organizational arrangements (e.g., the consulting teacher model, which provides help to an LD student in a regular classroom). We excluded those treatments that were at the top of the continuum. Although there are some gray areas in our selection, we did find it possible to identify instructional programs that are added to the typical instructional routine.

Key Constructs

Three constructs were important in our synthesis: learning disabilities, treatment, and outcome. First, although we took a nonjudgmental stance on the quality of the definition of learning disabilities reflected in intervention studies (e.g., operational vs. a school district definition vs. Federal Register definition), we held to a general parameter that such students must have at least normal intelligence (i.e., standardized intelligence scores at or above 85) or that the study states *explicitly* that participants are in the normal range of intelligence. The study must also state that the participants perform poorly (as indicated by teachers and/or psychometric tests) in at least one academic (e.g., reading) and/or behavioral domain (social skills). We coded the variations of definitions reflected in the database (discrepancy vs. cutoff scores; school identified vs. research identified; specific academic difficulty vs. multiple academic difficulties) to investigate the relationship between the definitional parameters related to learning disabilities and actual treatment outcomes.

Second, the term *treatment* or *intervention* was defined as the direct manipulation (assigned at will by the experimenter; see Campbell & Stanley, 1963, p. 200) by the researcher of psychological (e.g., metacognitive awareness), medical (e.g., drug), and/or educational (e.g., teaching, instruction, materials) variables for the purposes of assessing learning (1) efficiency (e.g., rate, time), (2) accuracy (e.g., percent correct), and/or (3) understanding (e.g., amount of verbal elaboration on a concept). In general, treatment was administered in the context of school as an extension of the regular classroom, special education classroom, and/or clinical services. This extension varied from three instructional sessions to several continuous instructional sessions over months or years.

Finally, treatment outcomes included six general categories of information. These categories were (1) article or technical report identification (authors, affiliation, funding sources, citations), (2) design and methodological characteristics (e.g., sampling procedure, single-subject vs. group design, reliability and validity of measures, internal and external validity; treatment integrity), (3) sampling characteristics (e.g., psychometric information, chronological age, gender, ethnicity, sample size, type of definition, marker variables), (4) parameters of intervention (e.g., domain, setting, materials, length of session, duration of intervention), (5) components of intervention (e.g., group vs. individual instruction, number and description of steps in intervention, level of student response to instruction, maintenance, and transfer), and (6) effect size (e.g., magnitude of treatment effects).

Comparison of Treatments

With the above parameters in mind, our major purpose in this synthesis was to identify effective intervention approaches for instructing students with learning disabilities. Based on the literature, studies were classified into two general approaches: strategy instruction and direct instruction.[1]

Prior to operationalizing these two models, however, it is critical to emphasize the commonalities of the two instructional approaches. The models overlap in two ways. First, both models (in one form or another) assume that effective *methods* of instruction include (1) daily reviews, (2) statements of an instructional objective, (3) teacher presentations of new material, (4) guided practice, (5) independent practice, and (6) formative evaluations (see Rosenshine, 1995; Rosenshine, & Stevens, 1986; and Slavin, Stevens, & Madden, 1988, for a review). Second, both strategy instruction and direct instruction follow a *sequence of events,* such as the following:

1. State the learning objectives and orient the students to what they will be learning and what performance will be expected of them.
2. Review the skills necessary to understand the concept.
3. Present the information, give examples, and demonstrate the concepts/materials.
4. Pose questions (probes) to students and assess their level of understanding and correct misconceptions.
5. Provide group instruction and independent practice. Give students an

opportunity to demonstrate new skills and learn the new information on their own.

6. Assess performance and provide feedback. Review the independent work and give a quiz. Give feedback for correct answers and reteach skills if answers are incorrect.
7. Provide distributed practice and review.

No doubt, the above sequence has some variations within a strategy or direct instruction model (e.g., Graham & Harris, 1996; Guthrie, VanMeter, McCann, & Wigfield, 1996). Graham and Harris (1993) outline a sequence from a strategy model to teach writing that includes some of the above steps. First, the teacher helps the student develop the prerequisite skills, including knowledge of the criteria for good writing (*Review the skills necessary to understand the concept*). Second, the teacher and the student examine and discuss current writing performance and the strategies used to accomplish specific assignments (*Assess performance and provide feedback*; *Pose questions [probes] to students and assess their level of understanding and correct misconceptions*). Third, the teacher models how to use the strategy employing the appropriate self-instructions (*Present the information, give examples, and demonstrate the concepts materials*). The self-instructions usually include a combination of problem definition, planning, strategy use, self-evaluation, error correction, and self-reinforcement. Fourth, there is a mnemonic for remembering self-statements. Fifth, students and teachers use a strategy of self-instructions collaboratively. Sixth, students use a strategy independently (*Provide independent practice*).

Several characteristics of this strategy model are different from the above sequence of events. For example, there is verbal interaction between the teachers and student in which the student is viewed as a collaborator in setting goals, completing the task, and modifying the procedures. In addition, the teacher provides individual tailored feedback and models the appropriate response based upon feedback.

Components of direct instruction are reviewed by Engelmann and Carnine (1982), Kameenui, Jitendra, and Darch (1995), Rosenshine (1982), Slavin (1987), and Spector (1995). Direct instruction emphasizes fast-paced, well-sequenced, highly focused lessons. The lessons are usually delivered in small groups to students who are given several opportunities to respond and receive feedback about accuracy and responses (see Kameenui, Jitendra, & Darch, 1995, for a review of model variations). Direct instruction methods fall roughly into two distinct categories. One might be called "master teaching models" (Rosenshine, 1982) because they are based on the practices of the most effective teachers. The other category of direct instruction might be called "systematic instruction" which is generally modeled after Distar. This approach includes specific instructional materials that are highly organized, and systematic methods of teaching and motivating students, managing a classroom, and assessing student progress.

Thus, both approaches involved the active presentation of information, clear organization, step-by-step progression from subtopic to subtopic, and use of many examples, demonstrations, and visual prompts. All emphasize conscious assessment of student understanding and altering the pace of instruction according to this information. That is, there is a focus on independent performance. Instruction is criterion-based rather than time-based. The student must master a particular stage before moving onto the next stage.

An example of an intervention study that tests the elements of both strategy instruction and direct instruction is provided by Lovett et al. (1994). They introduce a highly structured and graduated sequence of steps with multiple opportunities for overlearning all content and skills covered in a strategy and direct instruction reading program. Both instruction models include cumulative review routines, mass practice, and teaching all component skills to a defined mastery criterion. What varies between the models is that the strategy program focuses on process or global skills for a general approach to reading, whereas the direct instruction model focuses on word segmentation and "sound-getting skills." Both programs involve steps, isolating component skills, and mastery. Perhaps the contrast is that the strategy model focuses on teaching a few words at mastery, whereas the direct instruction model focuses on a level of subanalysis or segmentation (phonological awareness). For the strategy model, while students learn sound units, discussion concerns metacognitive issues, such as strategy implementation, strategy choice, and self-monitoring. The teacher explains *why* something is being used. A particular strategy is attached to a particular word. The teacher explains how it should be applied and how to check to see if the strategy is working. These strategies are practiced in a very structured, systematic manner with the training of words. There is usually a compare and contrast activity that explicitly trains the students on what they need to know to help them decode a new word. Thus, in their study the distinction between strategy programs and direct instruction programs may be the unit of information that is being emphasized. Direct instruction focuses on subskills (sound units, such as letter sounds, or linguistic units such as *mat-cat-hat*), whereas strategy instruction focuses on processes and rules of use.

In summary, the two models under investigation overlap on a number of instructional components. We assume, however, that each approach offers some independence in predicting treatment outcomes. Our assumptions are based on recent cognitive models of learning disabilities that suggest that such children suffer both metacognitive and phonological difficulties.

Model Testing

Three issues were of interest in our analysis. First, we test whether treatments that include components of strategy instruction (SI), direct instruction (DI), and/or both instructional models yield significant differences in effect size. The two models were operationally defined as the occurrence or nonoccurrence of specific instructional components (to be described) reflected in the treatment description. In addition to the components that are common to both approaches, *strategy instruction* was operationally defined as statements in the treatment condition that indicate: (1) verbal modeling by the teachers (or researcher) of steps or processes to solve a problem (e.g., writing an essay, comprehending text), (2) elaborate explanations (i.e., two or more statements by the teacher or researcher or visual prompts, e.g., refer to a flow chart and evaluate progress) to direct task performance, (3) reminders to use strategies or procedures (i.e., the student is cued to use taught strategies, tactics, or procedures), (4) multistep or multiprocess instructions (usually indicated by an acronym, e.g., PASS), (5) verbal dialogue (via questions between students or between students and teacher on when and where to use strategies), and (6) teacher provides only necessary assistance (i.e., individually tailored feedback). If the treatment conditions reflect two or more of the six components, it was labeled a strategy treatment. In addition to the components that are common to both approaches, direct instruction models were defined in the synthesis as follows: (1) the teacher models a skill (e.g., the teacher says "the sound the letter *c* makes is /*k*/ as in *C-A-T*"), (2) breaks down a task into small steps or skills or breaking the instruction down into simpler phases, (3) repeatedly administers probes and feedback, (4) provides set materials at a rapid pace, (5) asks directed questions (e.g., What sound does this letter make?) related to skills, (6) presents new (novel) materials (e.g., Corrective Reading Series) and/or provides a pictorial or diagram presentation, (7) allows for independent practice and individually paced instruction, and (8) instructs in a small group. If the treatment conditions reflect four or more of the eight components, it was labeled a direct instruction treatment.

One approach to testing the contributions of various instructional models to estimates of effect size is by a weighted regression modeling procedure (Hedges & Olkin, 1985). A number of configurations can be tested in this regression modeling, but most fall around four configurations: independence, redundancy, complementary, and suppression. The first model tested is the independence model. That is, direct instruction and strategy instruction make independent contributions to effect size. Support for this model is found when both direct instruction and strategy instruction contribute significant variance to the overall effect size.

The second model is the redundance model. This model assumes that direct instruction and strategy instruction correlate with each other and thus duplicate each other in treatment outcomes. Thus, prediction accuracy of effect size estimates is increased by minimizing this duplication or redundancy. For instance, if strategy instruction is merely a subcomponent of direct instruction, then this measure will *not* improve the accuracy of predictions when entered in a regression model after direct instruction.

A third model considers whether direct instruction and strategy instruction together exceed the sum of the individual contributions of each model. In this complimentary model (we refer to this as a combined model), the two predictors (direct instruction and strategy instruction) are complimentary if they both make positive contributions to effect size, but correlate weakly with each other.

A final test of contribution could be in the area of suppression. Given the publication bias toward reporting only successful interventions (e.g., Lipsey & Wilson, 1993), it is unlikely we will uncover an instructional approach that suppresses performance. It may be the case, however, that the type of information reported on the sample of students with learning disabilities could suppress outcome. For example, effect sizes may be predicted from the range of intelligence scores and the severity of the reading problem in the sample. The best prediction of treatment outcomes related to reading is obtained from the level of severity in reading, which in turn is negatively correlated with intelligence, in the sample with learning disabilities. Thus, the intelligence score is weighted negatively and the reading score positively in predicting treatment outcomes. This means that although the reading measure is a much better predictor of treatment outcomes than the intelligence measure, the intelligence measure is useful as a measure of a source of error in the former.

To test these models, a hierarchical regression analysis will be used to assess the contribution of direct instruction and strategy instruction to estimates of effect size. We will compare the alternative presentation orders of direct instruction and strategy instruction in predicting effect size. We will also determine which characteristics of the sample may suppress (weaken) estimates of effect size.

Two additional tiers of analysis will be used to identify models that best capture treatment effects. One tier to our analysis determines whether studies that overlap in direct instruction and strategy instruction components better predict outcomes than studies that have no overlap in the instructional components. A final tier to our analysis isolates the instructional components that make up each intervention model.

Second, we tested the assumption that certain intervention effects are more likely to emerge in some domains than in others. Children with learning disabilities are conceived to be poor information processors, primarily in areas of language (e.g., phonological coding), and on activities that make high demands on language skills (e.g., reading, writing). Based on several findings, students with learning disabilities are viewed as having inefficient strategies for compensating for low-order skills (e.g., awareness of the sound units of language). Thus, they experience difficulty meeting the complex requirements of several academic tasks in which efficient language processing is required and so are unable to effectively utilize generally intact intellectual abilities (see Swanson, 1990, for a review). The LD student is further described as an inefficient learner, one who either lacks certain strategies, chooses inappropriate strategies, and/or generally fails to engage in efficient self-monitoring behavior. In the present synthesis, we partially tested this general model by comparing intervention studies that include components of cognitive (or strategy) instruction with other approaches across treatment domains that clearly draw upon language skills, such as reading and writing. This was done by aggregating studies and examining the relationship between variables and effect sizes as a function of the range and scope of intervention (this is referred to as type A and type B theory testing, via meta-analysis; see Miller & Pollack, 1994). Based on a global framework that views LD students as (1) inefficient processors of verbal information and (2) responsive to explicit training in cognitive strategies, one would expect positive treatment results (high effect sizes) as a function of cognitive intervention across various academic domains that draw upon language skills. It is our assumption that only those studies that adequately define their sample and use vigorous methodology can contribute to any sort of theory testing that may emerge.

Finally, we tested the assumption that aptitude interacts with treatment outcomes. More specifically, we assessed whether variation in how the sample of LD students is defined interacts with treatment outcomes. A critical question is whether studies that include samples with intelligence and reading scores at a certain level yield different treatment outcomes than those studies in which such levels are not specified. Reading scores at or below the 25th percentile in reading recognition (see Siegel & Ryan, 1989; Stanovich & Siegel, 1994) and standardized intelligence performance at or above 85 have been considered as critical cutoff scores for defining learning disabilities (see Morrison & Siegel, 1991, for discussion of this issue). The rise of cutoff scores in the experimental literature has been made in response to the poor discriminant validity of discrepancy scores in defining LD children from generally poor achieving children (this issue will be discussed later under Implications). The treatment validity of such a cutoff score definition, however, has not been tested as a function of treatment outcomes. That is, we assume that the face validity of a definition is enhanced if one can show that such a definition is significantly related to treatment outcomes.

Practical Questions

With the above boundaries, assumptions, and theoretical concerns in mind, we also formulated six practical questions to direct our synthesis. First, Do the intervention studies reflect a primary domain of focus (e.g., reading), or are investigations distributed evenly over several domains (e.g., mathematics, reading, memory, etc.)? Second, Do studies that produce the largest effect sizes vary from other studies as a function of instructional parameters (e.g., length and number of sessions, instructional components, setting, type of materials) and type of intervention? Third, Is there a trend in treatment outcomes as a function of definition, demographic variables, age, and psychometric characteristics (e.g., standard scores related to intelligence, reading, math, language) in children and adolescents with learning disabilities? Fourth, Are some of the dependent measures (e.g., standardized reading scores vs. experimental comprehension measures) more susceptible to change, regardless of the type of intervention, than other treatment measures? Fifth, Is there is a relationship between the methodological procedures (e.g., treatment integrity and sampling procedures) and effect size? Finally, Which treatments, based on the methodological quality of the study, produce the largest effect sizes?

SUMMARY

In summary, this chapter has laid the groundwork for the current meta-analysis. A brief overview was provided for why a synthesis is necessary, what sort of contribution such an analysis could make toward the literature, and what shortcomings undermined a previous meta-analysis. We reviewed two major instructional models that have been influential in the field. Three research questions are of particular interest in directing this synthesis: one focused on comparison between direct instruction and strategy instruction, another focused on whether instructional effects are domain-specific, and the third focused on the influence of definitional characteristics of the sample on treatment outcome.

NOTE

1. In the literature, the term "strategy" has been used in reference to particular learning skills, such as rehearsal, imaging, and outlining; to more general types of self-management activities, such as planning and comprehension monitoring; and to complex plans that combine several techniques (see Borkowski & Turner, 1990; Levin, 1986; and Pressley & Ghatala, 1990, for a review). In this report we assume that strategies are made up of two or more goal-oriented tactics and sequential methods. A tactic is a single processing technique, such as self-monitoring, elaboration, or organization. Strategies depend on prerequisite learning of certain core skills and subskills. For example, organizing and monitoring information in a text is a strategy that requires the subskills representing word recognition, vocabulary, and spelling. However, the strategies are directed toward higher-order thinking such as problem solving, comprehending (e.g., reading comprehension), composing (writing prose), and rule learning (such as algorithms for word problems). In the present context, strategy instruction is assumed to direct students to focus on higher-order skills, such as metacognition, self-monitoring, rule learning, and/or awareness of task parameters to direct their problem solving, memory, and/or "information-handling" behavior. Strategy instruction is distinguished from other approaches because of instructions directing students to access information from long-term memory about procedural knowledge.

   As a point of contrast, we tested whether a direct instruction model (defined as a task-analytic, drill and repetition, individual, one-to-one instruction) provided a better account of the variance in treatment outcomes than strategy instruction. That is, in contrast to strategy instruction, effective instruction for students with learning disabilities may be best captured in studies that identify their orientation as a skills approach (drill-repetition and/or instruction focusing on low-order skills such as phonological coding, which in turn are reflected in such domains as word recognition and spelling). In this case, studies that yield high effect sizes may be isolated to specific skill domains, such as word recognition. Of course, it is possible that neither approach in isolation but instead both in combination predict effect sizes. To test these competing hypotheses, the instructional components of the various experimental interventions were coded into those that reflect cognitive strategies, those that reflect the remediation of specific skills, and those that do not focus on particular academic domains.

Chapter 2

Method

In this chapter we will review the methods used to conduct our meta-analysis. We discuss our procedures for data collection, data evaluation, and analysis. Particular attention is given to how studies were selected and coded. We finish with a general description of the studies included in the synthesis.

DATA COLLECTION

To begin our search for relevant materials on intervention, we systematically scanned several computer databases. The PsycINFO, MEDline, and ERIC on-line data bases were systematically scanned for studies from 1963 to 1997 that met the inclusion criteria described below. The computer search strategy used the following terms: "learning disabled (disabilities)," "reading disabled (disabilities)," "dyslexic," "educationally handicapped," or "slow learners," paired with variations of "intervention," "treatment," "training," "remediation," or "instruction." This search yielded approximately 2,900 abstracts of articles, technical reports, chapters, and dissertations. We examined all the abstracts prior to study selection to eliminate those studies that clearly did not meet the inclusion criteria (e.g., articles were reviews or position papers). Because the computer search procedures excluded unpublished studies and the most recent literature, researchers (as identified by journal board affiliations with the *Learning Disability Quarterly*, *Journal of Learning Disabilities*, and *Learning Disabilities Research and Practice* and/or membership in the International Academy for Research in Learning Disabilities) were sent letters requesting copies of unpublished and/or ongoing intervention studies. We also hand-searched the following journals for articles that did not emerge from the computer search: *Journal of Learning Disabilities*, *Journal of Educa-*

tional Psychology, Learning Disability Quarterly, Reading and Writing, Learning Disabilities Research and Practice, Exceptional Children, and the *Journal of Special Education.* In addition, every state department and 200 directors of educational research were sent a letter requesting technical reports on intervention studies for children and adolescents with learning disabilities.

DATA EVALUATION

The pool of relevant literature was narrowed down to studies that utilized an experimental design in which children or adults with learning disabilities received treatment to enhance their academic, social, and/or cognitive performance. This procedure narrowed the search to *913* data-based articles (or reports) that appeared potentially acceptable for inclusion in the quantitative review. After a review of these studies, each data-based report was evaluated on *five* additional criteria for study inclusion. These criteria include the following:

1. The study involved at least one between-instruction comparison condition (i.e., control condition) or within-design control condition (e.g., repeated measures design, or baseline as in a time-series analysis) that includes participants with LD. Thus, studies that included *only* a pretest and a posttest *without* an instructional control condition of LD participants were excluded.
2. The study provides sufficient quantitative information to permit the calculation of effect sizes. Effect sizes were calculated from the means and standard deviations of the performance outcomes for the experimental and control conditions, or from tests of the significance of the differences in performance between instruction conditions (e.g., t- or F-tests, χ^2, exact p values).
3. The recipients of the intervention were identified as children or adults with average intelligence, but with problems in a particular academic, social, and/or related behavioral domain. The mean IQ score reported for the LD participant sample could occur on any standardized verbal, nonverbal, intelligence test, or subtest. The cutoff score for inclusion in the synthesis was a reported mean IQ score of >84 for those in group design studies and for individuals in single-subject design studies. Studies that reported no IQ score, but stated that the group IQ or individual IQ scores (as in single-subject studies) were in the average range were included in the analysis. If a study did not report or state that IQ was in the average range, the study was not included in the general analysis.
4. The treatment group received instruction, assistance, or therapy that was over and above what they would have received during the course of their typical classroom experience. That is, the study focused on treatment, rather than merely a description of the child's current placement followed by an evaluation. The fine line between intervention and experimentation was drawn by requiring that the training or remediation had to have been dispensed over a minimum of 3 days.
5. The study has to be written in English.

The titles of articles accepted for analysis and of some of those rejected (other articles were rejected based on information presented in the abstract) are provided at the end of this report (Appendices A and B, respectively). Appendix B includes only those articles that could not easily be rejected from the abstract. Interrater agreement for article inclusion and exclusion exceeded 90%. Although design issues (no control or baseline condition) were the most frequent criteria for article exclusion, the inability to calculate effect sizes, lack of clarity about whether students with learning disabilities were included (e.g., IQ scores <84 or average IQ was not stated), the inability to separate the performance of students with learning disabilities from other ability groups, no information on sample size, and/or faulty statistical applications (e.g., incorrect degrees of freedom) were also frequent reasons for article exclusion.

CODING AND INTERRATER AGREEMENT

Because of the extensiveness to which the literature was coded, the coding form is provided in Appendix C. The general categories of coding reflected in the form include (1) sample characteristics, (2) demographics, (3) quality of research methodology, (4) components and parameters of instruction, (5) generalization/transfer, and (6) conditions of treatment.

Interrater agreement is reported for each category in Appendix C. Interrater agreements (i.e., two graduate students independently rated articles) across various items exceeded 80% in some areas (instructional components, key terms) and 95% in others (dependent measures, statistical information). Interrater agreement was also obtained on rejected articles. The principal investigator determined initial rejection of the article based on the reasons stated in the preceding sections.

Four doctoral students served as independent raters on the coding of each report. Raters were trained in coding of each category. Coding training was conducted during the first several months of this project. During this time, code definitions with low interrater agreement were refined and raters were provided feedback for coding both group and single-subject studies. Approximate time needed to code each article varied from 2 to 3 hours. Interrater agreement on the dependent measures was calculated by using the formula agreements divided by the number of agreements plus disagreements, multiplied by 100. Interrater agreements below 80% called for a redefinition of the particular code and the retraining of raters relevant to information in each report.

In the initial stages of the project, the interrater procedure involved randomly selecting approximately 25% of the completed coding sheets for review. Both the Kappa procedure and the agreements divided by the agreements plus disagreements procedure were used to determine interrater agreement. The criteria for interrater agreement were set at 80%. Feedback on disagreements was given directly to the graduate students, with retraining occurring if reliability fell below the criterion level. Although this procedure was relatively time-consuming, interrater agreement steadily increased over the duration of the project and remained at a high level (>90%). Sixty-nine qualified studies (25% of the total number of studies) were randomly selected for independent coding to determine the percentage of interrater agreement per study, per code. Per code item agreement is provided on the sample coding sheet found in Appendix C. Interrater agreement as calculated by agreements divided by agreements plus disagreements resulted in a mean agreement of 87% across studies with a range of 77–96%. Kappa agreement per study was .82.

CATEGORIZATION OF DEPENDENT MEASURES

The general categorical domains of the dependent measures were coded into 1 of 17 general categories. The categories are as follows:

1. The *Cognitive* domain included measures of self-monitoring, speed of processing, problem-solving processes, synthesis, cognitive style, problem-solving strategies, strategy use, and metacognition.
2. The *Word Recognition* domain included all measures of real word recognition.
3. The *Reading Comprehension* domain included all measures related to silent or oral reading comprehension.
4. The *Spelling* domain included all measures of word spelling.
5. The *Memory* domain included all measures of auditory and visual recall, free or serial recall, and/or retelling of information.
6. The *Mathematics* domain included all measures of computation accuracy and word-problem accuracy.
7. The *Writing* domain included all measures of prose, quality ratings, and grammar.
8. The *Vocabulary* domain included all measures of single word meaning.
9. The *Affective/Self-Concept* domain included all measures of attitude, attribution, and self-concept.
10. The *Intelligence* domain included all standardized measures of intelligence (e.g., from the Wechsler Intelligence Scale—Revised [WISC-R], Slosson Intelligence Test, the Kaufman Ability Scale for Children [K-ABC], etc.).
11. The *General Reading* domain included all composite scores that did not separate word recognition and comprehension into separate scores.
12. The *Word Skills/Phonological/Orthographic* domain included all component measures of word recognition, such as phonics, nonword (pseudoword) recognition, and orthographic (e.g., recognizing correct word patterns) coding.
13. The *General Achievement* domain included all global scores related to achievement subtests and overall classroom grades.
14. The *Creativity* domain included all measures from the Torrance Test of

Creativity, measures of convergent and divergent thinking, creative writing, or related creativity measures.

15. The *Social Skills* domain referred to all measures of social interaction (e.g., peer ratings) and behavior ratings.
16. The *Perceptual* domain included all dependent measures related to visual–motor skills (e.g., tracing), mazes, auditory and visual discrimination.
17. The *Language* domain included all measures of verbal communication, pragmatics, articulation, verbal expressive or receptive language, and speech.

Some dependent measures were not related to achievement (e.g., swimming) and were not used in the analysis. For the majority of the subsequent statistical analyses, only one effect size (average effect size within each study) as a function of each domain category (e.g., reading, mathematics, etc.) was computed (averaged). We thereby partially controlled for statistical independence within the meta-analysis. If a study had multiple dependent measures, those that assess the same constructs were combined and those that assess different constructs were reported in the appropriate categories. If statistical independence could not be achieved, for example, as when comparisons were made between domains (e.g., reading, mathematics), the subsequent analysis partialed out the overlapping variance (intercorrelation among domains within a study) via a weighted least squares regression analysis (to be discussed).

CATEGORIZATION OF TREATMENT VARIABLES

Forty-five instructional components were coded as present or not present in the study (see Appendix C). Based on a preliminary analysis of the frequency of representation of these components and the detail (or lack of detail) of information about the independent variables in the primary studies, two general models were identified: direct instruction and strategy instruction. These two models were operationally defined as the occurrence or nonoccurrence of specific instructional components reflected in the treatment description. Those components most frequently reported that reflect *direct instruction* were as follows (see Appendix C, the coding form): (1) breaking down a task into small steps, (2) administering probes, (3) administering feedback repeatedly, (4) providing a pictorial or diagram presentation, (5) allowing for independent practice and individually paced instruction, (6) breaking the instruction down into simpler phases, (7) instructing in a small group, (8) modeling a skill or behavior, (9) providing set materials at a rapid pace, (10) providing individual child instruction, (11) asking questions, and (12) presenting the new (novel) materials. Any procedure that included a minimum of four of these codes was labeled a direct instruction.

A second instructional variable, which we term *strategy instruction,* included at least three of the following instructional components: (1) elaborate explanations (i.e., systematic explanations, elaborations, and/or a plan to direct task performance), (2) modeling from teachers (including verbal modeling, questioning, and demonstration from teachers),[1] (3) reminders to use certain strategies or procedures (i.e., students were cued to use taught strategies, tactics, or procedures), (4) step-by step prompts or multiprocess instructions, (5) dialogue (in which teacher and student talk back and forth), (6) teacher asks questions, and (7) teacher provides only necessary assistance. Thus, the independent variables were dummy coded (1 = strategy and 0 = nonstrategy; 1 = direct instruction and 0 = nondirect instruction).

As a validity check on our classifications, we compared our classification of the treatment conditions with that of the primary author's general theoretical model and/or the label attached to the treatment condition. There was substantial overlap (involving approximately 70% of the studies) between those studies we classified as direct instruction and those classified as strategy instruction models and the primary authors' titles or descriptions of the independent variables. For example, terms frequently provided by the author included "strategy," "cognitive intervention," "monitoring," "metacognition," "self-instruction," and "cognitive-behavior modification" for the strategy model. The authors of studies that were classified as direct instruction by our criteria used such labels as "directed instruction," "advanced organizers," "adapting materials," "corrective feedback," or "direct computation." Authors of studies that used approaches other than direct instruction or strategy intervention typically used terms such as "perceptual processing," "multisensory instruction," "neuro-sensory condition," "CAI condition," or "social skills training."

Based on our reading of comprehensive reviews that identified instructional components that influence student outcomes (e.g., see Harris & Pressley, 1991; Rosenshine, 1995; Simmons & Kameenui, 1996; Vellutino & Scanlon, 1991), we reclustered (or reconfigured) from our coding sheets the 45 instructional codes into approximately 20 clusters of components. These components were dummy coded (i.e., clusters were coded as occurring or nonoccurring [coded as 1 and 0, respectively] within the treatment description). Based on several reviews that have identified salient factors in instructional outcomes (e.g., Adams, 1990; Becker & Carnine, 1980; Brophy & Good, 1986; Leinhardt & Greeno, 1986; Pressley & Harris, 1994; Resnick, 1987; Rosenshine, 1995; Rosenshine & Stevens, 1986; Slavin, Stevens, & Madden, 1988), we coded the occurrence or nonoccurrence of the following instructional components (note that the words "teacher" and "child" are used but the terms may also reflect "experimenter" and "adult," respectively):

1. *Sequencing.* Statements in the treatment description about breaking down the task, fading of prompts or cues, matching the difficulty level of the task to the child, sequencing short activities, and/or using step-by-step prompts.

2. *Drill–repetition* and *practice–review.* Statements in the treatment description related to mastery criteria, distributed review and practice, using redundant materials or text, repeated practice, sequenced reviews, daily feedback, and/or weekly reviews.

3. *Anticipatory or preparation responses.* Statements in the treatment description related to asking the child to look over material prior to instruction, directing the child to focus on material or concepts prior to instruction, providing information to prepare the child for discussion, and/or stating the learning objective for the lesson prior to instruction.

4. *Structured verbal teacher–child interaction.* Statements in the treatment description about elaborate or redundant explanations, systematically prompting children to ask questions, teacher and child talking back and forth (dialogue), and/or teacher asking questions that are open-ended or directed.

5. *Individualization + small group.* Statements in the treatment description about independent practice, and/or individual pacing, and/or individual instruction, and small group instruction.

6. *Novelty.* Statements in the treatment description about the use of developed diagrams or picture presentations, specialized films or videos, instruction via computers, specification that new curriculum was implemented, and/or emphasis on teacher presenting new material from the previous lesson.

7. *Strategy modeling + attribution training.* Statements in the treatment description about processing components or multisteps related to modeling from the teacher; simplified demonstrations modeled by the teacher to solve a problem or complete a task successfully; teacher modeling; teacher providing child with reminders to use certain strategies, steps, and/or procedures; think-aloud models; and/or the teacher presenting the benefits of taught strategies.

8. *Probing reinforcement.* Statements in the treatment description about intermittent or consistent use of probes, daily feedback, fading of prompts and cues, and/or overt administration of rewards and reinforcers.

9. *Nonteacher instruction.* Statements in the treatment description about homework, modeling from peers, parents providing instruction, and/or peers presenting or modeling instruction.

10. *Segmentation.* Statements in the treatment description about breaking down the targeted skill into smaller units, breaking it into component parts, or segmenting and/or synthesizing component parts.

11. *Advanced organizers* Statements in the treatment description about directing children to look over material prior to instruction, directing children to focus on particular information, providing prior information about task, and/or the teacher stating objectives of instruction prior to commencing.

12. *Directed response/questioning.* Treatment description related to dialectic or Socratic teaching, in which the teacher directs children to ask questions, the teacher and child or children engage in dialogue, and/or the teacher asks questions.

13. *One-to-one instruction.* Statements in the treatment description about activities related to independent practice, tutoring, instruction that is individually paced, and/or instruction that is individually tailored.

14. *Control difficulty or processing demands of task.* Treatment statements about short activities, level of difficulty controlled, teacher providing necessary assistance, teacher providing simplified demonstration, tasks sequenced from easy to difficult, and/or task analysis.

15. *Technology.* Statements in the treatment description about utilizing formal curriculum, newly developed pictorial representations, uses specific material or computers, and/or uses media to facilitate presentation and feedback.

16. *Elaboration.* Statements in the treatment description about additional information or explanation provided about concepts, procedures, or steps, and/or redundant text or repetition within text.

17. *Modeling by teacher of steps.* Statements or activities in the treatment description that involve modeling from the teacher in terms of demonstration of processes and/or steps the children are to follow.

18. *Group instruction.* Statements in the treatment description about instruction in a small group, and/or verbal interaction occurring in a small group with children and/or teacher.

19. *A supplement to teacher involvement besides peers.* Statements in the treatment description about homework, about parent helps reinforce instruction, and the like.

20. *Strategy cues.* Statements in the treatment description about reminders to use strategies or multisteps, of the teacher verbalizing steps or procedures to solve problems, use of "think-aloud models," and/or teacher presenting the benefits of strategy use or procedures.

As the reader can see after reading this list, there is some overlap in how the 45 codes were sorted into the instructional components.[2] Further, if only one of the appropriate codes emerges related to the component, then the study is given credit for that component (coded as 1). Thus, our focus was not on the amount of information in the treatment (i.e., the saturation of information), but on whether the information available reflected qualitatively different information. The independence of instructional components will be addressed in Chapters 3 and 4.

These 20 components, however, do capture an array of intervention approaches. For example, the *Segmentation* component would be a characteristic of analytic and synthesis approaches (e.g., phonics instruction), whereas the *Anticipatory or preparation responses* component characterizes treatment approaches that activate prior knowledge or provide a precursor to the main instructional activity (e.g., Meichenbaum's [1977] cognitive–behavioral model). The component that reflects the *Control of difficulty or processing demands of task* addresses the variations in teacher support (e.g., a teacher provides necessary assistance, tasks are sequenced from easy to difficult, i.e., help is provided to the student that covaries with his or her ability) of the student and are reflective of activities such as mediated scaffolding (e.g., Palincsar & Brown, 1984). Following an explicit set of steps and prompting the use of these steps are important activities that underlie strategy instruction (Rosenshine, 1995). The *Strategy cues* component reflects some of these activities, with reminders to children to use multiple step procedures.

In short, we coded the occurrence or nonoccurrence of these particular codes within the treatment description. Although we will test the contribution of global models, such as direct instruction or strategy instruction, to treatment outcomes, it is at the component level that we think we will be best able to identify effective treatment procedures.

CONTROL GROUP PARAMETERS

The control conditions were identified based upon the study's designation. However, in a few instances no such designation was made within the study, and therefore we made decisions about coding a condition as a control treatment were made based on the hypothesis of the study. If no hypothesis was given, the preferred treatment, based on the review of literature in the primary study, was assigned to the control condition. The coding of the control condition focused on the degree of treatment overlap between the experimental and the control conditions. Thus, we coded the control condition by the similarities with the experimental group in terms of teachers, setting, materials, dependent measures, exposure (e.g., length of time) to instruction, primary focus (e.g., reading, math, etc.), and method overlap (number of steps in treatment vs. control condition that overlap or are the same).

EFFECT SIZE CALCULATION

Group Design

Cohen's *d* (Hedge & Olkin, 1985) was the primary index of effect size (ES). Cohen's *d* is calculated as the difference between control and experimental treatment posttest mean scores (partialed for the influence of pretest scores if that information is available), or baseline and treatment mean scores (for single- subject design studies) divided by the pooled standard deviation of posttest (average of control and experimental posttest standard deviations), or baseline and treatment conditions (Cohen, 1988; Hedges & Olkin, 1985).

To provide a common standard deviation across various group design studies, we calculated the *pooled* (average) standard deviation from posttest performance. When posttest standard deviations could not be calculated (such as with repeated measures, covariance, and gain scores), adjustments were made in standard deviations. For example, a few studies present gain scores without pre- or posttest data. The standard deviations of gain scores for the experimental and control groups are often substantially smaller than the standard deviation of posttest scores (see Rosenthal, 1994, p. 241, for a discussion). ESs from achievement gains are typically inflated, and therefore standard deviations of gain scores are less than those of posttest scores to the degree that the pre–post correlations often exceed .50. Thus, consistent with Rosenthal's (1994; see p. 241) review, we calculated the ES for gain as follows:

$$S_p = S_g/\sqrt{2(1-r)}$$

where S_g is the standard deviation of gain scores and S_p is the standard deviation of the posttest scores. If the pre–post correlations were not reported, ESs from gain scores were transformed to a scale using the following multiplier:

$$\text{Corrected ES} = (\text{ES}_{\text{gain}}) \sqrt{2(1 - R)}$$

where R is the pretest and posttest correlation. The pretest–posttest correlation was assumed to be .80 (see Glass, McGraw, & Smith, 1981, for a discussion). Substituting .80 in the formula, a multiplier of .632 deflates the ES estimates from the gain score data (see Glass et al., 1981, for a discussion). This procedure puts all ES scores on the same metric.

Similarly, in the studies that statistically adjusted posttest scores for one or more covariates, effect sizes were calculated on both adjusted and unadjusted mean scores divided by the unadjusted pooled group's standard deviations. Hedges (1994, p. 241) has suggested that when adjustments in the standard deviations are employed, the synthesis should report both the adjusted and the unadjusted ESs. Thus, where the ESs are discrepant (>.10), we reported both adjusted and the unadjusted ESs. When means or standard deviations are omitted in the studies that *do* meet the inclusion criteria, ESs were estimated from t, F, χ^2, r, or exact p values.

Single-Subject Design

Single-subject design studies in which there is no separate control group (subjects serve as their own controls) were separated from group design studies in our analysis. Although there is no consensus on procedures for calculating ES for single-subject design studies (see Busk & Serlin, 1992; then see Faith, Allison, & Gorman, 1997), the primary index of increase or decrease in behavior was a difference between the mean scores on the baseline (last three sessions) and treatment phases (last three sessions) divided by the pooled standard deviation (last three sessions of baseline and treatment). Thus, for a single-subject design study to be included in the synthesis, both the baseline and the treatment must include a minimum of three sessions. We calculated ESs on the last three sessions in each phase so that a judgment could be made concerning subject improvement at the termination of an instructional phase. Although we coded all observation sessions, we relied on the calculation of ESs from the last three sessions to establish some stability and consistency in the comparisons across studies. That is, some reviews suggest that (1) the number of sessions used to calculated ESs either inflate or deflate the magnitude of ES (Franklin, Allison, & Gorman, 1996), (2) a statistical analysis (regression analysis) assumes an equal time interval across data points (i.e., observations presented in a graph are assumed to be equally spaced across time intervals; see Scruggs & Mastropieri, in press, for discussion), and (3) variations in time-series data are susceptible to cyclicity (fluctuations in the dependent variable that are not direct results of the independent variable treatment; see Franklin et al., 1996, for a discussion). We assumed that one means of addressing some of these artifacts was to decide a priori how long the observations in each phase should be in the calculation of effect size. A visual inspection of the single-subject design studies in this synthesis suggests some stability in the last three sessions (minimal variability) within each phase when compared to the stability across all observation sessions. Further, the mean intercorrelation between baseline and the first treatment phase is high (.796), suggesting some shared performance patterns across observations. In addition, judgments on the magnitude of ESs were qualified by (1) coding the trend in the data, (2) comparing outcomes to the percentage of nonoverlapping data points between the baseline and treatment conditions, (3) determining whether the study meets a stated a priori criteria for behavior change, and (4) ranking the study in terms of its employment of a strong or a weak criterion for treatment effectiveness.

Because ESs from single-subject studies are typically inflated, we corrected for the correlation between baseline and treatment phases. Thus, consistent with the formula developed by Rosenthal (1994), discussed earlier, which takes into consideration the standard deviation of repeated measures (S_g), the average standard deviation for the baseline and treatment was converted to the following formula:

$$S_p = S_g / \sqrt{2(1 - r)}.$$

ESs from single-subject studies can also be transformed to a scale using the following multiplier:

$$\text{Corrected ES} = (\text{ES baseline and treatment}) \sqrt{2(1 - r)}$$

where r is the baseline and treatment correlation and ES is the ES of the last three baseline and treatment sessions. The mean intercorrelation between the baseline and the first treatment phase for the last sessions was .796. Thus, the correlation of all studies was set at .80. We varied the correlation between .65 to .95. The pattern in results was comparable, and therefore the correlation was set at .80 across all studies.

All phases were coded and comparisons were made between the first baseline and every treatment up to six treatment phases. That is, if a study included a baseline and six variations of treatments, these six ESs were calculated and then averaged for each subject. If the treatment phase had less than three observations, those ESs were not calculated. Because ESs have been shown to vary tremendously (e.g., Franklin et al., 1996; reported in Scruggs & Mastropieri, in press; reported ESs from –.5 to 11 standard deviations), all adjusted ESs greater than 3.00 were considered outliers and removed from the synthesis. This eliminated approximately 15 studies from the analysis.

Multiple Interventions

Some studies we coded involved multiple interventions. For these multiple treatment studies we utilized a composite score. Gleser and Olkin (1994) state that in multiple treatment studies, "the treatments may all be regarded as instances or aspects of a common treatment construct" (p. 351). In addition, they state that "there is strong reason a priori to believe that a composite effect size of treatment obtained by combining the end point ESs would adequately summarize the effect of treatment" (p. 351). Thus, although we coded ESs for individual treatment aspects, we relied primarily on an overall composite of ES to reflect the treatment construct of each study.

Unit of Analysis

ESs were calculated on all dependent variables in each study with positive signs given to the ES when the experimental condition was attributed to higher performance. Depending on the experimental design, both the control and the experimental group included LD students. ESs between experimental conditions that included LD participants and control conditions that included chronological age-matched NLD subjects were also calculated if they were included in the study.

ESs were averaged for each study or reported separately for each major dependent measure category (e.g., word recognition, cognitive processing, mathematics). For each outcome category, several ESs were often extracted from a single study. No doubt, multiple ESs extracted from a single study can be problematic because the methods of research integration normally assume that the ESs are independent. This problem is not as pronounced, however, when different subjects from a study provide separate measures of ESs. Such a condition arises in single-subject designs, for example, when different ESs are extracted for each participant. Obviously, ignoring such dependence and treating the within-group effects as independent ESs increases a Type I error rate of the homogeneity of effect size test (test of variability and ESs) (Gleser & Olkin, 1994). On the other hand, disregarding the data has the opposite effect, increasing the likelihood of committing a Type II error (see Cooper, Nye, Charlton, Lindsay, & Greathouse, 1996, for a discussion of these issues). In this meta-analysis, the problem of stochastically dependent ESs (see Gleser & Olkin, 1994) was partially addressed by (1) calculating the number of independent samples per feature (e.g., moderator variables) from each study and (2) by comparing treatment outcomes with differing units of analysis. These variations allowed for study features to be represented (indexed) without throwing away valuable data.

In terms of independent samples, the majority of studies coded included separate LD samples in the control and treatment condition who were administered the same battery of tests (dependent measures). The control group and treatment group were considered as two independent samples. If additional (different) subjects were in another treatment (i.e., treatment 2), this was also considered as a separate independent sample, and so on. Therefore, because studies vary in the number of independent samples, this information is presented in subsequent tables. It is important for the reader to realize, however, that there are multiple ways that independent samples could have been calculated: socioeconomic status (SES), age, gender, and so on. Further, high and low IQ scores were other possibilities. Thus, our analysis of independent samples is not as accurate as we would like it to be. However, it was the case in the majority of studies that included subgroups (e.g., age levels, math vs. reading disability) that such subgroups were infrequent or were not a priori defined (i.e., the sample was divided in a post hoc fashion for analysis). Therefore, we kept our analysis of independent samples at only the most general level. The maximum number of independent samples calculated for a single study was eight (two controls, six treatments) and the minimum was one (a repeated measure design that included the same sample in the control and treatment conditions).

Because there is some debate about what constitutes an independent estimate of ES, we also used a shifting unit of analysis (Cooper, 1989) to analyze main effects across studies. Two units of analysis were considered because multivariate ES data posed at least three problems. First, ESs calculated for any one sample within a particular study are correlated, and therefore it is difficult to treat them as independent (e.g., Gleser & Olkin, 1994). On occasion, however, a single treatment may have different effects on different outcomes. Therefore, it may be inappropriate to average ESs in these studies or to choose simply a single-outcome measure. Second, there are several methodological variations across studies that influence ES. Thus, it cannot be assumed that a particular intervention program will have the same effect on an outcome variable when methodology varies. Finally, studies vary in terms of their outcome measures. Some studies may focus on word recognition, whereas others measure word recognition and reading comprehension, and still others measure only reading comprehension. Thus, there must be some modification in a traditional multivariate linear model to analyze the units of outcome.

In our synthesis, the ES for each dependent measure category was first coded as if it were an independent event. Thus, if a study included word recognition and reading comprehension measures, these two effect sizes were coded separately. We also coded the average ES for each study. Thus, a study would contribute only one ES proportionately to the sample size. To determine the stability of various moderator variables on intervention outcomes, we compared the outcomes as a function of the two units of analysis. We assumed that if a moderator variable is stable in terms of its influence on outcomes, then significant effects would occur for both units of analysis. Further, because a chi-square was used to assess moderators of ES, and because this procedure is sensitive to variations in sample size, the stability of the moderator variable must be evaluated across variations in sample size. However, Hedges and Olkin (1985; see pp. 1175–1183) report that simulations of the effect sizes in educational research are reasonably accurate across the number of dependent measures and studies reflected in this synthesis.

Analysis

To determine whether a set of *d*s shared a common ES (i.e., *d* was consistent across the studies), a homogeneity statistic, *Q*—which approximates chi-square distribution with $k - 1$ degrees of freedom, where k is the number of effect sizes—was computed (Hedges & Olkin, 1985). A homogeneity test (Hedges & Olkin, 1985) was performed using a Proc GLM computer program for the domain categories. When the homogeneity of the sample size was rejected (i.e., a significant chi-square was obtained), further exploration of the finding was done through analysis of the study features. A significant chi-square indicated that the study features significantly moderated the magnitude of effect sizes. When there were two or more levels of a study feature, a Scheffe post hoc comparison was performed to test for the significant differences between levels.

As suggested by Hedges and Olkin (1985), outliers were removed from the analysis of main effects and interactions. Outliers were defined as effect sizes lying beyond the first gap of a least one standard deviation between adjacent ES values in a positive or negative direction (Bollen, 1989). Seven studies were thus excluded from the group design analysis. Two of the studies included cognitive treatments. There did not appear to be any other particular pattern among these studies that we could discern. For reports of nonsignificant effects unaccompanied by any statistic, we followed a conservative procedure of estimating ES at 0.00.

For the general analysis of outcomes, two different procedures were used to estimate effect sizes. First, we analyzed main effects related to methodology, article characteristics, LD characteristics, and treatment variables. For each measure, an ES, based on the previous formula, was computed. Each ES was then weighted by the reciprocal in the sampling variance. The dependent measure for the estimate of ES was defined as

$$\text{Est} = d/(1/v)$$

where v is the inverse of the sampling variance,

$$v = (N_{\text{trt}} + N_{\text{crtl}})/(N_{\text{trt}} \times N_{\text{crtl}}) + d^2/[2(N_{\text{trt}} + N_{\text{crtl}})]$$

We conducted planned tests that focused on the area of primary interest related to the instructional approach (i.e., the way the sample was described in terms of reading and intelligence, child age, child gender, and methodological variables). For each of these variables, we tested a simple main effect. In cases where several comparisons were made, we preselected an alpha level based on the number of comparisons. As a follow-up for comparisons that were not statistically independent, we used a Scheffe method for a large number of contrasts or a Boole–Bonferroni Inequality Test which is less sensitive to the intercorrelation among multivariate measures when compared to other post hoc procedures.

Second, as a follow-up to main effects, we used a regression analysis. We tested the robustness of the main effect using a general linear model procedure to control statistically for each of the other variables. We tested the important main effects and whether they should be qualified by two- or three-way interactions. In order to characterize the relationships between study characteristics and outcomes, weighted least square fixed effects regression models were fitted to the empirical values, following methods recommended by Harwell (1992) and described by Hedges and Olkin (1985, pp. 168–174; see also Hedges, 1994, pp. 295–298). In the case of ES analysis, test model specifications do exist whenever the number of studies exceeds the number of predictors (see Hedges, 1994, for a review). These tests of model specifications are an important part of model building. Thus, we assumed that a regression model provides a useful framework for addressing some of the common problems in the meta-analysis (e.g., magnitude of effect sizes varies from study to study as a consequence of study methodology, diversity of treatment implementations, sampling errors, etc.; Bryk & Raudenbush, 1993).

The primary unit of analysis in the regression model was the average ES for each study (N = 180 for group design; N = 85 for single-subject design). Each study was weighted to its precision, giving more weight to the more precise estimates, weighing each study level according to the inverse of the sampling variance (attaching more weight to studies with larger samples). The regression was computed with the effect sizes as the dependent variable and with weights defined as the reciprocal of the sampling variance for each study. The procedure involved a weighted least square analysis that estimates the linear model parameters by *minimizing* the weighted sum of squared differences between observations and estimates. The weighted sum of squares due to the regression is the statistic $Q(\chi^2)$ that is also used for testing all components of β (beta), but not the intercept, are zero. The regression is computed with the estimated effect sizes as the dependent variable with weights defined as the reciprocal of the sampling variance. Thus, the F-tests in the analysis of variance for the estimates in the regression are ignored, but the weighted sum of squares about the regression is the chi-square statistic for testing model specification. The squared multiple correlation between the observed effect sizes and the predictors include two sources of variation (between-study effects) and within-study effects (nonsystematic or sampling effects). Only between-study effects are systematic and therefore can be used to interpret predictor variables. Thus, an R^2 of .38 would explain 62% of the variance (1.0 – .38), even though they explain only 38% of the total variance in effect estimates (see Hedges, 1994, p. 298, for a discussion).

In a model for a series of effect sizes, if it is found to be well specified, we hope to be in a strong position to draw inferences about model parameters. Whenever the number of case studies is larger than the number of predictors, we use a Q_e statistic (sum of squares related to the model error term) to test the model specifics. When the model is correctly specified, Q_e has the approximate chi-square distribution with k minus p degrees of freedom. If Q_e exceeds the critical value, we reject the model specification. Note that Q_e is analogous to the weighted sum of squares of the bottom regression line. Thus, the test for model specification corresponds to testing whether the residual variance is larger than expected. The test of statistic Q_r allows for testing that the slope and intercept are simultaneously zero. Unless otherwise specified, the degrees of freedom are 1.

We did not use a conventional ANOVA to test the influence of the moderator variables on ES because they lack two important features. First, the assumptions for the analysis of variance are not met by the ES data because ES estimates probably will not have an appropriate distribution between cells. The variance in the individual observations (ES estimates) is inversely proportional to the number of subjects in the study. Thus, when studies have different sample sizes, the individual error variances can differ by a factor of 10 to 20. Second, even if our between-class tests are accurate, according to Hedges and Olkin (1985), "the use of the ANOVA does not provide any indication whether or not studies within classes share a common effect size" (p. 148). Thus, even if an ANOVA could successfully detect studies that have different average ES, there is no guarantee that the average ES within each class is a reflection of common ES for that particular category.

SUMMARY

In summary, the key metric used in our synthesis of the literature is effect size. For interpretation purposes, the ES in the next chapter will be discussed in much the same way as a *z*-score. An ES of +1.00 indicates that the performance of the experimental group (in this case, students with learning disabilities receiving the experimental treatment) exceeded the control group's performance (students with learning disabilities receiving the control condition) on the dependent measure by one standard deviation. A negative effect size—for example, –1.00—indicates the superior performance of the control. For the purpose of interpretation, Cohen's (1988) distinctions on the magnitude of the ES will be used. A .20 in absolute value is a small size, .60 is moderate size, and .80 is a large ES.

To complete this chapter, we provide for the reader a table (Table 1) that summarizes the various studies. Table 1 provides a synopsis of the various interventions and effect sizes based on Cohen's *d* for both group and single-subject design studies used in the synthesis. The table lists by *broad* instructional categories the studies used in the meta-analysis (with outliers removed) and the instructional domains they cover. The right-hand column of Table 1 reports an overall mean treatment effect size found in each study and the sample size. The dependent measures (e.g., achievement measures) that were different than the focus of the study are *not* reported in this table (this will be provided in Table 3, in Chapter 3). As is evident in Table 1, a number of studies overlap in the various categories. Thus, some studies and some academic or cognitive domains are represented in more than one category of treatment.

It is important to note that the effect sizes cannot be taken at face value. This is because several variables influence the magnitude of effect sizes. These issues will be discussed further in the next chapter. We provide for the interested researcher effect sizes, averaged within studies for those using group design as a function of the 17 general categories of *dependent* measures, in Appendix D. Appendix D also provides effect sizes (based on the last three sessions in the baseline and treatment phases) for studies utilizing single-subject designs as a function of

TABLE 1. Synopsis of Studies Included in the Meta-Analysis

Category	Effect size	*N*
Attribution Training		
This experiment investigated how verbalization of subtraction with regrouping operations influenced LD Ss' self-efficacy and skillful performance and also explored how effort–attributional feedback affected these achievement behaviors. Ss in one treatment group verbalized aloud while solving problems. Ss in the second treatment group verbalized only during the first half of training. The control condition utilized no verbalizing (Schunk & Cox, 1986).	.49	90
Ss received attributional retraining through cognitive self-instructional methods and group-processing sessions that included controlled instruction and transition to direct instruction. One group was referred to as "Cool Catss are Stars" (Catss: Can do–Ability–Try Hard–Strategy–Success), while the second treatment group received "Stars" only (Stars: Stop–Think–Act–Review–Success). Subjects included math, reading, and written instruction (Morgan, 1991, Dissertation).	.36	81
Bibliotherapy		
This study focused on the use of bibliotherapy, a method through which adolescents can observe parallel stresses at an affective distance and incorporate change without a direct threat to personal independence. Ss read literature relevant to the problems they often faced. One group added a weekly discussion group (Lenkowsky, Barowsky, Dayboch, Puccio, & Lenkowsky, 1987).	1.70	96
Simultaneous and Successive Processing		
This study examined reading comprehension and information processing strategies, specifically successive and simultaneous synthesis and verbalization of the child during task performance (Brailsford, Snart, & Das, 1984).	.93	24
Intervention was based on whether the child with learning disabilities had difficulties with simultaneous or sequential processing. Tasks in the domain of interest (i.e., math, reading, self-concept) were developed to facilitate development of these cognitive processes (Balcerzak, 1986).	.44	40
Cognitive remediation of decoding deficit was attempted by following a theoretically based program. The theory identifies four major cognitive processes: planning, attention, simultaneous, and successive processing (PASS) (Das, Mishra, & Pool, 1995).	.34	51
Instructional Sequence		
Systematic math instruction using the concrete–semiconcrete–abstract teaching sequence was provided to students who were identified as having math disabilities. Data were collected via a 1-minute assessment probe at the end of each lesson for two purposes. The first purpose was to validate that this teaching sequence was effective for skill acquisition and short-term retention. The second purpose was to determine when during the instructional sequence the students would make the association between the concrete or semiconcrete lessons and the abstract probe presentation (Miller & Mercer, 1993).	1.80	9

(*continued*)

TABLE 1. (*continued*)

Category	Effect size	*N*
Computer-Assisted Instruction (CAI)		
CAI—Math		
The effectiveness of two drill and practice methods, computer-assisted instruction and workbook, was compared using six LD and six NLD students. Both instructional methods provided highly structured drill and practice of multiplication facts, but differed on several important dimensions: immediacy of feedback, individually tailored practice of problems, and mode of presentation (Foster, 1983, Dissertation).	4.21	12, 6
The study focused on the use of computer-assisted practice in achieving higher math computation skills through a mixture of visual and auditory modes (Kunka, 1984, Dissertation).	.24	110
The purpose of the study was to compare the effect of two types of instructional software on the math achievement of EMH, LD, and EH resource room students. The study also investigated the relationship between math achievement and attitude toward CAI for Ss learning math using the two types of math software (Whitman, 1986, Dissertation).	.13	72
The study utilized a single-subject design to investigate whether learning of multiplication tables via computer programs transfers to paper/pencil tasks. The baseline phase used flashcards, math games, and worksheets of math facts. The treatment phase used the computer program, which included a multiplication table, *A Treasure Hunt of Facts, Meteor Multiplication,* and a voice synthesizer (Chiang, 1986).	1.40	6
The study examined the efficacy of Teacher Net, an inexpensive computer networking system. The major question at issue was the extent to which Teacher Net could reduce the time teachers spend monitoring, grading assignments, and looking for error patterns. It was postulated that by automating these activities (at one-tenth the cost of a regular network), teachers would have a lot more time for direct teaching (Moore, Carnine, Stepnoski, & Woodward, 1987).	0.0	27
CAI—Reading		
This study examined reading and CAI at the secondary level. Attitudes toward reading and self-concept as impacted by CAI were investigated (Porinchack, 1984, Dissertation).	.43	51
In this study, computer-synthesized speech was incorporated into a reading program to improve the word recognition abilities of students with learning disabilities (Farmer, Klein, & Bryson, 1992).	.10	14
This study investigated the effects of presenting words to be read on a computer screen that represented the right or left visual field (VanStrien, Stolk, & Zuiker, 1995).	1.85	20
This alternating treatments design utilized computer-assisted instruction to aid in silent reading comprehension skills (Harper, 1986, Dissertation).	1.24	9

(*continued*)

TABLE 1. (*continued*)

Category	Effect size	N
The efficacy of computer-assisted training procedures with reading decoding were assessed in the training of children with three specific types of reading disability: oral reading, intermodal–associative, and sequential. The training involved an integration of current theoretical issues: application of the automaticity theory and a combination of the task-analytic and process-oriented models. It was hypothesized that improved performance in the trained skills would result in transfer of training to untrained reading subskills, as well as to reading in general (Fiedorowicz, 1986).	1.87	15
This study investigated the effectiveness of computer-assisted articulatory-based and nonarticulatory-based phonological analysis training on the reading and spelling of children with learning disabilities (Wise, Ring, Sessions, & Olson, in press).	.80	45
The relative efficacy of computer programs with and without synthesized speech support on the word recognition of children with learning disabilities was investigated (Farmer, Klein, & Bryson, 1992).	.11	14
This alternating treatments design compared computer-assisted instruction and teacher instruction in the area of reading comprehension. In both treatments, the S read a short story twice and answered a series of multiple choice questions (Van den Meiracker, 1987, Dissertation).	.87	9
Reading disabled students were trained on the Autoskill Component Reading Subskills Program (with computer) according to procedures specifically developed for three reading disability subtypes: oral reading, intermodel–associative and sequential (Fiedorowicz & Trites, 1987).	.44	91
A new computer program, *Hint and Hunt 1,* designed to increase decoding fluency in reading was evaluated with a sample of 20 LD students (Jones, Torgesen, & Sexton, 1987).	1.96	30
Segmented or whole word speech feedback (provided through a computer) was investigated. Speech feedback was hypothesized to be better for children in the early stages of reading (phonological recoding) than for children who were proficient readers (Van Daal & Reitsma, 1990).	1.33	17
This study presented an overview of a computer program directed toward the remediation of children's deficits in word recognition and phonological decoding. Ss read stories on the computer and were trained to request synthetic-speech feedback for difficult words. Groups received either whole word feedback or segmented word feedback (Olson & Wise, 1992).	.66	35, 149
This study determined the degree to which computer-mediated presentations of text influence LD Ss' reading comprehension, and whether cognitive factors related to metacognition, attribution, and working memory influence treatment effects. Ss were assigned to one of four treatment conditions: control, paper (offline), computer—no reread, and computer reread. Within each condition, traditional and cloze comprehension questions were presented at three levels of passage difficulty (Swanson & Trahan, 1992).	.46	120

(continued)

TABLE 1. (*continued*)

Category	Effect size	*N*
This study examined the effects of computer-based reading and spelling practice on the development of reading and spelling skills. Ss practiced hard-to-read words under three conditions: reading from the computer screen, copying from the screen, and writing from memory after presentation on the screen. For all words, whole word sound was available on call during practice. To assess learning effects, both a dictation and a read-aloud task were administered in which nonpracticed control words were also presented. During training, the computer kept record of several aspects of the pupils' learning behavior (Van Daal & Van der Liej, 1992).	1.39	28
The study investigated the connection between reading comprehension and decoding skills by using a computer-based text-to-speech system. The Ss read the text on the computer screen. When a difficult word was encountered, the S could target the word for the computer to provide speech feedback (Lundberg & Olofsson, 1993).	.44	33
Disabled readers and normal beginning readers were compared on requesting help in the form of speech feedback during computer-based word reading. It was also examined whether it was best to give feedback on all words or to allow the disabled readers to choose. Normal beginning readers and reading-age matched pupils with reading problems engaged in reading practice with speech feedback on call for both difficult and easy words. A set of both difficult and easy sums was completed as a control task. Another group of reading disabled pupils who were also matched on reading level practiced the reading of words with unsolicited speech feedback (Van Daal & Reitsma, 1993).	.09	46
Two CAI modes of instruction were compared. In the first condition, students read passages from a science textbook using a basic computer version (i.e., text, graphics, outline). In the second condition, the students read, with the aid of speech synthesis, an online glossary, links between questions and text, and highlighting of main ideas (MacArthur & Haynes, 1995).	.52	10
CAI—Reasoning skills		
This study evaluated the role of instructional design in the field test and revision process for CAI in drawing conclusions and critiquing syllogistic arguments: reasoning skills (Collins & Carnine, 1988).	1.48	26
CAI—Spelling		
The study investigated the use of computer-assisted instruction and feedback in attaining higher spelling skills (Kitterman, 1984, Dissertation).	.53	5
The study compared computer-assisted instruction and paper/pencil instruction as the means of delivering independent spelling practice in classes for LD students. Both groups utilized identical content and similar activities, but differed in instructional design features (MacArthur, Haynes, Malouf, Harris, & Owings, 1990).	.63	44

(*continued*)

TABLE 1. (*continued*)

Category	Effect size	*N*
The *SelfSpell* programs used in this study provide a multimedia environment for dyslexic children that uses synthesized speech to augment the written text. The *SelfSpell* treatment condition was compared with the *SpellMaster* in the control condition (Fawcett, Nicolson, & Morris, 1993).	.97	12
The purpose of this study was to determine the efficacy of three motoric conditions (writing, tracing, and computer keyboarding) on the spelling performance of 3rd- and 4th-grade students without learning disabilities and with learning disabilities. This study applied empirically based procedures for teaching spelling, examined student performance over time, and incorporated student interviews concerning their preference for motoric condition (Vaughn, Schumm, & Gordon, 1993).	.66	48
Two experimental studies examined the effects of different types of phonemic segmentation training on phonemic segmentation, reading, and spelling. Ss who were weak in phonemic segmentation were trained with the use of diagrams and alphabet letters, alphabet letters only, or with no visual support at all. The study incorporated computer-assisted instruction (Kerstolt, Van Bon, & Schreuder, 1994).	.31	48, 49
The purpose of this study was to investigate the impact of integrated proofreading strategy training, combining the use of a computer-based spelling checker and student strategies, on the proofreading performance of high school–aged students with learning disabilities (McNaughton, Hughes, & Ofiesh, 1997).	1.78	3
CAI—Writing		
Study participants generated text (story writing)and error monitoring and correction at microcomputers both alone and as members of dyads (Hine, Goldman, & Cosden, 1990).	.92	11
<u>Comprehension Monitoring Strategies</u>		
Error correction		
Two procedures for correcting oral reading errors during training in word attack strategies in a naturalistic setting were examined (Meyer, 1982).	.62	58
An alternating treatments design was used to investigate the relative effectiveness of two error correction procedures: word supply and phonic analysis on oral reading performance (Rose, McEntire, & Dowdy, 1982).	1.49	5
Study participants generated text (story writing)and error monitoring and correction at microcomputers both alone and as members of dyads (Hine, Goldman, & Cosden, 1990).	.92	11
Students were encouraged either to make active student responses during error correction, or, in the case of the control, they made no overt response. Effects of intervention on the acquisition and maintenance of geography facts was investigated (Barbetta & Heward, (1993).	.65	3

(*continued*)

TABLE 1. (*continued*)

Category	Effect size	*N*
Self-questioning strategies		
The study looked at the effects of cognitive monitoring, creative problem solving, and a combination of the two instructional programs on reading disabled 3rd graders' oral comprehension (Manning, 1984).	1.08	100
This study focused on reading comprehension, and provided cooperative skills training in reading with the strategies of self-questioning and paraphrasing, and in writing with the strategies of sentences and error monitoring. Cooperative skills training included four parts: orientation to types of goal structures, activation, skill training, and prestrategy training (Beals, 1985, Dissertation).	1.50	28
Ss were trained in one of four techniques while reading comprehension passages. The techniques were read–reread, self-questioning and underlining, self-questioning only, and underlining only. LD children were matched on reading age with regular children (Chan & Cole, 1986).	.97	72
The purpose of this study was to investigate the effects of using a questioning strategy with LD Ss to increase discussion participation and to increase reading comprehension (Dixon, 1984, Dissertation).	.58	60
The study investigated the use of dialogical thinking–reading lessons in which the S was engaged in reasoning and reflective thinking in order to decide what to believe about a central issue related to a story. Ss were asked to consider the evidence for two hypothesized explanatory conclusions regarding an important question (Commeyras, 1992).	1.34	14
This study investigated the hypothesis that insufficient metacomprehension is one possible cause underlying LD adolescents' comprehension problems, and that training them to monitor their understanding of important textual elements fosters metacomprehension and improves their comprehension performance. Half of the Ss received a five-step self-questioning training in which they learned to monitor their understanding of important textual units. The other half of the Ss received no training, but had the same materials as the experimental group (Wong & Jones, 1982).	.56	120
The study examined the effectiveness of two methods of teaching an efficient questioning strategy to Ss with learning disabilities. The study compared cognitive modeling alone in the use of constraint-seeking questions, and cognitive modeling plus verbalization in the use of constraint-seeking questions, involving explicit and consistent instruction and feedback (Simmonds, 1990).	.27	60
This study addressed the effectiveness of teacher acquisition and implementation of two methods for improving the comprehension skills of LD Ss: instruction in teaching specific questioning strategies (Question–Answer–Response; QARS) and selected traditional methods of reading comprehension instruction (Simmonds, 1992).	1.54	447
This study describes and evaluates an instructional program designed to help students with learning disabilities learn about the concept of theme, identify themes in stories, and apply themes to real life (Williams, Brown, Silverstein, & deCani, 1994).	1.36	69

(*continued*)

TABLE 1. (*continued*)

Category	Effect size	*N*
This study compared the effects of vocabulary instruction on reading comprehension. Students either were instructed about determining meanings of words in context or received vocabulary definitions (Pany & Jenkins, 1978).	3.11	6
<u>Consultative Services</u>		
This study tested the role of a child advocate and coordinator of services for LD children. Two treatment groups and one untreated control group were incorporated into the study. One of the treatment groups used the child advocate while the other was a school-informed group, but with no advocacy services given (Pihl, Parkes, Drake & Vrana, 1980).	1.14	90
The effects of a collaboration consultative model on the reading recovery of primary grade children with learning disabilities was investigated (Larson & Gerber, 1987).	1.74	5
This study compared the achievement of LD Ss in reading and written language across four conditions: one period of resource room instruction per day, two periods of resource room instruction per day, consultative services combined with in-class instruction, and consultative services to classroom teachers (Schulte, Osborne, & McKinney, 1991).	.46	67
This study describes the use of a consultation-collaboration model of intervention in which a psychologist and a teacher worked jointly to establish a remedial reading program for five special needs children placed in a regular primary school class (Cochrane & Ballard, 1986).	1.37	5
<u>Counseling</u>		
Adlerian		
The inclusion of group counseling was expected to facilitate the treatment of children involved in prescriptive remedial programs; specifically a significant increase in vocabulary and comprehension skills was anticipated. The therapeutic style was primarily Adlerian (McCollum & Anderson, 1974).	.29	48
Biofeedback		
This study examined the effects of biofeedback-induced relaxation training on attention to task, impulsivity, and locus of control (Omizo & Williams, 1982).	.56	32
In this study Ss were provided with long-term, symptom duration, sensorimotor rhythm biofeedback training for the remediation of learning disabilities (Tansey, 1985).	.80	8
Career counseling		
The study investigated the effects of a counseling program designed to promote career maturity among LD youth and other youth at risk of dropping out of school. Activities focused on self-awareness and an exploration of career options. Discussion, teacher modeling, and cognitive processing/thinking aloud were utilized in the treatment (Hutchinson, Freeman, Downey, & Kilbreath, 1992).	.58	16

(*continued*)

TABLE 1. (*continued*)

Category	Effect size	*N*
Rational–emotive (reality) therapy		
The purpose of this study was to determine the effects of Rational–emotive education (REE) counseling group sessions on LD Ss' self-concept and locus of control orientation. Ss met twice weekly in a peer-group situation for 12 consecutive weeks. Among other topics, Ss discussed problem-solving issues and skills, rational coping strategies, and how to give support, empathy, and encouragement to others in the group (Omizo, Cubberly, & Omizo, 1985).	.77	54
The authors investigated the effects of a rational–emotive education (REE) program on LD adolescents' self-concept and locus of control (Omizo, Lo, & Williams, 1986).	.82	50
Relaxation therapy		
Children participated either in a relaxation training session (listening to 30-minute audiotapes) or in a social skills group to reduce acting-out behavior (Amerikaner, 1982).	.44	46
This study compared two treatment groups; self-instruction (Meichembaum, 1977) and relaxation training (Jacobson, 1938), and a no-treatment control group. Treatment groups were given 10 half-hour sessions over 4 weeks and were assessed before and after the treatment on cognitive tasks requiring deliberation (Zieffle & Romney, 1985).	.56	30
Creativity Training		
The Purdue Creative Thinking Program was used to stimulate the LD experimental group's divergent thinking abilities (Jaben, Treffinger, Whelan, Hudson, Stainback, & Stainback, 1982).	1.38[c]	49
The Purdue Creative Thinking Program included two 45-minute sessions per week using a set of 28 audio tapes and printed materials designed to stimulate divergent thinking, figural and verbal fluency, flexibility, and originality.Separate studies were published in different journals (Jaben, 1983, 1985, 1986, 1987).	1.50 .39 .40 .58	49 52 98 50
This study examined whether intermediate-grade LD students could generalize creativity training to increase competency on a spontaneous writing task. Seven intact classrooms were used to analyze differences between groups on initial creative–productive–thinking level. Experimental Ss engaged in brainstorming activities where each child was free to share ideas, which were recorded and posted for observation (Fortner, 1986).	.37	51
Curriculum-Based Measurement—Programming		
The study examined the effectiveness of innovative curriculum-based measurement (CBM) in classwide decision-making structures within general education mathematics instruction, with and without recommendations for how to incorporate CBM feedback into instructional planning (Fuchs, Fuchs, Hamlett, Phillips, & Bentz, 1994).	.48	120

(*continued*)

TABLE 1. (*continued*)

Category	Effect size	*N*
Diagnostic–Prescriptive		
This study compared two treatment groups with a no-treatment control group. One treatment group included intense remediation of deficits through tutoring, while in the second treatment group teachers were instructed to teach to the Ss' strengths (Warner, 1973, Dissertation)	.59[b]	30
This study used ability measures to predict the most appropriate method or sequence of mathematics instruction for LD junior high school students (Glaman, 1974, Dissertation).	.23	33
This study examined the effects of psycholinguistic training on improving psycholinguistic skills. Training activities focused on 12 psycholinguistic areas and Ss received training in their deficit areas (Sowell, Parker, Poplin, & Larsen, 1979).	.25	63
The purpose of this study was to compare the effects of (1) remediation of hypothesized component deficits given prior to remediation of known academic deficiencies and (2) remediation of known academic deficiencies alone (Wade, 1979, Dissertation).	.22	76
Ten planned comparisons of pretest and posttest scores on the Slosson Oral Reading Test support the position that LD students regress in their reading skills when they experience extended breaks in their educational programs during the summer months. This study looked at a 5-week summer program during either the first or last half of the summer to see if such an intervention can prevent reading regression (Cornelius & Semmel, 1982).	.61	60
Ss received instruction based on an individualized remediation technique utilizing the deficits of the neuropsychological testing. The treatment included a more lively teacher presence, organized and structured sessions, frequent change of activities, success-oriented activities, and individualized and concrete instructional materials (DeBoskey, 1982, Dissertation).	1.06	23
Ss with major levels of retardation in reading were divided into two subgroups for intervention purposes. During the first phase of treatment one group (control) received diagnostic–prescriptive remediation and the other a direct instruction program (Distar Reading II, a phonetically weighted program), both delivered for equal amounts of time each day by the same teacher (Branwhite, 1983).	2.33	14
Three intervention programs were constructed for Ss with deficits in the areas of auditory closure and visual sequential memory. The first was designed to alleviate the specific disabilities in the areas of deficit. The second was based on a more general approach to language development. The third group (control) undertook a simple number program (Naylor & Pumfrey, 1983).	2.13	60
The purpose of the study was to compare the effects of remediation of ghypothesized component deficits given prior to remediation of known academic deficiencies, and remediation of known academic deficiencies alone. A corollary purpose was to study the immediate effect, if any, of the component deficit remediation on the criterion measure (Wade & Kass, 1987).	.42	76

(*continued*)

TABLE 1. (*continued*)

Category	Effect size	*N*
Direct Instruction		
Attention		
This study investigated improving attending behaviors and incorporated two treatment groups and a no-treatment control group. The first treatment group received training in attending behaviors by a direct instruction method. The second group was exposed to modeling of the attending behaviors but received no other formal training (Argulewicz, 1982).	.95	72
Math		
This study examined the influence of a modeling technique on the acquisition of long division computational skills by eight adolescents with learning disabilities (Rivera & Deutsch Smith, 1988).	1.66	8
This study examined the comparative effectiveness of direct instruction alone and direct instruction combined with supplemental homework assignments on the acquisition of basic mathematics skills among elementary school–aged students with learning disabilities (Rosenberg, 1989).	1.31	6, 4
This study employed direct instruction math and its components (strategy teaching and sequencing problems) in isolation to determine which was the most effective for teaching LD Ss to identify the correct algorithm for solving addition and subtraction word problems (Wilson, 1989, Dissertation).	.68	62
The effects of token reinforcement, cognitive behavior modification, and direct instruction on LD Ss' math skills were compared. Math skills were measured by 2-minute classroom timings of basic addition and subtraction problems (Ross & Braden, 1991).	.26	94
Reading		
This study compared the effectiveness of three instructional strategies that varied in the amount of direct instruction provided on reading comprehension. Specifically, the study measured recall of word meanings and recall of facts from a story (Pany & Jenkins, 1978).	5.32	6
During the first phase of treatment in this study one group (control) received diagnostic–prescriptive remediation and the other a direct instruction program (Distar Reading II, a phonetically weighted program), both delivered for equal amounts of time each day by the same teacher (Branwhite, 1983).	2.32	14
A comparison was made of the efficacy of metacomprehension (self-monitoring) plus direct instruction, direct instruction alone, and a control training condition in finding the main idea (Graves, 1986).	3.13	24

(*continued*)

TABLE 1. (*continued*)

Category	Effect size	*N*
Two approaches were used in teaching elementary LD students three critical reading skills (ability to detect faulty generalization, ability to detect false causality, ability to detect invalid testimonial). The experimental group utilized direct instruction and the control group used discussion and a workbook. The study had three major purposes: to evaluate whether a systematic direct instruction approach, found successful with nonhandicapped students, would be effective with LD students; to assess the relative effectiveness of two approaches to teaching critical reading; and to examine the effects of each instructional approach on several dependent measures to identify any differential effects of instruction (Darch & Kameenui, 1987).	1.22	25
Ss with reading difficulties were selected for this study. Three intervention conditions were utilized: psycho-motor, self-esteem enhancement, and direct instruction (Somerville & Leach, 1988).	1.24	40
The efficacy of instructional variables as examined comparing a progressive time-delay and trial-and-error strategy in teaching sight word acquisition. Observational learning versus direct instruction was also assessed by having children observe each other being taught different words (McCurdy, Cundari, & Lentz, 1990).	1.77	2
Children with reading disabilities were assigned to one of two word identification training programs or to a study skills control group. One treatment remediated deficient phonological analysis and blending skills and provided direct instruction of letter–sound mappings. The other program taught children how to acquire, use, and monitor four metacognitive decoding strategies (Lovett, & Steinbach, in press).	.77	122
Science		
The purpose of this study was to compare the effectiveness of two instructional approaches on mildly handicapped and nonhandicapped Ss' science achievement. Ss were assigned at random to one of two conditions: direct instruction or discovery teaching. The content of the lessons remained constant across conditions and focused on such concepts as displacement, flotation, variable, controlled experimentation, and scientific prediction (Bay, Staver, Bryan, & Hale, 1992).	2.41	68
Vocabulary		
This study examined the efficacy of a direct instruction corrective reading program that focused on vocabulary, sentence memory, logical reasoning, following directions, and common information (Lloyd, Cullinan, Heins, & Epstein, 1980).	.84	23
Goal Setting		
This study focused on a training program designed to teach LD junior high school Ss to set realistic achievement goals, to expend effort to reach those goals, and to accept personal responsibility for achievement outcomes (Tollefson, Tracy, Johnsen, Farmer, & Buenning, 1984).	.30	61

(*continued*)

TABLE 1. (*continued*)

Category	Effect size	*N*
This experiment tested the hypothesis that participation in goal setting enhances self-efficacy and skills. Included in the study were three groups: self-set goals, assigned goals, and no goals (Schunk, 1985).	1.14	30
The study examined the impact of a goal-attainment intervention related to the completion of project-type assignments. The study included seven steps: task evaluation, options generation, goal specification, plan identification, plan expansion, demands consideration, and self-monitoring (Lenz, Ehren, & Smiley, 1991).	1.69	6
This study was conducted to determine if a planning and writing strategy would improve the essay writing of LDSs. Four Ss were taught a strategy designed to facilitate the setting of product and process goals, generation and organization of notes, continued planning during writing, and evaluation of goal attainment. A multiple probe across subjects design was used (Graham, MacArthur, Schwartz, & Page-Voth, 1992).	1.66	4
This study extended previous research on components of effective strategy instruction operationalized in an approach referred to as self-regulated strategy development (SRSD). Comparisons were made among LD Ss on composition and self-efficacy in four conditions: SRSD, SRSD without goal setting and self-monitoring, direct teaching, and practice control (Sawyer, Graham, & Harris, 1992).	1.78	43
Hemispheric Stimulation		
Hemispheric stimulation of left hemisphere is attained by presenting target words to the right hand of the child as the child reads. Treatment begins at letter level and progresses to word level. Treatment varies according to whether one is P-dyslexic or L-dyslexic (Bakker, 1990).	2.26	56
Language Strategies		
Oral language		
This study examined paradigmatic language training. The effect that training paradigmatic language structures has upon the reading process was investigated with LD children. The effects of intelligence, special training, and training over time were analyzed in a pretest–posttest control group design (Cartelli, 1978).	2.25	46
Ss in this study received training either in word recognition and decoding skills, in oral and written language, or in classroom survival skills (Lovett, Ransby, & Barron, 1988).	.41	112
Ss in this study received training either in word recognition and decoding skills, in oral and in written language, or classroom survival skills (Lovett, Ransby, Hardwick, Johns, & Donaldson, 1989).	.39	178
Outcomes of minilessons in adverbial phrases was compared with results of minilessons on possessives for students in the intermediate grades (Dowis & Schloss, 1992).	1.58	4

(*continued*)

TABLE 1. (*continued*)

Category	Effect size	*N*
Language experience (reading)		
Individual classes were divided into three groups, an experimental group that focused on language experience,and two control groups (based on reading level) termed "action" and "double action." On a daily basis, each group alternated between working with the aide and worksheets, and working with the investigator and interactive instructional activities. Ss were graded on spelling, capitalization, punctuation, and English usage, and were encouraged to correct errors. Syllabication and phonics were used with vocabulary words (Lerner, 1978, Dissertation).	.11	60
Phoneme awareness		
This study examined the effects of psycholinguistic training (Minskoff, Wiseman, & Minskoff, 1972) on improving psycholinguistic skills. Training activities focused on 12 psycholinguistic areas. Ss received training in their deficit areas (Sowell, Parker, Poplin, & Larsen, 1979).	.25	63
The study analyzed the effect on literal reading comprehension of providing instruction in the application of psycholinguistic strategies used intuitively in apprehending meaning in discourse. A multiple-choice cloze procedure was used to implement the investigation (Vivion, 1985, Dissertation).	1.42	6
The study examined the possibility that phonemic discrimination training could improve the phonemic segmentation ability of children with reading disabilities (Hurford, 1990).	.40	48
Students with severe learning disabilities who received the Auditory Discrimination in Depth Program (Lindamood & Lindamood, 1975) on an intensive basis, in addition to a comprehensive remedial program, were matched for Verbal IQ, chronological age, reading, spelling, and phonological awareness abilities with 10 other students with severe learning disabilities who also received the comprehensive remedial program but not the Lindamood Program component. Progress in reading, spelling, phonological awareness, use of phonetic principles in spelling of real and nonwords, and phonetic reading of nonwords were documented in December and May (Kennedy & Backman, 1993).	.35	20
This study is one component of a 5-year program of research aimed at generating knowledge about the effectiveness of different approaches to the prevention and remediation of reading difficulties among children in the emergent stages of reading acquisition. Children with learning disabilities were assigned to one of two instructional groups: phonological awareness training (Auditory Discrimination in Depth Program; Lindamood & Lindamood, 1975) or implicit phonological awareness training plus phonics instruction embedded within real word reading and spelling activities (Torgesen, Wagner, Rashotte, Alexander, & Conway, 1997).	.27	31
Phonics		
The purpose of this research was to investigate rule learning in reading disabled and normal children when required to abstract phonetic rules independently and when required to use phonetic rules after instruction (Fletcher & Prior, 1990).	.51	20

(*continued*)

TABLE 1. (*continued*)

Category	Effect size	*N*
Vocabulary		
Three experiments were conducted to assess the effects of vocabulary instruction on word knowledge and reading comprehension. Treatments varied in the amount of direct instruction (Pany, Jenkins, & Schreck, 1982).	5.32	12, 6, 10
The study examined the effects of prior knowledge on the reading comprehension performance of Ss with learning disabilities. Instruction in information and vocabulary concepts was provided to junior high school Ss who lacked prior knowledge required. Reading comprehension performance on three types of reading passages was also examined: textually explicit, textually implicit, and scriptually implicit (Snider, 1989).	1.58	26
Memory Strategies		
The objective of this study was to utilize a mnemonic device to teach 10 letter cluster–sound associations to 17 reading disabled subjects. Direct instruction was incorporated into the intervention (Smith, 1989, Dissertation).	.74	34
Three classrooms of junior high school students with learning disabilities were taught U.S. history content over an 8-week period, in which mnemonic and nonmnemonic materials were alternated (Scruggs & Mastropieri, 1989).	1.01	26
Three classrooms of adolescent students with learning disabilities were taught U.S. history content alternatively using mnemonic and nonmnemonic materials to improve recall of chapter information (Scruggs & Mastropieri, 1989).	.99	20
The study investigated the effectiveness of predictable and unpredictable trial sequences during small group instruction in three experiments in teaching word and abbreviation identification to Ss with learning disabilities. The same Ss were used in each experiment (Ault, Wolery, Gast, Doyle, & Martin, 1990).	1.82	5, 4, 4
A count-by technique was taught to a 4th-grade student with learning disabilities. The procedure involved learning to translate a multiplication problem into a count-by problem as a way of quickly determining answers for difficult-to-master multiplication tables (McIntyre, Test, Cooke, & Beattie, 1991).	1.78	1
The use of mnemonics to learn and remember information holds promise for students with learning and memory problems. In this study keyword mnemonics were used in two of three instructional procedures taught to Ss with mild handicaps. Ss were required to learn and remember definitions of previously unfamiliar science terms. Systematic teaching, an imposed keyword method, and an induced keyword method were compared (King-Sears, Mercer, & Sindelar, 1992).	1.80	37
This study evaluated the effectiveness of classroom mnemonic instruction of science content (Scruggs & Mastropieri, 1992).	1.12[b]	20

(*continued*)

TABLE 1. (*continued*)

Category	Effect size	*N*
This investigation was intended to determine the effects of metamemory training on both metamemory knowledge and related memory performance, as well as its effects on other metacognitive and cognitive domains. The first experiment focused on metamemory training, while the second experiment focused on a metamemory training group, a metacognitive reading group, and a control group (Lucangeli, Galderisi, & Cornoldi, 1995).	.64	166
The purpose of the study was to evaluate the effects of instructing Ss to use a mnemonic strategy to identify and remember pairs or small groups of information (Bulgren, Hock, Schumaker, & Deshler, 1995).	1.77	12
This study investigated whether LD adolescents would transfer the use of four study rules from instructed materials (pictures) to a prose recall task. Two groups of LD Ss received extensive direct instruction that was informed, varied, explicit, extended, and included problem isomorph recognition training (Gelzheiser, 1984).	.54	80
<u>Multisensory Approach</u>		
The study examined word recognition. Via a whole word approach that used a multi-sensory technique for developing reading skills, including the Fernald Method of tracing letters and a Total Body Movement Learning Game (Waterman, 1974, Dissertation).	.96	34
Sight words and letter sounds were taught, tested and reviewed. VAKT (visual, auditory, kinesthetic, tactile) procedures were used and compared with an equated visual–auditory procedure (Bryant, 1979, Dissertation).	.39	42
This study examined the effectiveness of the Tomatis Program plus direct instruction in comparison to a direct instruction alone control on the general academic achievement of children with learning disabilities (Kershner, Cummings, Clarke, Hadfield, & Kershner, 1990).	.32	26
Multisensory instructional approaches have been used in teaching handicapped children for many years, but have never been adequately validated. Using a multiple baseline design and direct measurement of words read and spelled as the dependent variable, this study evaluated the effects of the kinesthetic–tactile component in VAKT (visual, auditory, kinesthetic, tactile) instruction (Thorpe, Lampe, Nash, & Chiang, 1981).	1.22	3
<u>Neurological Impress Method (NIM)</u>		
The Neurological Impress Method (NIM) was used to teach reading skills by having the pupil and the teacher read aloud in unison. The study examined whether the use of NIM would increase comprehension and word recognition abilities among LD Ss, and if the NIM method would work less effectively with Ss who have auditory rather than visual or unidentified learning disabilities (Lorenz & Vockell, 1979).	.27	54

(*continued*)

TABLE 1. (*continued*)

Category	Effect size	*N*
Peer Mediation (PM)		
PM—Behavior		
This study utilized a single-subject design to help a 14-year-old LD student overcome extreme use of obscenities. Peers in the math class participated by refraining from laughter and from responding to the S's obscenities (Salend & Meddaugh, 1985).	1.80	1
The study used a multiple baseline design and evaluated the effects of four 5th-grade LD students tutoring one 3rd-grade and three 2nd-grade LD students on word recognition skills (Chiang, Thorpe, & Darch, 1980).	1.77	8
This study examined the feasibility of an instructional management program for LD incarcerated youths. It compared peer tutors and learning disabilities teachers as implementers of a computational mathematics program for incarcerated, LD juvenile delinquents (Kane & Alley, 1980).	.26	38
The study evaluated the effectiveness of social skills training and cross-age tutoring for improving academic skills (specifically spelling) and social communication behaviors. The treatment groups included social skills training and tutoring, social skills training only, and a no treatment control group (Trapani & Gettinger, 1989).	.17	20
The authors investigated the combined effects of direct instruction and precision teaching by peer tutors in a high school driver education curriculum (Bell, Young, Salzberg, & West, 1991).	1.48	1
The study focused on classwide peer tutoring involving instructional procedures (provision of frequent, immediate feedback) that are known to be successful for children with attention-deficit/hyperactivity disorder (ADHD) (DuPaul & Henningson, 1993).	1.46	1
PM—Math		
The impact of grouping, learning handicap, locus of control, and self-esteem on students' performance on a math problem-solving program was assessed. Students worked alone in one group and worked in dyads in the treatment group taking turns at the computer (Cosden & English, 1987).	2.58	12
PM—Reading		
The study used a multiple baseline design and evaluated the effects of four 5th-grade LD students tutoring one 3rd-grade and three 2nd-grade LD students on word recognition skills (Chiang, Thorpe, & Darch, 1980).	1.77	8
This study investigated the efficacy of an intervention that involved parents as reading tutors at home during the summer (Duvall, Delquadri, Elliott, & Hall, 1992).	1.16	3
The study examined the effects of using repeated-reading and sustained-reading methods as classwide peer-mediated learning activities while manipulating and testing the effect of the level of text difficulty. Special education resource room teachers were assigned randomly to three conditions: peer-mediated repeated reading, peer-mediated sustained reading, or control (Mathes & Fuchs, 1993).	.61	6

(*continued*)

TABLE 1. (*continued*)

Category	Effect size	*N*
Piracetum, a drug thought to enhance learning and memory consolidation, was given in a 3,300 mg daily dose to half of a group of 55 dyslexic boys aged 8 to 13 years, in a 12-week, double-blind, placebo-controlled study (Chase, Schmitt, Russell, & Tallal, 1984).	.30	54
A double-blind, parallel experiment was conducted to determine the effects of Piracetum on reading speed and accuracy among elementary school–aged boys with reading disabilities (Wilsher, Atkins, & Manfield, 1985).	.25	46
Reinforcement Procedures		
Two types of learning environments were compared, an intensive, behavior-engineered resource room program with the regular classroom, for LD Ss who were observed as spending low percentages of time on task (O'Connor, Stuck, & Wyne, 1979).	1.84	108
The purpose of this study was to investigate, through an applied behavior analysis model, the interrelationships of three reading variables: correct oral reading rates, error oral reading rates, and percentage of comprehension. The intervention package included a combination of instructional and reinforcement procedures (Roberts & Smith, 1980).	.94	8
This study examined the relative efficacy of self- and externally imposed schedules of reinforcement on improving oral reading fluency (Billingsley, 1977).	.81	8
In this study, the operant technique of errorless discrimination training of digraphs was investigated (Schimek, 1983).	1.62	1
This study was aimed toward non-self-controlled problem children. It involved two treatment groups, cognitive–behavioral and behavioral, and an attention-control group. The treatment involved individual therapist contact focusing on psychoeducational, play, and interpersonal tasks and situations, including self-instruction, modeling, and contingencies for the cognitive–behavioral group and modeling and contingencies in the behavioral group (Kendall & Braswell, 1982).	.42	54
In this study of oral reading oral reading, beginning reading was taught to four LD Ss using a direct instruction program, Distar. The teacher systematically varied the rate of instructional presentation (rapid vs. slow pace) and frequency of praising (praise vs. no praise) (Darch & Gersten, 1985).	1.51	4
In this study an interdependent group-managed response–cost system mediated by fee tokens was employed to decrease the inappropriate verbalizations of two groups of students with learning disabilities (Salend & Lamb, 1986).	1.80	6
The effects of using a daily report card system on inappropriate verbalizations were examined using a combination ABAB and changing criterion design (Burkwist, Mabee, & McLaughlin, 1987).	1.02	1
Ss were taught planning, organizing, and writing paragraphs by using four steps. Modeling, interactive guided practice, and independent practice were also used along with verbal reinforcement and tokens (Boyer, 1991, Dissertation).	1.68	3

(*continued*)

TABLE 1. (*continued*)

Category	Effect size	*N*
The effects of token reinforcement, cognitive behavior modification, and direct instruction on LD Ss' math skills were compared. Math skills were measured by 2-minute classroom timings of basic addition and subtraction problems (Ross & Braden, 1991).	.26	94
This investigation was intended to evaluate the effects of teacher enthusiasm as an alterable variable on the academic and behavioral performance of LDSs. Ss with learning disabilities in two junior high school special education classrooms were given instruction in science over a 2-week period with levels of teacher enthusiasm manipulated in a crossover design (Brigham, Scruggs, & Mastropieri, 1992).	3.51	16
The efficacy of a dependent group evaluation system was examined in a class of students with disabilities using a reversal design. The group evaluation system involved giving each group member evaluation forms; having each group member rate the group's behavior during a specified time period; randomly selecting a group member whose rating represented the group's rating; comparing the selected group member's rating to the teacher's rating; and delivering reinforcement to all members of the group based on the group's behavior and the selected individual's accuracy in rating their behavior (Salend, Reeder, Katz, & Russell, 1992).	1.76	9
The relative effectiveness of the motivational system on hyperactivity and academic performance in math and reading was evaluated as an alternative to drug control of hyperactive children (Ayllon, Layman, & Kandel, 1975).	1.37	3
<u>Self-Monitoring</u>		
The effects of self-monitoring of attention (on-/off-task behavior) on handwriting and math achievement was investigated for a 7-year-old boy with learning disabilities and attention problems (Hallahan, Lloyd, Kosiewicz, Kauffman, & Graves, 1979).	1.67	1
The effects of self-monitoring on attention to task during small group instruction were investigated. Three LD Ss with severe attentional problems were taught to self-monitor their on-task behavior while participating in oral reading tasks. A reversal design demonstrated marked increases in attention to task for all three Ss (Hallahan, Marshall, & Lloyd, 1981).	1.50	3
Two experiments investigated the effects of self-recording, tokens, and contingent free time on the reading comprehension of elementary school–aged children with learning disabilities (Swanson, 1981).	1.34	3, 5
This study investigated the effectiveness of self-monitoring procedures on increasing on-task behavior among adolescents with learning disabilities (Prater, Joy, Chilman, Temple, & Miller, 1991).	1.29	4
This study investigated the effects of self-graphing on improving the reactivity of self-monitoring procedures for two students with learning disabilities (DiGangi, Maag, & Rutherford, 1991).	1.30	2
Self-monitoring of attention was compared with self-monitoring of productivity on on-task behavior and rate of academic response for children with attention difficulties (Harris, 1986).	1.32	4

(*continued*)

TABLE 1. (*continued*)

Category	Effect size	*N*
Students were taught to use self-monitoring and self-recording for on-task performance (Blick & Test, 1987).	1.33	12
This study extended previous research on components of effective strategy instruction operationalized in an approach referred to as "self-regulated strategy development" (SRSD). Comparisons were made among LD Ss on composition and self-efficacy in four conditions: SRSD, SRSD without goal setting and self-monitoring, direct teaching, and practice control (Sawyer, Graham, & Harris, 1992).	1.78	43
The study compared the effects of two types of self-monitoring on attention and academic performance. LD Ss were taught a spelling study procedure (SSP), followed by instruction in self-monitoring of performance (SMP) and self-monitoring of attention (SMA) (Reid & Harris, 1993).	.48	28
The effectiveness of two self-monitoring interventions on the attentional and academic performance of Ss with learning disabilities was compared in two separate experiments. The first experiment investigated if attention and performance monitoring had differential effects on the spelling study behaviors of four students. The second experiment used the same design and procedures with self-monitoring applied to story writing.	1.54	4, 4
The skills used in this study included behavior contracting, self-recording, self-monitoring, and self-reinforcement. Self-instructional materials in reading, writing, and math were used as the curriculum, and the dependent variables in the study were the number of lessons completed per student per day in the three academic areas (Seabaugh & Schumaker, 1994).	1.29	11
The effects of self-monitoring alone and self-monitoring in combination with external contingent reward on sight word acquisition were compared across two groups of LD students (Lalli & Shapiro, 1990).	1.77	8
In this study three forms of self-monitoring (attention, productivity, and accuracy) were investigated (Maag, Reid, & DiGangi, 1993).	1.28	6
In this study, the first experiment was designed to test the effects of self-instructional procedures on the academic performance of children with learning disabilities (Swanson & Scarpati, 1985).	1.51	3
The effects of overt, semiovert, and covert self-instructional procedures on reading comprehension was examined in this study (Weidler, 1986).	1.03	4
Social Skills Training		
The purpose of this study was to measure the impact of resource interventions upon the level of peer acceptance and self-concept (Sheare, 1978).	.75	82
The efficacy of training adolescents with learning disabilities in social and problem-solving skills was evaluated by conducting a group skills-training program that emphasized giving positive and negative feedback,accepting negative feedback, resisting peer pressure, negotiation, and problem solving in social situations (Hazel, Schumaker, Sherman, & Sheldon, 1982).	1.67	7

(*continued*)

TABLE 1. (*continued*)

Category	Effect size	*N*
The study used a posttest-only control group design to test the relationship between a nonverbal-oriented social acceptance training method and social ratings. The goal was to sensitize the Ss to appropriate use of nonverbal behaviors (Straub & Roberts, 1983).	.83	33
Social skills training was based on a human development program (16 weeks). Discussion was a primary focus of the intervention. Media (e.g., video) was used to support concepts introduced in discussion (Wanat, 1983).	.34	30
Behavioral instruction procedures designed to teach the skills involved in completing employment application materials were evaluated using a multiple baseline design (Mathews & Fawcett, 1984).	1.68	3
The effects of training procedures in the area of social skills were evaluated in this study. The study focused on positive styles of interaction in the workplace, specifically, explaining a problem to a supervisor, providing constructive criticism, accepting criticism, accepting a compliment, accepting an instruction, and providing a compliment (Whang, Fawcett, & Mathews, 1984).	1.52	2
The study evaluated the effectiveness of social skills training and cross-age tutoring for improving academic skills (specifically spelling) and social communication behaviors. The treatment groups included social skills training and tutoring, social skills training only, and a no-treatment control group (Ruhl, Hughes, & Gajar, 1990).	.64[b]	30
Public Law 101-467, the Individuals with Disabilities Education Act of 1990, specifies that students with disabilities,especially secondary-level students, should have an opportunity to participate in IEP conferences. This study investigated the effectiveness of strategy instruction designed to foster Ss' active participation in IEP conferences. High school students and their parents participated in either strategy instruction or an orientation lecture/discussion(Van Reusen & Bos, 1994).	.59	21
<u>Strategy Instruction (SI)</u>		
SI—Behavior		
The impact of alternative thinking on overt behavior of learning impaired 2nd and 3rd graders was examined. Measures of alternative problem solutions, classroom behavior, and reading proficiency were obtained before and after subjects participated in a therapeutic tutoring program. Some Ss received formal training in interpersonal problem solving as well as tutoring, while others received only tutoring (Helper, Farber, & Feldgaier, 1982).	.28	86
Special education resource teachers trained impulsive LD children to use verbal self-instruction (VSI) to decrease the children's impulsivity. Ss were identified as impulsive by the Matching Familiar Figures Test and ratings by regular classroom teachers (Graybill, Jamison, & Swerdlik, 1984).	.56	16
Verbal self-instruction (VSI) procedures were used to modify impulsivity in boys with learning disabilities (Nelson, 1985).	.62	18

(*continued*)

TABLE 1. (*continued*)

Category	Effect size	*N*
This study compared two treatment groups, self-instruction (Meichembaum, 1977) and relaxation training (Jacobson, 1938), and a no-treatment control group. Treatment groups were given 10 half-hour sessions over 4 weeks and were assessed before and after the treatment on cognitive tasks requiring deliberation (Zieffle & Romney, 1985).	.56	30
This study focused on enhancing Ss' roles as control agents for overall strategic functioning in the classroom. The goal was to increase the ability of Ss to generate new strategies or adapt previously learned task-specific strategies for meeting varying demands of the regular classroom. The SUCCESS Strategy (Ellis, 1985) was highlighted (Ellis, Deshler, & Schumaker, 1989).	1.48	13
SI—General problem solving		
LD students were trained to use planful strategic behavior in a tgame-instruction situation. Three strategies were taught: main ideation, subordinate ideation, and sequencing (Olsen, Wong, & Marx, 1983).	1.47	30
The study used a strategies intervention model that focused on Ss being taught *how* to learn instead of mastering specific content material. Ss learned a problem-solving strategy for word identification, paraphrasing to improve recall of main ideas, and sentence construction skills (Losh, 1991, Dissertation).	.20	64
SI—Handwriting		
This study examined the effect of allowing a student to choose among two handwriting strategies in comparison to teacher-determined choices of strategies on the handwriting performance on a paragraph copying task. The first strategy emphasized review of typical handwriting rules (such as punctuation, staying on the line, and correct proportioning of letters) prior to copying the paragraph. The second strategy emphasized circling quality work on the paper immediately following the copying task (Kosiewicz, Hallahan, & Lloyd, 1981).	1.69	1
SI—Health		
This study investigated the effectiveness of an explicit strategy as a means of linking facts, concepts, and problem solving in an unfamiliar domain of learning. Ss were learning disabled and were taught health facts and concepts,which they then applied to problem-solving exercises presented through computer-simulation games (Hollingsworth & Woodward, 1993).	.67	37
SI—Math		
Instruction focused on strategies for solving word problems. Ss were trained in computational selection that included strategies for identifying when to use addition and subtraction. Ss were also trained in five problem-solving steps (Fantasia, 1982, Dissertation).	1.19	6
Two experiments were designed to test the effects of self-instructional procedures on the academic performance of educationally handicapped children. Experiment 1 focused on reading/spelling; Experiment 2 focused on math (Swanson & Scarpati, 1985).	1.41	2, 1

(*continued*)

TABLE 1. (*continued*)

Category	Effect size	*N*
This study investigated the effect of an eight-step cognitive strategy on the verbal math problem-solving performance of six LD students. The cognitive strategy was designed to enable students to read, understand, carry out, and check verbal math problems that are encountered in the general math curriculum at the secondary level. During treatment, Ss received strategy acquisition training, strategy application practice, and testing. The eight steps included reading the problem aloud, paraphrasing it, visualizing by graphically displaying it, stating the problem, hypothesizing how many steps to the problem, estimating the answer, calculating it, and self-checking (Montague & Bos, 1986).	1.62	6
This investigation was conducted to test the effectiveness of strategy teaching and sequencing practice problems in teaching LD Ss to identify the correct algorithm for solving addition and subtraction word problems (Wilson & Sindelar, 1991).	.68	62
Participants were taught a strategy for comprehending math problems and devising an appropriate solution. Ss learned to apply the strategy first to addition word problems, then to subtraction word problems (Case, Harris, & Graham, 1992).	1.12	4
The study examined the effects of cognitive and metacognitive strategy instruction on the mathematical problem solving of six middle school Ss with learning disabilities. The cognitive strategy was combined with direct instruction (Montague, 1992).	1.34	6
The study investigated the effects of a two-phase cognitive strategy on algebra problem solving of LD adolescents. The strategy was designed to enable students to represent and solve three types of word problems. The study used a modified multiple baseline with 11 replications as well as a two-group design. Conditions of the multiple baseline design included baseline, instruction to master, transfer, and maintenance (Hutchinson, 1993).	3.97	20
The effects of cognitive strategy instruction on mathematical problem-solving performance was examined. The study included three treatment conditions and two cycles of treatment: direct instruction in cognitive strategies, metacognitive activities for solving mathematical word problems, and a combination of cognitive and metacognitive strategy instruction (Montague, Applegate, & Marquard, 1993).	.35	96
The effects of tape-recorded cues on the mathematics performance of students with learning disabilities were investigated. The conditions included SIT—Ss received self-instruction training; and Ss observed SIT, but did not partake (Wood, Rosenberg, & Carran, 1993).	1.39	1
In this study, the efficacy of using manipulatives in teaching elementary school-aged students with learning disabilities to identify the correct operation to use when solving math problems was investigated (Marsh & Cooke, 1996).	1.82	3

(*continued*)

TABLE 1. (*continued*)

Category	Effect size	*N*
SI—Reading		
This study investigated the hypothesis that insufficient metacomprehension is one possible cause underlying LD adolescents' comprehension problems, and that training them to monitor their understanding of important textual elements fosters metacomprehension and improves their comprehension performance. Half of the Ss received a five-step self-questioning training in which they learned to monitor their understanding of important textual units. The other half of the Ss received no training, but had the same materials as the experimental group (Wong & Jones, 1982).	.56	120
A comparison was made of the efficacy of metacomprehension plus direct instruction, direct instruction alone, and a control training condition in finding the main idea (Graves, 1986).	3.13	24
This study reported two interrelated, exploratory training studies to promote word knowledge and textual comprehension through elaboration in poor readers compared with their controls (Leong, Simmons, & Izatt-Gambell, 1990).	1.04	30, 41
The participants in the study were taught to use a self-questioning strategy for the identification of main ideas. They were randomly assigned to either a standard instruction or a generalization induction condition. In the latter,informed training and self-instructional training techniques were employed to promote generalization of strategy use. The study aimed to examine the effects of strategy generalization instruction on the comprehension performance of students with reading disabilities (Chan, 1991).	.81	60
The study investigated the use of dialogical thinking–reading lessons in which the S was engaged in reasoning and reflective thinking in order to decide what to believe about a central issue related to a story. Ss were asked to consider the evidence for two hypothesized explanatory conclusions regarding an important question (Commeyras, 1992).	1.34	14
The study utilized a comprehension procedure that makes visible to students their prior knowledge about a topic and the structures in expository text. The procedure used reciprocal-like teaching formats for the design of group interactions during instruction, as well as semantic mapping to make text structures apparent to students (Englert & Mariage, 1991).	1.32	28
The study used a strategies intervention model that focused on Ss being taught *how* to learn instead of mastering specific content material. Ss learned a problem-solving strategy for word identification, paraphrasing to improve recall of main ideas, and sentence construction skills (Losh, 1991, Dissertation).	.20	64
This author investigated using self-instruction to aid readers in looking for clues in reading (Reilly, 1991, Dissertation).	.32	39
The Interactive Teaching Project tested an instructional model designed to facilitate text comprehension and content learning for LD Ss. Semantic mapping and charting of concepts were compared (Bos & Anders, 1992).	.70	73

(*continued*)

TABLE 1. (*continued*)

Category	Effect size	*N*
This study examined the effectiveness of a summarization strategy for increasing reading comprehension of LDSs. Direct instruction was used (Gajria & Salvia, 1992).	4.46	30
This study addressed the effectiveness of teacher acquisition and implementation of two methods for improving the comprehension skills of LD Ss: instruction in teaching specific questioning strategies (Question–Answer–Response; QARS) and selected traditional methods of reading comprehension instruction (Simmonds, 1992).	1.54	447
This study investigated an instructional program designed to help students with learning disabilities learn about the concept of theme, identify themes in stories, and apply themes to real life (Williams, Brown, Silverstein, & deCani, 1994).	.94	30
This study investigated the effectiveness of an interactive vocabulary instructional strategy, semantic feature analysis, on the content–area text comprehension of adolescents with learning disabilities (Bos, Anders, Filip, & Jaffe, 1989).	1.63	50
In this study, the effects of a story mapping procedure on reading comprehension was investigated among intermediate-level students with learning disabilities (Idol & Croll, 1987).	1.63	4
Five 8–10-year-old children with dysphonetic and dyseidetic dyslexia were given instruction in reading comprehension using a story grammar strategy in which story instruction was differentially designed to match the simultaneous or sequential mental processing strengths of each dyslexia subtype (Newby, Caldwell, & Recht, 1989).	1.21	5
The purpose of this study was to determine whether adolescent students with learning disabilities could effectively be taught a reading comprehension strategy within a mainstreamed educational environment. The strategy emphasized steps to identify key information in content-area text, depict how that information is related or organized, and apply that information (Scanlon, Deshler, & Schumaker, 1996).	.80	17
This study examined the unique and combined contributions of instruction in goal setting and self-instructions on the acquisition, maintenance, and generalization of a reading comprehension strategy by 4th- through 6th-grade students with learning disabilities (Johnson, Graham, & Harris, 1997).	.47	59
The efficacy of a package of cognitive self-control procedures for decreasing the attention deficits and increasing academic productivity among 12-year-old students with learning disabilities was investigated (Brown & Alford, 1984).	.65	20
Writing		
The purpose of this study was to determine the effect of teaching LD adolescents an error-monitoring learning strategy with spelling, capitalization, punctuation, and appearance errors. The *COPS* (Capitalization, Overall appearance, Punctuation, Spelling) system was used (Schumaker, Deshler, Alley, Warner, Clark, & Nolan, 1982).	1.50	9

(*continued*)

TABLE 1. (*continued*)

Category	Effect size	*N*
This single-subject experiment explored the effect of providing an additional oral prompt to "write as many words and ideas as you can about a picture" on the amount of writing produced during a writing activity (Kraetsch, 1981).	1.58	1
This study involved writing. LDSs received cooperative skills training in reading with the strategies of self-questioning and paraphrasing, and in writing with the strategies in sentences and error monitoring. Cooperative skills training included four parts: orientation to types of goal structures, activation, skill training, and prestrategy training (Beals, 1985, Dissertation).	1.50	28
Ss were taught the three stages of writing (five steps of prewriting, drafting, revision). Ss wrote about topics in which they could express an opinion. Two revision strategies were taught: *COPS* (Capitalization, Overall appearance, Punctuation, Spelling) and Evaluative and Directive Phrases (Reynolds, 1986, Dissertation).	.52	54
This study focused on handwriting. A card showing seven self-instructional questions designed to prompt Ss to think about important aspects of handwriting was provided to two LD elementary students in a multiple baseline design. Daily assessments were made regarding letter formation, letter proximity to the line, letter height, and word spacing (Blandford & Lloyd, 1987).	1.66	2
Self-instructional strategy was the focus of this study with Ss exhibiting composition deficiencies. Incremental effects of explicit self-regulation procedures were examined in terms of writing performance measures (Graham & Harris, 1989).	.40	33
The effects of mechanical interference, rate of production, and contentless production signals to write more on the quantity and quality of 4th- and 6th-grade LDSs' compositions were examined (Graham, 1990).	1.19	23
The study investigated the impact of a reciprocal peer editing strategy on students' knowledge about writing and revising, their actual revising activity, and the quality of their writing. Ss learned to work in pairs to help each other improve their compositions. The process approach to writing instruction was used with word processing to support the writing process (MacArthur, Schwartz, & Graham, 1991).	.59	29
This study was conducted to determine if a planning and writing strategy would improve the essay writing of LDSs. Four Ss were taught a strategy designed to facilitate the setting of product and process goals, generation and organization of notes, continued planning during writing, and evaluation of goal attainment. A multiple-probe across-subjects design was used (Graham, MacArthur, Schwartz, & Page-Voth, 1992).	1.66	4
The study examined the effects of a socially mediated instructional program, Cognitive Strategy Instruction in Writing (CSIW). The program emphasized talk about the writing process, strategies, and text structures, and incorporated the four features of strategy instruction (Englert, Raphael, & Anderson, 1992).	1.26	63

(*continued*)

TABLE 1. (*continued*)

Category	Effect size	*N*
This study investigated the effectiveness of a metacognitive strategy, the *PLEASE* Strategy (P—*Pick* a topic, audience, format; L—*List* information regarding the topic to used in the organizational planning; E—*Evaluate* how to best organize information; A—*Activate* the paragraph with a topic sentence; S—*Supply* supporting sentences; E—*End* with a concluding sentence and evaluate [check work]), for teaching Ss with LD to write paragraphs. (Welch, 1992).	2.11	18
The study investigated the effectiveness of an instructional intervention that was designed to teach LD students to write a sequential expository paragraph (i.e., a set of directions) through strategy instruction and the use of a set of structured writing frameworks (Cole, 1993, Dissertation).	1.78	12
The study examined the effectiveness of embedding strategy instruction in the context of a process approach to writing in inclusive classrooms. Through a series of extended minilessons during writers' workshop, both Ss with and without learning disabilities were taught a previously validated writing strategy and procedures for regulating the strategy and the writing process (Danoff, Harris, & Graham, 1993).	1.57	6
This study investigated the effects of procedural and substantive , instruction in character development—on the quality and length of narratives written by nine junior high school students with learning disabilities. A multiple baseline design across triads was used to determine the effects of treatment (Montague & Leavell, 1994).	.96	9
Instruction in how to dictate plans for writing persuasive essays was compared with instruction in how to make handwritten plans. Of interest were the effects of intervention on time for advanced planning, number of propositions in students plans, transformations, composing rate, and coherence and quality of essays (De La Paz, 1995).	1.57	42
The study examined the effects of a self-management procedure designed to teach Ss with learning and behavior problems to improve the completeness (inclusion of identified story elements) and quality (organization and coherence) of their story compositions. The procedure was based on two strategies: teaching the students to plan stories composed in a narrative style, and teaching them to monitor the inclusion of elements from the plan with a check-off system (Martin & Manno, 1995).	1.34	3
Students were taught how to use a prestructured web to assist them in planning narrative writing. Of interest was the effects of intervention on planning time and quality of writing for children in the intermediate grades (Zipprich, 1995).	1.33	13
The purpose of the study was to determine whether a self-control strategy training procedure was effective in improving the quality of compositions generated by adolescents with learning disabilities (Harris & Graham, 1985).	1.44	2
This study investigated the effects of teaching a metacognitive text structure strategy upon the paragraph writing skills of 8th-grade students with learning disabilities. The technique, called Statement-Pie (Hanau, 1974),teaches students to understand the relationship of supporting details to a main idea (Wallace & Bott, 1989).	1.45	4

(*continued*)

TABLE 1. (*continued*)

Category	Effect size	*N*
Adolescent students with learning disabilities were taught how to plan, write, and revise opinion essays using interactive dialogue and compared to a no-treatment control (Wong, Butler, Ficzere, & Kuperis, 1996).	1.90	38
The efficacy of the self-regulated strategy development model of writing instruction as an approach to planning persuasive essays before and during composing was investigated (De La Paz, 1997).	1.76	2
Study Skills Training		
Ss were given eight 20-minute sessions of training in test-taking skills particular to the Stanford Achievement Test. Eight scripted lessons for each grade were provided in a direct instruction format. Specific test-taking strategies were taught for each reading subtest in the SAT (Scruggs & Tolfa, 1985).	.56	16
Experimental Ss received training in how to take the Math and Reading Subtests on the Stanford Achievement Test (SAT). Training included deductive reasoning strategies, checking their work, monitoring their place on the answer sheet, and more. The treatment was compared with a no-treatment control group (Scruggs, Mastropieri, & Tolfa-Viet, 1986).	.33	85
The purpose of this study was to design and evaluate the effects of teaching a comprehensive test-taking strategy to LD adolescents. The strategy, which comprised a carefully sequenced set of cognitive and overt behaviors designed for the test-taking task, was taught to six secondary Ss using a seven-stage instructional methodology including description, modeling, verbal rehearsal, initial practice, advanced practice, posttesting, and generalization. A multiple-probe across-subjects design was used to assess the Ss acquisition of the strategy (Hughes & Schumaker, 1991).	1.83	6
The study investigated a test-taking strategy that included writing mnemonic symbols (Letter Mnemonic Strategy and Paired Associates Strategy) and incorporated self-instruction and goal setting for learning the strategy (Kim, 1992, Dissertation).	1.26	8
The effects of explicit and implicit training of test-taking skills was examined for 4th grade Ss classified as learning disabilities. Both the Explicit and the implicit groups received 4 hours of scripted training exercises involving worksheet activities and completion of simulated tests (Maron, 1993, Dissertation).	.49	13
Visual Display		
Graphic organizers		
The study examined the relative effectiveness of two approaches to teaching LD Ss literal comprehension during content area instruction in social studies and science. One approach utilized an advanced organizer as a visual spatial display and was compared to a method in which Ss were presented content via text. Both groups were provided with study strategies (Darch & Carnine, 1986).	1.43	24

(*continued*)

TABLE 1. (*continued*)

Category	Effect size	N
This study examined the relative effectiveness of visual spatial displays to enhance comprehension of important information during science instruction with adolescent LD Ss. The treatment group utilized a graphic organizer as a visual spatial display and was compared to a method in which Ss were presented content via text (Darch & Eaves, 1986).	1.26	22
Two direction-setting activities designed to increase high school LD students' comprehension of important concepts during content area instruction were compared. One group was taught with prereading activities based on a basal approach to teaching comprehension. The major focus was on developing student interest and motivation, highlighting the relevance of the passage to the students' past experience, and offering a general introductory discussion. The second group received instruction using an advanced organizer in the form of a text outline designed to help Ss process information from the text (Darch & Gersten, 1986).	1.13	24
Graphic organizers were examined as a means for increased acquisition and recall on science content (Griffin, Simmons, & Kameenui, 1991).	.41	28
Semantic mapping		
The semantic mapping technique, with three different types of semantic maps, was compared with the verbal readiness approach for reading comprehension (Sinatra, Stahl-Gemake, & Berg, 1984).	.22	27
The focus of instruction was on semantic mapping to aid in memorization of information read (Carter, 1985, Dissertation).	.55	8
In this study of reading comprehension, semantic feature analysis (SFA) was used with a content area vocabulary and reading comprehension instructional strategy. The control group used a vocabulary look-up approach (Bos, Anders, Filip, & Jaffe, 1985).	1.63	50
This study examined the potential of a specific strategy, text structure recognition and use, for increasing LD high school students' recall of expository prose (Smith & Friend, 1986).	2.52	54
The study employed semantic mapping to aide in memorization and reading comprehension of information read. "Thinking aloud protocols" were used to identify cognitive processes during prose recall (Swanson, Kozleski, & Stegink, 1987).	.92	2
The study evaluated the effectiveness of concept diagrams and a related concept teaching routine. Ss were evaluated relative to performance on tests of concept acquisition, regular classroom tests, and notetaking before and after implementation of the concept teaching routine (Bulgren, Schumaker, & Deshler, 1988).	.63[b]	64
This study compared the effectiveness of three interactive vocabulary strategies: semantic mapping, semantic feature analysis, and semantic/syntactic feature analysis. The control group received definition instruction (Bos & Anders, 1990).	.66	61
The Interactive Teaching Project tested an instructional model designed to facilitate text comprehension and content learning for LD Ss. Semantic mapping and charting of concepts were compared (Bos & Anders, 1992).	.89	73

(*continued*)

TABLE 1. (*continued*)

Category	Effect size	*N*
Visual imagery		
This study was designed to examine the extent to which Ss with reading disabilities would benefit from instruction in the use of a visual imagery strategy for word recognition and reading comprehension relative to younger average readers with comparable word recognition skills (Chan, Cole, & Morris, 1990).	.37	78
<u>Word Discrimination Strategies</u>		
Phoneme discrimination		
1. *Spelling*		
The investigation of this study looked at the degree to which varying varying the number of spelling words taught relates to the percentage of words spelled correctly by LD children. Ss were divided into three treatment groups that differed only in the number of phonemically irregular spelling words taught (three, four, or five per day) across 3 days of instruction (Bryant, Drabin, & Gettinger, 1981).	.84	64
The study investigated the effects of instructing Ss in a strategy for spelling new words by using spelling patterns from known words. This method was contrasted with Ss who learned to read and spell sight word vocabulary (Englert, Hiebert, & Stewart, 1985).	.77	22
The study utilized the Simultaneous Oral Spelling (SOS) method. The study had two purposes. The first was to evaluate both the short- and long-term effectiveness of the SOS procedure for a group of children with long-standing unremediated reading disability. The second was to investigate the validity of the dysphonetic/dyseidetic (Chinese/Phonecian) classification among a group of disabled readers in terms of differential effects of the remedial procedure (Prior, Frye, & Fletcher, 1987).	1.24	27
Blending and spelling training were compared in this experiment to determine which intervention would improve the decoding skills of two 1st-grade boys with learning disabilities who were in the phonetic cue stage of reading. Additionally, the two boys received pre- and posttest administrations of a phonemic segmentation task (DiVeta & Speece, 1990).	.59	2
2. *Reading*		
The study focused on the use of an intensive phonetic teaching program for reading remediation over 4 months in comparison with nonspecific academic tutoring (Gittelman & Feingold, 1983).	.50	56
The study was designed to increase an adult male's oral reading performance. A direct instruction approach was used to teach lacking phonics skills (Idol-Maestas, 1981).	.67	1

(*continued*)

TABLE 1. ***(continued)***

Category	Effect size	*N*
Two experiments using pseudowords as stimuli were reported, showing that poor readers from 3rd grade were inferior to good readers in the utilization of intraword redundancy (Experiment 1) and that poor readers' performance with redundant stimuli can be increased when the stimuli are grouped into syllables (Experiment 2). A reading intervention program was then presented in which the children were taught how to segment words into syllables (Scheerer-Neumann, 1981).	1.23	30
Ss in this study received training either in word recognition and decoding skills, in oral and written language, or in classroom survival skills (Lovett, Ransby, & Barron, 1988).	.41	112
College students diagnosed as learning disabled were studied to determine whether they would make more progress in a summer program if taught by an adaptation of the Orton–Gillingham phonics approach (Guyer & Sabatino, 1989).	0	30
Ss in this study received either training in word recognition and decoding skills, in oral and written language, or in classroom survival skills (Lovett, Ransby, Hardwick, Johns, & Donaldson, 1989).	.39	178
The objective of this study was to utilize a mnemonic device to teach 10 letter cluster–sound associations to 17 reading disabled subjects. Direct instruction was incorporated into the intervention (Smith, 1989, Dissertation).	.74	34
The study included two experiments. Experiment 1 examined disabled and nondisabled readers' ability to discriminate between combinations of two-syllable, phoneme pairs with varying intersyllable intervals. Experiment 2 Ss were those who performed poorly in Experiment 1. They were trained on phonemic stimuli that became increasingly complex (Hurford & Sanders, 1990).	.40[b]	52, 32
The study included two word recognition and spelling training programs and a problem-solving and study skills training program. One word-training program taught orthographically regular words by whole word methods alone; the other trained constituent grapheme–phoneme correspondences. The word-training groups made significant gains in word recognition accuracy and speed and in spelling (Lovett, Warren-Chaplin, Ransby, & Borden, 1990).	.76	54
Children identified in kindergarten as being at risk for reading disability were taught in grades 1 and 2 using one of two strategies for word recognition, a structured phonics code-emphasis approach or an approach emphasizing use of context (Brown & Felton, 1990).	.50	48
Ss in this study included delinquents in two detention facilities. The treatment group received remedial reading instruction using an Orton–Gillingham approach (Simpson, Swanson, & Kunkel, 1992).	.54	63
This study compared two forms of word identification training to promote transfer of learning by children with dyslexia. One program trained phonological analysis and blending skills and provided direct instruction of letter–sound correspondences. The other trained the acquisition, use, and monitoring of four metacognitive decoding strategies (Lovett, Borden, DeLuca, Lacerenza, Benson, & Brackstone, 1994).	.56	62

(continued)

TABLE 1. ***(continued)***

Category	Effect size	*N*
Whole word discrimination		
1. Spelling		
The study investigated the effects of instructing Ss in a strategy for spelling new words by using spelling patterns from known words. This method was contrasted with Ss who learned to read and spell sight word vocabulary (Englert, Hiebert, & Stewart, 1985).	.77	22
2. Reading		
This study examined word recognition, with a whole-word approach that used a multisensory technique for developing reading skills, including the Fernald Method of tracing letters and a Total Body Movement Learning Game (Waterman, 1974, Dissertation).	.95	34
The Oralographic Reading Program (Kobler & Kobler, 1979) was compared with the progress of disabled learners in current special reading programs. The components of the program included printed lessons sheets and sound disks or tapes, used with a Talking Typewriter, printed extended reading selections and record-keeping materials (Ratekin, 1979).	.88	89
Written reproduction technique to increase word recognition. Student looks at a target word on a computer and copies the word using pencil and paper (Berninger, Lester, Sohlberg, & Mateer, 1991).	1.19	28
The study evaluated the effect of applying a mastery learning model to sight word instruction for LD elementary school children. Ss were taught 30 sight words in nine lessons which incorporated mastery learning strategies, and a comparison group with methods that are typically used in the teaching of sight words (Bryant, Fayne, & Gettinger, 1982).	1.59	48
The study included two word recognition and spelling training programs and a problem-solving and study skills training program. One word-training program taught orthographically regular words by whole word methods alone; the other trained constituent grapheme–phoneme correspondences. The word-training groups made significant gains in word recognition accuracy and speed and in spelling (Lovett, Warren-Chaplin, Ransby, & Borden, 1990).	.76	54
The effect of varying rates of practice on learning sight words was compared among students in the intermediate grades (Cuvo, Ashley, Marso, & Zhang, 1995).	1.81	5
Oral reading practice		
In this study two oral reading previewing procedures were investigated: Silent reading previous to reading aloud and listening to the teacher read the passage aloud previous to reading aloud (Rose & Sherry, 1984).	1.72	5
The relative efficacy of three error-correction techniques on the oral reading of adolescent students with learning disabilities was investigated. The three procedures were drill, word supply, and phonics drill (Rosenberg, 1986).	1.05	3

(*continued*)

TABLE 1. (*continued*)

Category	Effect size	*N*
This study examined the effects on reading fluency of two interventions involving rereading of passages (Weinstein & Cooke, 1992).	1.75	3
The study used the instructional hierarchy to compare the effects of three instructional interventions (listening passage preview, subject passage preview, and taped words) on subjects' oral reading performance on word lists and passages (Daly & Martens, 1993).	1.00	4

Note. Effect sizes (ESs) are not weighted by the reciprocal of the sampling variable nor have outliers been removed. ESs reported are the absolute average ESs using LD comparison groups for each study. ESs for maintenance conditions are not included in the average ESs. Studies were categorized according to the *primary* focus of intervention. Some studies are reported under more than one category if they addressed more than one type of intervention in the study.

[a]Due to missing data, maintenance data were used in the calculation of the ES.

[b]LD control group outcomes were used to calculate ES.

[c]ES was calculated using adjusted means

the general categories of dependent measures. The reader is referred to Appendix E for greater detailed descriptions of studies used in the subsequent analysis. Thus, Table 1 and Appendix E should be reviewed by the reader before proceeding to Chapter 3. They provide a context for the diversity of approaches used in the field. Again, I emphasize that the difficulty with reviewing these studies is that most yield positive outcomes, and therefore it is necessary to isolate the biases that exist across the various studies. That is, no study should be viewed in isolation, but rather attempts should be made to determine the common ingredients of success across all treatments. This problem will be addressed in the subsequent chapters.

In summary, we have provided the criteria for selecting the studies in this synthesis. We have also discussed the procedures for analysis. For the subsequent analysis, the next two chapters provide an in-depth analysis of group design and single-subject design studies, respectively. That is, although Table 1 and Appendix E provide a rich array of descriptive information, they are not informative about what moderates the treatment outcomes. Thus, we move to the heart of our analysis in Chapters 3 and 4.

NOTES

1. One flaw in our coding of studies is that weak interrater agreement emerged on measures of self-monitoring (>80%). We then coded whether children charted their behavior or evaluated their behavior in some fashion (e.g., children were directed to ask themselves a question about how they were doing). This information overlapped with the verbal dialogue code, and therefore was not separated in the analysis.
2. As the reader can easily tell, there is overlap in the listing of activities that reflect certain instruction components (more than one of the 45 codes can occur in several cate-

gories; for example, see #3 and #11). Treatments were coded as reflecting one of 19 components (component 5 required two activities) if at least one of the appropriate instructional activities was stated in the treatment section. However, once an instructional activity was not to be used for another instructional component. In rare cases where only one instructional activity was stated and that instructional activity could be applied to more than one category, preference was given to categories 1, 2, 3, 8, 17. These categories reflected a basic instructional core outlined by Rosenshine and Stevens (1986) and Slavin, Stevens, and Madden (1988) shared by both DI and SI models. The components in our synthesis that match these practices are orientation to a task (component 3, see methods section), drill-repetition-practice (component 2), teacher modeling of steps (component 17), sequencing (component 1), and systematic probing (component 8). However, it is important to note that the categories were not intended to be mutually exclusive, but rather capture an array of components identified in the literature. The independent contribution of each component was addressed in the subsequent regression analysis.

Although our codes were based on reviews of instructional literature, we did not code the independent variables by *what* aspect of instruction was addressed (e.g., phonological awareness, inferential comprehension, etc.), but instead focused on *how* it was taught. We focused on how the independent variable was delivered for two reasons. First, effect sizes for the experimental conditions are collapsed in the analysis for statistical reasons (see Hunter & Schmidt, 1994). Multiple-experimental treatment studies are regarded as instances of a common treatment construct. Variation in content variables reflect two or more experimental treatment comparisons *within* studies. Second, because of the bias related to positive outcomes in the synthesis of treatments, it is critical that the commonalities of effective treatments are identified. That is, one cannot adequately assess the "what" of instruction unless we clearly identify the "how." As shown by our previous synthesis, there are tremendous differences in instructional activities, as well as a host of other methodological variables, that moderate treatment outcomes. Unless these variables are identified and their influence on outcomes clearly delineated, testing the subtle aspects of content becomes a moot point.

Chapter 3

Group Design Studies

In this chapter we will review in detail the findings from our meta-analysis regarding studies that use group designs. An example group design would be one in which a treatment group (that includes children with LD that are taught with a new instructional program) is systematically compared to a control group (that includes children with LD who are taught with a typical or traditional model). The chapter has four parts. First, we review the main findings and characteristics of group design studies. Second, we isolate instructional methods and components that influence the magnitude of treatment outcome (ESs). Third, we analyze the influence of instructional domain (reading) and sample characteristics on treatment outcomes. Fourth, we examine those studies that compare children with LD and those without LD (non-LD students; NLD) in the experimental condition.

PROTOTYPE STUDY

Table 2 provides a summary of the most frequent (or average) characteristics of group design studies. The table is divided into characteristics related to articles, instruction, sample, and methodology. The analyses yielded 1,537 effect sizes comparing LD students in the experimental condition with LD students in the control condition. With outliers removed, the unweighted mean ES (ES that does not take into consideration sample size) across the 180 studies was .56 (*SD* = .67) and the absolute value was .79 (*SD* = .52).

The important characteristics of the studies reported in Table 2 can be quickly summarized. A prototypical intervention study includes 22.47 minutes (*SD* = 29.71) of daily instruction, and is given 3.58 times a week (*SD* = 1.58), over 35.72 (*SD* = 21.72) sessions. The mean sample size for the study is 27.06 (*SD* =

TABLE 2. Characteristics of Group Design Studies in Synthesis (Total N = 180; Outliers Removed)

	M	*SD*
Effect size (Cohen's *d*)	.56	.67
Effect size—absolute	.79	.52
Article characteristics		
Year of publication	1987	5.41
	M	*SD*
Number of authors	1.32	1.23
Number of citations	1.80	3.37
Citations (%)	57% not cited	
Author gender (%)	41% male	
Funding source (%)		
No funding cited	64%	
U.S. Department of Education	12%	
NICHD	4%	
State/province	4%	
Other	10%	
Publication outlets (%)		
Dissertation	13%	
Journal of Learning Disabilities	16%	
Learning Disability Quarterly	13%	
Learning of Disabilities Research and Practice	7%	
Exceptional Children	7%	
Journal of Special Education	4%	
Journal of Educational Psychology	4%	
Other	36%	
Most frequent affiliation		
1. Columbia University	15% (each contributed 3% or more)	
University of Arizona		
University of Houston		
University of Maryland		
Michigan State University		
2. Purdue University	14% (each contributed between 1.5 and 3%)	
Simon Frasier University		
University of Southern California		
University of Miami		
Arizona State University		
University of Toronto (The Hospital for Sick Children)		
Instructional parameters		
Time of instruction	*M*	*SD*
Number of instruction sessions	22.47	29.71
Length of session (minutes)	35.72	21.72
Number of sessions per week	3.58	1.58

(*continued*)

TABLE 2. (*continued*)

Setting of intervention (%)			
No information	56%		
Self-contained (other)	18%		
Resource room	23%		
Regular class	2%		
Primary focus of intervention (%)			
Reading	54%		
Math	10%		
Written language	11%		
Language	2%		
Information processing abilities	6%		
Behavior	1%		
Problem solving	1%		
Perceptual	1%		
Other	14%		
Sample parameters (%)			
Most frequent reason for participant exclusion from study			
• (Those who reported reasons; $N = 30$)			
• Other than normal intelligence	20%		
• No reading problems	10%		
• No reading or math problems	3%		
• Achievement consistent with general ability	10%		
• Other	57%		
Of those not reporting reasons for study exclusion	85% ($N = 153$)		
Geographic location of sample (%)			
No information	30%		
Midwest	12%		
Southeast	8%		
Non U.S.	20%		
Educational history (%)			
No information	50%		
Resource room	28%		
Other	22%		
	M	*SD*	
Sample size	27.06	40.15	
Number of males	15.54	10.42	(84)[a]
Number of females	6.66	8.33	(88)
Ethnicity reported	*M*	*SD*	
Asian American	4.71	6.01	(7)
African American	7.42	7.97	(25)
Anglo American	11.67	8.45	(36)
Hispanic American	9.36	10.11	(11)
Native American	1.0	—	(2)
Other	2.46	2.07	(2)

(*continued*)

TABLE 2. (*continued*)

	M	*SD*	
Chronological age	11.16	3.22	
Grade range (%)			
Elementary	54%		
Secondary	18%		
Mixed	28%		
Socioeconomic status (%)			
No information	40%		
Middle income	30%		
Mixed	30%		
Psychometric standardized	*M*	*SD*	
Intelligence	93.51	16.85	(104)
Reading	71.44	26.65	(82)
Math	75.36	25.38	(12)
Methodology parameters			
Internal validity	*M*	*SD*	
Rating scale (Abbr.) (4–12 high to low internal validity)	7.32	1.95	
Complete scale (10–30)	22.16	2.64	
Variation of control from treatment (%)			
% Similarity of overlap			
Same teacher	24%		
Same materials	27.8%		
Same setting	34.5%		
Same instructional focus	61.9%		
Group design (%)			
% Studies pre–post control group design	70%		
Measure of treatment integrity	18%		
Sampling procedure (%)			
Intact sample—no random assignment of treatment	35%		
Intact sample and random assignment of treatment	42%		
Other (or no information)	23%		
Type of design (%)			
A. Pretest–posttest control group design	70%		
B. Posttest-only design with random assignment	10%		
C. Factorial variations of pretest–posttest control group design (e.g., repeated measures design)	18%		
D. Other	2%		
Number of experiments reported for article (%)			
One experiment	95%		
Two experiments	4%		
Three experiments	1%		
Type of hypothesis (%)			
Directional	34%		
Null	15%		
Nonstated	51%		

(*continued*)

TABLE 2. (*continued*)

	M	*SD*
Dependent measures for treatment effects		
Mean number experimental measures	3.53	4.30
Mean number reliability information	1.73	1.51
Number standardized measure	2.57	5.73
Frequency reporting social validity information (%)	20%	

Note. Some percentages for categorizing comparisons are less than 100% because item examples from 1% to 5% were not listed.

[a]Parentheses indicate number of studies that report information. If left blank, the number of studies reporting information is >80%.

40.15). The mean treatment age is 11.16, with a standard deviation of 3.22. The most frequent sampling and treatment assignment procedures use (1) participants from an intact sample (a nonrandomly selected sample) with no random assignment to treatment conditions (35% of studies), or (2) an intact sample with random assignment to treatment and control conditions (42% of studies). Approximately 30% of the studies do not indicate the geographic region from which the sample is drawn. For the articles that do report the geographic region where the sample was drawn, 20% included non-U.S. samples of children (e.g., from Canada) and 12% samples drawn from the Midwest.

Although the majority of studies had samples identified as learning disabled, studies varied tremendously on the criteria and detail for participant selection. In terms of reporting group mean scores on psychometric information, 104 studies (64%) reported group mean scores for intelligence, 84 studies (50%) reported group mean scores on achievement scores in reading, and 22 studies (12%) reported group mean scores in mathematics. Beyond IQ, reading, and mathematic scores, psychometric information on other characteristics of the sample was infrequently reported (<3% of the studies). In terms of those studies that reported scores, 83.7% of the studies that reported IQ scores used the WISC-R as the measure of intelligence, and 20% of the studies that reported achievement scores used the Wide Range Achievement Test as the measure of reading achievement. The mean reported treatment IQ for the LD sample was 93.51 (*SD* = 16.51, range of 85 to 115). Of those studies reporting standardized reading scores (42%), the mean reported standard score was 71.44 (*SD* = 25.38).

The average year of publication for studies was 1987 (*SD* = 5.41), with publication dates ranging from 1972 to 1997. The most frequent year of publication was 1992 (12% of the studies). The most frequent publication outlets were the *Journal of Learning Disabilities* (16%), *Learning Disabilities Research and Practice* (7%), *Learning Disability Quarterly* (13%), and *Exceptional Children* (7%). Thirteen percent of the studies in the synthesis analysis were drawn from dissertations.

Approximately 57% of the published articles are not cited in the scientific literature. Approximately 64% of the studies do not report a funding source. Approximately 12% of the studies were funded by the U.S. Department of Education. Approximately 90% of the studies have authors affiliated with institutions of higher education. A typical group design study includes only one experiment (95%).

In terms of subject description, of the studies that report some criteria for subjects identified as learning disabled, more than 50% mention the concept of a discrepancy between achievement and IQ, and/or differences in IQ and achievement scores, and/or that LD children were presently placed in a special education class (e.g., a pull-out classroom). Approximately 56% of the studies do not report the setting in which treatment occurred; 23% report that interventions occurred in some variation of resource rooms. Approximately 60% of the studies do not report the time of day that the intervention occurred. Based on our coding criteria, approximately 60% of the studies do not report enough detail for replication. Less than half the studies (42.8%) make recommendations for teachers, students, or instruction. Approximately 57% of the studies fail to report the degree of accuracy to which treatment was implemented (referred to as "treatment integrity" or "treatment fidelity").

The internal validity ratings (see the coding form in Appendix C) in Table 2 include measures of (1) subject mortality; (2) Hawthorne effects and selection bias; comparable exposure of (3) materials; (4) instruction time; and (5) experimenter between treatment and controls; (6) procedural validity checks; (7) practice effects on the dependent measure; (8) floor and ceiling effects; (9) interrater reliability; (10) regression to the mean ruled out as an alternative explanation of findings; and (11) homogeneity of variance between groups. The internal validity Rating Scale included an abbreviated form (items 1, 2, 4, 8) and a complete form (items 1–11)]. A score of 1 reflects internal validity control, a score of 2 reflects no validity control, and a score of 3 reflects no validity information on each of the 11 items. As Table 2 indicates, most studies on the abbreviated form yield moderate internal validity ratings (a rating score around 7; a score of 4 reflected high internal validity). In terms of reporting reliability of dependent measures, studies provide on average reliability information on about one of three dependent measures used.

Materials for the experimental conditions were commercial (33% of the studies), novel (i.e., materials developed by the researcher; 54% of the studies), a combination of commercial and novel (9% of the studies), or were not classifiable (4% of the studies). The most frequent commercial materials (N = 54) were related to direct instruction (e.g., Corrective Reading, Distar, SRA, 8%), Houghton Mifflin series (4%), Orton–Gillingham approach (4%), Lindamood–Bell (4%), and Purdue Perceptual Motor activities (8%). For those studies that primarily utilized commercial materials, 25 of the 54 studies (46%) did not report the materials used (or used no commercial materials) in the control condition. In terms of student activities, 30 studies had participants monitor or evaluate (via recording, counting, charting, checking, graphing, and/or verbalizing) their academic behavior.

DOMAINS OF INSTRUCTION

Prior to the analysis of effect sizes, it was necessary to separate the effect sizes into categories of dependent measures. The 17 categories discussed earlier reflect a broad array of treatment domains (e.g., reading, writing, etc.). Appendix D provides the mean *d* effect sizes for each study, as a function of 17 categorical domains. Only the first author is cited in Appendix D, with the complete citation at the end of the report. In Appendix D, *k* refers to the number of dependent measures used in the calculation within a particular category domain for each study. The *k* also reflects multiple treatments compared to the control condition within a particular categorical domain. That is, if a study had multiple dependent measures across several categories and treatments, those that assess the same construct were combined (averaged) into one category and those that assess different constructs are reported in a separate category.

Table 3 provides the weighted means and standard deviations of effect sizes (absolute value of *d*) as a function of the dependent measures across studies. Typically, no intervention study yielded a negative ES. Some negative effect sizes emerged on the social skill measures (consistent with the expected direction of change for these interventions), and therefore *d* was converted to an absolute value. If the number of dependent measures (*k*) within a category exceeded 50, we attempted to subgroup the categories by standardized (normed referenced measures) and experimental (researcher developed) measures. This was not possible for all categories, however, because of the infrequent use of standardized measures. For example, the cognitive processing category was divided into metacognitive, attribution, and "other" because few standardized measures were reported in the primary studies.

Table 3 illustrates two findings of primary interest. First, the most frequent dependent measures reflected across the various studies are measures of reading. These studies include measures of word recognition, word skills, reading comprehension, and general reading. Also frequently represented are measures of cognitive processing. Dependent measures of categories infrequently represented include measures of intelligence, vocabulary, global achievement (grades), creativity, language processing, and memory.

Second, the magnitude of the estimates of ES related to treatment impact vary considerably across categorical domains. Table 3 shows the unweighted and weighted mean Cohen's *d* effect sizes for the general categories and subcategories. Based on the weighted effect sizes reported in Table 3, effect sizes considered marginal according to Cohen's criteria (effect sizes below .45) occurred in the domains of spelling, mathematics, attitude, intelligence, social skills, perceptual processes, and language processes. Those areas that approached Cohen's (1988) threshold of .80 for a "large effect" are reading comprehension (.72), vocabulary (.78), and creativity (.70). When the categories are divided into subcategories, the high effect sizes related to reading comprehension emerged on experimental ($M = .84$) measures when compared to standardized measures ($M = .45$). The subcategory related to metacognition also yielded an ES (.80) that met Cohen's criteria.

TABLE 3. Weighted Mean Effect Sizes for Group Design Studies as a Function of Dependent Measure Category

			LD treatment vs. LD control					
			Effect size *d*		95% confidence interval for weighted effects			
	N	*k*	Unweighted*	Weighted	Lower	Upper	Standard error	Homogeneity (*Q*)
1. Cognitive processing	41	115	.87 (.64)	.54	.48	.61	.03	311.67**
1a. Metacognitive	9	27	.98	.80	.66	.94	.07	83.91**
1b. Attribution	7	17	.79	.62	.44	.79	.08	31.99*
1c. Other processes	25	71	.65	.46	.38	.53	.03	176.07**
2. Word recognition	54	159	.71 (.56)	.57	.52	.62	.02	431.45**
2a. Standardized	23	79	.79	.62	.54	.69	.04	205.61**
2b. Experimental	35	80	.72	.53	.48	.60	.03	223.073**
3. Reading comprehension	58	176	.82 (.60)	.72	.68	.77	.02	565.95**
3a. Standardized	16	38	.45	.45	.36	.54	.05	33.87
3b. Experimental	44	138	.84	.81	.75	.86	.02	489.54**
4. Spelling	24	54	.54 (.53)	.44	.37	.52	.04	100.4**
4a. Standardized	8	20	.61	.45	.34	.57	.06	34.45
4b. Experimental	18	34	.48	.44	.33	.54	.05	65.94**
5. Memory/recall	12	33	.81 (.46)	.56	.43	.70	.06	42.72
6. Mathematics	28	71	.58 (.45)	.40	.33	.46	.04	128.28**
6a. Standardized	9	22	.41	.33	.23	.46	.05	25.72
6b. Experimental	21	49	.59	.42	.34	.51	.04	101.43***

(continued)

TABLE 3. (*continued*)

			LD treatment vs. LD control					
			Effect size *d*		95% confidence interval for weighted effects			
	N	*k*	Unweighted*	Weighted	Lower	Upper	Standard error	Homogeneity (*Q*)
7. Writing	19	67	.84 (.60)	.63	.54	.72	.05	157.45**
7a. Standardized	3	7	.37	.36	.14	.58	.11	5.01
7b. Experimental	16	60	.80	.68	.59	.78	.04	145.27**
8. Vocabulary	11	20	.79 (.44)	.78	.66	.89	.05	38.58**
9. Attitude/self-concept	25	86	.68 (.69)	.39	.33	.45	.03	210.65**
10. Intelligence	9	32	.58 (.59)	.41	.30	.52	.06	54.37**
11. General reading	15	31	.60 (.50)	.52	.41	.65	.06	55.15*
12. Phonics/orthographic skills	29	175	.70 (.36)	.64	.60	.69	.02	453.70**
12a. Standardized phonics	8	60	.72	.67	.62	.73	.03	275.87**
12b. Experimental phonics	21	78	.76	.60	.52	.67	.04	175.22**
13. Global achievement (grades, total achievement)	10	21	.91 (.76)	.45	.31	.58	.07	56.64**
14. Creativity	3	11	.84 (.49)	.70	.52	.87	.09	33.61**
15. Social skills	13	36	.46 (.22)	.41	.30	.51	.05	28.46
16. Perceptual processes	10	37	.74 (.65)	.26	.17	.35	.04	46.64
17. Language	9	52	.54 (.48)	.36	.28	.44	.04	75.53*

Note. Parentheses indicate standard deviation.

*$p < .01$; **$p < .001$; ***$p < 0001$.

The relationship between the year of publication and the type of dependent measure was analyzed to determine if some domains have been researched more recently. The point biserial correlations between the domain of the dependent measures (scored dichotomously as 1 and 0; e.g., word recognition measure = 1 and other measures = 0) and year of publication were all weak in magnitude, all *r*s < .20. The two coefficients of the highest magnitude indicate that the year of publication and nonstandardized word skill measures were positively related, ($r = .17$, $p < .05$), whereas a decrease in the use of standardized real word recognition measures has emerged over the years ($r = -.19$, $p < .01$).

Overall, the striking feature of the categories of dependent measures (data reported in Table 3) is the strong skew toward high effect sizes across all academic domains. It appears that most experimental treatments have a bias for positive effects, and therefore it seems implausible that we have presented a valid picture of the efficacy of interventions for students with learning disabilities. Further, these effect sizes are difficult to interpret because comparisons are not really being made between a treatment and a nontreatment condition, but instead reflect a treatment of interest to the researcher (typically the experimental treatment) and "treatment as usual" which includes typical classroom instruction (see Lipsey & Wilson, 1993, for further discussion of this issue). Because the homogeneity tests were significant across the majority of dependent measures, the subsequent analysis requires interpretations beyond the mean level of effects. The subsequent analyses will attempt to identify some variables that mediate the effect sizes.

MAIN EFFECTS

Table 4 provides a comparison of weighted and unweighted effect sizes as a function of study variations in methodology, article characteristics, setting, sample characteristics, and general instructional models. The weighted mean ES estimate is the primary measure used to compare studies across the various contrasts. To assess the stability of the results, two units of analysis were considered in the calculation of ES for the 180 group design studies. One unit calculates effect size estimates for each dependent measure as if it all the measures were independent of each other. The second averages the effect sizes across dependent variables within each study (i.e., each study contributes only one ES to the analysis).

As Table 4 indicates, the number of independent samples was also computed (see discussion in Chapter 2; also see Cooper, Nye, Charlton, Lindsay, & Greathouse, 1996, for the complete rationale). When the number of independent samples exceeds $2k$ (the number of studies), then the studies included more than one experimental treatment. When the number of independent samples is lower than $2k$, the intervention used the same participants in multiple treatments. In cases of repeated measures, effect sizes were recalculated using the aforementioned formula, which takes into consideration the correlation between the con-

TABLE 4. Effect Size Estimates as a Function of Unit of Analysis, Methodological, Instructional, and Sampling Variables (Outliers Removed)

All studies	Sample size	*k*	Mean	*SD*	Weighted mean	Independent sample	χ^2
	33,845	1207	.66	.59	.54		—
	4,871	180	.79	.52	.61	362	
I. Methodology							
Number of treatment sessions							
3 to 10	8,103	353	.66	.57	.51	—	
	1,750	72	.77	.53	.71	138	
11 to 30	7,137	330	.72	.63	.62	—	
	1,462	64	.85	.53	.78	126	
>31	16,885	507	.62	.57	.57	—	15.72**
	1,411	41	.74	.50	.66	88	3.32[a]
Treatment integrity (procedural validity)							
Reported	18,714	722	.62	.58	.47		
	2,209	67	.81	.51	.74		
Not reported	12,635	411	.72	.60	.59	132	37.29**
	2,330	103[b]	.82	.55	.69	104	.60
Internal validity rating (includes 5 variables)							
Low	24,668	927	.67	.60	.56		
	3,629	135	.83	.55	.74	274	
High	6,681	206[c]	.63	.54	.48		8.81**
	913	35	.74	.74	.62	66	2.97

Total sample size							
1. <25	8,643	588	.77	.63	.63		
	1,672	116	.88	.55	.78	232	
2. >24 and <50	15,366	508	.55	.55	.48		
	1,624	52	.64	.47	.55	102	
3. >49 and <100	5,167	85	.56	.41	.50		
	409	6	.49	.14	.47	12	94.49**
4. > 99	4,566	28	.60	.50	.79		49.68**
	1,165	6	.80	.43	1.12	16	(4 > 1 > 2 = 3)
Variation of teacher (researcher) in the administration of treatment							
1. Different teacher—CTRL + EXP	6,254	218	.60	.42	.64		
	1,447	41	.66	.35	.76	80	
2. Same teacher—CTRL + EXP	12,927	506	.64	.57	.49		
	1,487	70	.77	.47	.62	136	38.92**
3. Cannot determine (no information)	14,561	483	.71	.67	.55		6.03*
	1,936	69	.90	.63	.75	132	(1 = 3 > 2)[d]
Variation of setting between CTRL and TRT							
1. CTRL + TRT occur in *different* classroom/setting/school	11,786	413	.69	.63	58		
	1,505	60	.82	.53	.69	110	
2. CTRL + TRT occur in *same* classroom	8,849	368	.61	.56	.50		22.08**
	775	39	.70	.45	.59	64	(3 = 1; 3 > 2,2 = 1)
3. No information	13,107	426	.67	.57	.60		6.31*
	2,509	81	.82	.54	.71	188	(3 = 1 > 2)

(continued)

TABLE 4. *(continued)*

All studies	Sample size	*k*	Mean	*SD*	Weighted mean	Independent sample	χ^2
Variation of materials							
Same materials used (booklets, commercial materials)	5,079	240	.70	.55	.74		
	880	44	.81	.50	.67	78	
Different materials used	24,165	835	.64	.60	.52		
	3,283	112	.84	.56	.73	224	
No information	4,498	132	.70	.59	.63		28.85**
	708	24	.65	.33	.62	58	2.34
Domain (instructional) focus of control group							
1. Same domain as TRT	16,248	680	.69	.61	.60		
	2,862	108	.82	.33	.74	198	
2. Different domain	14,209	410	.58	.54	.47		
	1,439	48	.74	.51	.64	108	
3. Cannot determine	3,284	117	.74	.63	.53		
	659	24	.78	.42	.69	54	44.93**
							3.77
Standardized testing included in pretest and posttest							
1. No	9,058	387	.86	.65	.75		
	2,883	86	.92	.52	.87	166	
2. Yes	20,249	714[b]	.55	.53	.45		208.38**
	1,991	79	.69	.50	.57	190	30.37**
Variation of control from treatment in the number of instructional components and/or steps							
High overlap (>4 sequences, steps)	10,823	405	.56	.54	.45		
	1,767	67	.71	.51	.58	134	
Low overlap (<5 sequences, steps)	22,919	802	.71	.61	.59		31.06**
	3,104	113	.85	.53	.78	228	12.75**

Type of treatment assignment							
1. No random assignment	7,703	354	.72	.66	.52		
	1,317	61	.67	.53	.67	100	
2. Random assignment	17,965	611	.58	.51	.51		
	2,215	69	.69	.43	.69	138	
3. No information	5,851	242	.78	.63	.66		46.22**
	1,338	50	.77	.59	.77	112	2.73
Methods composite variable (maximum score = 14)							
1. <7	16,620	631	.77	.64	.59		
	3,399	126	.83	.55	.74	244	
2. >6 but <11	15,483	528	.55	.51	.50		
	1,358	51	.72	.45	.62	108	
							157.57**
3. >10	1,639	48	.37	.43	.35		11.33**
	113	3	.46	.11	.41	10	(1 > 2 > 3)
II. Publication characteristics							
Funding (stated)							
No	16,658	641	.68	.63	.58		
	2,945	117[b]	.84	.57	.75	220	
Yes	15,468	549	.64	.55	.55		3.20
	1,678	60	.70	.41	.65	134	3.71
Publication outlet							
Journal	31,013	1,065	.68	.60	.59		
	4,416	155	.83	.54	.76	308	
Dissertation/technical report	2,729	142	.52	.48	.34		36.45**
	454	25	.57	.32	.42	54	21.59**

(continued)

TABLE 4. (continued)

All studies	Sample size	*k*	Mean	*SD*	Weighted mean	Independent sample	χ^2
III. Setting of treatment							
Reported information							
Setting reported	8,430	397	.77	.64	.62		
	1,956	78	.87	.57	.79	162	
Setting not reported	20,613	711	.59	.55	.53		15.12**
	2,915	102	.74	.48	.66	200	7.09*[a]
Type of classroom							
1. Self-contained	2,789	161	.72	.57	.57		
	590	33	.84	.57	.69	80	
2. Resource room	4,638	203	.86	.69	.80		
	1,213	41	.90	.59	.89	72	
3. No information	20,613	711	.59	.55	.49		
	2,032	86	.76	.50	.64	160	
4. Regular class	1,002	33	.48	.51	.35		16.93**[a]
	151	4[b]	.78	.50	.66	8	(2 > 1 = 3 = 4)
IV. Sample characteristics							
Discrepancy							
Reported >1 year	7,769	347	.55	.49	.51		
	1,355	29	.76	.43	.74	62	
No information or <1 year	21,252	759[b]	.70	.63	.59		9.58**
	3,356	136	.82	.55	.72	164	.02

Amount of reported psychometric information on sample							
1. No information on intelligence and reading	15,460	517	.75	.66	.62		
	2,560	73	.83	.50	.82	144	
2. Information on both intelligence	6,776	295	.61	.58	.48		
	1,111	55	.80	.58	.62	112	
3. Information on both intelligence and reading	6,290	245	.60	.54	.52		
	849	39	.76	.54	.63	74	58.19**
4. Information on intelligence and reading, and mathematics	5,215	150	.53	.41	.46		13.50**
	349	13	.66	.28	.60	32	(1 > 2 = 3 = 4)
Age of subjects							
1. Young (<12)	15,080	543	.56	.55	.52		
	1,077	51	.79	.63	.72	96	
2. Adolescent (>11 but 17)	5,421	250	.60	.68	.52		
	770	40	.84	.57	.64	92	
3. Adult (>16)	713	49	.72	.67	.51		
	155	9	.76	.41	.61	18	
4. Multiage (elementary to secondary)	6,847	257	.88	.67	.71		68.77**
	2,867	80	.78	.48	.75	162	3.53
Gender ratio in sample							
1. Low male ratio (<70%)	780	330	.58	.51	.48		
	645	31	.65	.42	.66	70	
2. High male ratio (>69%)	7,559	303	.64	.61	.52		
	1,034	48	.69	.54	.65	86	
3. Cannot calculate ratio	18,374	574[b]	.71	.62	.59		31.10**
	3,072	96	.80	.55	.74	196	3.43

(continued)

TABLE 4. ***(continued)***

All studies	Sample size	*k*	Mean	*SD*	Weighted mean	Independent sample	χ^2
Intelligence							
1. >84 but <92	4,703	159	.69	.69	.66		
	1,464	69	.77	.57	.63	154	
2. No information	17,490	597	.72	.66	.59		
	2,822	86	.82	.50	.77	166	71.48**
3. >91	11,549	451	.56	.51	.45		7.43*
	584	25	.79	.48	.66	50	(2 > 3 = 1)
Reading severity							
1. <85	7,776	261	.66	.52	.55		
	771	35	.86	.52	.71	70	
2. >84 but <91	979	51	.47	.46	.43		
	127	9	.57	.39	.51	10	
3. No score	22,571	800	.69	.62	.57		
	3,629	122	.80	.54	.73	254	35.96**
4. >90	2,415	95	.53	.57	.38		6.36*
	293	14	.69	.44	.55	22	(1 = 3 > 1 = 4)

V. Independent variables (general models)							
Strategy instruction							
Strategy instruction	11,889	423	.76	.60	.66*		
	2,489	83	.86	.51	.84	194	
Nonstrategy instruction	21,854	784	.60	.58	.52		35.57**[d]
	2,382	97	.74	.52	.67	168	9.59**[e]
Direct instruction							
Direct instruction	11,950	519	.68	.58	.60		
	2,725	102	.82	.53	.82	198	
Nondirect instruction	21,792	688	.64	.60	.54		8.05**
	2,145	78	.76	.52	.66	164	7.92**[f]

Note. Top row is unit of analysis calculated across all studies and dependent measures; bottom row is unit of analysis averaged within each study. The variation between setting not reported ($N = 102$) and no information for the type of classrooms ($N = 86$) is because some studies partialed for separated age. *k*, number of dependent measures; CTRL, control condition; EXP, experimental condition. Underscoring indicates significant results for both units of analysis.

[a]Chronological partialed out.

[b]Not all comparisons add to 180 because of missing or unclear information.

[c]Composite score related to control and experimental comparability on materials, instructional time, administration consistency, subject mortality, random assignment, reliability of measures, and ceiling and floor effects.

[d]Read as 1 and 3 ("Different teacher" and "cannot determine") are statistically comparable but both are significantly larger in effect sizes than 2 (same teacher).

[e]Methodology composite scores are partialed out in the analysis.

[f]Also partialed for methodology composite score and age.

*$p < .05$; **$p < .01$.

trol and the treatment condition. A chi-square based on the weighted least square (WLS) analysis is presented for all independent measures for both types of units of analysis. When the degrees of freedom were greater than 1, a Scheffe test was used to make comparisons between the estimates of the mean effect size. We will now discuss the findings reported in each section of this table.

Methodology

We analyzed the methodological characteristics of each study first because several of these measures were used in computing a methodological composite score. The methodological composite score (to be discussed) was used to qualify treatment outcomes (effect sizes). As Table 4 illustrates, studies that include from 11 to 30 sessions yield higher effect sizes than those that include between 3 and 10 sessions. No significant differences in effect sizes were found between studies that lasted over 31 sessions and those that lasted between 3 and 10 sessions. However, when the unit of analysis includes averaging ES estimates within studies, no significant differences emerge in ES as a function of the number of sessions. Those studies that report treatment integrity (i.e., the degree to which an independent variable is carried out as designed) yield lower effect sizes than those that do not report treatment integrity, but the differences in ES were not significant when effect sizes were averaged within studies.

Because internal validity was moderately weak across the majority of the studies (see Table 2), we categorized studies into high and low internal validity on the variables of setting, different materials, comparability of teachers across conditions, reporting of reliability, procedural validity, and random assignment (scores ranged from 6 to 18, with a score of 6 reflecting high internal validity). As Table 4 indicates, studies with high internal validity (scores <10) yield lower effect sizes than studies with low internal validity. However, when effect sizes are averaged within each study there is no significant difference in estimates of ES in studies with high and low internal validity.

One variable of interest was whether the studies that randomly assign treatments to subjects yield higher ES than those that did not. As shown, when the type of treatment assignment was classified into (1) nonrandom assignment, (2) random assignment, or (3) those studies that reported ambiguous information or no information about how groups were assigned to treatment, differences in estimates of ES emerged. When the unit of analysis was averaged within study, however, there were no significant differences in effect sizes related to how treatments were randomly assigned. Those studies that included standardized testing as part of the pre- and posttest measures had significantly lower effect sizes when compared to studies that relied on experimental measures (.92 vs. .69). Those studies that had a high degree of overlap between the control group and the treatment group in terms of the number and types of instructional components yielded significantly lower effect sizes than those studies with minimal overlap (.71 vs. .85). As we expected, those studies that included larger samples sizes reported lower effect sizes than those that included small samples. A Scheffe test showed that studies that had a total sample of less than 25 yielded higher effect sizes than those with samples below 100. However, 6 studies that had sample sizes that totaled greater than 100 yielded an effect size of 1.12.

Because some methodological variables clearly separated out effect sizes, whereas others did not, it was decided to create a methods composite score related to internal validity (methodological sophistication). Studies that included (1) instructional sessions greater than 10 (selection of this variable was based on the assumption that the intensity of instruction—as reflected by the number of sessions—yields more reliable and stable outcomes than shorter intervention sessions), (2) random assignment to treatment, (3) measures of treatment integrity, (4) utilization of standardized tests, (5) internal validity scores on the abbreviated scale of 5 (number reflects highest possible score items including the variables of comparability of setting, materials, and teachers across conditions and the reporting of [a] reliability on dependent measures and [b] procedural validity), and (6) high control and treatment condition overlap in steps and procedures (at least three steps and/or procedures overlap) were assigned a score. The amount of psychometric data reported was also included in the methodological composite score (if additional psychometric information beyond an IQ score was reported, e.g., reading scores, the study was weighted positively). For each of the seven variables weighted positively and negatively, a score of 2 or 0 was assigned for each variable, respectively. For each study, the weighted score thus varied from 14 to 0, with 14 reflecting methodologically superior studies. As Table 4 indicates, effect sizes for studies receiving the highest ratings on the methods composite score were significantly lower than for those studies with lower methods composite scores. Thus, a total composite score close to the maximum of 14 was considered to reflect those studies of high methodological sophistication (or internal validity), whereas scores close to 0 reflected studies low in methodological sophistication. Based on the methodological composite score, studies were divided into three classifications, high (score >10), medium (score between 6 and 11), and low methodological sophistication (score <6). As Table 4 illustrates, studies that achieved higher methodological sophistication had a significantly lower effect size estimate than those studies weak in methodological sophistication. Regardless of whether the unit of analysis was averaged within studies or each dependent measure was considered as a separate ES, significant differences in ES estimates occurred between studies as a function of ratings on the methodological composite score. A Scheffe test indicated that higher effect sizes occurred for those studies with low methodological composite scores, followed by those studies that received medium ratings. The lowest ES occurred for those studies with higher methodological sophistication. This methodological composite score was used in the subsequent analysis to qualify the outcomes related to ES estimates. A methodological composite score was computed for each study. The mean score across studies for this methodological composite score was 7.25 (SD = 2.92).

A comparison was made between the 17 dependent measure categories (also referred to as *domains*; see Table 3) with the methodological composite score partialed from the analysis. The average ES per study as a function of domain was the unit of analysis. Significant differences in ES were found between the 17 general categories, $\chi^2(16, N = 377) = 45.71, p < .001$. The WLS mean effect sizes, with the influence of the methodological composite score partialed out, that approximated Cohen's threshold were reading comprehension (.81), vocabulary (.73), and creativity (.78). Those WLS means of moderate magnitude (>.60 but <.70) were the categories of cognitive processing (.69), word recognition (.65), memory (.66), writing (.65), intelligence (.61), attitude/self-concept (.60), phonics/orthographic skills (.60), and global achievement (.64). Those categories of relatively weak (<.55) magnitude were spelling (.51), mathematics (.45), general reading (.46), social skills (.47), perceptual processes (.53), and language processes (.50). A Scheffe test indicated that significant differences ($p < .05$) emerged between studies that included measures of ES near Cohen's threshold and those of weak magnitude (<.55). No significant differences emerged between those categories of dependent measures of moderate magnitude when compared to those measures near Cohen's threshold and those of weak magnitude. These results qualify the weighted means reported in Table 3 by partialing out the influence of variation in methodological sophistication.

Article Characteristics

Table 4 shows the mean outcomes on ES as a function of the characteristics of studies in terms of funding and the type of publication. No significant differences emerged in the magnitude of ES for studies that reported a funding source and those that did not. Those studies that were published in dissertations had significantly lower effect sizes than those published in journals.

Setting of Intervention

Studies were sorted by those that reported the setting in which treatment occurred and those that did not. As Table 4 indicates, those studies that do not report the setting ($N = 102$) in which the intervention occurred yield lower effect sizes than those that do report the setting. Setting information was further divided into those studies that reported that treatment occurred in a self-contained classroom, a resource room, or a regular classroom, or that failed to report the type of classroom setting where the treatment occurred. As Table 4 indicates, the number of studies reporting no information ($N = 102$) was reduced ($N = 86$) in the comparisons between the type of classrooms because 16 of these studies failed to report a mean age score (age or grade ranges were provided instead) of the sample. Because the influence of age and the methodological composite score were partialed out in the analysis of WLS means, the number of studies in the comparison was reduced. As Table 4 demonstrates, significant differences related to setting occurred whether the unit of analysis was averaged within study or each dependent measure was considered as a separate independent event. As shown, larger effect sizes occurred in resource rooms when compared to other settings. As shown, however, only four studies, with a total sample size of 151 participants, provided information on effect sizes related to the regular classroom.

Sample Characteristics

Several ES differences emerged related to information on sample characteristics. The general pattern was that those studies that fail to report psychometric information on participants with learning disabilities yield significantly higher effect sizes than those studies that report psychometric information. For example, studies were categorized by the amount of psychometric information reported. Four categories were developed for comparisons (no information, standardized intelligence test scores, standardized intelligence scores + standardized reading test scores, and standardized intelligence test scores + reading scores + mathematics scores). As Table 4 illustrates, a significant chi-square emerged for both units of analysis. The Scheffe test indicated that those studies that provided no psychometric information on the LD sample produced larger effect sizes than those studies that report intelligence, reading, and/or mathematics scores. No significant differences were found between those studies that reported intelligence scores and those that reported standardized intelligence scores and reading and/or math scores.

Given that psychometric information is related to ES, the sample characteristics were further categorized by the reported range in intelligence scores and the range of reading scores. Three categories for comparison were created for intelligence: those studies that reported mean standard scores between 85 and 92, those that reported mean standardized intelligence scores greater than 92, and those that did not report standardized information. If studies provide multiple IQ scores (verbal, performance, nonverbal, etc.), these scores were averaged within studies. As Table 4 illustrates, the highest effect sizes occurred when no information is presented.

The next category considered in our sample analysis was reading severity. If multiple standardized reading measures were provided in the study, reading scores were averaged across word recognition and reading comprehension. Four categories were created for comparisons: scores below 85, scores above 84 but less than 91, scores greater than 90, and no standardized scores reported. Significant chi-squares emerged between the four categories of reading for the two types of unit of analysis. When we examined the differences using the WLS method, high effect sizes emerged when no IQ and reading scores were reported when compared to the other condition. However, when methodology was partialed out in the analysis, effect sizes for studies that reported scores below 85 were comparable to those studies that reported no scores. The lowest effect sizes occurred between studies that reported reading scores between 84 and less than 91 and those studies that reported scores above 90.

Because the discrepancy between intelligence and achievement was a frequent way of defining samples, we categorized studies that "stated" that the sample has a discrepancy between potential or IQ and achievement (or some specific academic domain) versus those that did not. Although we placed no restrictions on the type of discrepancy reported, we decided that the study must use the term *discrepancy* and also state that the participants were at least 1 year behind in some achievement domain. This variable was analyzed because the majority of the studies included school-identified LD groups that relied on discrepancy criteria for classification. As Table 4 demonstrates, the influence of the discrepancy variable is only significant when the unit of analysis was not averaged within studies. Higher effect sizes occurred when no discrepancy information is presented when compared to those studies that report discrepancy information. However, no significant differences were found in effect sizes when averaged within studies.

Sample characteristics that failed to emerge as significant when we considered the main effects were the age and gender of the participants. When we examined the age differences using the WLS method and effect sizes were averaged within studies, we found larger mean effect sizes in studies that included both elementary and secondary age children ($N = 80$, mean =.75) than for studies treating adults ($N = 9$, mean = .61), adolescents (12 years of age and older; $N = 40$, mean = .64), and children 11 years of age and younger ($N = 51$, mean = .72), but the differences were not significant, $p > .05$.

As Table 4 illustrates, few studies provided information that allowed us to investigate the effects of gender on treatment outcome. Thus, we calculated the median ratio of those studies that reported the number of males and females in each study. We computed a gender ratio (number of males/total in the sample) and divided the studies by the median ratio (.70) across the 180 studies. Those studies that report male and female samples but include greater than 69% males in the sample were compared to those studies that report less than 70% males in the sample. These two categories were compared with those studies in which the gender ratio of the sample could not be computed. As Table 4 demonstrates, only 31 studies were considered to have a low male ratio. When examining the effect sizes differences using the WLS method, we found that larger effect sizes occurred for those studies in which we could not calculate the gender ratio. However, the results indicated that no main effects emerged related to gender ratio when the unit of analysis included effect sizes averaged within studies.

Type of Intervention

The final analysis of main effects considered the type of intervention. Studies that reflected the components of strategy instruction discussed earlier were assigned a 1 (dummy coded) and those studies that included instructional components below the threshold (less than three of the components) were assigned a 0. The same dummy coding procedures were used to classify those studies that utilized direct instruction (studies that included at least four of the possible eight components were coded as 1, and those studies that included less than four of the possible eight components were dummy coded as 0) and nondirect instruction methods. Prior to our analysis, however, we found it necessary to partial the influence of methodology from the WLS analysis. This variable was then used to partial estimates of ES related to the two treatments.

As shown in Table 4, studies that include strategy instruction produce larger effect sizes than those studies that do not. This occurs whether the unit of analysis is averaged within studies or each dependent measure is considered as an independent ES. In addition, the magnitude of the ES is maintained even when the effects of the methodology composite score are partialed from the main effects. The least square mean effect size, weighted by the reciprocal of the sampling variance, is .84 versus .67 for strategy versus nonstrategy studies, respectively. Also provided in Table 4 are the effect sizes related to direct instruction and nondirect instruction. Similar to the strategy instruction models, the direct instruction model is more powerful than the nondirect instruction model. Least square mean ES, partialing the influence of methodology, yields an ES of .82 for direct instruction studies and .66 for studies that do not use direct instruction.

In summary, regardless of the unit of analysis, studies that include components related to strategy instruction or direct instruction yield larger effect sizes than studies that use nonstrategy and nondirect instruction models. Both models appear to yield the same approximate magnitude in ES estimates, and therefore the independent contribution of each model will be investigated in the subsequent analysis.

INTERVENTION MODELS AND OUTCOMES: A THREE-TIER ANALYSIS

The previous analysis of main effects does not allow for a qualification of treatment outcomes. For example, we have no idea about what are the effective ingredients of instruction. That is, we have isolated several important methodological variables that influence outcomes, but we have not uncovered the components of effective instruction. Thus, to isolate the locus of treatment effects on outcome measures, a three-tier structure was used to investigate the various instructional approaches. The unit of analysis was the aggregated (averaged) ES of each study.

For the first tier, as in the previous analysis on treatment main effects, we determined if the broad categorization of studies that were classified as strategy instruction models contributed independent variance to estimates of ES when compared to direct instruction models. It could be argued, based on the comparable magnitude of effect sizes (.84 for strategy instruction and .82 for direct instruction; see last section of Table 4), that these two intervention approaches overlap in a number of studies, and therefore that the two approaches are not independent of each other. To determine the independence of these two models, phi coefficients were calculated on the two dummy variables. The phi coefficient showed a weak but significant correlation, $r = .179$, $p < .05$. Thus, the two approaches are not completely independent. To further address the independence issue, however, a WLS hierarchical regression model was employed to assess whether the general instructional models contributed independent variance to estimates of ES. The analysis is shown in Table 5.

As Table 5 indicates, methodology and age were forced to enter the equa-

TABLE 5. Hierarchical Regression Model with Weighted Least Squares for Effect Size Estimates

	df^a	χ^2	R^2	Increment in R^2
1. Forced entry				
Methodology Chronological age	158[b]	309.27**	.07	—
1. Forced entry				
Methodology Chronological age Direct instruction	157	304.04**	.08	—
2. Strategy instruction	156	298.70**	.10	.02
1. Forced entry				
Methodology Chronological age Strategy instruction	157	301.58**	.10	—
2. Direct instruction	—	ns	—	—

[a] *df* is $k - p$.
[b] *df* includes a total of 160 studies because 20 studies included only ranges in age or grade and not means.
$^{**}p < .01$.

tion first, followed by the alternating order of direct instruction and strategy instruction. As Table 5 illustrates that, strategy instruction was the only instructional approach that contributed significant (independent) variance to ES estimates. When direct instruction was entered after strategy instruction (also forced first in entry were the methodological composite score and chronological age), no significant variance emerged in predicting ES. In contrast, when strategy instruction followed direct instruction, strategy instruction contributed significant variance (2% of the variance) to ES estimates. Thus, support is found for the idea that the general model of strategy instruction contributes significant variance to ES estimates that is independent of direct instruction. However, it is important to note that not all studies reported mean age scores (some reported grade ranges rather than ages), and that such studies were excluded from the analysis. In addition, some studies could be classified as both direct and strategy instruction, and thus there is a partial overlap in variance that predicts ES. More importantly, a contribution of 2% of the variance to effect sizes would not be considered meaningful in practical terms. Thus, making a further refinement of our analysis of the contribution of treatment to ES estimates became necessary.

Those studies that overlapped in components between strategy and direct instruction were separated for analysis. Studies that included at least three components of the direct instruction model and three components of strategy instruction were considered as a separate model (referred to hereafter as the Combined Model). Thus, four general interventions models were compared. The four general models are direct instruction alone (DI Alone; direct instruction components, but no strategy components), strategy instruction alone (SI Alone; strategy components, but no direct instruction components), direct instruction coupled with strategy instruction (*Combined Model,* or DI + SI; both direct and strategy instruction components), and those studies that do not include or do not report a critical threshold of direct or strategy instruction components (NonDI + NonSI Model).

The mean effect sizes and standard deviations for the four models of this first tier of analysis are shown in Table 6. As shown, the four models were compared by partialing out the influence of the methodological composite score (top row) and partialing out the influence of the methodological composite score and age (bottom row). A Scheffe test indicated that the Combined Model (combination of direct [DI] + strategy instruction [SI]) yielded significantly higher effect sizes (all *p*s < .05) than the other models (DI + SI > DI Alone = SI Alone = NonDI + NonSI).

The next tier refines the four models into instructional components because it is unclear how many of the components in the NonDI + NonSI Model were comparable to the *Combined Model* (DI+SI). Thus, this second tier of analysis included a fine-grain description of the components of instruction that underlie the four models. This tier of analysis is important because it determines which of the instructional components within the four models are different. Such a determination would establish the discriminant validity of the four general models. Chi-squares ($df = 3$) were computed across the four instructional approaches on the 20 instructional components discussed earlier in the methods section.

The 20 components are listed in Table 7 as a function of the four instructional models. Also reported in Table 7 are the percentage of studies in each model that include each instructional component (first column under each treatment heading). Also included is mean Cohen's *d* for each study that includes the component. A chi-square analysis ($df = 3$) of the *frequency* of components was computed for each of the 20 components between the four models. To facilitate

TABLE 6. Four General Conditions as a Function of Effect Size Estimates

Instructional components	DI Alone			SI Alone			DI + SI			NonDI + NonSI			
	N	*M*	*SD*	*N*	*M*	*SD*	*N*	*M*	*SD*	*N*	*M*	*SD*	χ^{2a}
Total model	47	.79	.51	28	.78	.47	55	.85	.54	43	.69	.53	21.77*
Weighted least square mean with method and age partialed out		.68			.72			.84			.62		12.79*[b]

Note. Seven studies could not be included because of inability to determine mean age.

[a]χ^2 assesses whether weighted *d* is significantly different.

[b]Scheffe ($p < .05$) indicated DI + SI > SI = DI; SI > NonDI + NonSI; DI = NonDI + NonSI.

*$p < .01$.

TABLE 7. Four General Treatment Conditions as a Function of the Percent of Instructional Components and Effect Size Estimates (Total N = 180)

	DI Alone			SI Alone			DI + SI			NonDi + NonSI			
Instructional components	%	*M*	*SD*	%	*M*	*SD*	%	*M*	*SD*	%	*M*	*SD*	χ^2
1. Sequencing (e.g., process or task analysis to goal, shaping)	<u>91</u>[a]	.79	.52	64	.95	.52	<u>87</u>	.86	.56	25	.78	.54	68.50***
2. Drill–repetition–practice–feedback	<u>48</u>	.85	.55	<u>53</u>	.89	.29	<u>47</u>	.89	.64	20	.74	.59	14.91**
3. Orienting to process or task (e.g., preparatory to task, Meichenbaum)	<u>40</u>	.91	.56	<u>42</u>	.92	.37	30	.97	.68	6	1.27	.78	18.75***
4. Question/answer sequence (e.g., structured verbal interaction, Socratic questioning)	6	.40	.25	<u>42</u>	.92	.47	21	.81	.43	11	.58	.23	18.90***
5. Individual and group instruction	<u>97</u>	.81	.51	57	.84	.42	<u>98</u>	.86	.54	<u>88</u>	.71	.56	19.13***
6. Novelty (pictorial presentation, flow chart, related visual presentation, mapping, new material or curriculum)	<u>87</u>	.80	.80	<u>82</u>	.96	.47	<u>80</u>	.84	.48	39	.67	.53	37.79***
7. Attributions/benefits to instruction (e.g., This approach works when . . . , This will help you . . .)	2	.72	—	57	.82	.42	<u>92</u>	.82	.54	4	.29	.10	136.22***
8. Systematic probing (CBM, daily testing)	<u>38</u>	.77	.49	14	1.46	.63	<u>40</u>	.78	.40	11	.72	.59	17.29**

9. Peer modeling/mediation (e.g., peer tutoring)	4	.69	.18	10	3.62	.31	10	.62	.34	2	.72	—	4.51
10. Segmentation (e.g., sounds divided into units then synthesized)	74	.76	.49	42	.79	.37	82	.81	.49	13	.82	.66	62.04**
11. Advanced organizer (overview of task)	40	.91	.56	42	.92	.37	30	.97	.68	6	1.27	.78	18.75***
12. Directed response/questioning (child directed to summarize, asked what's the thing to do)	6	.40	.25	32	.87	.53	18	.69	.33	11	.58	.23	10.60*
13. One-to-one instruction	89	.81	.51	42	.97	.59	87	.85	.56	48	.57	.53	43.14***
14. Control task difficulty (adapting material to reading level)	55	.88	.55	67	.90	.52	36	.92	.55	13	.78	.59	30.40***
15. Technology (computer-mediated, highly structured materials)	57	.87	.51	53	.83	.54	60	.75	.41	.34	.64	.65	11.38*
16. Elaboration (additional information, examples, rely on context)	—	—	—	16	1.09	.13	5	1.12	.60	—	—	—	8.84*
17. Teacher models directly (models problem solving, steps, correct sounds)	21	.66	.51	71	.94	.50	72	.89	.51	62	.72	.56	16.46**
18. Small interactive groups (reciprocal, directive, therapy groups)	36	.85	.51	71	.94	.50	72	.89	.51	62	.72	.56	16.46**
19. Mediators other than peers or teacher (homework, parents)	4	1.10	.18	—	—	—	—	—	—	2	1.94	—	3.36
20. Strategy cuing (reminders to use strategies or tactics)	—	—	—	39	.73	.28	43	.87	.56	0	—	—	51.01***

Note. Underlining indicates significant results for both units of analysis.

[a] Read as 91% of the studies labeled as DI Alone include this component.

*$p < .05$; **$p < .01$; ***$p < .001$.

your visual analysis of the table, please note that when the chi-squares were significant, we have underlined the highest percentiles that separated one model from another. If more that one percentile score is underlined across the rows, differences were not found between those treatments, but those treatments were significantly higher than the remaining treatments.

Three very important findings are reported in Table 7. First, we are able to isolate those instructional components that primarily make up the NonDI + NonSI Model. As shown, this model reflects an emphasis on individual and/or small group instruction (component 5). No other components (the remaining components are less than 50%) characterized this condition. Second, based on the number of significant chi-squares (18 of 20), there is discriminate validity among the treatments. As shown in Table 7, significant effects emerged on all components as a function of the four models except for peer modeling (see #9) and nonteacher mediation (#19).

Finally, some components are unique to the Combined Model. Because of the classification procedures, it was expected that the Combined Model would reflect more components than either of the remaining three approaches. However, it was not clear which components overlapped or which components were most characteristic (no overlap) of the competing models. As shown in Table 7, a high representation (>70%) of components that occurs for the Combined Model includes the following instructional components: 1, 5, 6, 7, 10, 13, 17, and 18 (refer to Table 7 to attach labels to the numbers), when compared to DI Alone (components 1, 5, 6, 10, 13), SI Alone (6, 18), and NonDI + NonSI (component 5) models. Significant differences in the components represented occurred between the Combined Model and the DI Alone Model. Components 4, 7, 17, 18, and 20 were more frequent in the Combined Model than the DI Alone Model. The DI Alone Model was more frequent in its representation of component 14 (control of task difficulty) than the Combined Model.

Significant differences in component representation occurred between the Combined Model and SI Alone Model (i.e., components 1, 5, 7, 8, 10, and 13 were more frequently represented in the Combined Model). Component 4 (structured verbal teacher–student interaction) was more frequent in the Combined Model than in the DI Alone Model. Components 4, 12, 14, and 16 were more frequent in the SI Alone Model than in the Combined Model.

In sum, the previous analyses suggest that the instructional models vary in the frequency of components represented in treatment. The Combined Model appears distinct from the other approaches because of its inclusion of attributions (#7), teacher modeling of problem-solving steps (#17), and emphasis on small interactive groups (#18). In general, the Combined Model primarily reflects (see underlined percentiles >50% in Table 7) the components related to sequencing, individual and/or group instruction, segmentation, highly structured material (technology), and teacher modeling of problem-solving steps when compared to the other models.

What we don't know from our analysis as reported in Table 7 is whether the magnitude of ES for each of the instructional components vary as a function of the four general models. To address this issue, we computed, via WLS analysis, differences among effects sizes for each component as a function of the four instructional models. The influence of the methodological scores was then partialed from the analysis. As Table 8 illustrates, the magnitude of the effect sizes as a function of each component varied across the four general models. As shown, the significant estimates of effect size in favor of the Combined Model are isolated to the components of sequencing, drill–repetition–practice, segmentation, one-to-one instruction, control of task difficulty, technology, teacher modeling of strategies, and small interactive groups.

It was of interest to us in this second tier of analysis to also determine whether the treatment approaches and instructional components varied in their emphasis in studies over the 30-year period. That is, Are treatments better now (more robust) than they were at the inception of the field? The answer to this question appears to be No. The correlation between the overall unweighted ES ($M = .79$, $SD = 52$) averaged across studies and year of publication ($M = 1987$, $SD = 5.41$) was not significant, $r\ (178) = .05$, $p > .45$. In addition, none of the correlation coefficients between year of publication and the 20 instructional components were of sufficient magnitude (all *r*s $< .16$) to be of interest. The point biserial correlation between year of publication and direct instruction (coded as 1 for direct instruction and 0 for studies not including direct instruction) was not significant, $r\ (178) = .09$, $p > .20$. We did find that the emergence of strategy models has increased positively over the years. A significant positive point biserial correlation (although moderate) emerged between year of publication and strategy instruction (coded as 1 for the occurrence of strategy instruction and 0 for nonstrategy instruction), $r\ (178) = .23$, $p < .01$.

Our final (third) tier of analysis attempted to determine which of the 20 components, either in isolation or in combination with other components, best predicted effect sizes. As indicated earlier, those components that made up the Combined Model that yielded the highest effect sizes when compared to the competing models included sequencing, segmentation, one-to-one instruction, teacher modeling, and small interactive groups (components 1, 5, 7, 10, 13, 17, and 18, shown in Table 8). However, as Table 8 clearly illustrates, several components (16 of 20) yield effect sizes above the .80 threshold, suggesting that the instructional components may not be independent. In addition, we have not identified the instructional components most important in predicting ES, or those components that when combined account for most of the variance in treatment outcomes.

We used a WLS regression analysis to isolate the instructional components that play a significant role in predicting ES. All instructional components were dummy coded (coded 1 for occurrence of components and 0 for nonoccurrence) for the subsequent analysis. Because mean age was not reported in 20 studies and the grade ranges were 3–7, we assigned an age of 10.6 so as not to delete those studies from the analyses. Further, based on the previous analysis, age was not a significant predictor of ES, and therefore the assignment of a constant score for missing values was appropriate. To determine the relationship between the 20 in-

TABLE 8. Weighted Least Square Means for Instructional Components as a Function of the Four General Interventions (N = 180)

	1	2	3	4			
Instructional components	DI Alone	SI Alone	DI +SI	NonDI + NonSI	N	Difference[b]	χ^{2a}
1. Sequencing (e.g., process or task analysis to goal, shaping)	.72	.76	<u>.89</u>	.65	119	3 > 2 = 1 = 4[b]	8.03*
2. Drill–repetition–practice–feedback	.66	<u>.83</u>	<u>.96</u>	.68	72	3 = 2 > 1 = 4	11.13*
3. Orienting to process or task (e.g., preparatory to task, Meichenbaum)	.93	.81	.83	1.20	50	—	2.93
4. Question/answer sequence (e.g., structured verbal interaction, Socratic questioning)	.57	.74	.72	.45	31	—	3.41
5. Individual and group instruction	.69	<u>.80</u>	<u>.86</u>	.63	156	2&3 > 1&4	12.76**
6. Novelty (pictorial presentation, flow chart, related visual presentation, mapping, new material or curriculum)	.78	.69	.91	.60	117	3 > 1 = 2, 2 = 4	5.19
7. Attributions/benefits to instruction (e.g., This approach works when . . . , This will help you . . .)	69	1.19	<u>.87</u>	.30	76	2 > 3 > 1 > 4	11.44**
8. Systematic probing (CBM, daily testing)	.65	1.23	.67	.69	48	—	5.82
9. Peer modeling/mediation (e.g., peer tutoring)	.90	.59	.49	.74	11	—	1.79

10. Segmentation (e.g., sounds divided into units then synthesized)	.68	.62	<u>.85</u>	.55	97	3 > 1 = 2 = 3	9.46*
11. Advanced organizer (overview of task)	.92	.81	.83	1.20	50	—	2.93
12. Directed response/questioning (child directed to summarize, asked what's the thing to do when . . .)	.51	.64	.62	.45	26	—	1.41
13. One-to-one instruction	.68	.69	<u>.86</u>	.49	122	3 > 1 = 2 > 4	19.16**
14. Control task difficulty (adapting material to reading level)	.80	.73	<u>1.07</u>	.66	70	3 > 1 = 2, 2 = 4	13.42**
15. Technology (computer-mediated, highly structured materials)	.77	.61	<u>.88</u>	.53	89	3 > 2,3 = 1,2 > 4	13.92**
16. Elaboration (additional information, examples, rely on context)	1.09	1.09	1.03	—	5	—	.001
17. Teacher models directly (models problem solving, steps, correct sounds)	.52	.76	<u>.89</u>	.44	75	3 > 2 > 1 = 4	21.55**
18. Small interactive groups (reciprocal, directive, therapy groups)	.80	.79	<u>.93</u>	.65	103	3 > 1 = 2 > 4	12.56**
19. Mediators other than peers or teacher (homework, parents)	1.06	—	—	2.03	2	—	2.08
20. Strategy cuing (reminders to use strategies or tactics)	—	.69	.74	—	34	—	.11

Note. N = total number of studies that report information. Total possible N = 180. Underlining indicates significant results for both units of analysis.

[a]χ^2 partialed for methodological composite score.

[b]Post-hoc Scheffe.

*$p < .05$; **$p < .01$.

structional components and ES estimates, WLS fixed effects regression models were fitted to the empirical values, following methods recommended by Harwell (1992) and described by Hedges and Olkin (1985, pp. 168–174; see also Hedges, 1994, pp. 295–298). Three approaches were used to control partially for preselection bias (control for order) of the instructional components and our capitalization on chance in the WLS regression analysis. Our goal was to identify those components that when combined and/or in isolation contribute important variance to the prediction of ES.

First, we used a stepwise selection procedure in which the order of entry is determined via a mathematical maximization procedure. That is, after the methodological composite score and age are entered, the component with the largest correlation to ES is entered, followed with the second component with the largest semipartial coefficient correlation, and so on. The results indicated that methodological composite score and age contributed approximately 6% of the variance in predicting ES, $R^2 = .058$, $\chi^2(2, N = 180) = 20.81$, $p < .001$. The first instructional component to enter the regression model was control of task difficulty; increment in $R^2 = .056$, $\chi^2(3, N = 180) = 40.80$, $p < .001$, followed by small interactive groups with an increment in $R^2 = .049$, $\chi^2(4, N = 180) = 58.49$, $p < .001$, followed by directed response/questioning; increment in $R^2 = .022$, $\chi^2(5, N = 180) = 66.22$, $p < .001$ The complete model was significant, $R^2 = .18$, $\chi^2(174, N = 180) = 290.34$, $p < .001$. Thus, three components (control of task difficulty, small interactive groups, and directed response/questioning) contributed approximately 12% of the variance in predicting ES estimates. No other components entered significantly into the model.

Second, we identified those components that when combined yield the highest adjusted R^2 in predicting ES estimates. The squared multiple correlation, adjusted for the number of explanatory variables, was used to quantify the predictive power of the given model. The SAS regression program (SAS Institute, 1992a) was used to conduct the statistical analysis using the "best model" option. The adjusted R^2 procedure was used to find the model with the highest R^2 within the ranges of effect sizes. The adjusted R^2 was .04 when the methodological composite score and age were used to predict effect sizes across studies. The adjusted R^2 was improved to .20 when methodological composite score and age included sequencing (#1; see Tables 7 and 8), drill–repetition–practice (#2), segmentation (#10), directed response/questioning (#12), control of task difficulty (#14), technology (#15), small interactive groups (#18), mediation other than peers or teacher (#19), and strategy cuing (#20). Thus, nine instructional components (sequencing, drill–repetition–practice, segmentation, directed response/questioning, control of task difficulty, technology, small interactive groups, mediation other than peers or teacher, and strategy cuing) contribute 16% of the variance in predicting ES estimates.

The final analysis attempted to identify those components that in isolation (i.e., when the contributions of the remaining components are partialed out) contribute to effect sizes when all variables are entered into the equation simultaneously. Based on the question we proposed, a Type III sum of squares (which corresponds to Yates's weighted squares of means analysis) was used. A Type III sum of squares is used because the calculation adjusts for the effects of other variables. The Type III sum of squares partials the influence of variables on a single variable, that is, the results when the variable is entered last in the equation.

Table 9 shows the independent contribution of the instructional components, as well as the methodological composite score on ES estimates as a function of the total studies. As shown, the results indicate that when all dependent measures were averaged within studies, the component that positively predicted ES estimates at the .05 alpha level was controlling task difficulty. The isolated component that was significantly (alpha = .05) related to lower effect sizes (negative beta weight) included one-to-one instruction. The interpretation of negative beta weights (as well as positive) when dummy variables are used in a partial re-

TABLE 9. Weighted Least Square Regression on Effect Size Estimates to Determine Independent Influence of Isolated Instructional Components

	χ^{2a}	β	*SE*
I. Methodology	13.80***	–.03	.01
Age	.21	–.005	.02
II. Instructional components			
1. Sequencing	3.39*	.17	.12
2. Drill–repetition–practice–feedback	1.83	.08	.08
3. Orienting to process or task	.01	.02	.09
4. Question/answer sequence	.36	.24	.52
5. Individual plus group instruction	3.43*	.23	.16
6. Novelty	.12	.02	.10
7. Attributions/benefits to instruction	2.14	.12	.11
8. Systematic probing	.27	–.03	.08
9. Peer modeling/mediation	.93	–.11	.15
10. Segmentation	3.44*	–.15	.10
11. Advanced organizers	.01	.001	.01
12. Directed response/questioning	1.14	–.43	.52
13. One-to-one instruction	5.00**	–.17	.10
14. Control task difficulty	6.65**	.16	.08
15. Technology	.20	.02	.09
16. Elaboration	.02	–.004	.47
17. Teacher models problem solving	.12	–.02	.09
18. Small interactive groups	2.74	.11	.09
19. Mediators other than peers or teacher	1.59	.36	.37
20. Strategy cuing	3.48*	–.16	.11
R^2	.25		
N	179		
df	158		
Q_e	267.30**		

Note. R^2 for methods and age is .06.

[a]Type III sum of squares.

*$p < .10$; **$p < .05$; ***$p < .01$.

TABLE 10. Weighted Least Square Regression on Effect Size Estimates to Determine Partialed Influence of Independent Instructional Components as a Function of Types of Dependent Measure (Type III Sum of Squares)

	Real word recognition χ^2	Real word recognition		Word skills χ^2	Phonological	Reading compre-hension χ^2	Reading compre-hension	
Predictor variables	Total	Exp.[a]	Stand.	Total	Exp.	Total	Exp.	General reading[a]
I. Methodology ($R^2 = .10$)	1.08	–6.95**[b]	1.20	1.30	–3.61	–4.27*	–12.92**	1.93
II. Instructional components								
1. Sequencing	.53	.10	2.95	1.86	3.83**	.05	.004	(.10)
2. Drill–repetition–practice–feedback	.35	7.52**	3.45	2.87	1.57	.02	.001	4.49**
3. Orienting to process or task	.000	.00	.00	.00	.00	.00	3.14	
4. Question/answer/sequence	.36	.00	.00	.00	.00	.01	.00	—
5. Individual + group instruction	.02	.08	.77	.02	.04	.009	4.72*	—
6. Novelty	2.64	.21	.16	.91	.12	.00	.00	—
7. Attributions/benefits to instruction	1.47	6.47**	.26	.27	.13	1.05	.23	—
8. Systematic probing	1.05	3.33	1.18	.25	.53	.78	.46	—
9. Peer modeling	.008	.00	.02	1.74	.00	.20	.00	—
10. Segmentation	2.64	4.39*	1.10	2.18	4.10*	.05	.97	—
11. Advanced organizers	.00	.00	.01	.00	.00	.00	.00	—
12. Directed response/questioning	.00	.00	.00	.00	.00	.01	.00	—
13. One-to-one instruction	.01	1.72	.12	1.61	.78	.41	3.96*	—
14. Control task difficulty	.14	3.03	.48	.43	.67	.04	3.86*	—
15. Technology	.94	.02	.29	1.11	.06	2.03	5.70*	—
16. Elaboration	.00	.00	.00	.43	.00	.00	.00	—
17. Teacher models directly	1.80	.52	.84	.42	1.79	3.55*	8.37**	—
18. Small interactive groups	.00	3.40	.005	1.28	.36	2.08	.35	—
19. Mediators other than peers or teacher	.01	.00	.00	.00	.58	.00	.00	—
20. Strategy cuing	.48	.16	.17	1.18	1.25	<u>6.72</u>**	.36	—
R^2	.23	—	.30	—	—	.41	.52	—
df[a]	31	6	17	11	4	39	26	15
N	53	22	34	28	20	57	43	—
$\chi^2(Q_e)$	76.87**	12.20*	49.80**	8.42	1.71	103.60**	70.29**	—
Weighted mean ES	.59	.61	.61	.58	.64	.82	.90	.42

Note. Unit of analysis = ES averaged within each study by domain. Underlining indicates significant results for both units of analysis.

[a] $df = k$ (number of studies) – p (number of predictors).

[b] Reflects direction of beta.

*$p < .10$; **$p < .05$

Predictor variables	Spelling χ^2 Total	Writing[a] χ^2	Mathematics χ^2 Total	Mathematics Exp.	Cognitive processes Total	Metacognitive processes Exp.
I. Methodology (R^2 = .10)	−10.01**	1.44	2.66	1.82	19.31**	−22.04***
II. Instructional components						
1. Sequencing	14.21**	—	.23	1.23	3.14	1.16
2. Drill–repetition–practice–feedback	1.52	—	.73	1.22	.14	1.36
3. Orienting to process or task	.00	22.30**	.00	.00	.00	1.52
4. Question/answer/sequence	.00	—	.00	.00	.00	.16
5. Individual + group instruction	2.50	—	3.08	.47	7.83**	.00
6. Novelty	2.32	—	.11	.15	1.01	3.21
7. Attributions/benefits to instruction	.00	—	1.66	.19	2.08	1.87
8. Systematic probing	2.06	4.20*	1.26	.53	.98	.12
9. Peer modeling	.00*	—	.27	.72	.34	.07
10. Segmentation	−11.99**	—	.02	1.24	1.67	.16**
11. Advanced organizers	.08	—	.00	.00	.00	4.80*
12. Directed response/questioning	.00	—	.00	.00	.29	.00
13. One-to-one instruction	.28	—	.02	.12	.95	.00
14. Control task difficulty	.55	—	.33	.53	.93	.29
15. Technology	4.00*	3.51	3.41	.39	1.48	.01
16. Elaboration	.00	—	.00	.00	.90	.20
17. Teacher models directly	.00	—	.00	.05	1.64	.00
18. Small interactive groups	.51	—	5.99*	2.56	2.33	4.91*
19. Mediators other than peers or teacher	6.24*	—	.00	.00	2.52	2.53
20. Strategy cuing	.13	—	.01	2.70	.21	10.85**
R^2	—	—	.56	—	.40	—
df^a	7	—	10	3	20	7
N	23	19	27	21	40	24
$\chi^2(Q_e)$	3.45	—	15.11*	9.01*	64.26**	19.47*
Weighted mean ES	.46	.66	.45	.49	.68	.60

Note. Unit of analysis = ES averaged within each study by domain.

[a]Could not model general reading and writing because. . . . $k < p$.

*$p < .05$; **$p < .01$; ***$p < .001$.

gression coefficient (β) must be done carefully (see Cohen & Cohen, 1983, pp. 193–198, for a discussion). For example, one-to-one instruction is not compared to non-one-to-one instruction, but rather to all other studies. Thus the βs are dutifully recorded in Table 9, "but in the context of nominal scale coding they are not particularly useful" (Cohen & Cohen, 1983, p. 194). Thus, the χ^2 test is of singular importance in our analysis. Our important finding was that only two components significantly contribute to ES estimates. However, this finding merely capitalizes on chance (a Bonferroni-adjusted per-comparison alpha level would be .05/22 = .002). In addition, only one of these components (control of task difficulty) overlaps with the stepwise regression model and the regression model that specifies the maximum number of components that yield the highest R^2.

The 20 components were next analyzed as a function of the dependent measure category (domain). Not all domains could be analyzed because the number of predictors clearly exceeded the number of ES estimates. Table 10 includes the χ^2 and the direction of beta weights (all beta weights are positive unless followed by a negative sign for each variable), the adjusted R^2 (adjusts for the variables that adequately predict effect size), degrees of freedom on the adjusted R^2 and chi-square test, and weighted means effect size. Because of the number of effect sizes, we were able to analyze word recognition and reading comprehension as a function of experimental and standardized measures. The R^2 is not reported for those studies that reported degrees of freedom less than 10. Although the table shows significance at alpha .05 and .01, because of the multiple comparisons we used only a preselected alpha at .001 (chi-square > 7.88) to interpret the findings.

The important findings include:

1. *Word recognition.* None of the components in isolation predict effect sizes for the general category of real word recognition.
2. *Reading comprehension.* None of the components in isolation predict effect sizes for the general category of reading comprehension. When experimental measures are considered, teacher modeling of strategies is predicative of ES.
3. *Spelling.* Sequencing of lessons and segmentation play a major role in predicting effect sizes.
4. *Mathematics.* None of the components in isolation predict effect sizes for the general category of mathematics.
5. *Writing.* There were not enough studies to model all instructional components. However, in a reduced regression model, components predictive of treatment outcomes included orientation to process or task.
6. *Cognitive processing.* Interestingly, the best predictor of general cognitive processing is individual and group instruction. When process measures (e.g., metacognitive) are considered, strategy cuing emerged as on important predictor.

What does this analyses tell us? At least two answers appear obvious. First, good instruction within a particular domain cannot be boiled down to a single component. Good instruction interacts with several components. Although we were able to isolate some components that independently predict effect sizes, instruction is best reflected by (as suggested by the amount of variance that predicts ES) variance shared across several components. Second, the variance was restricted by the small number of studies represented in each domain.

SPECIFICITY OF TREATMENT EFFECTS

Given the dismal results reported in the previous component analysis, we are left with an important question: Do treatments have broad effects across all domains or are they specific to an academic domain. This is a difficult question to answer because in some cases outcomes measures are highly similar to treatment activities (see Weisz, Weiss, Han, Granger, & Morton, 1995, for discussion of this issue), and therefore confound conclusions that can be drawn about the independent effects of treatment. For example, when one treats a child's poor word recognition with phonics instruction, the most valid test of the child's ability to read is a test of real word recognition, not a test of performance on pseudowords or phonics measures. Or, when one treats a child's poor writing ability with metacognitive training, the ability to write a coherent essay rather than metacognition is probably the most valid test of the training. Thus, isolating the specific effects of treatment requires control of confounds related to the dependency between the domain (category of dependent measures) of the estimated ES and treatment.

To address this issue, in this study we used as outcomes measures those considered appropriate for transfer (i.e., general performance categories of reading, mathematics, spelling, writing), as well as those that may be closely related to treatment activities (cognitive processes, word skill training). A WLS regression has been suggested as one approach to handle a wide variety of these multivariate statistical problems (Gleser & Olkin, 1994), and therefore was utilized in this analysis. Thus, the overlapping variance related to various treatments (global vs. specific), correlations between treatment and outcome measures, and the correlation between multiple outcome measures were partialed out in the subsequent analysis.

To address the issue of whether treatment influences broad or specific domains of dependent measures, contrast variables were created between broad and specific outcome domains and the four general instructional models (Combination, DI Alone, SI Alone, NonDI + NonSI).

Four domain contrast variables were created. (The coding of contrast variables follows the regression model outlined by Cohen & Cohen, 1983, pp. 196–217.) The first general contrast variable separated the 17 dependent measure categories (see Table 3) into *language domains* (referred to as *high language,* which includes the domains of word recognition, reading comprehension, cognitive processing, memory, writing, vocabulary, general reading, word skills, and language) versus other (referred to as *less or low language domains,* i.e., the remaining seven categories), coded 1 versus –1, respectively. The second focused on the general domain of *reading* (this included the domain categories of word recognition, reading comprehension, general reading, and word skills) versus nonreading measures (all other domains). The reading contrast variable was also coded 1 versus –1, respectively.

Thus, the first contrast variable reflects a broad domain of instructional behaviors and the second isolates the general area of reading. Because reading is the most thoroughly investigated domain, we refined our comparison to include more specific areas of reading. A third contrast variable was created within the domain of reading to compare real word recognition and reading comprehension. This variable was coded +1 reading comprehension, –1 word recognition, and 0 for the other domains. (Note: For this trichotomy, 1, –1, 0, the 0 coded groups are omitted in the β coefficients of the regression model. We will follow up potential interactions that emerge in the regression modeling, however, by only describing properties of the 0 coded group.)

A fourth contrast variable focused on the skills or processes that underlie the transfer measures (e.g., real word recognition and reading comprehension). The word skill and cognitive process categories of dependent measures were contrasted because we assumed they underlie transfer to words, comprehension, writing, and the like. We created a variable to compare the word skill domain and the cognitive process domain. Thus, the fourth variable assessed *skill* (i.e., word skills, category related to phonics, orthographic) and process (category related to cognitive processes) coded 1 and –1, respectively. A code of 0 was assigned to the other categories.

Three contrast variables were created related to instruction. The first contrast variable included the composite scores related to a *generally effective instruction* that draws upon the various components of direct and strategy instruction (direct instruction, strategy instruction, direct instruction + strategy instruction) vs. other approaches (coded 1, 1, 1, vs. –3, respectively). We termed the SI Alone and DI Alone Models and the Combined Model contrast as an *undifferentiated* model. Thus, the three generally effective models (undifferentiated models) were compared with a model that primarily includes one-to-one and small group instruction (NonDI + NonSI Model). The second contrast variable directly compares a bottom-up approach (DI Alone) to a top-down (SI Alone) approach. The second contrast variable compares SI Alone versus DI Alone. The DI Alone and SI Alone Models were coded +1 and –1, respectively. The high overlap model (Combined Model) and the weak overlap model (NonDI + NonSI Model) were coded 0 (these are irrelevant models and therefore were omitted in the regression analysis). The third contrast compared the *Combined Model* with DI Alone or with SI Alone (coded 3 for the Combined Model, and –1 for the SI Alone Model, –1 for the DI Alone Model, and 0 for the NonDI + NonSI Model, respectively).

In general, we sought to determine if the contrasts related to instructional domains (language vs. other; reading vs. other; recognition vs. comprehension; and skills vs. processes) and to instruction interacted with each other. Because comparisons were made between categories or domains of dependent measures, we changed the unit of analysis from the averaging of all effect sizes within studies to one ES, to averaging effect sizes within each study as a function of the category of the dependent measure. Because the coding scheme did not necessarily yield independent effect sizes within studies, it was necessary to partial the effects of all the variables, via a Type III sum of squares. The variables (main effects and interactions) used to predicted estimates of ES are shown in Table 11. The methodological composite score, type of setting (e.g., treatment occurred in a regular classroom, treatment occurred in a special education classroom), and sample variables were also entered into the equation to partial out their influence on potential interactions. Because it was necessary to consider ESs across categories, the unit of analysis reflects the number of studies plus the number of categories reflected in each category.

The results of the regression analysis are shown in Table 11. The critical alpha level (prespecified alpha per comparison, chi-square > 7.88) was .001. For the main effects (see Table 11), the important findings were: (1) the significant positive beta weight reflects higher mean effect sizes for reading comprehension versus word recognition measures and (2) the Combined Model yields higher mean effect sizes than the competing models. The significant negative beta weight indicates that studies of low methodological sophistication yield higher effect sizes than those with higher methodological composite scores. As Table 11 indicates, a significant treatment × domain interaction (word × general approach) emerged, and therefore qualifies the main effects. There are two other interactions (read × combined, word × general) that approach the preselected alpha.

Table 12 provides a follow-up of these interactions by reporting the weighted least square mean effect sizes. Because our analysis is exploratory, we investigated all three interactions, as illustrated in Table 12. As the bottom of each section shows, we captured each interaction in terms of a research question. Also shown in Table 12 are the mean scores for the variables coded as 0 (e.g., *word* in the regression model reading comprehension was coded +1, word recognition/spelling –1, and other domains 0). However, it is important for the reader to remember that the variables coded 0 are not important to interpreting the direction of the interactions that emerged, as portrayed in Table 11. Figures 1, 2, and 3 illustrate the important interactions. Only the findings of theoretical interest will be discussed. Figure 1 clearly shows the advantage of the Combined Model on reading measures (this included the categories of word recognition, reading comprehension, general reading, and word skills) when compared to nonreading measures. As shown, the Combined Model yields significantly higher effect sizes on reading measures when compared to nonreading measures. No differences were found between various instructional models on the nonreading measures.

Figure 2 shows the interaction related to various combinations of SI and DI Models (labeled as general or undifferentiated SI and DI Models) versus a model that includes minimal components related to strategy instruction and direct in-

TABLE 11. Weighted Least Square Analysis of Effect Size Estimated on Treatment Domain and Treatment Approach to Determine Target Domain × Treatment Interactions[a]

Predictors	$\chi^2(df = 1)$	β	*SE*[b]
1. Method composite	21.59***	−.03	.009
Setting			
2. State setting	.21	.02	.09
3. Type of setting	.26	−.01	.05
4. Unit of instruction	2.81	.07	.06
Instructional domain			
5. *Lang*uage vs. nonlanguage	1.41	.03	.03
6. *Read*ing vs. nonreading	.07	−.006	.03
7. Comprehension vs. word (*Word*) 8.15**	.09	.04	
8. *Skill* vs. process	.02	−.009	.08
Type of instruction			
9. *Undifferentiated* vs. other (*General*)	.58	−.0093	.01
10. Bottom-up vs. top-down (*Orientation*)	5.33*	.090	.05
11. SI + DI (*Combined*) vs. DI Alone or SI Alone	10.17**	.07	.03
Sample characteristics			
12. Age	6.70*	−.02	.01
13. Gender ratio	.00	.00	.04
14. Discrepancy	2.91	.08	.07
15. Intelligence	.001	−.001	.03
16. Reading severity	1.47	−.03	.04
Interactions			
17. Lang * general	1.40	.01	.01
18. Lang * orient	1.03	−.04	.06
19. Lang * combined	1.86	−.03	.03
20. Read * general	3.06	−.01	.03
21. Read * orient	.83	.03	.05
22. Read * combined	6.83**	.03	.03
23. Word * general	4.12*	.03	.02
24. Word * orient	7.95**	−.13	.06
25. Word * combined	2.47	.04	.04
26. Skill * general	.05	.005	.03
27. Skill * orient	.02	.01	.11
28. Skill * combined	.27	.02	.07
df	306		
χ^2	660.24**		
R^2	.14		

Note. The italicized words reflect the contrast variables discussed in the text and are used as predictor variables in the main effects and interactions. All individual predictors have a $df = 1$.

[a]Type III sum of squares (partials influence of all variables).

[b]Standard errors are approximations because the Proc GLM program does not correct by factors of $\sqrt{MS_e}$, a procedure suggested by Hedges and Olkin (1985) where MS_e is the error or residual mean square of regression.

*$p < .05$; **$p < .01$; ***$p < .001$.

TABLE 12. Follow-Up to Instruction × Domain Interactions for Group Design Studies

Reading instruction[a] Read × combined instruction	Sample size	*k*	Mean	*SD*	Weighted mean	Number of independent samples	Scheffe
I. Reading domain							
1. NonDI + NonSI[b]	1,615	51	.67	.49	.67	92	
2. DI + SI	1,344	34	.84	.67	.98	78	
3. DI Alone or SI Alone	2,116	71	.74	.50	.59	164	
II. Nonreading domain							
4. NonDI + NonSI	2,368	76	.60	.61	.58	122	
5. Combined (DI + SI)	1,235	62	.74	.56	.65	148	
6. SI Alone or DI Alone	2,004	83	.76	.54	.63	204	(2 > 3 = 5 = 6)

Word × general interaction[c]	Sample size	*k*	Mean	*SD*	Weighted mean	Number of independent samples	Scheffe
I. Word recognition							
1. General (combinations of SI or DI in isolation or combined)	1,280	50	.71	.59	.58	108	
2. NonDI + NonSI	862	28	.57	.48	.63	48	
II. Nonreading (coded as 0)							
3. General	3,530	149	.76	.52	.63	354	
4. NonDI + NonSI	2,378	77	.64	.61	.60	120	
III. Reading comprehension							
5. General	1,889	51	.82	.60	.82	130	
6. NonDI + NonSI	737	22	.68	.54	.66	44	(5 > 6 = 1 = 2)

(continued)

TABLE 12. *(continued)*

Word × general interaction[d]	Sample size	*k*	Mean	*SD*	Weighted mean	Number of independent samples	Scheffe
I. Word recognition							
1. DI Alone	589	27	.76	.52	.67	50	
2. Combined + other approaches	127	41	.58	.55	.62	82	
3. SI Alone	426	10	.75	.67	.36	34	
II. Nonreading behavior (coded as 0)							
4. DI Alone	1,093	54	.80	.59	.65	104	
5. Combined + other approaches	3,606	39	.68	.56	.62	278	
6. SI Alone	1,209	33	.74	.44	.54	102	
III. Reading comprehension							
7. DI Alone	379	16	.64	.45	.56	28	
8. Combined + other approaches	1,824	43	.85	.67	.86	100	
9. SI Alone	423	14	.71	.43	.68	40	(8 > 1 = 2 = 7 = 9 > 3)

[a] Reading domain includes measures of word recognition, word skill, and reading comprehension. *Question:* Does it matter if combinations of both direct or strategy instructions are compared with each model in isolation? *Answer:* Yes, but only in the domain of reading.

[b]Variables coded as 0 are ignored in the regression analysis.

[c]*Question:* Does undifferentiated instruction (general combinations of the Direct and Strategy Models) produce larger ESs when compared to various combinations of competing models? *Answer:* No, but a positive treatment effect emerges for reading comprehension.

[d]*Question:* Does direct instruction in isolation yield higher ES estimates than strategy instruction in isolation? *Answer:* Yes, but only on word recognition measures. The reverse effect emerges for strategy instruction on reading comprehension measures.

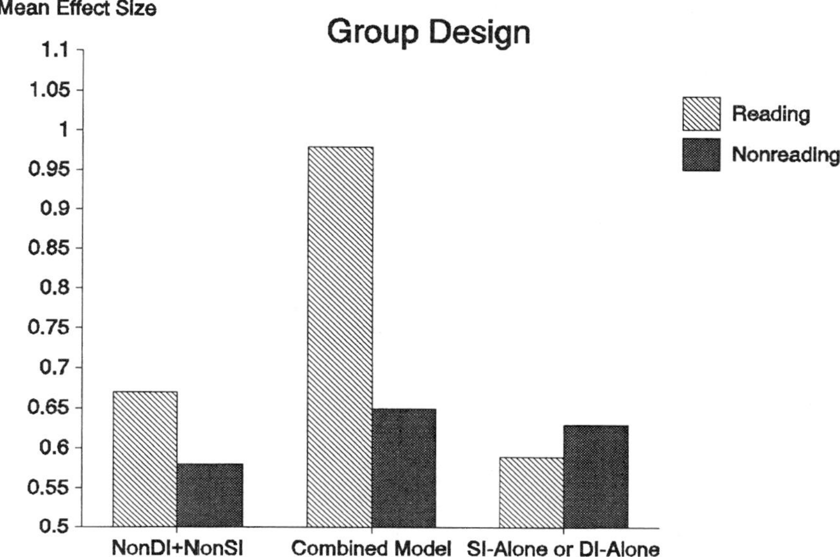

FIGURE 1. Effect size as a function of domain (reading vs. nonreading domains) and variations in treatment.

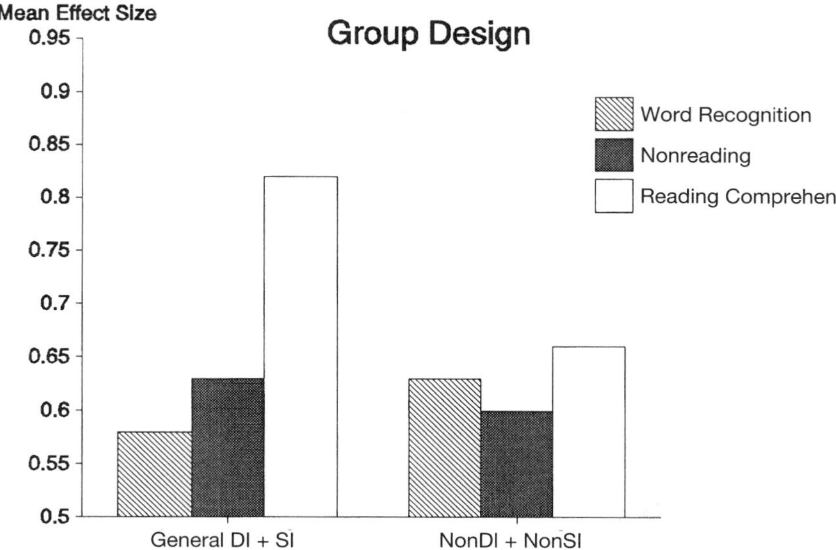

FIGURE 2. Effect size as a function of reading domain (word recognition vs. reading comprehension vs. other domains) and variations in treatment.

struction (NonDI + NonSI Model). As shown in Figure 2, high effect sizes emerged on reading comprehension measures for undifferentiated (general) models when compared to word recognition measures. No differences emerged between reading measures for the NonDI + NonSI Model. Figure 3 illustrates the reading skill × orientation (top-down vs. bottom-up; i.e., SI Alone vs. DI Alone) interaction. As shown, the results indicated that strategy instruction models yield higher effect sizes on reading comprehension measures than on word recognition measures (the nonreading measures were ignored in the analysis). In contrast, the DI Alone Model yields comparable effect sizes across reading measures. As shown, the DI Alone Model and the SI Alone Model produced comparable effects on reading comprehension measures. The DI Alone Model yields significantly higher effect sizes than on the SI Alone Model for the word recognition measures.

The results support the notion that treatment specificity emerges *between* reading and nonreading domains, as well as *within* the reading domain. The Combined Model has its most pronounced effect on measures of reading comprehension. The SI Alone Model yields substantially lower effect sizes on word recognition when compared to the comprehension measures. The comparisons of outcome measures show no significant difference in ES between treatments at a global level (high language vs. low language demand measures) or at a skill or process level (word skill vs. the cognitive process category).

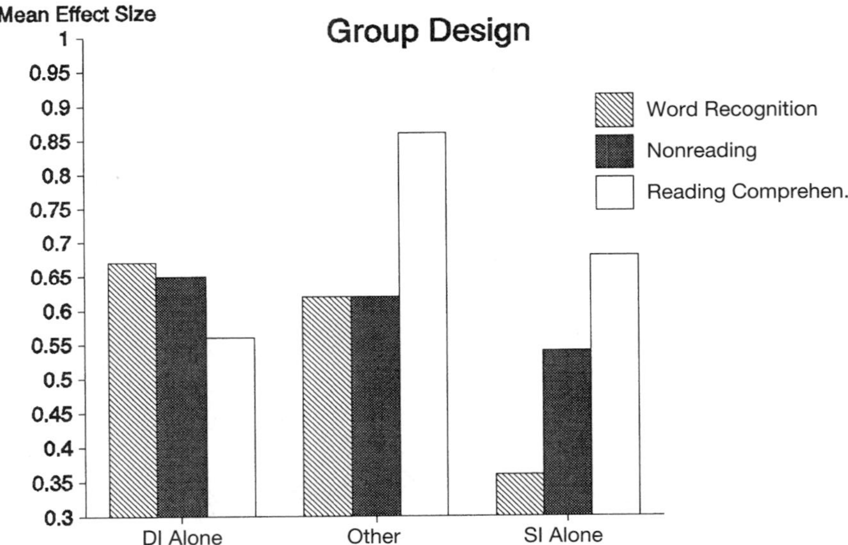

FIGURE 3. Effect size as a function of reading domain (word recognition vs. reading comprehension vs. other domains) and variations in treatment.

DOMAIN AND TREATMENT OUTCOMES AS A FUNCTION OF APTITUDE

As a preliminary analysis exploring the role of aptitude on effect sizes, we isolated two aptitude measures reflected across studies as a means of identifying the LD sample: standardized measures of intelligence (primarily a Full Scale IQ score on the Wechsler Intelligence Scale for Children) and reading (primarily word recognition on the Wide Range Achievement Test). Categories related to intelligence and reading were selected because they are the most commonly used operational criteria for classifying children as learning disabled (see Swanson, 1991, for a review). The independent results of the intelligence and reading severity variable on outcomes for the two primary interventions (direct instruction, strategy instruction) as a function of intelligence and reading deficiency were provided in Table 4. The present analysis focused on the interaction of the two aptitude variables on the magnitude of ES.

ES estimates, averaged within each of the 180 studies, were analyzed to determine whether combinations of intellectual and reading level influenced treatment outcomes. This analysis was done because standardized scores at or below the 25th percentile in reading recognition (see Siegel & Ryan, 1989; Stanovich & Siegel, 1994), along with standardized intelligence scores above 84, are considered reasonable cutoff scores toward operationalizing the term "learning disabilities" (See Morrison & Siegel, 1991, for a discussion of this issue). Four levels of reading severity (no information, <85, >84 but <91, >90) and three levels of intellectual performance (no information, low-average [<92], average [>91]) were analyzed, via a WLS analysis with the methodological composite score partialed from the analysis. Direct instruction and strategy instruction were analyzed separately because some cell sizes for intelligence and reading were too small (<5 studies) for the complete analysis. Studies that did not report mean ages of the sample ($N = 20$) were excluded from the analysis.

A 2 (direct vs. nondirect) × 3 (intelligence: high vs. low vs. no information) × 4 (reported reading severity: <85, >84 but <91, >90, and no information) WLS (analogue to an ANOVA and ANCOVA), which partials the influence of methodology and chronological age, was computed. The main effects of reading severity, $\chi^2(3, N = 160) = 9.78, p < .05$; intelligence, $\chi^2(2, N = 160) = 9.43, p < .05$; direct instruction, $\chi^2(1, N = 160) = 14.39, p < .001$; reading severity × intelligence, $\chi^2(6, N = 160) = 17.13, p < .05$, intelligence × direct instruction, $\chi^2(2, N = 160) = 9.08, p < .05$; and reading severity × direct instruction interaction, $\chi^2(3, N = 160) = 7.10, p < .10$, were significant. No other effects were significant. When methodology and age were partialed from the analysis, however, significant effects were isolated to the severity of reading × intelligence interaction, $\chi^2(6, N = 160) = 13.95, p < .05$, and the partialing influence of the methods composite score, $\chi^2(1, N = 160) = 14.12, p < .001$. The WLS means, when partialed for age and methodology for the intelligence categories of no formation, high scores, and low scores, were .89, .61, and .64 for studies that include no reading scores; .58, .72, and .74 for studies that report standardized reading scores below 85; .31, .55, and .90 for studies that report scores between 85 and 90; and .62, .68, and .18 for studies that report scores above 89, respectively. Thus, no aptitude × treatment interaction emerges when the results are partialed for the influence of methodology and age. An interaction emerges, however, related to intelligence and reading severity.

A 2 (strategy vs. nonstrategy) × 3 (intelligence: high vs. low vs. no information) × 4 (reported reading severity: <85, >84 and <91; >90, and no information) WLS (which partials the influence of methodology and chronological age) was again computed of ES estimates. The main effect of reading severity, $\chi^2(3, N = 160) = 9.78, p < .05$; intelligence, $\chi^2(2, N = 160) = 9.43, p < .05$, strategy instruction, $\chi^2(1, N = 160) = 16.29, p < .001$, and the reading severity × intelligence interaction, $\chi^2(6, N = 160) = 12.38, p < .05$, were significant. No other effects were significant. When methodology and age were partialed from the analysis, a significant effect occurs for severity of reading × intelligence, $\chi^2(6, N = 160) = 14.08, p < .05$, and the partialing influence of methods, $\chi^2(1, N = 160) = 14.72, p < .001$. Thus, the results are similar to those of direct instruction. Chronological age contributed no significant variance in ES estimates.

In sum, across direct instruction and strategy instruction studies, we found that the magnitude of effect sizes interacted with intelligence and reading severity level. Figure 4 shows the interaction related to intelligence and reading severity across the group design studies. Three findings emerged related to this

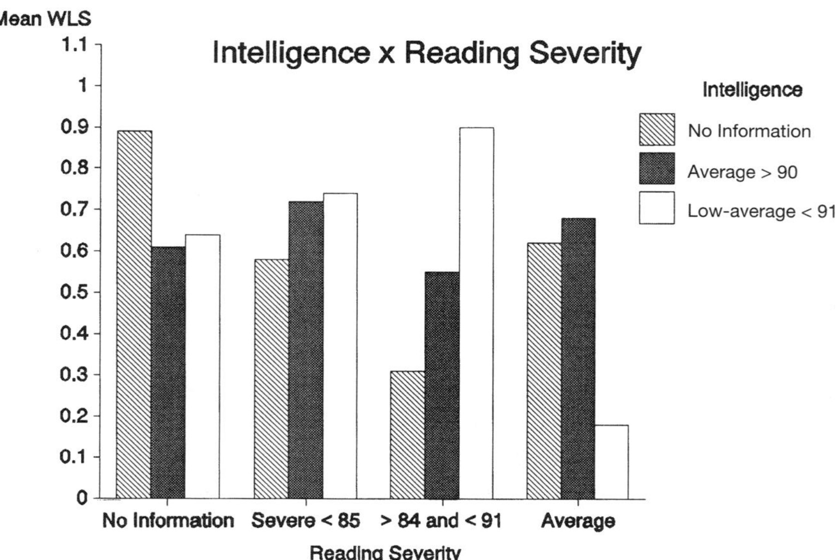

FIGURE 4. Effect size as a function of intelligence and reading.

interaction. First, studies that produced the highest effect sizes had (1) no psychometric information on intelligence or reading *or* (2) reported a minimal discrepancy between intelligence and reading (low-average intelligence scores [<92] and comparable reading scores [between >84 but <91]) when compared to other conditions. Second, studies that yield the lowest effect sizes reported (1) reading scores that were slightly higher than intelligence scores (i.e., reading scores above a standard score of 90 and intelligence scores in the standard score range of 84 to 90), or (2) reported reading scores between 84 and 90 with no information on intelligence. Finally, the results suggest a pattern related to reading for studies that report intelligence scores below 90. Effect sizes were significantly higher when reading scores were in the 84 to 90 range when compared to the severe (<85) and average range (>90). Thus, when intelligence scores approximate reading scores (i.e., both intelligence and reading scores are comparable and are in the 84 to 90 range), effect sizes are higher when compared to other conditions.

INFLUENCE OF OPERATIONAL DEFINITIONS ON DOMAIN AND TREATMENT OUTCOMES

There are two problems with the previous analyses on the influence of intelligence and reading severity. First, we did not take into consideration the issue of domain generality and domain specificity. As shown in our previous analysis, some combinations of treatment (Combined Model) interact with treatment domain (reading vs. nonreading domains), and thus aptitude × treatment interactions emerge when domain is taken into consideration. Second, the combinations of intelligence and reading scores are not placed within a context of operational definitions of learning disabilities. For example, there has been debate on whether intelligence has any influence on outcome measures when groups are primarily deficient in reading (see Stanovich & Siegel, 1994, for discussion of this issue). Thus, in the next analysis we compared various configurations of IQ and reading scores that have application to the definitional issues of learning disabilities. We assumed that the face validity of a definition is enhanced if one can show that such a definition is significantly related to treatment outcomes. To this end, we created three contrast variables related to the definition of learning disabilities.

The first contrast variable compares studies that report psychometric information (report reading and/or intelligence scores) with those studies that fail to report psychometric information. This contrast variable was defined as those studies that reported psychometric *criteria* versus those studies that reported no psychometric information (i.e., no reported psychometric criteria); these studies were coded as 1 and –1, respectively. Thus, this first contrast compares those studies that report psychometric information (reading and/or intelligence scores; 57% of the studies) to those that fail to report any psychometric information (43%).

A second contrast variable was defined as "meets *cutoff* criteria vs. does not meet cutoff criteria." A cutoff score in reading at or below the 25th percentile (i.e., the 25th percentile is a standard score of 90) and intelligence scores at or above 85 is considered one possible operational definition of learning disabilities (see Morrison & Siegel, 1991; Stanovich & Siegel, 1994). For the second contrast variable, studies were coded as meeting cutoff criteria (20% of the studies) and those that met other criteria (coded as +1 and –1, respectively).

A final contrast variable compares discrepancy-defined samples in which IQ is above 90 (IQ scores >90 and reading scores <91; 13.5% of the studies) and discrepancy-defined samples in which intelligence is below 90 (intelligence and reading <91; 17 % of the studies). We were unable to make comparisons between nondiscrepancy-defined groups because many of these children were excluded from the synthesis (i.e., the majority of studies include school-identified LD samples, and thus most of the studies include samples placed in special education related to some form of discrepancy criteria). Coding of the studies was +1 for discrepancy-defined samples with high IQ mean scores, –1 for low IQ discrepancy-defined samples, and 0 for the remaining samples.

To test the robustness of potential interactions related to the sample definition, two units of analysis were used in WLS analysis. One unit considers every ES in a study as independent and the other averages effect sizes within the 17 domains (see Table 3) for each study. The results of this analysis are presented in Table 13. Because setting and gender were not significant predictors in the previous analysis, they were removed from the analysis so that they would not take variance from the primary variables of interest.

As Table 13 indicates, several significant interactions emerged. However, when effect sizes were based on averages within studies for each domain, only the language × reported criteria, orientation of instruction × reported criteria, combined instruction × reported criteria, and combined instruction × cutoff score interactions remained significant. Table 14 provides the least square means for the various interactions when the unit of analysis is averaged within domain and within study, as well as the mean IQ and reading scores across studies. To facilitate reader interpretation, we have underlined the high and low score of the weight least square mean. Figures 5 through 11 illustrate the interactions.

The interactions reveal a general pattern: high effect sizes emerge in the areas of language and reading when compared to other domains when studies fail to report psychometric information on the sample. As shown in Figure 5, the important finding was that no significant differences in ES emerged between language and low language academic domains for studies that reported psychometric information. No differences in ES emerge between criteria and noncriteria definitions for nonreading tasks (see Figure 6). However, no criteria studies (those that fail to report psychometric information) inflate ES on reading tasks (see Figure 6), especially measures of reading comprehension (see Figure 7). As Figure 7 illustrates, no differences in ES emerge on reading comprehension and reading recognition for studies that report psychometric criteria.

TABLE 13. WLS Regression Analysis of Aptitude Interactions Related to Domain and Instruction for Group Design Studies

Predictors	χ^{2a}	β	χ^{2b}	β
1. Method composite	26.71***	–.02	14.77***	–.02
Main effects				
Instructional domain				
2. *Language* vs. nonlanguage	9.58***	.06	2.83	.06
3. *Reading* vs. nonreading	1.98	.02	.60	–.02
4. Comprehension vs. *word* recognition	2.69	.03	5.16**	–.08
5. *Skill* vs. process	10.67***	–.11	.94	–.06
Type of instruction				
6. *General* (undifferentiated) vs. other	27.74***	.07	8.40***	.068
7. Bottom-up (DI) vs. top-down (SI) *orientation*	1.92	.03	5.74**	.08
8. SI plus DI (*Combined*) vs. SI or DI in isolation	15.68***	.05	9.61***	.07
Sample				
9. Age	.70	–.004	2.29	–.013
10. Report psychometric *criteria* vs. no criteria	.96	–.01	1.68	.03
11. Report *cutoff* scores vs. no information	1.13	–.02	.90	–.04
12. *Disc*repancy-high IQ vs. discrepancy-low IQ	.01	.0001	.00	.005
Interactions by domain				
13. Lang * criteria	12.63***	–.04	7.83***	–.05
14. Read * criteria	.58	.01	5.97**	.05
15. Word * criteria	.82	–.01	9.19***	–.09
16. Skill * criteria	25.25***	.14	2.17	.07
17. Lang * cutoff	2.04	.02	.13	.01
18. Read * cutoff	4.96*	–.03	.19	–.01
19. Word * cutoff	.76	.02	.13	.01
20. Skill * cutoff	6.73**	–.09	1.98	–.09
21. Lang * disc	.06	.009	.38	.04
22. Read * disc	.002	.001	.007	–.004
23. Word * disc	5.29**	–.081	.75	–.05
24. Skill * disc	4.91*	.12	1.06	.10
Interactions by instruction				
25. General * criteria	1.29	–.007	.14	–.004
26. Orient * criteria	26.02***	–.13	12.06***	–.16
27. Combined * criteria	9.77**	–.04	10.10***	–.68
28. General * cutoff	7.56**	.04	2.93	.04
29. Orient * cutoff	11.49***	.10	6.83**	.13
30. Combined * cutoff	2.08	.02	4.29*	.05
31. General * disc	10.69***	–.08	3.33	–.08
32. Orient * disc	1.16	.04	.36	.03
33. Combined * disc	1.53	–.02	.05	–.009
df	1140		310	
N	1173		343	
χ^2	2510.63*		709.81*	
R^2	.17		.16	
Mean ES	.54		.61	

Note. Underlining indicates significant results for both units of analysis.

[a]Unit of analysis considers all dependent measures as independent.

[b]Unit of analysis aggregated across study and category.

$*p < .05$; $**p < .01$; $***p < .001$.

TABLE 14. Interactions Related to Domain and Instruction as a Function of LD Definition: Group Design

						Intelligence			Reading		
	Sample size	*k*	Mean	*SD*	Weighted mean	*M*	*SD*	*k*	*M*	*SD*	*k*
	Domain as a function of reported and nonreported psychometric information										
I. Language × criteria											
High language demands											
1. Criteria	4,112	162	.69	.51	.61[a]	97.53	6.67	145	82.83	10.81	90
2. No criteria	3,899	110	.83	.61	.57	—	—	—	—	—	—
Low language demands											
3. Criteria	1,305	52	.62	.56	.71	97.01	8.20	45	84.16	11.63	21
4. No criteria	1,249	52	.65	.57	.50	—	—	—	—	—	—
II. Reading × criteria											
Reading											
1. Criteria	2,427	97	.74	.55	.65[b]	97.00	6.67	87	83.57	10.64	55
2. No criteria	2,643	59	.94	.70	.56	—	—	—	—	—	—
Nonreading											
3. Criteria	3,102	118	.62	.48	.70	97.74	1.04	104	82.57	11.29	55
4. No criteria	2,505	103	.79	.62	.61	—	—	—	—	—	—
III. Word × criteria											
Reading comprehension											
1. Criteria	1,044	46	.74	.61	.64[c]	96.26	6.83	39	86.29	10.28	27
2. No criteria	1,582	27	.82	.55	.90	—	—	—	—	—	—

Other (score as 0)											
3. Criteria	3,122	117	.65	.49	.59	97.55	7.05	104	82.30	9.80	52
4. No criteria	2,786	109	.79	.60	.60	—	—	—	—	—	—
Word recognition											
5. Criteria	1,363	52	.67	.52	.62	98.00	7.16	48	81.33	12.83	32
6. No criteria	780	26	.64	.66	.46	—	—	—	—	—	—
				Instruction interactions with definitions							
I. Orientation × criteria											
SI Alone											
1. Criteria	672	22	.80	.47	.73[d]	95.57	5.43	22	75.04	10.11	16
2. No criteria	1,385	35	.69	.49	.48	—	—	—	—	—	—
Other (coded as 0)											
3. Criteria	3,296	127	.65	.55	.59	98.32	6.00	111	84.37	8.36	62
4. No criteria	3,261	96	.75	.62	.68	—	—	—	—	—	—
DI Alone											
5. Criteria	1,560	66	.67	.47	.60	96.35	8.95	58	84.53	13.86	33
6. No criteria	501	31	.93	.65	.73	—	—	—	—	—	—
II. Combination × criteria											
Combined SI + DI											
1. Criteria	1,221	61	.73	.55	.62[e]	97.27	6.25	56	84.89	8.47	20
2. No criteria	1,358	35	.86	.67	.95	—	—	—	—	—	—
Other (coded as 0)											
3. Criteria	2,075	66	.58	.54	.56	99.38	5.59	55	84.13	8.40	42
4. No criteria	1,903	61	.68	.61	.57	—	—	—	—	—	—

(continued)

TABLE 14. (*continued*)

						Intelligence			Reading		
	Sample size	*k*	Mean	*SD*	Weighted mean	*M*	*SD*	*k*	*M*	*SD*	*k*
DI Alone or SI Alone											
5. Criteria	2,233	88	.70	.47	.62	96.13	8.11	80	81.44	13.42	49
6. No criteria	1,887	66	.81	.58	.58	—	—	—	—	—	—
III. <u>Orientation × cutoff scores</u>											
SI Alone											
1. Cutoff score	544	15	.61	.31	<u>.67</u>[f]	93.50	3.11	15	73.94	9.36	15
2. No cutoff score	1,514	42	.78	.52	<u>.52</u>	100.00	6.88	7	92.00	—	1
Other (coded as 0)											
3. Cutoff score	1,073	37	<u>.67</u>	.50	.67	97.79	4.15	37	80.51	5.70	37
4. No cutoff score	5,484	186	.70	.60	.63	98.58	6.75	74	90.09	8.47	25
DI Alone											
5. Cutoff score	535	23	<u>.76</u>	.46	.77	92.42	4.99	23	77.85	8.18	23
6. No cutoff score	1,527	74	.75	.57	.59	98.93	10.60	35	99.88	11.96	10

IV. Combination × cutoff scores											
Combined DI + SI											
1. Cutoff	367	14	.90	.61	.81[g]	97.84	5.93	14	82.58	5.93	14
2. No cutoff	2,212	82	.75	.60	.72	97.08	6.41	42	90.28	11.47	6
NonDI + NonSI											
3. Cutoff	706	23	.52	.37	.58	97.75	2.71	23	79.25	5.30	23
4. No cutoff	3,271	104	.65	.60	.57	100.56	6.77	32	90.04	7.70	19
DI Alone or SI Alone											
5. Cutoff	1,079	38	.70	.41	.70	92.85	4.31	38	76.31	8.76	38
6. No cutoff	3,041	116	.76	.55	.59	99.11	9.54	42	99.17	11.60	11

Note. All weighted means are partialed by the methodological composite score and age. Total *k* possible for 17 domains averaged within studies is 376. Underlining indicates significant results for both units of analysis.

[a]Scheffe 3 > 2&4; 3 = 1; 3 > 4.

[b]Scheffe 1 > 2; 1 = 3&4; 2 = 4.

[c]Scheffe 2 > 1 = 5 = 6.

[d]Scheffe 1 = 6 > 5 > 2.

[e]Scheffe 2 > 1 = 5 = 6.

[f]Scheffe 5 > 2; 1 > 2, 3 = 4 = 5; 5 > 6.

[g]Scheffe 1 > 5 > 3; 2 > 4 = 6.

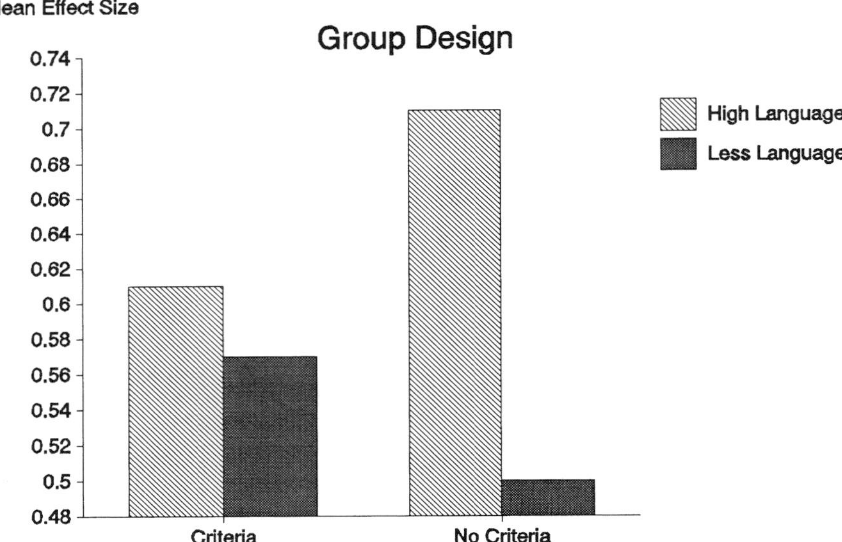

FIGURE 5. Effect size as a function of domain (high language vs. low language tasks) and variations in definition.

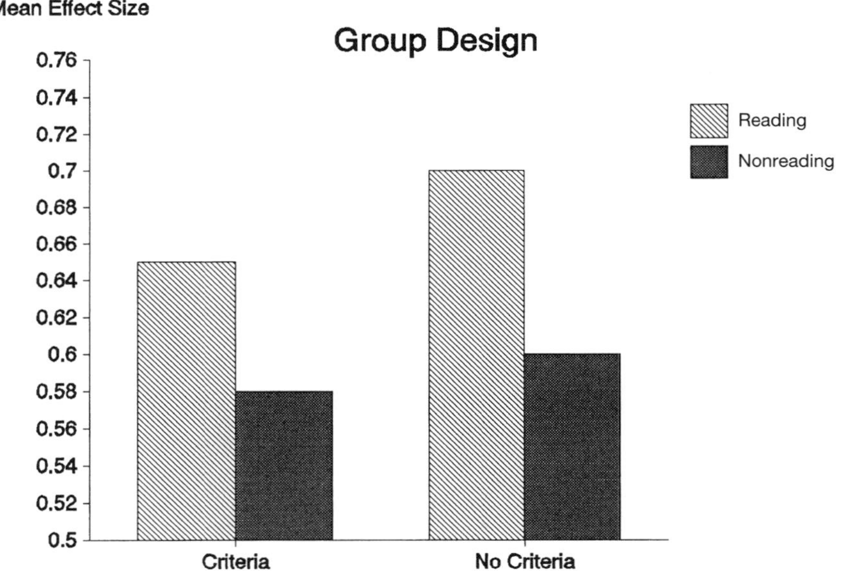

FIGURE 6. Effect size as a function of domain (reading vs. nonreading tasks) and variations in definition.

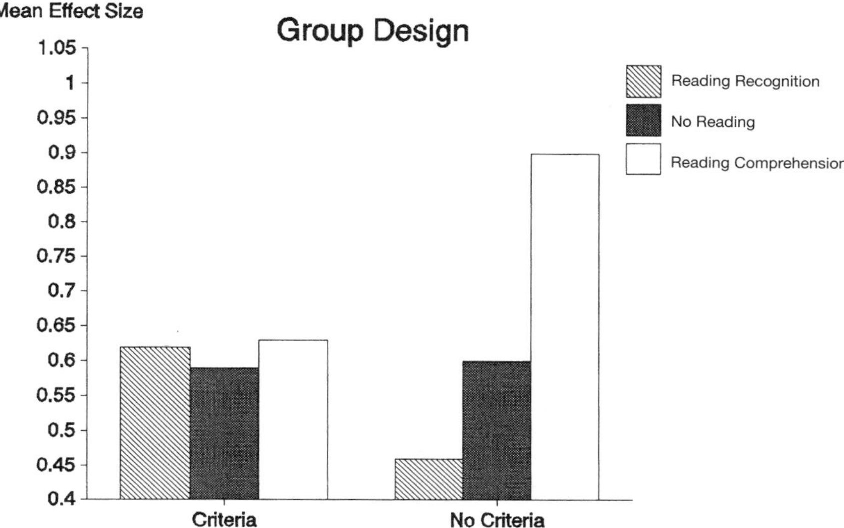

FIGURE 7. Effect size as a function of domain (reading recognition vs. reading comprehension vs. nonreading tasks) and variations in definition.

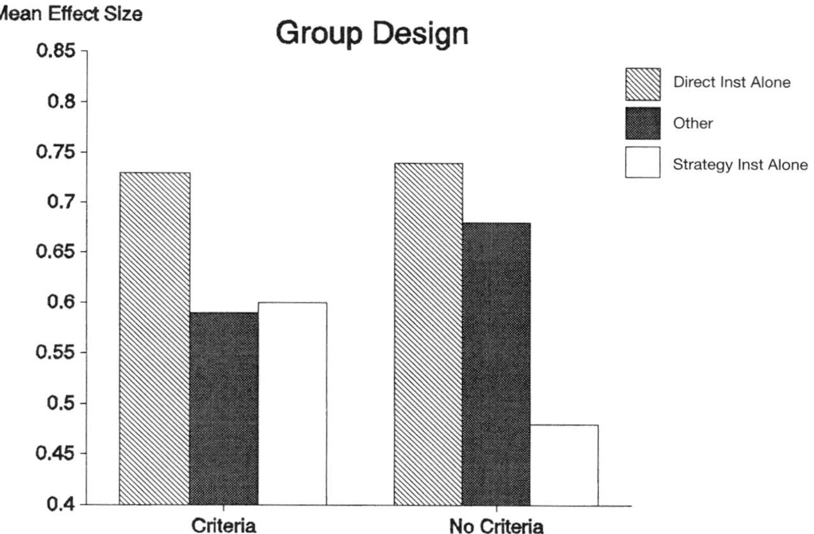

FIGURE 8. Effect size as a function of instruction (DI Alone vs. other vs. SI Alone) and variations in definition.

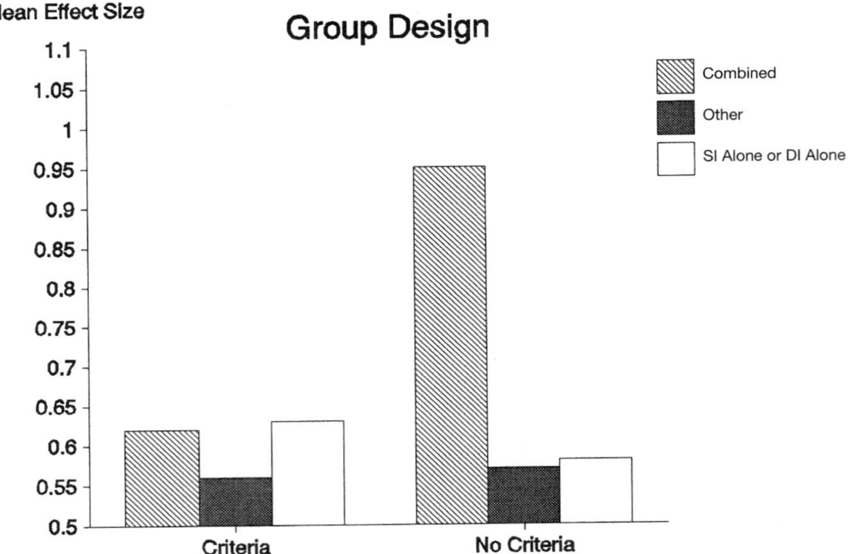

FIGURE 9. Effect size as a function of instruction (Combined Model vs. other vs. SI Alone or DI Alone) and definition.

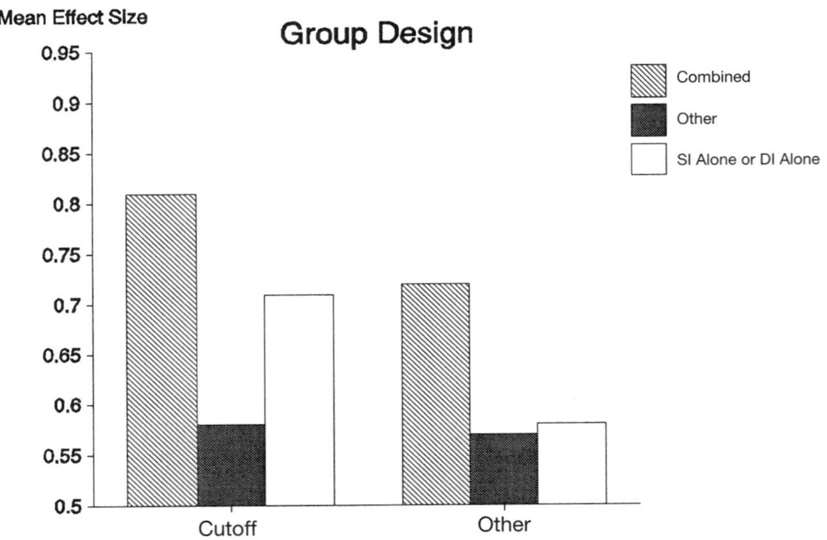

FIGURE 10. Effect size as a function of instruction (Combined Model vs. other vs. SI Alone or DI Alone) and definition.

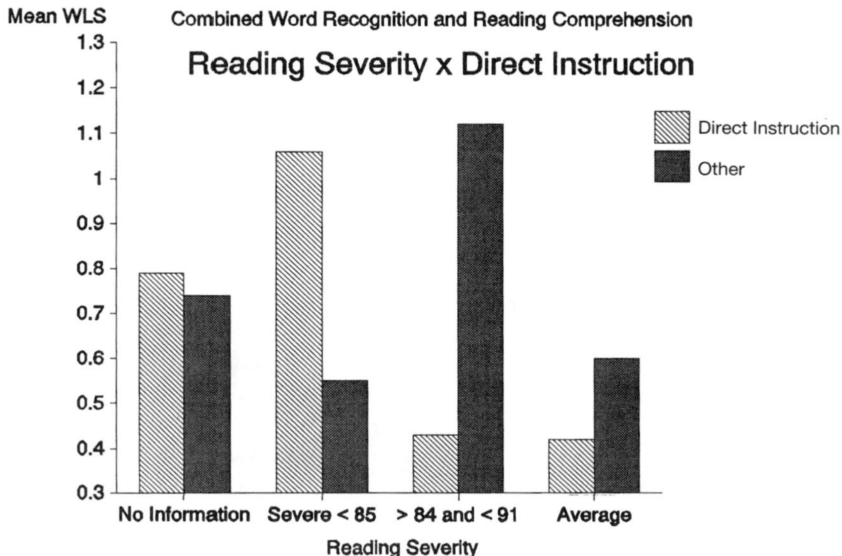

FIGURE 11. Effect size as a function of instruction (DI vs. other) and reading severity.

Figures 8 through 10 illustrate the interactions related to instruction. Our important findings illustrated across these figures follow:

1. As Figure 8 demonstrates, DI Alone yields higher effect sizes than SI Alone whether or not psychometric information is presented. SI Alone is significantly lower when no psychometric information is presented than when it is *not* reported, whereas DI Alone yields approximately the same magnitude in effect sizes as SI Alone under both reported and nonreported psychometric conditions. Figure 8 also shows that SI Alone is statistically comparable to DI Alone conditions when criteria are specified.

2. As Figure 9 illustrates, the Combined Model yields substantially higher effect sizes than competing models (SI Alone, DI Alone, NonDI + NonSI) when no psychometric information is reported. No significant differences emerged in effect size between instructional models for those studies that report some form of psychometric information.

3. As Figure 10 indicates, when cutoff scores (IQ >91 and reading <91) are computed, there are smaller differences between the Combined Model and SI Alone and DI Alone models when compared to studies where cutoff scores cannot be computed.

APTITUDE × TREATMENT ANALYSIS WITHIN GROUP DESIGN STUDIES

The LD literature reflects growing interest in subgrouping ability groups on isolated psychological parameters to (1) reduce the heterogeneity within samples and therefore better interpret ability group differences and (2) to match different subtypes to various instructional approaches (earlier diagnostic prescriptive models of LD research operated on these assumptions, e.g., instruction is one of matching visual learners to visual material, auditory learners to auditory presentations of material, etc.). Because results of research efforts in search of aptitude × treatment interactions (ATI) among children (either with or without disabilities) have been equivocal, and few studies have shown that children are differentially responsive to teaching methods (Brinker, 1990; Brophy, 1986; Cronbach & Snow, 1977; Tobias, 1981), we tried to determine whether the notion that individual differences within LD groups may be important sources of variation in response to treatment. Thus, within the data set, Maureen Hoskyn reviewed the LD intervention research that focused on the dimension of aptitude as so defined within the primary studies. Aptitude, in this analysis, was defined broadly, and included cognitive as well as noncognitive sources of variation among children. This approach is consistent with recent theories of aptitude, such as the ones described by Cronbach and Snow (1977) and Snow (1994). According to Snow and Swanson (1992), aptitude is defined as "a multivariate mixture, . . . a complex of person and treatment characteristics that promotes the person's benefit in a given situation. Different treatment situations will involve different mixtures. New aptitude constructs will thus need to be particularized to the local situations of interest" (p. 270). The focus of this analysis is to determine whether evidence is suggestive of ATI in LD intervention research. Articles in this review are a subset of the studies in this synthesis.

Within the criterion for article selection for the group design studies (N = 180), 19 studies were selected for further analysis based on meeting one of the following criteria: (1) study samples were divided into treatment *subgroups* on the basis of cognitive, affective, or conative attributes; or (2) study measures of aptitude (attributes) were analyzed as potential mediator variables in the analysis of treatment outcome (i.e., variables were either post hoc, a priori, or covariates in the analysis of posttest scores). Selection of articles as meeting one of the two criteria is analogous to analyzing aptitude as a categorical (i.e., subgroups) or continuous variable (aptitude is allowed to covary). For the first criterion, LD groups are assumed to be categorically distinct from one another; in the second case, individual variation among LD children is conceptualized along a continuum.

Tables 15, 16, 17, and 18 summarize the descriptive characteristics of the studies selected as meeting criteria 1 or 2, respectively. Overall, two studies were conducted in 1972 and the remaining studies were conducted during the period 1981–1996. Sample sizes ranged from 8 to 128 children. The average number of children in each treatment group was 8 (SD = 4.1). Two investigations included children in the primary grades (ages 7 years) in the study sample, nine studies in-

TABLE 15. Characteristics of Studies That Examined LD Subgroups

Author/year of study	Sample size	Average IQ	Range IQ	Average achievement	Range achievement	Gender	Age of children (yrs)	Grouping characteristic
Ayres, A. J. (1972)	128	Generalized dysfunction group = 94.6	Not reported	GE = 7.7	Not reported	Not reported	7.5–8.3	Generalized dysfunction vs. auditory language disorder
		Auditory language disorder = 92.5		GE = 4.5				
Fiedorowicz, C. (1986)	15	Oral reading group (O) = 93.0	85–104	Reading lag of 2.6 grades	Not reported	15 males	8.1–13.8	Oral reading deficit vs. intermodel–associative vs. sequential relations deficit
		Intermodel–associative group (A) = 96.8	86–107	2.5 grades				
		Sequential relations group (S) = 91.6	82–101	1.9 grades				
Lovett, M. W., Ransby, M. J., & Barron, R. W. (1988)	112	Accuracy-disabled group = 94.1	Not reported	Not reported	Not reported	2.3:1 and 3.4:1	8–13	Accuracy-disabled vs. rate-disabled
		Rate-disabled group = 98.5						
Prior, M., Frye, S., & Fletcher, C. (1987)	61	Not reported	Not reported	Dysphonetic group = 62.3	52.7–84.3	44 males, 17 females	Mean = 13.5	Dysphonetic vs. dyseidetic spellers
				Dysdeidic group = 70.2	49.3–86.0			
Smith, P. L., & Friend, M. (1986)	54	Not reported	Not reported	GE = 6.8 (total sample)	GE = 4.0–10.0	38 males, 16 females	14–18 years	Good vs. poor readers[a]
Sullivan, J. E. (1972)	82	107.3	Not reported	35th percentile	Not reported	Not reported	8.3–18.00	Binocular fusion difficulties vs. no visual difficulties
VanStrien, J. W., Stolk, B. D., & Zuikers, S. (1995)	40	P-dyslexic group[b] = 90.3	Not reported	Reading lag of 24.1 months	Not reported	24 males, 16 females	Mean = 8.0	P-dyslexic vs. L-dyslexic[b]
		L-dyslexic group = 92.7		25.5 months	Not reported			

[a]Students in the good reader group were children with disabilities who scored above the median in reading achievement; those in the poor reader group were children who scored below the median.
[b]Students in the P-dyslexic group were children who were *accurate but slow* readers; children in the L-dyslexic group were *slow but accurate* readers.

TABLE 16. Study Results

Author/ year of study	Grouping characteristic	Treatment	Dependent variables	Effect size[a]	Results/interpretation
Ayres, A. J. (1972)	Generalized dysfunction vs. auditory language disorder	Sensory integration therapy	Reading achievement Math achievement Perceptual motor skills	Unable to compute ES	The magnitude of treatment effects for children with auditory language disorders was similar to those for children with more generalized problems.
Fiedorowicz, C. (1986)	Oral reading deficit vs. intermodel–associative vs. sequential relations	Diagnostic prescriptive approach	Reading comprehension Word recognition Reading accuracy Reading rate	Unable to compute ES	Groups were differentiated by rate of response and by accuracy of response. Type S subjects were significantly faster ($p < .01$) than Type A and Type O subjects on responding to stimuli and training procedures. Type O and Type A subjects were more accurate in their responses than Type S subjects. No significant transfer effects across trained or untrained stimuli were specific to sub types.
Lovett, M. W., Ransby, M. J., & Barron, R. W. (1988)	Accuracy-disabled vs. rate-disabled	Decoding skills program (DSP) vs. Oral and Written Language Program (OWLS)	Spelling	Unable to compute ES	Treatment gains in spelling achievement were similar for both groups.
			Reading (exception word test)—DSP		The magnitude of DSP treatment effects on reading exception words was greater for the rate-disabled group than for the accuracy-disabled group.

			Reading (exception word test)—OWLS		Only the rate-disabled group benefited from an oral language program to improve exception word reading, suggesting that a threshold of language integrity may be a prerequisite for success in an oral language program.
			Reading (regular word test)—DSP		Only the accuracy-disabled group benefited from a DSP program to improve regular word reading.
			Reading (regular word test)—OWLS		Treatment gains in reading regular words were nonsignificant for both the accuracy- and rate-disabled groups.
Prior, M., Frye, S., & Fletcher, C. (1987)	Dysphonetic vs. dyseidetic spellers	Oral spelling procedure (SOS)	SOS-trained words correctly spelled	Unable to compute ES	Treatment effects on spelling achievement was the same for both groups (no significant differences found).
			Reading achievement (Schonnell)		Reading achievement gains were greater for the dyseidetic group than for the dysphonetic group.
			Regular word reading (Baron word list)		Regular word reading gains were greater for the dysphonetic than for the dysdeidic group.
					The authors explain differential improvement in group performance could be due to (1) lexical access of groups or (2) ceiling effects on the Baron word list for the dysdeidic group.

(continued)

TABLE 16. (*continued*)

Author/ year of study	Grouping characteristic	Treatment	Dependent variables	Effect size[a]	Results/interpretation
Smith, P. L., & Friend, M. (1986)	Good readers vs. poor readers[b]	Use of text structure to aid recall of instructional prose	Structure recognition Main idea units recalled	Unable to compute ES	The magnitude of treatment effect on structure recognition was similar for both groups of readers.
Sullivan, J. E. (1972)	Binocular fusion difficulties vs. no visual difficulties	Kephard Perceptual Motor Training	Reading comprehension	Unable to compute ES	Treatment gains were greater for the group with adequate vision compared to the group with binocular fusion difficulties.
VanStrien, J. W., Stolk, B. D., & Zuikers, S. (1995)	P-dyslexic vs. L-dyslexic	Hemispheric stimulation through use of anxiety-laden words in text	Substantive errors	L-dyslexic ES = .91 P-dyslexic ES = 1.96	The magnitude of positive change in the number of substantive errors was greater for the L-dyslexic than the for P-dyslexic group.
			Fragmentation	L-dyslexic ES = .71 P-dyslexic ES = 1.82	
			Reading time	L-dyslexic ES = 3.56 P-dyslexic ES = 2.85	The magnitude of change in the number of fragmentations was greater for the L-dyslexic than for the P-dyslexic group. Treatment effects on reading time were the same for both groups.

[a]ES was calculated between treatment subgroups.

[b]Students in the good reader group were children with disabilities who scored above the median in reading achievement; those in the poor reader group were children who scored below the median.

TABLE 17. Characteristics of Studies That Included Factors to Explain Treatment Effects

Author/year of study	Sample size	Average IQ	Range IQ	Average achievement	Range achievement	Gender	Age of children (yr)
Bos, C. S., & Anders, P. L. (1990)	61	91.97	Not reported	81.30	Not reported	41 males, 20 females	Mean = 13.8
Bos, C. S., Anders, P. L., Filip, D., & Jaffee, L. E. (1985)	50	Not reported	Not reported	Not reported	Not reported	Not reported	High school students
Brailsford, A., Snart, F., & Das, J. P. (1984)	24	>85	Not reported	<35 percentile	Not reported	19 males, 5 females	9–12
Cosden, M. A., & English, J. P. (1987)	28	88.6	Not reported	GE = 3.69	Not reported	23 males, 5 females	Mean = 9.9
Graham, S., & Harris, K. R. (1989)	22	95.0	85–113	>2 yr below grade level	Not reported	14 males, 8 females	10.2–13.7
Kerstholt, M. T., VanBon, W. H. J., & Schreuder, R. (1994)	50	Not reported	Not reported	Not reported	Not reported	35 males, 15 females	Not reported
MacArthur, C. A., Schwartz, S. S., & Graham, S. (1991)	29	95.4	Not reported	82.6	Not reported	25 males, 4 females	10.9–11.2
lor, J. G., & Pumfrey, P. D. (1983)	60	97.3	Not reported	Not reported	Not reported	Not reported	Not reported
ub, R. B., & Roberts, D. M. (1983)	33	Not reported	Not reported	Not reported	Not reported	26 males, 7 females	7–12
te, C. W., Pascarella, E. T., & um, S. W. (1981)	30	Anagram treatment = 88.6	Not reported	GE = 2.5 (reading comprehension)	Not reported	10 males, 5 females	Mean = 11.37
		Sentence study treatment = 91.87		GE = 2.6 (reading comprehension)		11 males, 4 females	Mean = 10.87

TABLE 18. Studies That Included Factors to Explain Treatment Effects

Author/ year of study	Factor that may explain treatment effects	Treatment	Dependent variables	Mean effect size for study	Analyses of treatment effects
Bos C. S., & Anders, P. L. (1990)	Prior knowledge of topic Prior interest in topic	Interactive vocabulary learning	Vocabulary use Reading comprehension Written recall	.76	No significant treatment effects on the acquisition of scriptal knowledge was reported immediately posttest. Followup analyses showed students in interactive vocabulary learning treatments generated a higher quality of scriptal knowledge than students in a definition instruction condition. No interaction between scriptal knowledge or prior interest in topic was reported.
Bos, C. S., Anders, P. L., Filip, D., & Jaffee, L. E. (1985)	Prior knowledge of content	Semantic feature analysis vs. looking up words in dictionary	Conceptual comprehension Vocabulary	1.15	Semantic feature analysis treatment was superior to looking up words in a dictionary on both measures of comprehension. Prior knowledge had a statistically significant effect on multivariate test of group differences, $F(2,46) = 5.92, p < .005$, but no interaction was reported.
Brailsford, A., Snart, F., & Das, J. P. (1984)	Planning, attention, successive, and simultaneous cognitive processing	Strategy use to aid in reading comprehension	Reading comprehension	.93	Main effects of treatment are discussed only. There was no attempt by authors to link treatment with aptitude variables associated with cognition and reading.

Cosden, M. A., & English, J. P. (1987)	Self-esteem Locus of control	Computer-assisted instruction	Productivity Help-seeking behavior Response accuracy	3.26	Individual skill levels had more impact on treatment outcomes than measured personality characteristics of self-esteem and locus of control. Scores on dependent measures did not vary as a function of self-esteem or locus of control.
Graham, S., & Harris, K. R. (1989)	Self-efficacy	Self-regulation strategies	Writing quality	.29	The main effects of strategy instruction and strategy instruction plus self-regulation on measures of self-efficacy were not significant. No treatment by aptitude interactions were reported.
Kerstholt, M. T., VanBon, W. H. J., & Schreduer, R. (1994)	Prior knowledge of grapheme–phoneme correspondences	Phoneme segmentation training with visual support	Word recognition	.35	Visual support in the form of alphabet letters or diagrams did not have supplementary value in remedial phonemic segmentation training. This finding contrasts with previous research that shows that children in the early stages of reading benefit from visual support. The authors explain this discrepancy in research findings in terms of individual differences (i.e., older children with learning disabilities vs. typical preschoolers).
MacArthur, C. A., Schwartz, S. S., & Graham, S. (1991)	Metacognitive awareness about knowledge structures	Reciprocal peer revision and strategy instruction	Writing quality	.74	Results of the study showed students learned to use strategies and used these strategies to help each other during the writing process. Relatively few comparisons between areas of metacognitive functioning and treatment condition were significant. Significant differences between treatment and control groups were found on social process ($p < .04$) in the category of substantive criteria).

(continued)

TABLE 18. (*continued*)

Author/ year of study	Factor that may explain treatment effects	Treatment	Dependent variables	Mean effect size for study	Analyses of treatment effects
Naylor, J. G., & Pumfrey, P. D. (1983)	Psycholinguistic abilities	Diagnostic prescriptive approach	Reading comprehension Language functioning	2.64	The Kirk Program and the Peabody Language Program were both effective in improving achievement scores of children with learning disabilities. The Kirk strategies, however, were not consistent with the theoretical model posed by the IPTA, and therefore interpretation of results is limited to discussion of main effects. No interaction between treatment and psycholinguistic ability profiles was reported.
Straub, R. B., & Roberts, D. M. (1983)	Nonverbal sensitivity	Social skills training in nonverbal awareness	Peer acceptance Social affect rating	.56	Results of regression analyses indicated nonverbal sensitivity did not have a differential effect on peer acceptance or social affect ratings. No aptitude–treatment interactions reported.
White, C. W., Pascarella, E. T., & Pflaum, S. W. (1981)	Age, gender, IQ, sentence comprehension	Sentence construction training	Sentence construction Reading cloze	.62	Anagram treatment was superior to sentence study in producing positive change in sentence construction and reading cloze. Results of multiple regression analyses (holding sex, IQ, age, pretreatment cloze, or sentence construction constant) suggest greatest treatment effects occurred among students with highest level of cloze achievement prior to intervention. No aptitude–treatment interactions reported.

vestigated treatment efficacy for children in the middle grades (age range: 8 to 13 years), and four studies used study samples from high school populations (ages: >13 years). The ratio of boys to girls was on average 6:4 among the studies that reported gender ratios.

Studies of Subgroups

As shown in Table 15, seven studies subgrouped children with learning disabilities. Treatments within the domain of reading were most frequently investigated (four studies). The remaining studies examined treatment effects on spelling performance, perceptual motor skills, and general achievement. As shown in Table 16, effect sizes related to each subgroup could only be calculated for one study. Computation required pretest means and standard deviations in the calculation, which eliminated all except the VanStrien, Stolk, and Zuiker (1995) study. As shown in Table 16, the criteria for subgrouping within the studies vary as a function of the learning model that directs the study, as a function of models that were in contention at the time of the study, and as a function of various methodological artifacts. For example, Sullivan (1972) investigated the influence of binocular fusion subgroups and found no differences related to perceptual motor treatment, thus calling into question the basis for perceptual–motor interventions that were popular at the time.

There is suggestive evidence that subgrouping children in terms of rate and accuracy in word recognition predicts treatment outcome. VanStrien, Stolk, and Zuiker (1995) subgrouped LD children according to dominance of hemispheric function under conditions of reading. Based on word accuracy and reading rate, children with P-type dyslexia were hypothesized to use a visual–perceptual reading strategy primarily involving the right hemisphere of the brain. Children with L-type dyslexia were thought to use a linguistic reading strategy that involves left-hemispheric stimulation. The authors suggested that stimulation of the right hemisphere through the use of text-based anxiety-laden words would result in treatment gains for the accuracy-disabled group because reading strategy use is altered. No improvement was expected for the rate-disabled group. Their results supported this position. Compared to an accuracy-disabled control group, the accuracy-disabled experimental group made fewer substantive errors and more repetitions and corrections after treatment. Furthermore, the investigators found the opposite effect for the rate-disabled group: performance on reading measures decreased after stimulation of the right hemisphere through the reading of anxiety-laden words.

Similar findings were described by Lovett, Ransby, and Barron (1988) in their study of reading interventions for LD groups. Accuracy-disabled readers responded positively to a decoding skills (i.e., visual-perceptual) intervention and made nonsignificant gains after receiving an oral and writing (i.e., linguistic) program. In contrast to the VanStrien et al. results, however, the performance of rate-disabled groups, on measures of reading increased with intervention from both a decoding skills and a language program. Lovett et al. interpreted these results as suggesting that children with severe language impairments (i.e., severe deficits in accuracy of phonological and orthographic processing) are less likely to benefit from a global language intervention when compared to children with intact linguistic abilities.

Prior, Frye, and Fletcher (1987) also subgrouped children according to word skill. Dysphonetic and dyseidetic (Boder, 1973) spellers were identified, based on the strategies (phonetic word analysis vs. memory for visual gestalts) used by the children to spell lists of phonetically regular and irregular words. No reliable differences were found between groups in response to intervention. A serious problem expressed by the authors was that the classification procedure was unreliable. Most academic tasks require proficiency in several cognitive skills: when given a problem-solving task, children will likely use a combination of skills to reach a solution. Fiedorowicz (1986) subgrouped children into oral reading (O), intermodel–associative (A), and sequential relations (S) deficits. As would be expected, the results showed that the A and O groups responded more positively than the S group to oral reading and auditory–visual match tasks designed to remediate these specific problems.

In summary, several flaws related to methodological differences among studies prevent a systematic analysis of ATIs within studies. Given these flaws, however, it is possible that defining aptitude in terms of word accuracy and rate fluency may play an important role in predicting treatment outcomes. That is, one implication of the Lovett et al. (1988) and the VanStrien et al. (1995) studies is that accuracy-disabled and rate-disabled groups are differentially responsive to treatment. This analysis is consistent with current information-processing models of reading in which phonological and orthographic processing are postulated as sources of individual variation in decoding skill and linguistic ability (see Share & Stanovich, 1995, for review).

Aptitude as a Continuum

Twelve studies in this review investigated the relation between posttest treatment performance and aptitude. Table 17 summarizes the information on the demographic and psychometric characteristics of the sample with learning disabilities. Table 18 summarizes the aptitude and treatment characteristics of the studies. As shown in Table 18, three studies examined the effects of cognitive process variables, four studies examined the effects of prior knowledge, and five studies examined the effects of affective variables on the magnitude of treatment outcome. In each case, pretest and posttest measures of the aptitude were administered and then statistical analyses were conducted to investigate interactions among variables. A synopsis of the results related to each of the aptitude categories follows:

1. *Cognitive processing.* Information-processing models of cognition guided three studies that investigated the role of cognitive processing variables on treat-

ment outcomes. Osgood's (1957) language-processing model was used by Naylor and Pumfrey (1983); the Information-Integration Model (Das, Kirby, & Jarman, 1979) was used by Brailsford, Snart, and Das (1984). Naylor and Pumfrey (1983) relied on the Illinois Test of Psycholinguistic Abilities (ITPA) to operationalize the linguistic processing components of Osgood's (1957) theory. Despite the theoretical appeal of the ITPA, it received much criticism in the early 1970s for both its statistical properties and its educational validity as a diagnostic-prescriptive tool (Cohen, 1970). Results of Naylor and Pumfrey's (1983) study corroborated these concerns. Although the Kirk program was superior to a global-based language program (Peabody) in improving reading performance, these results were tempered when the treatment included multiple component, and the components in some cases did not match the theoretical underpinnings of the ITPA.

2. *Prior knowledge.* The degree or the conditions under which prior knowledge is activated plays a role in treatment outcomes. For example, MacArthur, Schwartz, and Graham (1991) showed that children with learning disabilities who participated in a reciprocal peer revision strategy group produced written expression of higher quality and demonstrated a greater awareness of criteria to evaluate writing than alternative treatment controls. In another study, Kerstholt, Van Bon, and Schreuder (1994) suggested that older children with learning disabilities did not benefit from visual support on a phoneme segmentation intervention in the same way as younger children (from previous analyses) because the older children may have had difficulties that are different from normal reading development exhibited by preschoolers. Bos, Anders, Filip, and Jaffe (1985) proposed the "aptitude" hypothesis, which postulates that the relation between vocabulary and reading comprehension is based on a reader's underlying verbal ability. Unfortunately, no interaction was reported between prior knowledge and treatment of content.

3. *Affect.* Self-efficacy, self-esteem, and locus of control are variables that have potential to moderate treatment results (Bandura, 1989; Schunk, 1985). Graham and Harris (1992) found that a self-regulation strategy improved children's feelings of self-efficacy while performing on a composition task, which in turn impacted positively on evaluation of written expression. Cosden and English (1987), however, found prior competence (i.e., knowledge) in math proved to be a more reliable predictor of accuracy than the affective variables.

In summary, the findings related to potential aptitude predictors (or qualifiers) of treatment outcomes are inconclusive. Studies that determine the role and conditions for accessing prior knowledge appear promising, but cannot be assessed adequately because the aptitude variable was not partialed from posttest scores and/or aptitude × treatment interactions were not reported. Not enough studies have investigated the role of cognitive processing and attributions on treatment outcomes in LD samples to draw substantive conclusions. Thus, research on the relationship between typology (subgroup) and treatment outcomes is at best inconclusive and at worst suffers from a weak database.

READING INTERVENTION STUDIES

It is clear from our analysis of domains of study (see Table 3) that the domain of reading is the most frequent intervention focus for samples of children with learning disabilities. This makes sense because reading problems are the most frequent basis for referring children suspected of a learning disability (Moats & Lyon, 1993). Because a number of policy and instructional issues emerge related to reading and learning disabilities, we isolated for analysis all intervention studies that included measures of word recognition and reading comprehension.

Prototypical Studies

As shown in Table 19, 55 studies included measures of word recognition and 57 studies included measures of reading comprehension. Seventeen studies included both word recognition and reading comprehension measures. Articles were comparable in terms of the year of publication, number of authors, and number of citations. Some variations emerged in the sources of funding. Of those studies that were funded, approximately 44% of the reading comprehension studies were funded by the U.S. Department of Education. As shown in Table 19, approximately 15% of the word recognition studies and 11% of the reading comprehension studies were published in dissertations. Approximately 18% of the word recognition studies used as their primary outlet the *Journal of Learning Disabilities*. The primary outlet for reading comprehension studies was the *Learning Disability Quarterly*.

In terms of instructional parameters, word recognition studies are more likely to have a larger number of instructional sessions (M = 38 vs. M = 22). Sample sizes tended to be larger in reading comprehension studies than in word recognition studies, but there was a comparable distribution in the number of males and females across the two types of studies. Children tended to be slightly older (M = 11.62) in reading comprehension studies than in word recognition studies (M = 10.03). There was a trend, although not significant, in which word recognition studies have slightly higher intelligence scores, and slightly lower reading and math scores, when compared to reading comprehension studies. When comparing the control condition to the treatment condition, reading comprehension studies are more frequent in their use of the same teacher, materials, and setting when compared to word recognition studies.

Main Effects

Table 20 shows the weighted means for comparisons on methodology, article characteristics, sampling characteristics, and the independent variables for studies that include reading measures. The unit of analysis is the average ES for word recognition and comprehension within each study. When the studies are compared, we find a number of methodological, setting, sampling, and instructional variations that influence effect sizes. Because the pattern of results is comparable when the 17 overlapping studies (studies including both word recognition and

TABLE 19. Group Design Studies for Studies That Include Reading Recognition and Reading Comprehension Measures ($N = 112$)

	Word recognition			Reading comprehension		
		M	*SD*		*M*	*SD*
Absolute effect size (*N* = 112); overlap (*N* = 17)[a]	(*N* = 55)	.71	.56	(*N* = 57)	.82	.60
Article characteristics						
Year of publication		1987	6.82		1987	5.32
Number of authors		1.33	1.25		1.31	1.21
Number of citations		1.97	3.89		1.60	2.42
Author gender (%)		56%			62%	
Funding sources (%)						
No funding cited		52% (*N* = 29)			68% (*N* = 18)	
U.S. Department of Education[a]		15.3%			44.2%	
NICHD		15.3%			5.6%	
State/province		23%			11.2%	
Other		46.4%			39%	
Publication outlets						
Dissertation		14.5%			10.7%	
Journal of Learning Disabilities		18.2%			10.7%	
Reading and Writing		5.5%			1.8%	
Brain and Language		3.6%			1.8%	
Learning Disabilities Research and Practice		5.5%			10.7%	
Journal of Child Psychology and Psychiatry		1.8%			1.8%	
Learning Disability Quarterly		9.1%			17.9%	
Journal of Educational Psychology		1.8%			1.8%	
Developmental Psychology		1.8%			1.8%	
Exceptional Children		1.8%			7.1%	

	Word recognition			Reading comprehension		
	k[b]	*M*	*SD*	*k*	*M*	*SD*
Instructional parameters						
Time of instruction						
Number of instruction sessions		38.60	42.12		22.78	23.30
Length of session (minutes)		38.94	29.20		43.14	26.45
Number of sessions per week		3.50	1.27		3.84	1.20

(continued)

TABLE 19. (*continued*)

	Word recognition			Reading comprehension		
	k^b	*M*	*SD*	*k*	*M*	*SD*
Sample parameters						
Sample size		28.23	16.23		46.90	65.81
Number of males	44	16.71	9.24	24	19.17	14.04
Number of females	46	8.62	13.96	25	8.12	7.30
Ethnicity reported						
Asian American	1	—	—	3	3	—
African American	11	4.75	2.48	7	7.71	10.60
Anglo American	18	16.22	9.16	9	18.11	10.49
Hispanic American	8	19.00	24.00	2	1.00	—
Native American	2	—	—	2	—	—
Other	2	4.0	—	1	1	—
Chronological age		10.03	1.62		11.62	3.11
Psychometric standardized						
Intelligence	62	97.33	7.14	30	95.74	6.55
Reading	44	79.97	11.78	24	85.92	10.78
Math	12	88.31	11.46	5	91.58	12.80
Methodology parameters						
Internal validity						
Rating scale (Abbr.) (4–12 high to low internal validity)		7.63	1.79		7.14	1.76
Variation of CTRL from treatment						
% Similarity of overlap						
Same teacher		21.8%			37%	
Same materials		19.1%			21.2%	
Same setting (e.g., classroom)		29.1%			31%	
Same instructional focus		57.4%			66.7%	
Group design						
% Studies pre–post control group design		85%			79%	
Measure of TRT integrity		23%			21.5%	
Dependent measures for treatment effects						
		M	*SD*		*M*	*SD*
Mean number experimental measures		3.68	4.62		4.05	4.82
Mean number reliability information		1.05	2.67		1.52	2.64
Number standardized measures		5.42	9.49		4.19	9.22

Note. TRT, Treatment; CTRL, control group; %, read as percent of studies reporting information.
[a] Overlap of word recognition and comprehension studies.
[b] When *k* is blank all studies reported information.

reading comprehension measures) are removed from the analysis, all studies are included in the subsequent analysis. As Table 20 indicates, shorter instructional sessions are more likely to yield higher effect sizes than longer instructional sessions. Those studies that use a random assignment of treatment, as well as those studies that include some variation of random assignment, are more likely to have higher effect sizes than those studies that do not use random assignment. No differences were found in ES estimates between studies classified as reflecting (1) high and low internal validity, or between studies that (2) reported or did not report measures of treatment integrity (procedural validity).

As expected, those studies that included experimental conditions that report different teachers, different materials, or different settings; provide no information on the setting in which intervention occurred; and have the same instructional focus as the control group produce large effect sizes when compared to the contrasting conditions. Those studies that have a high overlap in the number of instructional components between the control and treatment condition yield significantly lower effect sizes than those studies that report low overlap. Those studies that have small sample sizes (<25) or sample sizes greater than 100 subjects yield larger effect sizes than those studies that have sample sizes between 25 and 100. Those studies that primarily include experimental measures to assess outcomes have larger effect sizes than those studies that primarily rely on standardized tests. One important finding is that the methodological composite score (i.e., each study was weighted by treatment integrity, internal validity, use of standardized tests, amount of psychometric information, number of treatment sessions, overlap of instructional steps) indicated that studies that receive a low methodological weighting yield larger effect sizes than those studies that receive a high methodological composite score.

In terms of article characteristics, those studies that report a funding source yield lower effect sizes than those studies that do not report a funding source. Those studies that are published in dissertations or technical reports yield significantly smaller effect sizes than those studies that are published in journals. In terms of setting, studies that report the setting in which the treatment occurs have higher effect sizes than those that do not report the setting. As a follow-up to this analysis, those studies that report implementing treatment in the regular classroom have higher effect sizes than those studies reporting treatment that occurred in the resource room. This finding should be interpreted cautiously because only two studies reported implementation of experimental procedures (training) in the regular classroom. Those studies that report the lowest effect sizes took place in self-contained or clinical settings or report no setting information. Another setting variable coded was whether treatment occurred in multiple instructional units. Those studies that occurred in multiple instructional units (i.e., one-to-one settings, small group settings, and large group settings) yield significantly higher effect sizes than those studies that occurred in only a single unit (i.e., one-to-one instruction).

In terms of sample characteristics, those studies that report subjects were at least 1 year behind their peers yield lower effect sizes than those studies that report

TABLE 20. Word Recognition and Reading Comprehension on Effect Size Estimates Averaged within Studies (N = 112; Outliers Removed)

	Sample size	k^a	M	SD	Weighted mean	Independent samples	χ^2
All studies	3,895	112	.77	.58	—	—	
I. Methodology							
Number of sessions							
1. 3 to 10	1,115	34	.85	.62	.85	66	
2. 11 to 30	745	33	.81	.68	.74	74	
3. >31	1,820	43[a]	.67	.48	.60	98	18.49** (3 < 1 = 2)
Type of treatment assignment							
1. No random assignment	943	38	.73	.61	.55	77	
2. Random assignment	1,873	45	.68	.42	.75	102	
3. Other (no information)	1,078	29	.95	.72	.79	70	9.98* (3 = 2 > 1)
Internal validity (based on rating scale)							
Low	2,905	85	.80	.60	.75	142	
High	665	17[a]	.87	.52	.67	80	2.49[a]
Treatment integrity							
Reported	1,630	30	.53	.37	.73	44	
Not reported	2,265	82	.85	.62	.70	176	.17
Variation of control from treatment							
High overlap	1,386	41	.69	.61	.61	92	
Low overlap	2,508	71	.81	.57	.76	132	5.63*

Sample size (total)							
1. <25	848	59	.92	.66	.78	142	
2. >24 but <50	1,061	32	.56	.47	.52	60	
3. >49 but <100	494	8	.52	.14	.51	14	
4. >99	1,331	7[a]	.83	.48	1.09	20	49.90*** (4 > 1 > 2 = 3)
Standardized posttest measures							
No	1,514	43	.98	.61	.96	90	
Yes	1,624	55[a]	.69	.56	.59	122	33.56***
Variation in administration between treatment and control							
1. Different teacher or researcher	1,112	26	.63	.36	.83	52	
2. Same teacher or researcher	1,207	43	.70	.52	.56	90	
3. No information	1,575	43	.91	.71	.75	92	13.72*** (1 = 3 > 2)
Variation in materials between treatment and control							
1. Same materials (focus on methods)	510	20	.91	.65	.71	42	
2. Different materials	2,788	75	.82	.59	.76	168	
3. No information	597	17	.38	.27	.39	32	15.00*** (1 = 2 > 3)
Variation in setting between treatment and control							
1. Different setting	1,285	38	.76	.55	.65	80	
2. Same setting	567	24	.58	.41	.50	42	
3. No information	2,091	50	.86	.66	.82	120	16.94*** (3 > 1 > 2)
Control group has same domain focus as treatment							
1. Yes	2,146	67	.82	.62	.79	134	
2. No	1,418	33	.68	.53	.60	88	
3. Cannot assess focus of control group	330	12	.71	.49	.68	22	8.29** (1 > 2; 2 = 3; 1 = 3)

(continued)

TABLE 20. ***(continued)***

	Sample size	*k*	*M*	*SD*	Weighted mean	Independent samples	χ^2
Methodological weighting (max. score 14)							
1. <7	2,552	69	.84	.66	.81	138	
2. >6 but <11	1,137	38	.64	.44	.55	90	
3. >10	205	5	.66	.27	.69	16	16.82*** (1 > 3 > 2)
II. Publication characteristics							
Funding							
No	2,091	67	.84	.69	.78	136	
Yes	1,590	43[a]	.67	.47	.62	102	6.43*
Publication outlet							
Journals	3,615	98	.80	.61	.77	196	
Dissertations/technical reports	280	14	.50	.26	.39	30	16.15***
III. Setting of treatment							
Setting information							
Setting reported	1,250	40	.96	.66	.91	92	
Setting not reported	2,644	72	.66	.51	.62	152	20.77***
Specific setting in which treatment occurred							
1. Self-contained (or clinic)	277	16	.90	.68	.76	46	
2. Resource room	864	22	.97	.68	.99	38	
3. No information	2,644	72	.72	.54	.60	120	
4. Regular classroom	109	2	1.20	.16	1.14	6	31.42*** (4 > 2 > 1 > 3)

Multiple instructional units							
1. Single units (e.g., one-to-one group or small group)	2,358	78	.72	.60	.61	94	
2. Multiple units (e.g., one-to-one and small group and large group)	1,537	34	.87	.54	.90	70	22.12***
IV. Sample characteristics							
Reported discrepancy							
>1 year	518	22	.65	.45	.61	58	
<1 year or no information	2,635	77[a]	.86	.62	.78	158	4.43*[b]
Amount of psychometric information reported							
1. No information	2,070	41	.73	.57	.80	80	
2. Intelligence	652	30	.87	.66	.68	64	
3. Intelligence and reading	892	35	.77	.57	.64	84	
4. Intelligence, reading, and mathematics	279	6	.47	.11	.44	16	11.75** (1 > 2 = 3 > 4)
Gender ratio							
1. Low male ratio (<70%)	397	16	.56	.32	.50	42	
2. High male ratio (>69%)	632	26	.70	.61	.58	52	
3. No information	2,812	68[a]	.86	.61	.80	136	21.09*** (3 > 1 = 2)
Intelligence							
1. >84 but <92	654	22	.72	.47	.61	54	
2. No information	2,250	50	.73	.55	.80	100	
3. >91	990	40	.83	.67	.65	90	7.48** (2 > 1 = 3)
Reading severity							
1. <85	761	28	.83	.60	.66	58	
2. >84 but <91	51	3	.62	.49	.63	8	
3. No scores	2,778	68	.77	.60	.76	136	
4. >92	304	13	.64	.46	.60	30	3.54

(continued)

TABLE 20. (*continued*)

	Sample size	*k*	*M*	*SD*	Weighted mean	Independent samples	χ^2
Age (years)							
1. <12	866	36	.82	.61	.73	70	
2. >11 but <17	520	23	.91	.76	.70	52	
3. >16	80	4	1.01	.69	.67	8	
4. Multiage (elementary–secondary)	2,428	49	.64	.44	.73	114	.20
V. Independent variable (instruction)							
Strategy							
Strategy	1,910	43	.84	.60	.85	114	
Nonstrategy	1,985	69	.72	.53	.63	130	6.53*
Direct instruction							
Direct instruction	1,966	57	.82	.62	.83	120	
Nondirect	1,928	55	.71	.54	.66	124	6.93**
Combination							
1. Combined DI + SI	1,195	24	.90	.73	.90	58	
2. DI Alone	771	33	.77	.66	.68	62	
3. SI Alone	714	19	.76	.55	.58	56	
4. NonDI + NonSI	1,214	36	.58	.54	.64	66	22.14***[b] (1 > 2 = 3 = 4)
V. Dependent variable							
Word recognition	1,523	54	.71	.56	.59	108	
Reading comprehension	2,372	58	.82	.60	.81	138	13.43**[b]

Note. Underlining indicates significant results for both units of analysis.

[a]Because of missing, no specific, or unclear information, *k* does not always total 112.

[b]WLS means with methods partialed.

that the participants are 1 year or less behind their peers. Those studies that report more psychometric information (i.e., intelligence, reading, and mathematic scores) yield significantly smaller effect sizes than those studies that do not report such information. Those studies that report no information on the gender ratio of the sample yield higher effect sizes than those studies that report a high male ratio or a low male ratio. Those studies that report no psychometric information on intelligence yield a significantly higher ES than those studies that report average or low average intelligence scores. In addition, studies that report no scores on reading severity yield higher effect sizes than those studies that report reading severity scores, but the differences are not significant. No significant differences were found between age groups in the magnitude of ES.

In terms of instruction, as the last section of Table 20 shows, those studies that use strategy models yield higher effect sizes than those that do not use strategy models. In addition, those studies that utilize direct instruction models yield higher effect sizes than those that do not use direct instruction models. When strategy instruction and direct instruction are divided into four general models, the Combined Model yields larger effect sizes than the DI Alone, the SI Alone, or NonDI + NonSI Models. No differences in effect size were found between direct instruction and strategy instruction alone. In terms of the dependent variable, those studies that utilize reading comprehension scores yield higher effect sizes than those studies that use word recognition scores.

Regression Modeling

In an attempt to qualify the main effects, we entered several variables into a WLS regression analysis. The results are reported in Table 21. As shown in Table 21, the regression analysis (Type I sum of squares; see left column) uses a preorder entry of variables. The right column shows the results when controls are made on presentation order (Type III sum of squares). The dependent measure was the weighted ES for each study. The methodological composite score was entered first. The following variables were entered next in a predetermined order. Three setting variables one related to reporting the setting in which treatment occurred (dummy coded +1 and –1), are related to type of setting (regular vs. special education), and one related to the instructional unit—were entered into the equation. The type of setting was coded as a contrast variable in which –2 pertains to a self-contained setting, -1 refers to resource room, and +3 refers to regular classroom. A score of 0 was assigned when the study did not indicate the setting in which the treatment occurred. The instructional unit variable measures whether treatment occurred in a one-to-one context or setting, and/or in a small group (with five or fewer students) setting, and/or in a large group (a group greater than five) setting. The instructional unit variable was a continuous variable that ranged from 0 to 3, with a 3 indicating treatment occurred individually, in a small group, and in a larger group.

The next set of variables entered were the two general instructional models: direct instruction and strategy instruction. These were scored as dummy variables (+1 and –1 for occurrence and nonoccurrence, respectively). The next sets of variables entered were the chronological age and aptitude measures. Chrono-

TABLE 21. Weighted Least Square Hierarchical and Nonhierarchical Regression Analysis on Effect Size Estimates of Word and Reading Comprehension Measures ($N = 98$)

	χ^2	β	*SE*	χ^2 (partial)[a]
1. Method composite	16.13**	–.02	.02	2.42
Setting				
2. Stated vs. not stated	11.49**	.16	.17	2.54
3. Special vs. regular education	3.49	.04	.10	.46
4. Instructional unit	4.68*	.27	.16	8.02**
Instruction method				
5. Direct instruction (DI)	3.24	.04	.12	.43
6. Strategy instruction (SI)	1.19	.05	.14	.37
Age				
7. Age	1.04	–.04	.03	4.17*
Type of dependent measure (DV)				
8. Reading recognition vs. comprehension (*DV*)	1.73	.06	.06	2.63
Aptitude				
9. Discrepancy	3.45	.05	.16	.36
10. Intelligence (IQ)	2.85	.06	.14	.41
11. Severity of reading (*Read*)	.26	.04	.14	.05
12. IQ × read	2.8	.03.	.15	.11
Aptitude × instruction interactions				
13. IQ × DI	1.32	.07	.18	.41
14. IQ × SI	.37	.10	.22	.62
15. IQ × Read × DI	.72	–.09	.34	.20
16. IQ × Read × SI	3.63.	.32	.39	1.82
17. Read × SI	.75	.13	.21	1.18
18. Read × DI	5.98*	–.29	.18	6.76**
19. IQ × Read × DI × SI	.01	–.008	.54	.00
20. DV × IQ × Read	2.64	.14	.12	3.80
21. DV × DI × IQ	1.81	.08	.14	1.13
23. DV × SI X IQ	.30	–.01	.21	.01
24. DV × DI × IQ × Read	.002	.019	.30	.01
25. DV × SI × IQ × Read	.60	–.15	.34	.53
26. DV × SI × DI × IQ × Read	.01	.02	.45	.01
df	72			
χ^2	202.11**			
R^2	.25			

[a] Type III sum of squares.

$*p < .05$; $**p < .01$.

logical age was entered first and was the mean reported age of the sample (or for each subject, if provided). A new variable was created that directly compared the type of dependent variables (coded as 1 for reading comprehension and –1 for word recognition). The next variable was the reported discrepancy in achievement (scored as a dummy variable 1 for >1 year or more behind classmates and –1 for all other categories). The next variable entered was the reported range of IQ scores. The range was coded as +1 if the reported means were within the range of 91 to 115, and –1 if the reported mean IQ score was in the range of 85 to 90. Scores in which psychometric information was *not* reported were assigned a score of *0*. The last variable entered in the regression model was the severity level for *reading* based on the reported standard score. This was coded 1.5 for scores above 90, –.5 for scores 85 to 90, –1 for scores below 85, and 0 for no reported scores. The interaction variables were entered last. Because we were interested in the presentation order as well as in the unique contribution of each variable after partialing the influence of other variables to ES, both a hierarchical and a nonhierarchical model were analyzed.

As shown in Table 21, the methodological composite score and setting effects are significant when entered into the model first. The unit of instruction was significant, as was the reading severity × direct instruction interaction. When the variables are partialed for presentation order, several important findings emerged. As found earlier, the combination of instructional units (one-to-one + group instruction) yielded higher effect sizes than instruction that occurs in only one context (e.g., one-to-one instruction). In addition, younger children yielded higher effect sizes than older children. Only one reliable interaction emerged. Figure 11 (p. 133) illustrates the reading severity × direct instruction interactions for the weighted effect sizes. As shown, the highest effect sizes for direct instruction occurred for studies that included participants with severe reading problems or in those studies that failed to report reading severity. Those studies that reported reading scores in the moderate or average range yielded lower effect sizes with direct instruction models when compared to the competing model. Because reading is such a critical domain of instruction with the field of learning disabilities, we decided to provide a descriptive analysis of some of the studies. Two doctoral students (Bonnie Krammer, Brian Murrey) were particularly helpful in bringing the following studies to my attention.

Descriptive Analysis

Several studies within the present analysis included word recognition measures that resulted in extremely high positive effect sizes (e.g., ES >2.0). One of these studies was by Branwhite (1983). In this study, the treatment condition included direct instruction (DISTAR). This intervention approach is based on the premise that reading programs should be derived from the nature of the skills to be mastered. In this study, the mean age of the treatment sample ($N = 14$) was 8.7 years, and the mean IQ was 91. The intervention was conducted within a typical resource classroom, with teaching implemented by an experienced remedial specialist. The mean ES resulting from this study was 2.32, indicating a rapid and substantial acceleration in word recognition for the children who received the direct instruction treatment. In this study, the control group (*N* = 7) received a method of instruction that typically occurred in the resource classroom.

A second study that yielded an extremely high ES (2.27) is reported by Fiedorowicz (1986). In this study, reading intervention was conducted using a microcomputer. Instruction involved the subjects reading aloud stimuli presented on the screen, matching an auditory sample with the correct visual item presented in an array of three visual choices, and matching a visual sample with the correct visual items selected from an array of three visual choices. Feedback was provided on the computer with a "+" if correct, and when incorrect the correct item was presented again on the screen. Treatment occurred within the school setting and took place for 30 minutes a day, 4 days a week, for a total of 43 sessions. Results indicated a significant improvement on the reading of words and syllables for the trained group, with little or no change for the untrained group. In addition, follow-up results indicated that performance remained fairly stable after 4 months. It is important to note, however, that although this study involved computer-based instruction, it did not involve speech feedback, the primary component of the other computer intervention studies evaluated in the present meta-analysis. This may be one reason why this particular study resulted in high effect sizes, whereas the other computer-based intervention studies (Farmer et al., 1992; Olofsson, 1992) resulted in low and/or negative effect sizes.

Another study that produced high effect sizes is reported by Hurford (1990). In this study, two experimental groups (one consisting of nine 2nd graders and one consisting of seven 3rd graders) were given phonemic discrimination training for 30–45 minutes a day for 3 to 4 days. The control groups (*N* = 9 and 7 for 2nd- and 3rd-grade control groups, respectively) did not receive the phonemic discrimination training. Results from the 3rd grade treatment group on the dependent measure of phonemic segmentation ability (a combined measure of word and nonword recognition) resulted in an effect size of .26 (note: controls were NLD children), whereas results from the 2nd-grade experimental group resulted in an effect size of –2.08. These results indicate that phonemic discrimination is important to phonemic awareness, which in turn impacts word decoding and word recognition performance. It was postulated by the authors of the study that the reason the older children in the study (3rd graders) showed greater gains on the dependent measure, as compared to the younger children (2nd graders), is because younger children with learning disabilities have had less experience with learning to read and therefore less experience with phonemic awareness.

A fourth study that resulted in high effect sizes (ES >2.0) for each experimental group on several measures of word recognition was reported by Lovett et al. (1990). This study involved two experimental groups. One group received phonics-based reading instruction for regular word and whole word reading instruction for exceptional words. The other group received whole word reading instruction for both regular and exceptional words. The control group engaged in social skills training. The results from the study indicated high effect sizes for both experimental groups on several measures of word recognition. However, the highest ES (1.94) was obtained by the whole word experimental group on a measure of reading *exception* words (i.e., words that do not conform to predictable grapheme–phoneme correspondence rules). When words to be read followed predictable grapheme–phoneme rules (regular words), whole word instruction appeared to be only slightly more effective (ES = 1.31) as compared to the phonics method (ES = 1.15).

The studies that resulted in the smallest effect sizes involved reading instruction via the computer and synthesized speech feedback. Both the Olofsson (1992) study and the Farmer et al. (1992) study resulted in average mean effect sizes less than .20. In fact, the majority of treatment groups in the Olofsson study resulted in large negative effect sizes, indicating that the treatment had a negative effect on word recognition skills. This finding may have occurred because the control group was less severely disabled than the treatment group. Apparently, computerized speech feedback (verbal output of unknown words within reading passages) does not facilitate word recognition performance among children with learning disabilities. According to Farmer et al. (1992), "There was no evidence from the results that the use of a computer-assisted reading program with speech feedback under the conditions employed in this study might improve specific word recognition skill" (p. 56). Hence, when compared to phonics instruction, whole word instruction, and combined approaches, computerized instruction emphasizing speech feedback needs further investigation.

One study included reading comprehension measures that clearly produced a high ES, relative to all other studies. Gajria and Salvia (1992) conducted a study that yielded an overall mean ES of 6.60 related to reading comprehension. This measure was identified as an outlier in analysis and therefore was not included in the regression analysis. In this study, however, intervention involved training participants in the use of a summarization technique to facilitate the comprehension of written passages. The dependent measure was a five-item multiple choice questionnaire administered immediately after the training sessions were completed. The questionnaire contained questions that assessed the student's knowledge of main idea, cause and effect relationships, concepts, and inferences. In addition, a separate five-item multiple choice questionnaire was administered to assess the student's factual knowledge (mean ES = 2.89).

COMPONENT ANALYSIS

It is important to note that many studies use reading approaches that are not mutually exclusive of other approaches (Lovett et al., 1990). For example, many of the word recognition studies can be classified as "combined" methods that employ phonetic instruction in conjunction with whole word instruction. In addition, several strategy methods of instruction in the domain of reading comprehension involved behavioral principles, such as positive reinforcement and direct feedback, that are components of direct instruction. Hence, there is some overlap of techniques and strategies across all studies of word recognition and reading comprehension.

Table 22 shows the overlap in the instructional components for word recog-

TABLE 22. Frequency of Instructional Components and Effect Size Estimates for Reading Studies

	Word recognition				Reading comprehension					
	%	N	M	SD	%	N	M	SD	χ^{2a}	χ^{2b}
1. Sequencing (e.g., process or task analysis to goal, shaping)	69.1	38	.62	.55	69	40	.89	.65	.03	13.09**
2. Drill–repetition–practice–feedback	49.1	27	.60	.50	41.4	24	.98	.75	.51	16.77**
3. Orienting to process or task (e.g., preparatory to task, Meichenbaum)	18.2	10	.95	.64	24.1	14	.90	.68	.52	.04
4. Question/answer sequence (e.g., structured verbal interaction, socratic questioning)	5.5	3	.48	.71	24.1	14	.60	.41	8.06**	.33
5. Individual plus group instruction	90.9	50	.66	.56	91.4	53	.82	.62	.01	5.89*
6. Novelty (pictorial presentation, flow chart, related visual presentation, mapping, new material or curriculum)	50.9	28	.65	.48	67.2	39	.87	.59	2.76	7.01**
7. Attributions/benefits to instruction (e.g., This approach works when . . . , This will help you . . .)	29.1	16	.51	.57	41.4	24	1.03	.72	2.26	19.72**
8. Systematic probing (e.g., CBM, daily testing)	23.6	13	.42	.58	19.0	11	.67	.50	.43	2.23
9. Peer modeling/mediation (e.g., peer tutoring)	3.6	2	.62	.22	5.2	3	.42	.16	.14	.55

10. Segmentation (e.g., sounds divided into units then synthesized)	54.5	30	.55	.47	62.1	36	.86	.57	.80	14.57**
11. Advanced organizer (overview of task)	18.2	10	.95	.64	24.1	14	.91	.68	.52	.10
12. Directed response/questioning (child directed to summarize, asked what's the thing to do when . . .)	5.5	3	.44	.71	19.0	11	.48	.39	4.88*	.03
13. One-to-one instruction	74.5	41	.61	.57	67.2	39	.82	.66	1.03	8.11**
14. Control task difficulty (adapting material to reading level)	40	22	.78	.65	44.8	26	.88	.61	.19	.85
15. Technology (computer-mediated, highly structured materials)	50.9	28	.62	.62	44.8	26	.87	.48	.30	7.65**
16. Elaboration (additional information, examples, rely on context)	0	—	—	—	5.2	3	1.10	.11	4.05*	.00
17. Teacher models directly (models problem solving, steps, correct sounds)	25.5	14	.46	.60	48.3	28	.98	.72	6.04*	24.03**
18. Small interactive groups (reciprocal, directive, therapy groups)	38.2	21	.76	.57	65.5	38	.89	.57	9.20**	2.10
19. Mediators other than peers or teacher (homework, parents)	0	—	—	—	0	0	—	—	—	—
20. Strategy cuing (reminders to use strategies or tactics)	14.5	8	.55	.29	19.0	11	.80	.69	.75	.80

Note. Underlining indicates significnt results for both units of analysis.

[a]Compares frequency of components.

[b]WLS with the influence of the methodological composite score partialed out.

$*p < .05$; $**p < .01$.

nition and reading comprehension studies. The 17 studies that included both word recognition and comprehension measures were partialed from the analysis. Table 22 shows the frequency of instructional components (first column under main heading) and the WLS means (third column under each main heading) with the methodological composite score partialed from the analysis, as a function of word recognition and reading comprehension studies. As Table 22 indicates, reading comprehension studies were more likely to emphasize instructional components related to question/answer sequences, elaboration, teacher modeling of strategies, and small interactive groups. Generally, it appears that reading comprehension studies emphasize greater verbal interaction than do word recognition studies. In terms of ES, the weighted least square means are significantly higher for reading comprehension studies on components related to sequencing, drill-repetition-practice, group + individual instruction, novelty, attribution, segmentation (analysis), one-to-one instruction, technology, and teacher modeling. The patterns of results are comparable with or without the 17 overlapping studies removed from the analysis.

There was one particularly interesting finding. It is commonly assumed that intense one-to-one instruction, most directly in phonics, is the best approach to the remediation of reading problems. As shown in Table 22, effect sizes are higher in small interactive groups (M = .76) for word recognition and when one-to-one instruction is paired within small group instruction (M = .66) for word recognition than in one-to-one instruction alone (M = .61) for word recognition.

In general, the results suggest that orienting to task and advanced organizers yield effect sizes greater than the .80 threshold for word recognition. For reading comprehension, 15 of the 20 instructional components yield effect sizes greater in magnitude than Cohen's .80 threshold.

LD CHILDREN VERSUS CHRONOLOGICALLY MATCHED NLD PEERS

A comparison was made between effect sizes of those participants with learning disabilities in the *treatment* conditions to those without learning disabilities (NLD), but matched on chronological age. Of the 180 studies that did not include outliers, 17 of those studies included measures that allowed direct comparisons between LD and NLD children. The number of studies comparing LD and NLD participants is small because several studies failed to include an instructional control group of LD participants. The average effect size within the 17 studies served as the primary index for assessing the magnitude of treatment effects.

The mean weighted ES between LD and NLD participants was .97, with a standard deviation of .52 (the positive effect size is in favor of the NLD participants). The skewedness was .10 and the kurtosis was –.79. Table 23 provides mean ES estimates as a function of methodological, article, setting, sampling, and treatment characteristics. Of interest in this analysis was the identification of variables that significantly reduced the ES difference between LD and NLD stu-

TABLE 23. Effect Size Estimates Comparing LD and Chronologically Aged Matched Children on Treatment Conditions (N = 17 Studies)

	Sample size	k^a	M	SD	Weighted ES	Independent samples	χ^2
I. Methodology	367	17	.97	.52	.83	34	
Sessions							
<10	129	9	.86	.58	.60	18	
>9 but <30	64	4	1.04	.48	1.08	8	
>29	36	3	1.07	.53	1.47	6	$\chi^2(2) = 4.97$, NS
Sample size							
<25	166	14	.99	.55	.91	28	
>24 but <50	63	2	.64	.04	.63	4	
>49 but <100	—	—	—	—	—	—	
>99	138	1	1.45	—	1.45	2	$\chi^2(2) = 4.56$, NS
Type of treatment assignments							
1. Nonrandom	38	3	.93	.49	.85	6	
2. Random	54	4	.93	.89	.69	8	
3. Other	275	10	1.01	.43	.94	20	$\chi^2(2) = 1.06$, NS
Type of dependent measure							
Experimental only	181	12	.92	.58	.77	24	
Standardized and experimental	48	4	1.03	.38	1.03	8	$\chi^2 = 1.12$, NS
Treatment integrity							
Reported no	277	11	1.17	.46	.87	22	
Reported yes	89	6	.62	.47	.61	12	$\chi^2 = .84$, NS

(continued)

TABLE 23. (*continued*)

	Sample size	k^a	*M*	*SD*	Weighted ES	Independent samples	χ^2
Internal validity							
Low	97	7	.76	.35	.72	14	
High	270	10	1.12	.59	1.07	20	$\chi^2 = 2.09$, NS
Variation of instruction of experimental condition from control condition							
Low variation	89	6	.62	.47	.56	12	
High variation	277	11	1.70	.46	1.04	22	$\chi^2 = 5.27, p < .05$
Control variations							
Materials							
Same as experimental	92	6	.85	.70		12	
Different from experimental	116	8	1.08	.42		16	
No information	158	3	.93	.49		4	$\chi^2(2) = 1.90$, NS
Setting (6)							
Different setting	91	7	.90	.42	.85	14	
Same setting	52	3	1.14	.70	.84	6	
No information	224	7	.98	.61	.93	14	$\chi^2(2) = .14$, NS
Teachers (5)							
Different teacher	41	2	.56	.14	.62	4	
Same teacher	104	7	.93	.58	.78	14	
No information	228	8	1.11	.52	1.08	16	$\chi^2(2) = 3.45$, NS

Methods composite score						
Low methodological rating	349	15	.99	.54	.88	30	
High methodological rating	18	2	.89	.60	.82	4	$\chi^2 = .26$, NS
II. Article characteristics							
Funding							
No stated fund	156	11	1.07	.50	.96	22	
Funding	73	5	.68	.53	.53	10	$\chi^2 = 2.56$, NS
Publication outlet							
Dissertations	24	3	.82	.44	.84	6	
Journals	343	14	1.01	.55	1.19	28	$\chi^2 = .09$, NS
III. Setting							
Reported the setting in which treatment took place							
Yes	161	10	1.02	.48	.88	20	
No	67	6	.82	.62	.70	12	$\chi^2 = .53$, NS
Type of setting in which LD received treatment (NLD received treatment in regular class)							
No information on LD setting	87	6	.82	.62	.74	12	
Resource room	101	6	.98	.55	.70	12	
Self-contained/other (e.g., clinic, separate room)	60	4	1.08	.43	.97	8	$\chi^2 = .79$, NS
IV. Sample description							
Discrepancy							
>1 year	35	3	1.17	.31	1.43	6	
No information	193	13	.89	.56	.78	26	$\chi^2 = 3.69$, NS

(continued)

TABLE 23. (*continued*)

	Sample size	k^a	*M*	*SD*	Weighted ES	Independent samples	χ^2
Amount of psychometric information							
1. No information	173	5	1.41	.46	1.44	10	
2. IQ score only	149	9	.82	.48	.75	18	
3. IQ and reading scores	45	3	.69	.39	.67	6	
4. IQ, reading, and math scores	—	—	—	—	—	—	$\chi^2(2) = 8.74$, $p < .05$ (1 > 2 = 3)
Gender ratio							
Low male ratio (<70%)	42	3	.84	.78	.77	6	
High male ratio (>69%)	66	5	1.008	.61	1.03	10	
No information	259	9	.99	.45	.76	18	$\chi^2(2) = .89$, NS
Age							
Younger (<12)	18	2	.89	.60	1.21	4	
Adolescent (>11)	81	6	.92	.35	.75	12	
Adult (>16)	39	2	.57	.05	.72	4	
Multiage (elementary and secondary)	90	6	1.04	.81	.86	12	$\chi^2(3) = 2.34$, NS
Intelligence							
1. >84 but <92	63	2	.64	.04	.62	4	
2. No information	183	6	1.32	.47	1.27	12	
3. >91	121	9	.82	.52	.79	18	$\chi^2(2) = 4.95$, NS (2 > 1 = 3)

Reading							
<85	25	2	.80	.48	.89	4	
>84 <91	20	1	.46	—	.48	2	
0	312	13	1.05	.56	.89	26	
>91	10	1	.87	—	.48	2	$\chi^2(3) = 1.43$, NS
V. Independent variable							
Strategy instruction							
Nonstrategy instruction	173	5	1.12	.51	1.24	10	
Strategy instruction	194	12	.91	.54	.76	24	$\chi^2 = 3.28$, NS
Direct instruction							
Nondirect instruction	223	6	1.14	.47	.90	12	
Direct instruction	144	11	.88	.55	.80	22	$\chi^2 = .15$, NS
Combination							
DI + SI	130	9	.86	.59	.74	18	
DI Alone	14	2	1.08	.43	1.29	4	
SI Alone	64	3	1.09	.39	.81	6	
NonDI + NonSI	159	3	1.17	.64	1.21	6	$\chi^2(3) = 3.76$, NS

Note. NS, not significant. Positive ES reflects higher score by NLD participants.

[a]Unit of analysis = Effect size averaged within each study.

dents. In general, the results shown in Table 23 indicate that effect sizes in favor of NLD are pervasive across the majority of comparisons (i.e., very few variables reduced the magnitude of ES). Nondisabled participants have a general trend of "just doing better" than LD participants. The only moderator variables that influenced the magnitude of NLD and LD differences were the variations in the number of instructional components (overlap of steps and procedures) between treatment (LD) and control (NLD) and whether psychometric information was reported on the LD children.

Clear differences were found between effect sizes if the NLD group activities had a high degree of overlap to the LD treatment group, $\chi^2(1, N = 16) = 5.27, p < .05$. The weighted least square mean was 1.04 for a low degree of overlap and .56 for a high degree of overlap. Eleven studies represented a low degree of overlap and six studies represented a high degree of overlap. Another significant effect was how much psychometric information was provided on the LD children, $\chi^2(2, N = 16) = 8.74, p < .001$. The weighted least square mean was 1.44 when no IQ information was presented, .75 when IQ information was presented, and .67 when IQ plus reading information was presented. Five studies provided no information on IQ, nine studies reported IQ information, and three studies reported IQ plus reading information.

Because of the limited number of studies, the exploratory analysis of potential interactions, via a WLS regression analysis, was not considered. We were, however, able to do a hierarchical regression analysis without the interactions. Thus, the methodological composite score, whether the setting was reported, type of setting, size of instructional group, direct instruction (dummy coded 1 vs. O), strategy instruction (dummy coded 1 vs. 0), age, degree of discrepancy, intelligence, and severity of reading were entered in a predetermined order to predict effect size. As shown in Table 24, the order effects were also partialed from the analysis (see column under Nonhierarchical). For the hierarchical regression model, we entered the direct instruction model first because bottom-up processing probably has the richest database in the intervention literature. Further, it is assumed that a certain threshold or level of low-order skills is necessary before one can engage efficiently in high-order skills, such as strategy use.

As shown in Table 24, the only significant effect to emerge in predicting ES estimates was dummy variable related strategy instruction versus nonstrategy instruction, $\chi^2(1, N = 15) = 6.25, p <.01$. The direction of the beta weight for the dummy variable indicates that the ES differences between LD and NLD are significantly lower in studies that include strategy conditions when compared to other studies that do not include a sufficient number of strategy components. The total regression model was not significant, $\chi^2(5, N = 15) = 7.52, p > .05$.

Table 25 presents the mean effect sizes comparing LD versus NLD as a function of the 20 aforementioned instructional components. The analysis attempted to determine those components that reduce the ES difference between

TABLE 24. Weighted Least Squares General Linear Model on Effect Size Estimates of LD Participants in Preferred Treatments Compared to Chronological Age-Matched Nondisabled Children

Hierarchical model	Hierarchical model χ^2	β	Nonhierarchical model χ^{2a}
1. Methods composite score	1.50	–.14	3.07
Setting			
2. Stated setting of treatment	.53	.02	.00
3. Type of setting	.60	–.53	1.33
4. Unit of instruction	.76	.88	3.36
General instruction			
5. Direct instruction	.09	.32	.62
6. Strategy instruction	6.52	–1.26	7.27
Age and aptitude			
7. Chronological age	.001	.006	.01
8. Reported discrepancy	.28	.53	1.26
9. Intelligence	1.53	.34	1.54
10. Reading severity	.009	.03	.009
N^b	15		
df	5		
χ^2 (Q_e)	7.52		
Adj. R^2	.61		

[a]Type III sum of squares.

[b]Two studies had missing data on one or more variables and therefore could not be included in the analysis.

LD and NLD students. As shown, those components yielding effect sizes below .80 between LD and NLD were drill–repetition–feedback, systematic probing, peer mediation, and strategy cuing.

We further investigated whether the year of publication was related to treatment procedures. The average year of publication was 1987 (SD = 5.15). The year of publication was correlated with the dichotomous variables of strategy instruction and direction instruction, as well as with the 20 instructional components. Only five significant ($p < .05$) effects emerged. The year of publication correlated positively with strategy instruction, $r = .65$, and the instructional components related to attributions (benefits of strategy instruction) ($r = .45$), advanced organizers ($r = .42$), elaboration ($r = .59$), and small interactive groups ($r = .73$). No other significant relationships between instructional components or general instructional models emerged, ps > .05.

TABLE 25. Mean Effect Sizes of Instructional Components Comparing LD in Treatment Conditions to NLD Participants (*N* = 17)

Components	*N*	Mean	*SD*
1. Sequencing	13	.96	.55
2. Drill–repetition–practice–feedback	9	.78	.44
3. Orienting to process or task	8	1.13	.52
4. Question/answer verbal interaction	3	1.20	.46
5. Individual plus small group	16	.95	.53
6. Novelty	14	.94	.54
7. Strategy attributions (self-monitoring)	10	.80	.53
8. Systematic probing	6	.73	.38
9. Peer mediation (tutoring)	1	.52	—
10. Segmentation	10	1.04	.62
11. Advanced organizers	8	1.31	.52
12. Directed questioning	2	1.06	.55
13. One-to-one tutoring	12	.85	.54
14. Control for task difficulty	5	1.21	.43
15. Technology	6	.97	.74
16. Elaboration	1	1.50	—
17. Teacher modeling	9	.93	.57
18. Small group interaction	12	1.01	.56
19. Parents as mediators	1	1.68	—
20. Strategy cuing	5	.74	.72

Note. NLD served as a control group and did not participate in treatment. *N*, number of studies.

SUMMARY

This chapter reports the results related to an extensive analysis of group design studies. Our important findings will be discussed in greater detail in Chapter 5. In general, however, effect sizes for 180 intervention studies were analyzed across instructional domains (e.g., reading, mathematics), sample characteristics (e.g., age, intelligence), intervention parameters (e.g., number of instructional sessions, instructional components), methodological procedures (e.g., internal validity, treatment integrity, random assignment), and article characteristics (e.g., funding source). The overall mean ES of instructional intervention was positive and of high magnitude ($M = .79$). Effect sizes were more positive for a Combined Model that includes components of direct and strategy instruction than for competing models. Other important findings were that (1) interventions that included instructional components related to controlling task difficulty, small interactive groups, and directed responses and questioning of students were significant predictors of ES; and that (2) interventions that vary from the control condition in terms of setting, teacher, and number of instructional steps yield larger effect sizes than studies that fail to control for such variations. Other important findings were that variations in IQ and reading level are related to the magnitude of treatment outcomes. More importantly, it appears that an operational definition that takes into consideration these two aptitude variables has a better prognosis (yields higher effect sizes) than variations of other definitions for studies that use a combined model. The instruction approach that allowed for children with LD to do some catching up to NLD youngsters was a strategy instruction model. We know turn our attention to single-subject design studies.

NOTE

1. Ten additional studies were identified as meeting inclusion criteria prior to the submission of this report. Four of the studies were group design and six were single-subject design. Six of the studies yield effect sizes >.70 for strategy instruction. Thus, because studies may have been inadvertently left out of our synthesis (as well as the fact that published studies are biased), we calculated the number of studies necessary (i.e., studies that report null results) that would threaten our overall conclusions (i.e., the File Drawer Problem). We calculated the tolerance levels for null results (see Hunter & Schmidt, 1990, Table 22.2, p. 511, for the number of null results as a function of the number of studies). In the present synthesis, the mean effect size was .61 for group design studies (N = 180) and .90 for single-subject design studies (N = 85). Effect sizes were converted to r (i.e., $r = d/[d^2 + 4]$) and then to mean Z values ($Z = 1.15 \log[1 + r/1 - r]$; mean Zs were .31 and .42 for group and single-subject designs, respectively) to utilize a formula reported in Hunter and Schmidt (1990, p. 510). The number of studies required to indicate an inclusion bias for this synthesis is 971 (X = (180/2.706)[180(.31)^2 – 2.706]) for group design studies and 386 (X = 85/2.706)[85(.42)^2 – 2.706]) for single-subject design studies. Thus, 971 group design studies and 386 single-subject design studies meeting the synthesis criteria and reporting null results would have to been *not* retrieved before one could conclude that our selection of studies reflects a sampling bias.

Chapter 4

Single-Subject Design Studies

In this chapter we provide an overview of educational interventions for LD students that utilize single-subject designs across several academic domains. In contrast to Chapter 3, which focused primarily on pretest–posttest control group designs, this chapter focuses on studies that include successive time samples of behaviors across baseline (control conditional) and treatment phases of single subjects or groups of subjects. This chapter is unique in that very few previous syntheses have included single studies. This is unfortunate because approximately one-third of all data-based interventions conducted on students with learning disabilities use single-subject designs (Swanson, O'Shaughnessey, McMahon, Hoskyn, & Sachse-Lee, 1998). Our analyses reported in this chapter follow the general patterns of those reported in Chapter 3, except that we forgo the subgroup analysis and comparisons to NLD participants.

DEPENDENT MEASURES

Eighty-five single-subject design studies were included in our syntheses. When multiple experiments were included in a single study (e.g., experiment 1, experiment 2) and also included different subjects, they were analyzed as separate studies. As we noted in Chapter 2, effect sizes for single-subject design studies were calculated on the last three sessions of baseline and the last three sessions of treatment. Because several studies in the current synthesis involved multiple treatments (reflecting variations of reinforcement, instructional components, and/or contingencies), mean effect sizes were averaged across treatment phases.

Faith, Allison, and Gorman (1997) suggest averaging effect sizes across studies because separate effect sizes overestimate treatment effects (see their p. 266 for a discussion). Moreover, unless each study yields the same number of separate effect sizes, some studies may receive more weight than others. Table 26 provides the adjusted effect sizes (i.e., effect sizes partialed for the intercorrelation between baseline and treatment phase; see Chapter 2 for discussion) as a function of sample size and number of studies, and the heterogeneity analysis for the dependent measure category. As Table 26 indicates, most of the intervention studies were in the domain of reading. The next most frequently investigated domains were cognitive processing, mathematics, and writing.

In contrast to the group design studies (see Table 3), all domain categories for the single-subject design studies reported in Table 26 meet the assumption of homogeneity. This makes sense because, as indicated by Hunter and Schmidt (1990), repeated measures control for errors related to subjects; therefore the treatment effects are assumed to be the primary mediating variable. Because the effect sizes for each dependent measure category are homogeneous, the studies are assumed to be estimating a common parameter (e.g., treatment vs. baseline) and the variations among the observed effects are assumed to be due to sampling error (Hunter & Schmidt, 1990). Thus, it is appropriate to combine the studies under consideration and focus on the main effects of treatment. However, because the standard errors were particularly high in some domains (general reading, handwriting, word skills), our homogeneity tests must be qualified.

PROTOTYPE STUDIES

As Table 27 indicates, the 85 studies yielded 793 effect sizes across various treatment phases and categories of dependent measures. The unadjusted mean ES for the last three sessions of baseline and treatment was 1.41 (SD = .82) for absolute values and 1.04 (SD = .52) for nonabsolute values. As Table 27 shows, the adjusted ES, which partials out the correlation between the three baseline sessions and the final three treatment sessions, was substantially smaller than the unadjusted ES. The adjusted mean ES was also substantially smaller than the ES computed across all sessions (M = .87 vs. M = 5.30). When averaged within each study, the adjusted ES is .90, with a standard deviation of .23. Effect sizes were calculated for each subject (or sets of subjects if the study focused on groups of subjects) and averaged across studies. Based on Cohen's criteria, all dependent measure categories, except those that focused primarily on handwriting, were above the .80 threshold.

As Table 27 illustrates, the average year of publication was 1987. Approximately 21% of all published studies and dissertations originated at the University of Virginia, University of Maryland, and the University of Kansas. The average reported age of intervention is 11, with children scoring approximately 95 on a standardized IQ test and 80 on a standardized reading test. Most studies include an average of four subjects, with the majority of these participants being male.

TABLE 26. Single-Subject Design Studies

Dependent measures and domains ($N = 85$)	Sample size	Number of studies	Unadjusted effect size	Adjusted[a] effect size	*SD*	*SE*	Low[b]	High	*Q*
1. Cognitive processes	77	12	1.46	.87	.34	.06	.74	1.01	9.00
2. Word recognition	108	20	1.26	.82	.43	.06	.69	.96	20.29
3. Reading comprehension	69	11	1.36	.95	.45	.08	.78	1.13	13.86
4. Spelling	67	8	1.16	.77	.62	.07	.62	.93	25.41
5. Mathematics	195	14	1.31	.91	.61	.03	.83	.49	73.18
6. Writing	122	14	1.36	.82	.63	.05	.72	.92	48.30
7. General reading	3	2	1.78	.90	.09	.49	.06	1.87	.01
8. Word skills	10	4	1.42	.87	.22	.44	.03	1.75	.44
9. Global achievement	76	7	1.06	1.07	.38	.05	.95	1.19	10.89
10. Social skills	13	2	1.51	.85	.23	.29	.27	1.43	.63
11. Perceptual/motor (handwriting)	14	6	1.22	.58	.62	.20	.18	.98	4.68
12. Language	1	1	1.80	1.13	—	—	—	—	—
13. Other	37	5	1.17	.79	.52	.10	.59	.99	9.85

[a]Adjusted for correlation between last three baseline and last three treatment observations.

[b]95% confidence interval.

TABLE 27. General Characteristics of Single-Subject Design Studies

	Total (N = 85 studies)	
	M	*SD*
Effect sizes		
Effect size (N = 793)		
Effect size—unadjusted	1.05	.93
Effect size—absolute	1.36	.47
Effect size—adjusted	.87	.32
Averaged within studies (N = 85)		
Effect size—unadjusted	1.04	.82
Effect size—absolute	1.41	.82
Effect size—adjusted	.90	.23
All observation sessions (N = 85)		
Effect size—absolute	5.30	12.68
Article characteristics		
Year of publication	1987	5.08
Number of coauthors	1.45	1.25
Number of citations	2.05	7.77 (67)
Author gender (%)	44% male	
Funding source (%)		
No funding cited (those reporting N = 22)	74% (63)	
U.S. Department of Education	68%	
NICHD	—	
State/province	—	
Other	32%	
Most common publication outlets (%)		
Dissertations	10.6%	
Learning Disability Quarterly	30.6%	
Journal of Learning Disabilities	15.3%	
Journal of Applied Behavior Analysis	7.1%	
Learning Disabilities Research and Practice	4.7%	
Remedial and Special Education	3.5%	
Primary university affiliations (%)		
1. University of Kansas	21.3%	
University of Maryland		
University of Virginia		
2. Penn State	21%	
State University of New York		
University of Kentucky		
University of Miami		
University of North Carolina		
University of Northern Colorado		
University of Washington		
University of Wisconsin		

(*continued*)

TABLE 27. (*continued*)

	Total (N = 85 studies)	
	M	*SD*
Instructional parameters		
Time of instruction		
Number of instruction sessions	25.41	26.44
Length of session (minutes)	38.28	48.40 (57)
Number of sessions per week	4.78	2.83 (41)
Primary focus of intervention (%)		
Reading	33%	
Math	19%	
Written language	21%	
Most frequent reason for participant exclusion (%)		
No information	86%	
Emotional problems	6%	
Geographic location of sample (%)		
No information	47%	
Midwest	5%	
Educational history (%)		
No information	55%	
Resource room	28%	
Sample characteristics		
Sample size (per study)	3.83	3.22
Number of males	2.77	2.98
Number of females	1.05	.93
Ethnicity		
Asian American	1.0	— (1)
African American	2.35	1.64 (14)
Anglo American	4.05	3.07 (17)
Hispanic American	3.00	1.41 (4)
Native American	—	—
Other	—	—
Chronological age	10.91	2.09
SES		
No information	55%	
Middle class	30%	
Psychometric standardized		
Intelligence	95.22	8.16 (57)
Reading	77.48	22.29 (38)
Math	84.16	9.01 (16)

(continued)

TABLE 27. (*continued*)

	Total (N = 85 studies)	
	M	*SD*
Methodology parameters		
Internal validity rating scale (Abbr.) (4–15 high to low internal validity)	11.04	1.70
Complete scale (10–30)	28.85	2.75
Variation of baseline from treatment (%)		
% Similarity or overlap		
Same teacher	84.7%	
Same materials	69%	
Same setting	69%	
Same instruction focus	95%	
Single-subject design (%)		
% Studies using multiple baseline	65%	
Other	45%	
Number of experiments		
One experiment	90%	
Two experiments	6.0%	
Three experiments	3.0%	
Measure of treatment integrity reported	29%	
Dependent measures for treatment effects		
Number of experimental measures	4.81	3.79
Number with reliability	3.08	2.12
Number of standardized measures	0	0
Frequency reporting social validity information	<6%	

Note. Parentheses indicate number of studies from the 85 that reported information.

Most studies include the same teacher between baseline and treatment; they also utilize the same setting, materials, and instructional focus.

A frequent publication outlet of these studies is the *Learning Disability Quarterly*. Other frequent journal outlets include the *Journal of Learning Disabilities* and the *Journal of Applied Behavior Analysis*. Approximately 11% of the single-subject studies in the synthesis are from dissertations. Twenty-six percent of the articles had a single author, and another 31.3% had two authors. Of those articles that report funding, approximately 68% cite as their funding source the U.S. Department of Education. The gender of the first author is fairly evenly divided between female (56%) and male (44%). Sixty-nine percent (69%) of the studies are not cited and 13.2% of the studies received only one citation in the scientific literature.

Approximately 72% (72.3%) of the studies have no directional hypothesis. As expected, the most common (78%) sampling procedure is an intact sample with no random assignment of the order of presentation for intervention phases (assuming that the study has multiple phases). Forty-seven percent of the studies provide no information on the region of the country where the sample was tested; approximately 5% of the studies indicate that the sample was drawn from the Midwest. Sixty-two percent of the studies use a multiple baseline design (or variation) and 19% of the studies use an alternating treatment (or multielement) design to assess treatment effects. Approximately 16% of the studies use a reversal (or variation of reversal) design. The most common statistical analysis is descriptive (frequencies, percentages, or measures of central tendencies; 85.2%). The most common means of recording the dependent measure are a frequency count (31.9%) and the measurement of permanent products (e.g., arithmetic computation on a worksheet, 35%). Approximately 90% of the studies report only one experiment; 6% report two experiments.

In terms of criteria for determining a learning disability, approximately 31% of the studies report the following cluster of sample characteristics: a specific disability, a discrepancy, a difference between IQ and achievement scores, and a history of or current placement in special education. The most common reason for excluding subjects from the intervention study was because of emotional difficulty (6%). Ninety-seven percent of the studies do not indicate the year in which the study took place.

The most frequently reported difference between the treatment and the baseline phase is related to materials (30% of the studies). Forty-one percent of the studies report a measure of transfer to tasks or behaviors other than that which was trained. Seventy percent of the studies fail to report the conditions under which the transfer of skills occurred. Of those studies reporting such information ($N = 26$), 46.2% indicated that transfer occurred to a similar skill under the same instructional conditions and 30.8% of the studies ($N = 8$) indicated that transfer of the same skill occurred under different instructional conditions. Seventy-three percent (72.8%) of all the single-subject studies reported no information about how generalization of the instructed skill was assessed. Approximately 34% of the interventions occurred in the resource room. Ninety-nine percent (98.9%) of the studies include materials found in classrooms or available to regular or special education classes. Approximately 73.9% of the studies do not indicate the schedule in which maintenance data was collected. Seventy-eight percent of the studies indicate that the age range in the sample is between 9 and 14 years.

Only 28% of the studies provide a measure of treatment integrity. Of those that do, 71.2% failed to mention the steps used to measure treatment integrity. Independent observers were used in the studies that indicate that measures of treatment integrity were gathered (15.2%). Of those studies reporting treatment integrity, 20% indicate that the number of independent observations was three, and another 13.3% indicate that the number of observations was two. The most common means of social validation concerning the success or failure of the treatment were professionally (e.g., classroom teachers) stated criterion levels or rates of accomplishment (14.8%). Forty-five percent of the studies provide information on social comparisons of scores between the LD students and other students in the classroom.

Approximately 11.2% of the studies indicate instructional components in the treatment phase that include (1) breaking down the task, (2) conducting probes, (3) using a diagram or picture, and (4) independent practice. The most frequent independent variable tested was some variation of self-instruction, self-monitoring, or self-regulation (12.2%). The mean number of sessions (both baseline and instruction) was 25.41 (*SD* = 6.44); the mean length of each session was 38.28 minutes (*SD* = 48.40); and the mean number of sessions was approximately four per week (*SD* = 2.83).

Materials for the treatment phases were commercial (22 studies), novel (i.e., materials developed by the researcher; 55 studies), or a combination of commercial and novel (8 of the studies). The most frequent commercial materials (*N* = 22) were related to direct instruction (e.g., Corrective Reading, Distar, SRA, the Corrective Reading; 18%). In terms of student activities, 37 studies enjoined participants to monitor (via recording, counting, charting, checking, graphing, and/or verbalizing) or to evaluate their own behavior during the treatment phase.

The two graduate students who coded single-subject design studies indicated that 65.9% of the studies reported treatment information in three or more paragraphs in the Method's section, suggesting that there may be enough information for replication and application. However, approximately 95% of the studies provided *no* information on whether the intervention was adopted by the schools or the teachers. Approximately 23% of the studies made no recommendation for teachers, but did suggest the type of LD student and the type of instructional material that could benefit from the treatment.

MAIN EFFECTS

As Table 28 indicates, an analysis was made of single-subject design studies related to methodology, setting, sample, and independent variables. Because the unit of analysis is of concern for single-subject design studies, we report both (1) the average ES as a function of each participant or group of participants (whichever is the smallest unit), such that each dependent measure is considered as independent; and (2) the average ES within each study. For interpretation purposes, the average ES for each study was used as the primary unit of analysis. We must note that a weighted analysis was carried out because there were variations across studies in terms of (1) the number of subjects per study, and/or (2) some studies collapsed or aggregated all subjects onto a single graph; therefore our ES estimates reflect *group,* not *individual,* subject scores. In one study, for example, approximately 26 subjects were used in the multiple baseline design and averaged across sessions, whereas in other studies only 1 subject was used. Therefore, we weighted the ES by the reciprocal of the sampling variance in the subsequent analysis. Thus, the primary measure of interest in Table 28 was the weighted least square mean (LSM).

TABLE 28. Main Effects for Single-Subject Design Studies as a Function of Method, Article Characteristics, Setting, Sample Description, and Treatment ($N = 85$)

	k	Mean absolute	Adjusted means	*SD*	Weighted LSM	χ^2	Scheffe
I. Methods							
Number of sessions							
1. <11	286	1.41	.91	.33	.92		
	25	1.38	.89	.26	.89		
2. <30	379	1.30	.84	.34	.90		
	37	1.38	.89	.23	.92		
3. >29	128	1.45	.89	.28	.82	9.65	1 > 2; 1 = 3; 2 = 3
	23	1.47	.94	.21	.87	.33, NS	
Design							
Multiple baseline (or variation)	603	1.41	.91	.31	.92		
	54	1.44	.92	.19	.93		
Other	185	1.21	.77	.36	.77	25.54	
	30	1.35	.87	.29	.84	2.44, NS	
Internal validity (rating on 4 variables)							
Low	760	1.38	.88	.32	.90		
	83	1.40	.90	.23	.99		
High	33	.92	.63	.31	.57	44.20	
	2	1.52	.99	.03	.89	2.49, NS	
Treatment integrity (procedural validity)							
Not reported	540	1.42	.91	.31	.92		
	61	1.42	.91	.21	.90		
Reported	253	1.26	.80	.35	.82	12.28	
	24	1.36	.87	.27	.92	.13, NS	

Treatment variation (number of steps that vary) from baseline							
High variation (>3 steps)	736 74	1.39 1.44	.89 .92	.32 .21	.89 .92		
Low variation (<4 steps)	57 11	1.06 1.20	.67 .76	.38 .29	.62 .69	8.81 3.93	
Variations in setting							
1. Different setting	147 12	1.47 1.52	.97 .97	.31 .14	.95 .95		
2. No variation	499 55	1.28 1.36	.81 .87	.30 .25	.81 .88		
3. No information	147 18	1.55 1.47	1.00 .95	.25 .22	1.01 .94	59.87 .82, NS	3 = 1 > 2
Teacher variation in administration							
1. Different teacher administers baseline and control	7 5	1.73 1.73	1.09 1.10	.94 .04	1.09 1.09		
2. Same teacher administers baseline and control	677 72	1.34 1.38	.85 .88	.32 .23	.87 .89		
3. No information	109 8	1.46 1.48	.97 .95	.34 .24	.97 .97	12.46 .12, NS	1 > 3 > 2
Variations in instructional units							
One instructional unit[a]	657 94	1.35 1.39	.86 .88	.33 .24	.90 .87		
More than one instructional unit	136 15	1.45 1.45	.93 .94	.28 .13	.98 .95	.01 2.83	

(continued)

TABLE 28. (*continued*)

	k	Mean absolute	Adjusted means	*SD*	Weighted LSM	χ^2	Scheffe
Discussion given as to how participant was selected to enhance generalization							
No information	675	1.37	.87	.32	.89		
	81	1.43	.91	.22	.91		
Information	113	1.30	.88	.38	.88	.03, NS	
	3	.96	.65	.31	.77	2.38, NS	
Instructional materials same as baseline							
Same instructional materials	376	1.33	.84	.33	.82		
	54	1.41	.89	.25	.88		
Different instructional materials	354	1.38	.89	.32	.90		
	22	1.37	.89	.26	.91		
No information	63	1.47	.96	.29	.92	14.57	
	9	1.50	.99	.19	.13	.33, NS	(3 = 2 > 1)
The focus of methods in baseline was the same as treatment (i.e., baseline reflects systematic instruction and treatment adds to baseline)							
Same focus	675	1.36	.87	.32	.88		
	75	1.42	.91	.22	.90		
Different focus for baseline	16	1.09	.69	.34	.78		
	3	.87	.55	.26	.67		
No clear information	102	1.45	.93	.31	.90	1.16, NS	
	8	1.45	.96	.20	.92	1.21, NS	

Psychometric information on sample							
1. No information	247 28	1.37 1.36	.89 .87	.34 .20	.91 .87		
2. IQ	205 24	1.43 1.53	.92 .98	.30 .22	.91 1.01		
3. IQ plus reading	327 22	1.27 1.33	.81 .85	.36 .28	.86 .87		
4. IQ, plus reading, plus math	114 11	1.42 1.44	.86 .92	.26 .18	.85 .85	5.13, NS 7.63	(2 > 1 = 3 = 4)
Methodological composite score[b]							
Low composite score	760 82	1.38 1.42	.88 .91	.34 .22	.90 .91		
High composite score	33 3	.92 1.07	.63 .70	.32 .39	.57 .58	44.20 7.64	
II. Article characteristics							
Funding							
Funding reported	128 22	1.37 .43	.84 .89	.27 .21	.78 .83		
Funding not reported	665 63	1.36 1.40	.88 .91	.33 .24	.91 .92	13.67 2.42, NS	
Outlet							
Dissertation/technical report	208 9	1.19 1.27	.77 .85	.35 .25	.83 .93		
Journals	585 76	1.42 1.42	.91 .91	.31 .23	.93 .90	12.79 .50, NS	

(continued)

TABLE 28. (*continued*)

	k	Mean absolute	Adjusted means	SD	Weighted LSM	χ^2	Scheffe
III. Setting							
Reported information							
Reported	474	1.37	.88	.34	.92		
	52	1.35	.86	.23	.89		
Not reported	318	1.36	.86	.31	.84	10.67	
	57	1.44	.91	.23	.88	.02, NS	
Type of setting							
1. Regular class	18	1.51	1.01	.34	1.02		
	3	1.47	.98	.09	1.02		
2. Resource room	339	1.35	.87	.34	.92		
	22	1.31	.82	.25	.92		
3. No information	318	1.36	.86	.31	.85		
	42	1.44	.91	.25	.91		
4. Self-contained other	118	1.38	.88	.31	.8	8.55	(1 > 3 = 4; 2 = 3 = 4;1 > 2)
	18	1.38	.92	.21	.87	1.03, NS	
IV. Sample characteristics							
1. >1 year	70	1.19	.76	.34	.76		
	10	1.26	.80	.24	.83		
2. <1 year	12	1.33	.88	.23	.80		
	1	1.37	—	—	.85		
3. No information	643	1.38	.87	.34	.91	10.22	(3 > 1;3 = 2;1 = 2)
	74	1.40	.91	.22	.92	1.51, NS	
Age							
Young <12	28	1.20	.76	.39	.80		
	8	1.39	.88	.26	.91		

Adolescent >11	40	1.57	.99	.27	.96		
	10	1.59	1.01	.25	1.01		
Multiage (mixed grade range reported)	725	1.36	.87	.32	.90	.65, NS	
	67	1.38	.89	.22	.90	.67, NS	
Gender							
Males	68	1.42	.90	.34	.90		
	9	1.44	.91	.32	.90		
Not reported (e.g., gender uncertain because subject labeled by ID#)	68	1.36	.87	.32	.88		
	67	1.39	.89	.22	.90		
Females 40	1.26	.80	.37	.96	1.19		
	9	1.54	.99	.18	.99	.34	
Reading severity							
1. <85	176	1.33	.82	.32	.89		
	18	1.27	.80	.25	.95		
2. >84 but <91	127	1.38	.88	.34	.89		
	9	1.36	.86	.25	.85		
3. No reported score	422	1.40	.90	.32	.91		
	47	1.45	.94	.21	.78		
4. >92	68	1.22	.80	.33	.86	32.55	(4 < 1 = 2 = 3)
	11	1.47	.95	.24	.91	5.99, NS	
Intelligence							
1. >84 but <92	228	1.27	.80	.32	.81		
	20	1.42	.93	.22	.87		
2. No information	247	1.37	.89	.34	.91		
	28	1.36	.87	.20	.91		
3. >91	318	1.43	.91	.31	.92	14.91	1 < 2 = 3
	37	1.43	.91	.26	.94	1.28, NS	

(continued)

TABLE 28. (*continued*)

	k	Mean absolute	Adjusted means	*SD*	Weighted LSM	χ^2	Scheffe
V. Instruction							
1. SI	426	1.40	.89	.36	.83[a]		
	48	1.40	.89	.23	.88		
2. NonSI	367	1.32	.85	.35	.87[a]	4.96	
	37	1.41	.92	.23	.94	1.40, NS	
1. DI	586	1.37	.88	.32	.90[a]		
	49	1.41	.90	.21	.90		
2. NonDI	207	1.35	.85	.34	.89	.31	
	36	1.41	.90	.26	.90	.01, NS	
Treatment separated							
1. DI + SI	309	1.41	.90	.29	.90[a]		
	30	1.42	.91	.17	.88		
2. DI Alone	277	1.32	.86	.34	.91		
	19	1.38	.89	.23	.94		
3. SI Alone	117	1.37	.86	.33	.88		
	18	1.37	.86	.29	.87		
4. NonDI + NonSI (e.g., reinforcement only)	90	1.33	.83	.35	.82	.62, NS	
	18	1.45	.94	.22	.93	.47, NS[c]	

Note. Top row reflects number of individual effect sizes and the bottom row reflects the number of studies (aggregated by individual effect sizes).

[a]Either one-to-one *or* small group.

[b]This composite score reflects weightings of procedural validity, internal validity, psychometric characteristics of sample, sample size within study, and number of sessions.

[c]Partial out methods composite score and chronological age.

As Table 28 indicates, one of the few significant effects to emerge related to both units of analysis was the methodological composite score. This score included weighting of each study on measures of high treatment integrity, internal validity (e.g., control of ceiling and floor effects), amount of information on the sample in terms of psychometric characteristics, reported reliability of measures, number of steps that overlap between treatment and baseline, and number of instructional sessions. A score of 2 was assigned for the occurrence of each of the following items: (1) report of treatment integrity, (2) a score <5 on the internal validity rating scale (see previous discussion of group design studies; items include control of mortality, ceiling and floor effects, comparable daily duration of treatment with baseline, controls related to teachers, materials, and setting), (3) report of standardized scores on the sample, (4) treatment implementation greater than 29 sessions, (5) report reliability scores >85% on all dependent measurers, (6) report of high overlap between instruction procedures between baseline and treatment (less than four instructional steps vary between the baseline and treatment), and (7) report the representativeness of the sample (i.e., discussion regarding how the sample was selected). Methodological composite scores that could vary from 0 to 14 for each study. The mean methodological composite score was 3.37 (SD = 1.92). As shown in Table 28, studies with a high methodological composite score had significantly lower effect sizes than those with a low methodological composite score. Thus, there is support for using the composite scores as a covariate in the subsequent analysis.

Another significant finding was that studies with high variations in the instructional procedures between treatment and baseline (treatment has three or more steps, methods, or procedures) yield higher effect sizes than those studies that report low variation (less than three steps). Interestingly, the amount of psychometric information reported when the unit of analysis for ES was not averaged was not significant ($p > .05$), whereas a significant effect emerged when effect sizes were averaged within studies. When effect sizes are averaged within studies, those studies that only report IQs have higher effect sizes (LSM = 1.01) than those studies in the other three conditions: report no information (LSM = .87) = IQ + reading scores (LSM = .87) = IQ-reading-math scores (LSM = .85), $\chi^2(3, N = 81) = 7.63, p < .05$. As shown in Table 28, no other significant main effects emerged across sample, article, and treatment characteristics for effect sizes averaged within studies. No significant main effects related to the magnitude of ES emerged between the Combined Model, the DI Alone Model, the SI Alone Model, or the NonDI + NonSI Model.

A comparison was made between the 13 dependent measure categories reported in Table 26 with the methodological composite score partialed from the analysis. No significant differences in ES were found between the categories, $\chi^2(12, N = 109) = 11.94, p > .10$, when the average ES per study as a function of a domain was the unit of analysis.

The point biserial correlations between the domain of the dependent measures (scored dichotomously as 1 and 0, e.g., word recognition measure = 1 and other measures = 0) and the year of publication were weak in magnitude, all rs <

.30. The two coefficients of the highest magnitude indicate that word recognition was negatively related to the year of publication, ($r = -.23$, $p < .05$), whereas an increase in writing measures was more frequent over the years ($r = .26$, $p < .01$). The correlation between the weighted ES averaged across studies ($M = .90$, $SD = .23$) and the year of publication was not significant, $r\,(85) = .17$, $p > .05$.

INTERVENTION MODELS AND OUTCOMES: A THREE-TIER ANALYSIS

What can be generally concluded from the previous analysis? Because there were few significant moderators in our analysis of main effect, the most pessimistic answer is that every treatment worked. All treatment conditions were generally more effective than baselines, and only three methodological variables (amount of treatment variation from the baseline, reporting of IQ scores, and methodological composite scores) predict ES. Further, variations in the significant main effects are a function of the units of analysis (more significant effects emerge when the unit of analysis considers each subject's performance on a dependent measure as independent of other measures) as merely reflecting artifacts in the comparison (e.g., chi-square is sensitive to variations that increase *N*, i.e., the number of effect sizes). Fortunately, these global conclusions cannot be taken at face value because the previous analysis of main effects failed to qualify treatment outcomes by the variations in methodology. Thus, we have not directly answered the question of whether specific intervention approaches yield high effect sizes when compared to other approaches when the methodological composite score is partialed from the analysis.

A three-tier structure, similar to that used in our group design studies, was used to investigate the effects of various instructional approaches on treatment outcomes. As in the previous analysis of group design studies, one tier included a broad categorization of studies that include a component related to strategy instruction and those that did not. As shown in the last section of Table 28, this approach yields no significant differences among the general treatment models when the influence of the methodological composite score is partialed from the analysis.

Tier two included a finer grain analysis of the instructional components that make up the four general models and their relationship to ES. The mean effect size, standard deviations, and number of studies reporting information as a function of the 20 instructional components are provided in Table 29. As shown, peer tutoring yields the highest ES ($M = 1.03$) and strategy cuing the smallest ES ($M = .79$). However, all components approximated or were above Cohen's .80 threshold of a significant ES.

Prior to analyzing the contribution of these components to estimates of ES, we assessed trends related to the year of publication. We were interested in determining whether the general instructional models (SI and DI) and the 20 instructional components increased in emphasis over the 30-year period ($M = 1{,}987$,

TABLE 29. Adjusted Effect Size Estimates by Components Aggregated across Single-Subject Design Studies ($N = 85$)

	N	*M*	*SD*
1. Sequencing	58	.90	.22
2. Drill–repetition–practice–feedback	42	.89	.24
3. Orienting to process or task	19	.90	.27
4. Question/answer sequence	10	.85	.31
5. Individual plus group instruction	69	.91	.22
6. Novelty	51	.89	.24
7. Attributions/benefits to instruction	46	.90	.23
8. Systematic probing	59	.90	.22
9. Peer modeling (peer tutoring)	7	1.03	.09
10. Segmentation	42	.91	.21
11. Advanced organizer	19	.90	.27
12. Directed response/questioning	7	.87	.33
13. One-to-one instruction	64	.89	.22
14. Control task difficulty	25	.92	.25
15. Technology	42	.91	.24
16. Elaboration	5	.82	.29
17. Teacher models strategy steps	42	.93	.22
18. Small interactive groups	21	.99	.13
19. Mediators other than peers or teachers	3	.82	.22
20. Strategy cuing	15	.79	.23

Note. N = number of studies reporting information.

$SD = 5.08$) reflected in this synthesis. The point biserial correlation between the publication year and DI (coded as 1 for DI and 0 for studies not including DI) was not significant, $r(83) = .08, p > .05$, nor was year of publication and SI (coded as 1 for the occurrence of SI and 0 for NonDI), $r(83) = -.02, p > .05$. The correlations between publication year and the instructional components (20; scored as present or absent in the study) yield coefficients below .25. The only positive significant coefficient was related to drill–repetition–practice, $r = .25, p < .01$).

For the second tier of analysis, the correlation between the type of component (dummy coded variable) and ES was computed. In general, none of the correlation coefficients between ES and the 20 instructional components were of sufficient magnitude (all rs $< .25$) to be of interest. For the correlations between ES and type of components, the only significant coefficients to emerge were related to instruction in small interactive groups (#18; see Table 29), $r = .21, p < .01$), and reminders to use strategies (#20), $r = .23, p < .05$. No other significant coefficients emerged, ps $> .05$.

The third tier of analysis attempted to isolate those instructional components that best predicted effect sizes when the effects of methodology were partialed from the analysis. The weighted least squares regression analysis is shown in Table 30, which partials the effects of each variable (Type III sum of squares). Effect sizes were calculated across subjects as well as averaged within each study. The results indicate that when all dependent measures were averaged within

TABLE 30. The Independent Influence of Instructional Components on Effect Size Estimates in Single-Subject Studies, via a Weighted Regression Analysis That Partials the Influence of All Variables on a Single Predictor

	χ^{2a}	β	*SE*	χ^{2b}	β	*SE*
Methods composite	47.00	–.06	.008	8.63	–.04	.01
Age	12.90	.02	.007	2.43	.01	.01
Instructional components						
1. Sequencing (e.g., process or task analysis to goal, shaping)	.07	–.01	.05	.60	–.07	.08
2. Drill–repetition–practice–feedback	8.39	.09	.03	1.15	.05	.05
3. Orienting to process or task (e.g., preparatory to task, Meichenbaum)	.90	–.08	.03	.00	–.02	.06
4. Question/answer sequence (e.g., structured verbal interaction, socratic)	.37	–.13	.22	.01	.001	.26
5. Individual plus group instruction	1.21	–.14	.13	.28	–.07	.19
6. Novelty (pictorial presentation, flow chart, related visual presentation, mapping, new material or curriculum)	.03	–.01	.07	.45	–.04	.09
7. Attributions/benefits to instruction (e.g., This approach works best when . . . , This will help you . . .)	.42	.04	.06	.38	–.04	.10
8. Systematic probing (CBM, daily testing)	.04	–.008	.04	.15	–.02	.06
9. Peer modeling/mediation (e.g., peer tutoring)	1.84	.11	.08	.61	.10	.12
10. Segmentation (e.g., sounds divided into units then synthesized)	3.14	.06	.03	1.16	.09	.06
11. Advanced organizer (overview of task)	.00	.001	.22	.00	.00	.26
12. Directed response/questioning (child directed to summarize, asked what is the thing to do when . . .)	.01	.027	.15	.07	–.06	.29
13. One-to-one instruction	.31	.05	.09	.03	.006	.15
14. Control task difficulty (adapting material to reading level)	5.59	.08	.03	.20	.08	.06
15. Technology (computer-mediated, highly structured materials)	3.14	.12	.07	1.30	.10	.08
16. Elaboration (additional information, examples, rely on context)	.30	.08	.15	.04	–.02	.21
17. Teacher models directly (models problem solving, steps, correct sounds)	.83	–.05	.05	.12	.03	.08
18. Small interactive groups (e.g., reciprocal teaching, direct instruction groups)	18.67	.15	.03	7.10	.16	.06
19. Mediators other than peers or teacher (homework, parents)	1.81	.12	.08	.42	.03	.15
20. Strategy cuing (reminders to use strategies or tactics)	10.11	–.17	.055	2.39	–.14	.08
$R^2 = .17$, $\chi^2(21, N = 769) = 7.87$, $p > .05$						
$R^2 = .31$, $\chi^2(21, N = 63) = 1.36$, $p > .05$						

Note. Underlining indicates significant results for both units of analysis.

[a]Unit of analysis - individual subjects.

[b]Unit of analysis - ES averaged within study.

studies, only the component related to small interactive groups independently predicted ES estimates. However, the alpha did not meet a Bonferroni-adjusted per-comparison alpha level (.05/22 = .002, or $p < .001$), and therefore this finding may be capitalizing on chance. When the effect sizes are not averaged, the components that significantly ($ps < .001$) and positively predicted ES were drill–repetition–practice, small interactive groups, and strategy cuing.

The SAS regression program (SAS Institute, 1992a) was used to conduct the statistical analysis to determine the optimal model that yields the best combination (highest adjusted R^2) of instructional components for the 85 studies. The adjusted R^2 procedures were weighted by the number of subjects reported in each study. The adjusted R^2 was .0416 with the methodological composite score and age predicting effect sizes across studies. The adjusted R^2 was improved to .19 when the methodological composite score and age, plus drill–repetition–practice (see Table 29, #2, for description), segmentation (#10), small interactive groups (#18), and strategy cues (#20) were included in the model. Thus, four instructional components contribute 15% of the variance to ES estimates.

SPECIFICITY OF TREATMENT EFFECTS

As in the group design analysis, to address the issue of whether treatments influence broad or specific domains of dependent measures, we contrasted the four instructional conditions (DI + SI, DI Alone, SI Alone, NonDI + NonSI) with broad and specific outcome domains. As in the group design, four domain contrast variables were created that included *language versus low language domains* (word recognition, reading comprehension, cognitive processing, memory, writing, vocabulary, general reading, word skills, and language) vs. other [the remaining categories]), *reading* versus nonreading domains (word recognition, reading comprehension, general reading, and word skills) vs. all nonreading measures), *word* recognition versus comprehension domains (basic skills or low-order skills as an outcome measure [word recognition, spelling]) vs. high-order activities [reading comprehension, general reading]), and *skills* versus process domains (word skills vs. cognitive process domain). Three contrast variables were created related to instruction: *general* (or undifferentiated DI and/or SI instruction) instruction (DI Alone, SI Alone, DI + SI) versus other approaches; *orientation*, or a bottom-up approach (DI Alone) versus a top-down approach (SI Alone); and *combined* instruction (DI + SI) versus DI Alone and SI Alone. Because comparisons are made within studies as a function of categories of dependent measures, we changed the unit of analysis from the averaging of all effect sizes within studies to averaging effect sizes within each study by the categories of dependent measures. Because the coded schemes are not orthogonal, it was necessary to partial the effects of all the variables via a Type III sum of squares.

The variables used to predict estimates of weighted effect sizes are shown in Table 31. An SAS Proc Mixed (SAS Institute, 1992b) was used to identify significant parameters. In contrast to the SAS Proc GLM model procedure used in the

TABLE 31. Weighted Least Square Analysis of Effect Size Estimated on Treatment Domain and Treatment Approach to Determine Target Domain × Treatment Interactions for Single-Subject Studies

Predictors	$\chi^2(df = 1)$
1. Method composite	5.55*
Setting	
2. State setting	.61
3. Type of setting	.21
4. Unit of instruction	.04
Instructional domains	
5. *Lang*uage vs. nonlanguage	4.95
6. *Read*ing vs. nonreading	.11
7. Comprehension vs. word (*Word*)	7.53**
8. *Skill* vs. process	.01
Type of instruction	
9. *General* vs. other	.80
10. Bottom-up vs. top-down (*Orientation*)	4.14*
11. DI + SI (*Combined*) vs. DI Alone or SI Alone	4.60*
Sample characteristics	
12. Age	.89
13. Gender ratio	.76
14. Discrepancy	.02
15. Intelligence	.28
16. Reading severeity	.11
Interactions	
17. Lang × general	.14
18. Lang × orient	.02
19. Lang × combined	.24
20. Read × general	3.06
21. Read × orient	1.42
22. Read × combined	8.73**
23. Word × general	.05
24. Word × orient	2.42
25. Word × combined	9.83**
26. Skill × general	.03
27. Skill × orient	.07
28. Skill × combined	2.04
df	109
χ^2 (–2 log likelihood value)	92.78

Note. Type III sum of squares (partials influence of all variables).
$*p < .05$; $**p < .01$.

group design studies, the Proc Mixed procedure was selected because it provides a wider variety of covariance structures for time-series data. Methodological, setting, and sample variables were entered into the WLS regression to partial out some of the contextual variables that may underlie potential interactions. As can be determined from Table 31, the only variables to meet a critical Bonferroni-adjusted per-comparison level (*p*s < .001; chi-square > 7.88)) were the read × combined and word × combined interaction.

For the read × combined instruction interaction, the weighted least square means, partialed for methodology and age, for the NonDI + NonSI Model, Combined Model, and SI Alone or DI Alone Models for reading measures were .78 (*N* = 7), .76 (*N* = 15), .90 (*N* = 15), and .99 (*N* = 19), .91 (*N* = 28), and .90 (*N* = 25) for nonreading measures, respectively. As shown in Figure 12, lower effect sizes occurred for the NonDI + NonSI Model and the Combined model on reading than nonreading measures when compared to SI Alone or DI Alone Models. No significant differences (*p* > .05) were found between reading and nonreading measures for the DI Alone and SI Alone Models. No significant differences were found between treatment conditions on nonreading measures.

For the word × combination instruction interaction, the least square means, partialed for methodology and age, for the NonDI + NonSI Model, Combined

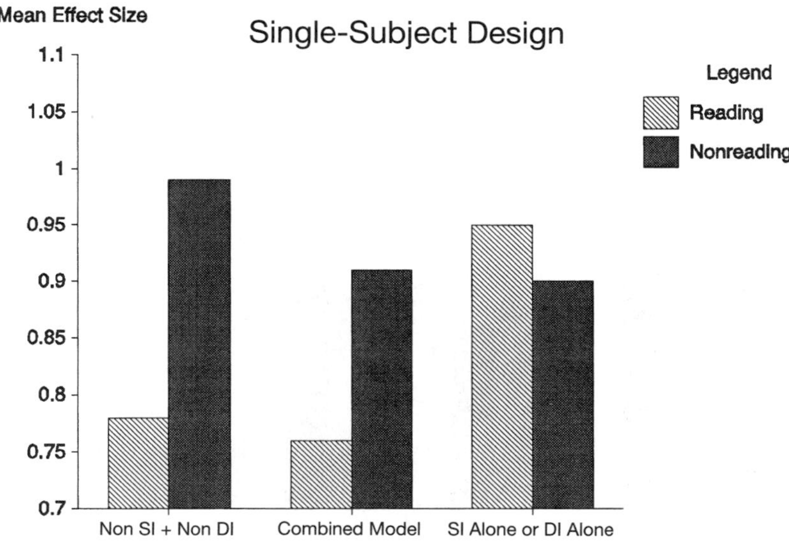

FIGURE 12. Effect size as a function of domain (reading vs. nonreading domains) and variations in treatment.

Model, and SI Alone or DI Alone Models for word recognition measures were .70 (*N* = 5), .87 (*N* = 13), .82 (*N* = 12), .99 (*N* = 27), .86 (*N* = 18), and .93 (*N* = 27) for nonreading measures, and .90 (*N* = 3), .68 (*N* = 5), and 1.07 (*N* = 4) for reading comprehension measures, respectively. Because nonreading measures were coded as 0 (ignored in WLS regression model), we only interpreted the interaction related to word recognition and reading comprehension. As shown in Figure 13, effect sizes for reading comprehension are higher than word recognition for the NonDI + NonSI and for the SI Alone/DI Alone Models, whereas the reverse effect occurred for the Combined Model. No differences were found in the magnitude of ES for word recognition across treatment conditions, whereas reading comprehension was lower in the Combined Model when compared to the competing models.

In sum, the results support the notion that a certain level of treatment specificity emerges, at least within the reading domain. The NonDI + NonSI Model and the Combined Model yield higher effect sizes for nonreading than reading measures. Thus, the level of specificity differs considerably from the group design studies. The group design studies found that the Combined Model was robust on reading measures, especially reading comprehension measures. The differences may be because of the focus of reading comprehension studies (e.g., literal vs. inferential comprehension) and/or the number of studies reflected in single-subject design studies as well as the limited number of studies in nonreading domain areas for group-design studies. Consistent with the group design

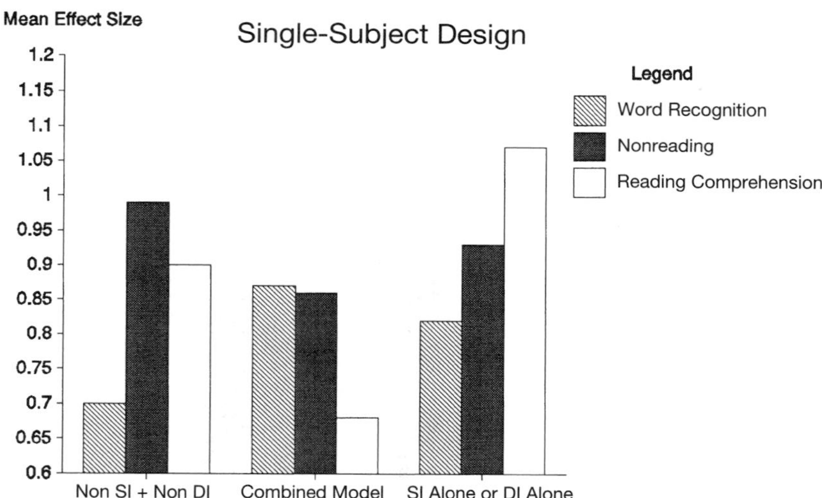

FIGURE 13. Effect size as a function of reading domain (word recognition vs. reading comprehension vs. other domains) and variations in treatment.

studies, however, treatment effects did not occur at the skill or process level. In contrast to group design studies, which suggest that the Combined Model has the most pronounced effect on reading comprehension, results of the synthesis for single-subject design studies suggest higher effect sizes for reading comprehension emerge with strategy or direct instruction in isolation when compared to the other treatment approaches.

TREATMENT OUTCOMES AS A FUNCTION OF INTELLIGENCE AND READING SEVERITY

As in the group design studies, we assessed whether the general instructional models that influence ES are moderated by intelligence and reading severity. ES estimates were averaged for each study (within each of the 85 studies) to determine whether the intellectual and reading level of the sample influenced treatment outcomes. The four levels of reading severity (no information, <85, >84 but <91, >90) and the three levels of intellectual performance (no information, low-average [<90], and average [>91]) were analyzed, via a WLS, with the methodological composite score partialed from the analysis.

Table 32 provides the variables included in the analysis. A Type III sum of squares was used to calculate the chi-square ratio, via the SAS Proc Mixed procedure (SAS Institute, 1992b). As shown, significant effects emerged for the main effect of strategy instruction and intelligence and the IQ × reading and the IQ × reading × strategy instruction interaction. No other significant interactions emerged. The significant main effect for strategy instruction indicates that higher effect sizes emerge for strategy than for nonstrategy instruction models. This finding was qualified, however, by the strategy instruction × reading severity × IQ interaction.

The three-way interaction is shown in Figures 14 and 15. The interactions must be interpreted cautiously because some cells had an infrequent number of studies. Although the Proc Mixed Procedure (SAS Institute, 1992b) provides estimators of least square means (LSM), the standard errors for the LSM were high in some cells. As shown in Table 14, the highest effect sizes for SI occur when reported reading scores are moderate (<85) and IQ scores low (<91) (LSM = 1.15), whereas the highest effect sizes for nonstrategy instruction emerge (see Figure 15) when intelligence scores are less than 91 and reading scores are not reported (LSM = 1.19). Figure 14 shows that the lowest effect sizes for strategy instruction occur when no information is provided on intelligence and reading (LSM = .79), and Figure 15 shows that lowest effect sizes for nonstrategy instruction occur when intelligence scores are not reported and reading is severe (<85; LSM = .37). Additional important patterns of results are revealed when the two figures are combined: (1) larger effect sizes occur for nonstrategy than strategy models when reading scores are not reported (LSM = 1.06 vs. .86), and (2) larger effect sizes occur for strategy instruction than nonstrategy instruction when reported

TABLE 32. WLS Regression Analysis of Effect Size Estimates for Single-Subject Design Studies

	χ^2
1. Methods composite	1.43
Setting	
2. Stated vs. nonstated	.49
3. Special vs. regular education	.36
4. Instructional unit	.30
Instruction	
5. Direct instruction (DI)	.03
6. Strategy instruction (SI)	8.89**
Age	
7. Age	.03[a]
Aptitude	
8. Discrepancy	.61
9. Intelligence (IQ)	4.02*
10. Severity of reading (Read)	2.19
11. IQ × Read	4.18*
Aptitude × instruction interactions	
12. IQ × DI	2.36
13. IQ × SI	2.16
14. IQ × Read × DI	.01
15. IQ × Read × SI	7.14**
16. Read × SI	2.62
17. Read × DI	.98
18. IQ × Read × DI × SI	.17
df	48
χ^2	59.30
N = 66 because of missing cells related to age	

Note. Type III sum of squares.
[a]Nineteen studies failed to report ages for LD participants.
$*p < .05$; $**p < .01$.

reading scores are severe (<85) (LSM = .90 vs. .68) or in the moderate (>84 and <90) range (LSM = 1.02 vs. .72). No differences emerge between instructional conditions when reading scores are in the average range (LSM for strategy instruction = .90 vs. .86 for nonstrategy instruction). Strategy instruction yields higher effect sizes than nonstrategy instruction when no information is available on intelligence (LSM = .87 vs. .66) or when intelligence is low (<91; LSM = .98 vs. .83). No differences in ES emerge between strategy and nonstrategy instruction conditions when reported IQ scores are greater than 91 (LSM = .91 and .90, respectively).

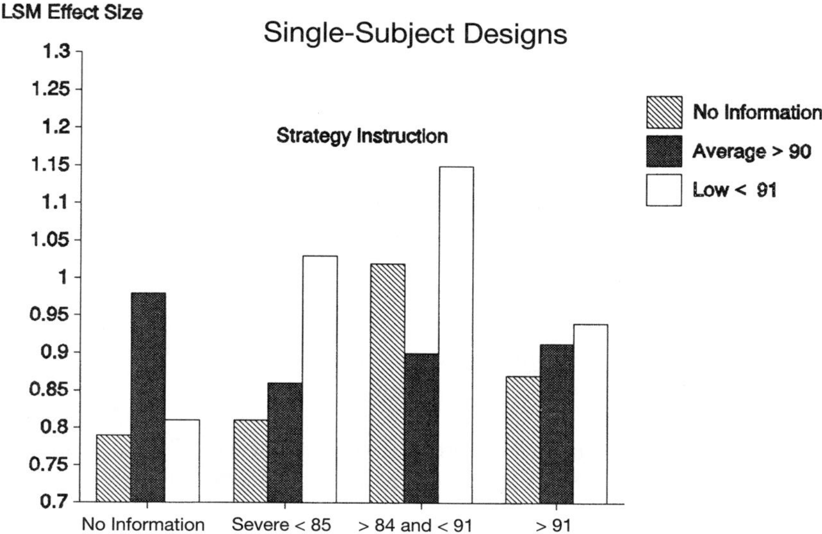

FIGURE 14. Effect size for strategy instruction as a function of intelligence and reading.

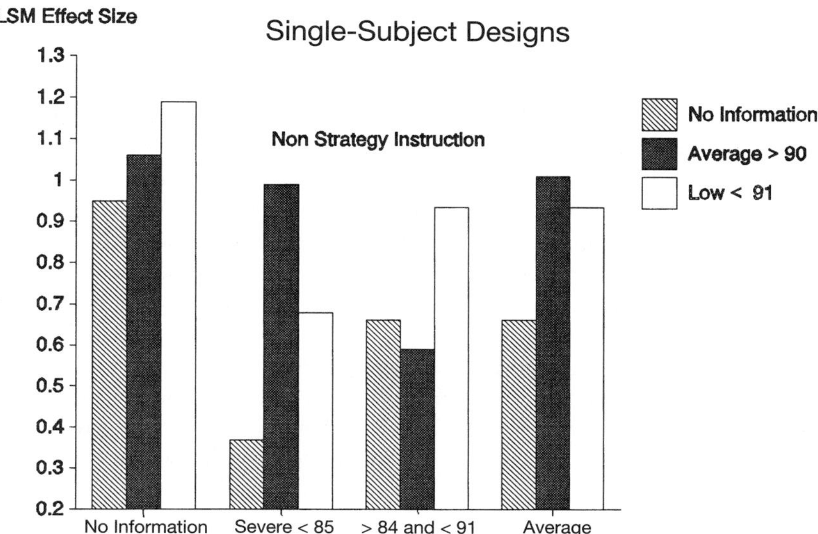

FIGURE 15. Effect size for nonstrategy instruction as a function of intelligence and reading.

DEFINITION × DOMAIN OF INSTRUCTION

As in the group design analysis, we assumed that the face validity of a definition of learning disabilities is enhanced if one can show that such a definition is significantly related to treatment outcomes. To this end, three contrast variables related to the definition of learning disabilities were created (see previous discussion). The first contrast variable compares studies that report psychometric information (referred to as some stated *criteria* definition, i.e., the study reports reading and/or intelligence scores) versus those studies that fail to report psychometric information. A second contrast variable (defined as meets *cutoff* criteria vs. no cutoff score) considers a cutoff score in reading at or below the 25th percentile (i.e., the 25th percentile is a standard score of 90) and intelligence scores at or above 85 versus studies in which cutoff scores could not be computed. A final contrast variable compares discrepancy defined samples (approximately a 15 standard score difference between IQ and reading) in which IQ is above 90 and discrepancy samples in which intelligence is below 90.

To test the robustness of potential interactions related to the sample definition, two units of analysis were used in a WLS regression procedure. One unit considers each ES as independent and the other unit averages effect sizes within the 13 domains (see Table 26) for each study. The results are presented in Table 33. Because setting and gender were not significant predictors in the previous analysis, they were removed from the analysis so that they would not take variance away from the primary variables of interest.

The important results related to both units of analyses can now be summarized. The unit of analysis that considers each ES as independent within each study yields several interactions related to the type of definition and domains/or type of instruction. However, when effect sizes where based on averages within studies for each domain, only the reading × IQ discrepancy, Combined Model × cutoff scores, and the Combined Model × IQ discrepancy score interactions remained significant. To facilitate the interpretation of these interactions, look at Table 34, which provides the weighted least square means for the various interactions when the unit of analysis is averaged within domain and study, as well as the reported mean IQ and reading scores across studies. To facilitate reader interpretation of this information, the high and low score of the weighted least square mean has been underlined.

Table 34 reveals an important finding related to the main effect for studies in which it was possible to calculate cutoff scores versus those in which cutoff scores could not be calculated. Significantly higher effect sizes emerged for studies that met the cutoff score criteria than for studies that did not meet the cutoff score criteria.

Figures 16 through 18 illustrate the interactions. As Figure 16 indicates, the low IQ discrepancy group yields higher effect sizes when compared to the high IQ discrepancy group on both reading and nonreading measures.

TABLE 33. WLS Regression Analysis of Aptitude × Domain and Aptitude × Treatment Interactions for Single-Subject Design Studies (Type III Sum of Squares)

Predictors	χ^{2a}	χ^{2b}	β	*SE*
1. Methods composite	61.66	15.44	–.05	.01
Main effects				
Instructional domain				
2. *Language* vs. nonlanguage	4.48	2.52	.07	.04
3. *Reading* vs. nonreading	.84	.47	–.02	.04
4. Comprehension vs. *Word* recognition	.10	.01	–.005	.05
5. *Skill* vs. process	7.18	2.94	.18	.10
Type of instruction				
6. *General* (undifferentiated) vs. other	.25	1.04	–.02	.02
7. Bottom-up (DI) vs. top-down (SI) *Orientation*	7.82	2.42	.07	.05
8. DI plus SI (*Combined*) vs. DI and SI in Isolation	.07	.01	–.002	.02
Sample				
9. Age	.30	.50	.009	.01
10. Report psychometric *criteria* vs. no criteria	.03	.01	–.003	.03
11. Report *cutoff* scores vs. no information	9.05	8.38	.12	.04
12. *Disc*repancy high IQ vs. Discrepancy low IQ	.49	1.01	–.06	.06
Interactions—domain				
13. Lang × criteria	2.86	2.96	–.07	.04
14. Read × criteria	.00	.56	–.02	.03
15. Word × criteria	.02	.07	–.01	.05
16. Skill × criteria	.13	.00	–.01	.09
17. Lang × cutoff	.87	1.34	–.04	.03
18. Read × cutoff	2.08	2.38	.04	.03
19. Word × cutoff	1.26	.54	.03	.04
20. Skill × cutoff	1.97	.56	.06	.90
21. Lang × disc	.87	.15	.02	.06
22. Read × disc	21.46	11.89	–.16	.04
23. Word × disc	.26	.47	.04	.06
24. Skill × disc	.78	.12	–.05	.15
Interactions—instruction				
25. General × criteria	.56	1.04	.01	.01
26. Orient × criteria	9.21	3.78	–.08	.04
27. Combined × criteria	.98	.15	.00	.02
28. General × cutoff	.55	.79	–.02	.02
29. Orient × cutoff	.39	.02	–.007	.04
30. Combined × cutoff	11.14	4.71	.05	.02
31. General × disc	.04	.01	.004	.04
32. Orient × disc	2.56	2.61	.12	.07
33. Combined × disc	21.92	7.93	–.11	.03
DF	757	65		
N	790	108		
χ^2	636.43	92.77		
R^2	.27	.33		
Mean ES	.89	.88		

Note. Underlining indicates significant results for both units of analysis.
[a]Unit of analysis computed for each dependent measure for each subject.
[b]Unit of analysis averaged within domain and study.

TABLE 34. Interactions Related to Domain and Instruction as a Function of LD Definition—Single-Subject Design

		Effect size				IQ			Reading		
	Sample size	*k*	Adjusted mean	*SD*	Weighted LSM	*M*	*SD*	*k*	*M*	*SD*	*k*
I. Domain × discrepancy (high IQ vs. low IQ)											
Reading × nonreading studies as a function of discrepancy and no discrepancy definitions with studies[a]											
Reading											
1. Discrepancy—High IQ	25	10	.65	.26	.72	98.88	6.06	10	78.26	11.47	10
*2. Other	7	24	.88	.21	.81	96.88	8.20	6	66.15	29.92	9
3. Discrepancy—Low IQ	15	3	1.02	.15	1.10	88.28	3.06	3	68.76	14.49	3
Nonreading											
4. Discrepancy—High IQ	46	7	1.00	.11	1.03	97.72	7.16	7	85.16	3.16	7
*5. Other	190	55	.92	.23	.90	97.67	9.03	35	96.92	3.84	9
6. No discrepancy—Low IQ	41	10	.84	.24	.84	87.19	4.74	10	68.19	25.28	10
k = Number of studies											
Scheffe = 3 = 4 > 6 > 1; 3 > 1; 4 > 6											
II. Instruction											
Instruction as a function of cutoff scores and other scores											
Combined DI + SI											
1. Cutoff score	48	8	.78	.23	.96	97.06	2.84	7	78.23	12.09	8
2. Other	122	29	.89	.21	.80	95.40	6.12	14	74.57	22.81	7

Other											
3. Cutoff score	13	3	.96	.25	<u>1.04</u>	88.66	2.08	3	71.66	10.21	3
4. Other	40	21	.91	.24	.90	100.44	11.52	12	96.86	5.42	3
DI Alone or SI Alone											
5. Cutoff score	54	13	.75	.28	.86	91.32	5.53	13	70.60	23.01	13
6. Other	104	30	.93	.23	.95	96.30	9.02	16	83.23	30.51	9
k = Number of studies that reported information											
Scheffe = 1 > 2; 3 > 4; 6 = 5											
Instruction as a function of discrepancy—high IQ and no discrepancy—low IQ											
Combined DI + SI											
1. Discrepancy—high IQ	48	8	.78	.22	.91	97.06	2.85	8	78.23	12.09	8
*2. Other	122	29	.89	.21	.80	95.04	6.12	14	74.57	22.81	7
3. Discrepancy—low IQ	13	3	.96	.24	<u>1.11</u>	88.66	2.08	3	71.66	10.21	3
Other											
4. Discrepancy—high IQ	10	4	.95	.18	1.03	104.23	10.65	4	85.69	3.76	4
*5. Other	40	21	.91	.24	.90	100.44	11.52	12	96.86	5.42	3
6. Discrepancy—low IQ	1	1	1.13	—	1.17	81.00	—	1	71.50	—	1
DI Alone or SI Alone											
7. Discrepancy—high IQ	13	5	.70	.38	.88	95.89	4.10	5	82.03	7.91	5
*8. Other	103	29	.93	.23	.95	97.26	8.46	15	81.88	32.33	8
9. Discrepancy—low IQ	42	9	.82	.23	.87	87.75	4.58	9	66.85	27.16	9
Scheffe = 3 > 1; 6 = 4; 7 = 9; 3 = 4 = 6 > 1 = 7 = 9											

Note. LSM, least square mean. Underlining indicates significant results for both units of analysis.

[a]Discrepancies are computed within studies. Thus, a discrepancy would occur when studies are averaged.

*Coded 0. Therefore ignore condition when interpreting interactions.

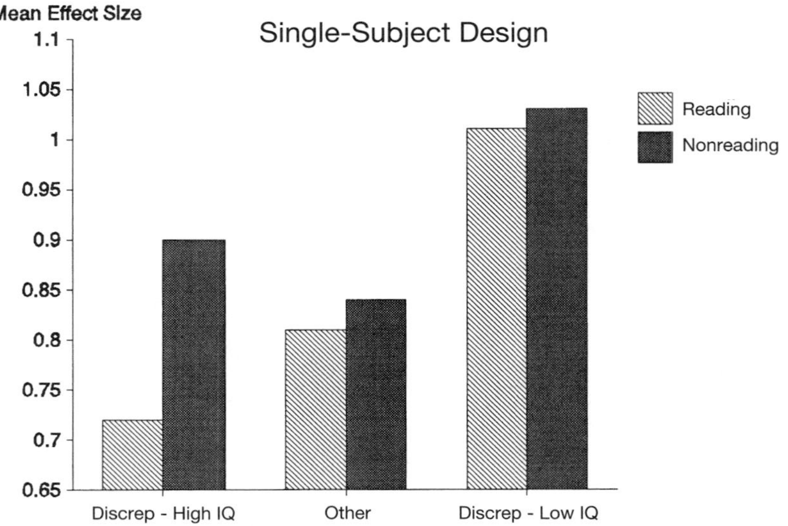

FIGURE 16. Effect size as a function of domain (reading vs. nonreading tasks) and variations in definition.

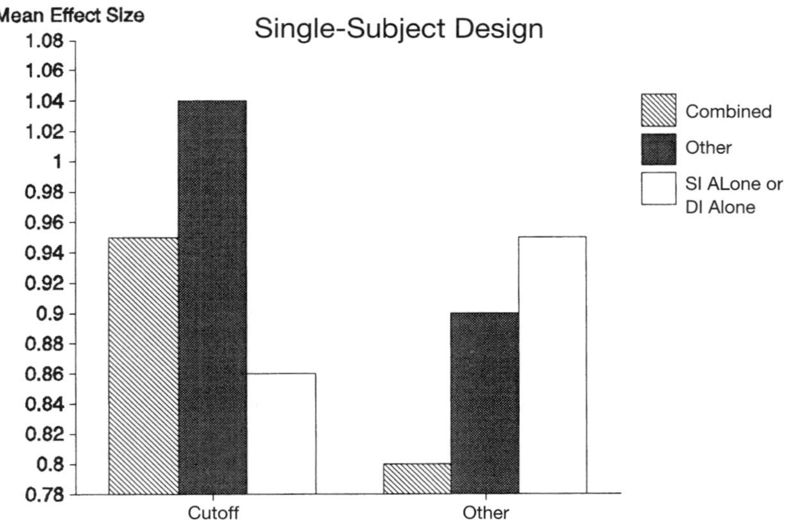

FIGURE 17. Effect size as a function of instruction (DI Alone vs. other vs. SI Alone) and variations in definition.

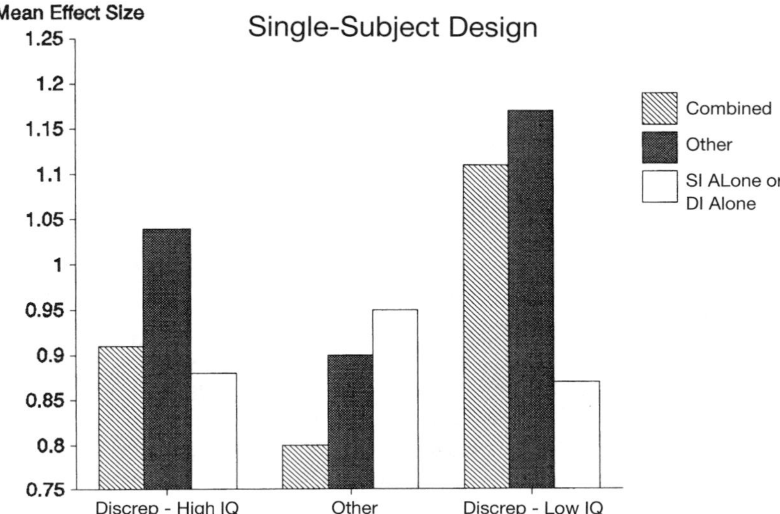

FIGURE 18. Effect size as a function of instruction (DI Alone vs. other vs. SI Alone) and variations in definition.

However, the high IQ group has higher ES estimates on nonreading than on reading measures when compared to the low IQ group. Figure 17 shows that studies that meet a cutoff score criteria yield high effect sizes for the non-strategy + nondirect instruction conditions when compared to the other conditions. This condition, as indicated from the group design studies, reflects components primarily related to small group interaction. The Combined Model yields higher effect sizes than models that reflect isolated components of DI or SI, whereas the reverse effect occurs when cutoff scores cannot be computed.

Figure 18 shows that the Combined Model yields higher effect sizes for low IQ discrepancy-defined groups when compared to discrepancy-defined groups with higher IQs. Thus, the Combined Model yields its highest effect sizes on studies that report low but average IQs ($M = 88.66$) and reading scores below an 85 standard score ($M = 77.66$). The results must be interpreted cautiously. As shown in Table 34, some cells had less than four studies.

In summary, the results suggest that cutoff scores and variations in IQ discrepancy scores qualify treatment effects. The general model that we defined as having few strategies or direct instruction components (i.e., the primary component of the 20 possible is small interactive groups) and the Combined Model yield higher effect sizes in studies where cutoff scores can be calculated and in studies that report discrepancy scores, but the IQ is below 90.

READING INTERVENTION DESCRIPTIVE ANALYSIS

As in the group design studies, reading deficit is the most frequently addressed problem in single-subject design studies. Tam O'Shaughnessey (former doctoral student) analyzed in some descriptive detail studies that focused on word recognition and basic word skills (e.g., phonics). Based on a review of articles using single-subject designs, she developed several broad categories of reading interventions to further organize the results: (1) oral reading practice, (2) whole word, and (3) phonics/direct instruction interventions. In addition, studies were grouped together based on type of dependent measure (i.e., passage reading, word list reading, or other) and age/grade level for analysis. Oral reading interventions focus on increasing the speed and accuracy of word recognition. In whole word instruction, students were trained to look at words as whole units rather than as sequences of phonemes. In phonics/direct instruction, students were systematically and explicitly taught to analyze words by their letter-sound and letter-cluster-sound subunits. Fifteen studies in the present meta-analysis compared the reading performance of individual students with reading disabilities before and during reading intervention. That is, at least one dependent measure within each study focused on a student's word recognition or oral reading skills before and during the implementation of a reading intervention. For descriptive purposes, *effect sizes were calculated from the means of all treatment phases defined as the mean score of all the baseline sessions/the pooled standard deviation.* It was decided to use this formula because the major synthesis has already reported conservative effect sizes, based on the last three sessions of each phase.

Tables 35, 36, 37, and 38 provide a summary of each study included in this descriptive meta-analysis. The author(s), age/grade of subjects, gender, ethnicity, and number of subjects are provided for each study. Table 35 also indicates the type of single-subject design, type of reading intervention, dependent variable, and mean ES. The 15 studies included in the meta-analysis produced 84 effect sizes, for an average of 5.6 ES comparisons per study. Table 36 provides the means and standard deviations of baseline and treatment phases for each study from which effect sizes were calculated. The average year of publication was 1984. Nine studies included only male subjects; one study included only female subjects; five studies consisted of both male and female subjects. However, only one study separated results as a function of gender. In addition, only 1 of 15 studies reported information on the ethnicity of subjects. Thus, reading performance as a function of gender and/or ethnicity could not be compared across studies. The average sample size per study was 3.47 (SD = .39; range 1–8; N = 52). The majority of studies (11 out of 15) involved elementary age students.

The most frequently used measure of general cognitive ability across all studies was the WISC/WISC-R (8 of 15 studies), and the most commonly used measure of reading achievement was the *Woodcock–Johnson Reading Test* (3 of 15 studies) (see Table 37).

Across all studies, students with learning disabilities improved their word recognition skills. (Because this was a descriptive analysis only, we calculated ef-

TABLE 35. Characteristics of Individual Studies

Author	*N*	Gender	Ethnicity	Age/ Grade	Single-subject design	Type of intervention	Condition	Dependent variable	Mean effect size
Billingsley (1977)	3	M	NR		ABAB reversal	Oral reading		CWPM (passages)	–0.94*
	1			3rd grade		practice	Self-reinforce		–0.98
							External reinforce		0.89
	1			2nd grade			Self-reinforce		–0.33
							External reinforce		–0.90
	1			2nd grade			Self-reinforce		–1.59
							External reinforce		–0.88
Chiang, Thorpe,	8	M & F	NR		Multiple baseline	Whole word	Peer tutoring	Number of correct	–3.85
& Darch (1980)	1			2nd grade		instruction	Tutee	words (word lists)	–4.74
	1			2nd grade			Tutee	–4.73	
	1			2nd grade			Tutee	–2.47	
	1			2nd grade			Tutee	–3.40	
	1			5th grade			Tutee	–4.15	
	1			5th grade			Tutee	–5.61	
	1			5th grade			Tutee	–2.95	
	1			5th grade			Tutee	–2.79	
Daly & Martens	2	M	NR		Multielement	Oral reading		CWPM (passages)	–1.89
(1994)	1			6th grade		practice	Listen/read preview		–3.49
							Silent preview		–1.23
							Listen preview		–0.98
	1			6th grade			Listen/read preview		–4.31
							Silent preview		–1.17
							Listen preview		–0.17

(continued)

TABLE 35. (*continued*)

Author	*N*	Gender	Ethnicity	Age/ Grade	Single-subject design	Type of intervention	Condition	Dependent variable	Mean effect size
Darch & Gersten (1985)	4	M & F	NR	2nd + 3rd grade	ABAB reversal	Direct instruction		Percentage of words/letters correct	–4.58
	1						Rapid pace		–3.01
							Rapid pace and praise		–6.06
							Praise only		–5.54
	1						Rapid pace		–1.08
							Rapid pace and praise		–5.36
							Praise only		–5.18
	1						Rapid pace		–2.08
							Rapid pace and praise		–3.48
							Praise only		–6.15
	1						Rapid pace		–2.96
							Rapid pace and praise		–6.36
							Praise only		–7.73
DuVall, Delquadri, Elliott, & Hall (1992)	3	M & F	NR		Multiple baseline	Oral reading practice		CWPM (passages)	
	1	M		3rd grade			Parent tutoring		–2.36
	1	M		3rd grade			Tutee		–3.00
	1	F		3rd grade			Tutee		–1.47
							Tutee		–2.60
Idol-Maestas (1981)	1	M	NR	adult (21 years)	Multielement	Direct instruction	Phonics instruction	Number of correct words (word list)	–0.67
Lalli & Shapiro (1990)	8	M & F	NR	1st–6th grade	Multiple baseline	Whole word instruction		Number of correct words (word lists)	–2.96
	1						Self-monitoring		–3.40
							Self-monitor and reward		–3.64
	1						Self-monitoring		–2.53
							Self-monitor and reward		–4.41

	1						Self-monitoring		–2.56
							Self-monitor and reward		–2.58
	1						Self-monitoring		–1.86
							Self-monitor and reward		–2.48
	1						Self-monitoring		–2.26
							Self-monitor and reward		–2.28
	1						Self-monitoring		–2.27
							Self-monitor and reward		–2.57
	1						Self-monitoring		–5.04
							Self-monitor and reward		–5.31
	1						Self-monitoring		–2.03
							Self-monitor and reward		–2.14
Roberts & Deutsch Smith (1980)	2	M	NR	5th and 6th grade	Multiple baseline	Whole word instruction	Modeling and drill	CWPM (passages)	–2.14
	1								–2.33
	1								–1.94
Rose & Sherry (1984)	5	M & F	NR	9th–11th grade		Alternating treatments	Oral reading practice	CWPM (passages)	–3.25
	1						Silent preview		–2.01
							Listen preview		–4.00
	1						Silent preview		–1.66
							Listen preview		–5.03
	1						Silent preview		–4.65
							Listen preview		–8.31
	1						Silent preview		0.32
							Listen preview		–0.74
	1						Silent preview		–3.25
							Listen preview		–3.17
Schimek (1983)	1	F	NR	1st grade	Multielement	Direct instruction	Phonics instruction	Number of correct words (word lists)	–3.35

(continued)

TABLE 35. (*continued*)

Author	*N*	Gender	Ethnicity	Age/ Grade	Single-subject design	Type of intervention	Condition	Dependent variable	Mean effect size
Thorpe, Lampe, Nash, & Chiang (1981)	3	M	NR	9th and 10th grade	Multiple baseline	Phonics instruction	Visual–auditory–kinesthetic–tactile instruction	Number of correct words (word lists)	–4.90
	1								–8.10
	1								–3.71
	1								–2.90
Weinstein & Cooke (1992)	4	M	3 white/ 1 black		ABAC reversal practice	Oral reading	Repeated readings	CWPM (passages)	–1.70
	1		white	3rd grade			Reread/improve		–0.45
							Reread/90% criterion		–0.92
	1		Black	2nd grade			Reread/improve		–0.27
							Reread/90% criterion		–0.96
	1		White	2nd grade			Reread/improve		–1.85
							Reread/90% criterion		–2.90
	1		White	2nd grade			Reread/improve		–4.06
							Reread/90% criterion		–2.19

Note. ES = (Baseline – treatment)/*SD* baseline across *all* sessions.

*Negative score reflects advantage for treatment when compared to baseline phase.

TABLE 36. Means and Standard Deviations of Baseline and Treatment Phases

Author	Subject[a]	Condition	Baseline		Treatment	
			Mean	*SD*	Mean	*SD*
Billingsley (1977)	4	Self-reinforce	29.0	9.7	37.6	8.0
	4	External reinforce	29.5	10.1	36.9	6.3
	5	Self-reinforce	39.9	7.6	42.9	10.9
	5	External reinforce	38.9	10.3	47.7	9.4
	6	Self-reinforce	44.1	7.9	56.2	7.4
	6	External reinforce	45.4	9.3	53.5	9.1
Chiang, Thorpe,		Peer tutoring				
& Darch (1980)	A	Tutee	57.1	7.7	93.9	7.9
	B	Tutee	61.3	3.0	76.4	4.3
	C	Tutee	28.8	4.2	68.9	12.7
	D	Tutee	39.0	5.4	67.0	4.6
	A	Tutor	13.7	6.6	29.3	6.0
	B	Tutor	12.7	5.3	43.7	15.7
	C	Tutor	25.3	4.4	47.7	8.8
	D	Tutor	44.2	9.9	63.3	3.8
Daly & Martens	3	Listen/read preview	17.7	4.1	57.4	18.6
(1994)	3	Silent preview			27.9	12.4
	3	Listen preview			23.9	8.4
	4	Listen/read preview	26.7	7.6	54.4	5.3
	4	Silent preview			44.7	15.4
	4	Listen preview			28.3	11.4
Darch & Gersten	1	Rapid pace	45.86	9.32	65.3	3.6
(1985)	1	Rapid pace and praise		82.5	2.8	
	1	Praise only			79.0	2.7
	2	Rapid pace	51.71	11.51	60.6	4.9
	2	Rapid pace and praise			88.3	2.1
	2	Praise only			86.0	1.7
	3	Rapid pace	54.00	3.21	63.4	5.9
	3	Rapid pace and praise			66.6	4.0
	3	Praise only			65.7	0.6
	4	Rapid pace	18.29	1.70	23.1	1.6
	4	Rapid pace and praise			30.5	2.1
	4	Praise only			29.3	1.2
DuVall, Delquadri,		Parent tutoring				
Elliott, & Hall	Steven	Tutee	65.6	13.2	118.7	22.2
(1992)	Dean	Tutee	19.4	11.8	35.9	10.6
	Janeen	Tutee	101.3	12.2	135.7	14.3
Idol-Maestas (1981)	1	Phonics instruction	70.2	34.4	88.9	21.2
Lalli & Shapiro	1	Self-monitoring	0.5	1.5	6.6	3.9
(1990)	1	Self-monitor and reward			8.2	3.8
	2	Self-monitoring	0.3	0.8	7.0	4.5
	2	Self-monitor and reward			9.5	3.4
	3	Self-monitoring	0.8	1.5	7.3	3.6

(*continued*)

TABLE 36. (*continued*)

Author	Subject[a]	Condition	Baseline Mean	Baseline *SD*	Treatment Mean	Treatment *SD*
	3	Self-monitor and reward			7.8	3.9
	4	Self-monitoring	1.4	2.5	7.8	4.5
	4	Self-monitor and reward			8.6	3.4
	5	Self-monitoring	0.6	1.2	7.8	5.2
	5	Self-monitor and reward			7.6	5.0
	6	Self-monitoring	0.9	1.8	4.6	1.5
	6	Self-monitor and reward			5.4	1.7
	7	Self-monitoring	0.1	0.3	4.6	1.5
	7	Self-monitor and reward			5.4	1.7
	8	Self-monitoring	0.8	1.8	7.8	5.2
	8	Self-monitor and reward			8.0	5.0
Roberts & Deutsch		Modeling and drill				
Smith (1980)	Dan		37.8	7.0	56.2	8.8
	Wade		23.4	5.9	31.4	2.4
Rose & Sherry	1	Silent preview	60.5	7.0	71.7	4.2
(1984)	1	Listen preview			87.2	6.4
	2	Silent preview	54.5	4.1	62.1	5.0
	2	Listen preview			75.3	4.2
	3	Silent preview	53.3	3.5	67.0	2.4
	3	Listen preview			81.8	3.4
	4	Silent preview	43.3	3.4	41.8	5.6
	4	Listen preview			45.7	3.1
	5	Silent preview	37.0	6.7	57.7	6.1
	5	Listen preview			63.9	10.3
Schimek (1983)	1	Phonics instruction	3.0	3.5	9.8	0.6
Thorpe, Lampe,	A	Visual–auditory–	4.8	0.5	8.8	0.5
Nash, & Chiang	B	kinesthetic–tactile	3.9	1.6	8.6	0.9
(1981)	C	instruction	5.8	2.0	9.5	0.6
Weinstein &		Repeated readings				
Cooke (1992)	1	Reread/improve	31.0	8.9	39.8	9.2
	1	Reread/90% criterion			50.6	12.7
	2	Reread/improve	42.7	4.3	50.5	15.1
	2	Reread/90% criterion			68.4	11.6
	3	Reread/improve	29.7	8.9	50.7	13.9
	3	Reread/90% criterion			60.3	12.3
	4	Reread/improve	37.7	8.5	68.0	6.4
	4	Reread/90% criterion			65.7	17.0

[a]Participant identified in study.

TABLE 37. Reading Achievement and Intelligence Measures Used to Define Learning Disability

Author	Subject	Reading test	Grade level	Intelligence test	IQ
Billingsley (1977)	4	Diagnostic Reading Scales (reading delay)	1 year 9 months	WISC VIQ	92
	5		2 year 4 months		100
	6		2 year 6 months		109
Chiang, Thorpe, & Darch (1980)	All	Slosson Oral Reading Test (reading delay)	>1 year	Not given	Average IQ
Daly & Martens (1994)	3	KTEA–reading decoding (standard score)	66	WISC-R	95
	4	Diagnostic Achievement Battery Reading Quotient (standard score)	61	WISC-R	89
Darch & Gersten (1985)	All	Not given (reading delay)	>1 year	Not given	101
DuVall, Delquardi, Elliott, & Hall (1992)	Steven	Woodcock–Johnson Psycho-Educational Battery Reading Cluster (reading delay)	0.4 year	WISC-R	130
	Dean		0.7 year	WISC-R	92
	Janeen		1.4 year	WISC-R	112
Idol-Maestas (1981)	Adult	Sucher–Allred Reading Inventory (independent reading level)	2nd grade	Not given	Average IQ
Lalli & Shapiro (1990)	All	Curriculum-Based Reading (reading delay)	2.1 years	WISC-R Stanford–Binet	102
Roberts & Deutsch Smith (1980)	All	Gilmore Oral Reading Test (reading delay)	>2 years	Not given	Average IQ
Rose & Sherry (1984)	All	Gilmore Oral Reading Test (reading delay)	>4 years	WISC-R	Average IQ (range 85–92)
Schimek (1983)	1	Not given (reading delay)	1 year	WISC-R	Average IQ
Thorpe, Lampe, Nash, & Chiang (1981)	A	Woodcock–Johnson Psycho-Educational Battery Reading Cluster (reading delay)	>5 years	WISC-R	86
	B		>5 years	WISC-R	93
	C		>5 years	WISC-R	91
Weinstein & Cooke (1992)	All	Brigance Word Recognition Test (reading delay)	>1 year	WISC-R	85

TABLE 38. Categorization of Reading Intervention Studies

Domain	No. of studies	No. of effect sizes	Mean effect size (absolute value)	Standard deviation
Overall studies	15	84	2.98	1.89
Phonics/direct instruction	5	18	4.18	2.22
Whole word instruction	3	26	3.17	1.15
Oral reading practice	6	39	2.34	1.88
Letter naming instruction	1	1	1.36	NA
Dependent variable[a]				
1—Passage reading	7	35	2.17	1.80
2—Word list reading	5	29	3.34	1.48
3—Other	3	20	3.74	2.43
Age/grade level				
Elementary (grades 1–6)	11	64	2.83	1.72
High school (grades 9–12)	3	19	3.60	2.30
Adult	1	1	0.67	NA

[a]1, number of words read correctly per minute; 2, number of words read correctly; 3, number of letter-naming errors, % words/letters/sounds read correctly, number of words read correctly per minute on word list.

fect sizes using this formula for the mean of the treatment minus the mean of the baseline divided by the standard deviation of the baseline across all sessions. Thus, the effect sizes are *substantially* higher than our general analysis.) The average ES (absolute value) across all studies was 2.98 (SD = 1.89). In terms of Cohen's criteria, this is a *very* large ES. In excess of 90% of the treatment data points could be differentiated from the mean baseline data points. The standard deviation, however, indicates some variability in the studies. This can be seen in the range of individual effect sizes, which shows that individual students varied in the degree to which specific reading interventions improved their reading skills (see Table 36).

As shown in Table 38, phonics/direct instruction produced a larger ES (mean ES = 4.18, SD = 2.22) than whole word instruction (mean ES = 3.17, SD = 1.15) or oral reading practice (mean ES = 2.34 SD = 1.88). However, based on Cohen's distinctions, all three reading interventions substantially improved the word recognition performance of children with learning disabilities in reading. A single study using letter-naming instruction also demonstrated improvement in letter recognition performance (mean ES = 1.36).

The studies included in the meta-analysis primarily used two types of dependent measures (see Table 38). Seven studies measured oral reading fluency (i.e., number of words read correctly per minute on reading passages) as the dependent measure of treatment effectiveness, while five studies measured oral reading accuracy (i.e., number of words read correctly from word lists). Three studies used idiosyncratic dependent measures: for example, number of letter-naming errors, percent words, letters or sounds read correctly, and number of words read correctly from word lists. All three categories of dependent measures yielded large mean effect sizes: 2.17 (*SD* = 1.80), 3.34 (*SD* = 1.48), and 3.74 (*SD* = 2.43), respectively.

Overall, reading interventions had a greater impact on older students (mean ES = 3.60, *SD* = 2.30) than it did on younger children (mean ES = 2.83, *SD* = 1.72). A single study with a 21-year-old male with severe reading disabilities achieved only a moderate effect (mean ES = 0.67) on word recognition.

SALIENT STUDIES

Several reading studies within the present analysis which resulted in extremely high effect sizes (i.e., ES > 3.0). For example, Thorpe, Lampe, Nash, and Chiang (1981) studied the effects of a phonics instruction technique that employed simultaneous input through multisensory channels. Using a multiple baseline across subjects design, their results indicated that their subjects, three high school students with learning disabilities, read more words correctly after the introduction of multisensory phonics instruction than during phonics instruction utilizing visual–auditory input alone, which was the baseline condition (ES = 4.90). In this intervention, students not only looked at and read the sounds of phonemes in isolation and within words, but also underlined and traced words to provide kinesthetic and tactile components.

A second study that resulted in an extremely high ES (ES = 4.58) was conducted by Darch and Gersten (1985). In this study, four students with learning disabilities were taught beginning reading with a direct instruction program. The teacher systematically varied the rate of instruction and the frequency of praise during the 25 days of the intervention. The results indicated that increases in teacher presentation rate and increased use of praise lead to an increase in the percentage of correct letter and letter combination sounds, sounded-out words, and whole words read. When one examines individual effects, however, a more precise picture emerges. For two students, the most effective reading intervention involved a faster pace of reading instruction along with more frequent praise (ES = 6.06 and ES = 5.36, respectively). In contrast, the other two students in this experiment responded best to more frequent praise alone while learning to read (ES = 6.15 and ES = 7.73, respectively).

Another salient study was implemented by Freeman and McLaughlin (1984). In their study the effects of modeling vocabulary words using a tape recorder on six high school boys' with learning disabilities in sight word reading was examined. Response rates were first recorded during baseline without tape-recorded word practice. Later, response rates were measured immediately following treatment in which students read along with the teacher-modeled words on a tape recorder. Response rates were measured from the same word list used during treatment. The effect sizes for the six students ranged from 1.08 to 6.80. Thus, although all students improved their reading fluency, some students appeared to benefit more than others from this type of reading intervention.

A fourth study that resulted in high effect sizes (mean ES = 3.85) was a cross-age tutoring reading intervention conducted by Chiang, Thorpe, and Darch (1980). Using a multiple baseline design, the researchers evaluated the effects of four 5th-grade students with learning disabilities tutoring 2nd- and 3rd-grade students with learning disabilities on word recognition skills. Results of this study suggest that cross-age tutoring can be mutually beneficial for both tutees and tutors. The reading intervention consisted of 15–20 minutes of daily tutoring. In each session, the tutor modeled correct pronunciation of each word in a stack of flashcards, the tutee repeated it, the tutor asked the tutee to say each word alone, and the tutor praised the tutee for correct responses and corrected errors. Next, the misread word flashcards were separated into a separate stack and the tutor repeated the tutoring process for these words only. During the intervention all tutees improved their reading performance on reading 60 monosyllable words such as "ham" or "nap," while all tutors showed gains in reading multiple syllable words containing one or more of the monosyllables they had taught.

A final study in the current meta-analysis that resulted in high effect sizes was implemented by Rose and Sherry (1984). In this study, an alternating treatment's design was used to determine the relative effects of two oral reading previewing techniques: (1) *silent*—the student reads silently prior to reading a passage out loud, and (2) *listening*—the student reads silently along while the teacher reads a passage out loud, then the student reads the passage out loud. Results from this study showed that in four out of five cases systematic previewing resulted in increased reading fluency over oral reading without previewing. In addition, listening and reading in combination were related to higher rates of words read correctly (ESs: 4.00, 5.03, 8.31, 0.74, 3.17) than was the silent previewing procedure (ESs: 2.01, 1.66, 4.65, 0.32, 3.25).

The study that resulted in the smallest ES (ES = 0.67) involved a 21-year-old male with severe reading disabilities. This study utilized a direct instruction approach to teach to the deficit phonic skills. The intervention consisted of tutorial instruction over a period of 3 months. Instructional targets involved four classes of vowel patterns: R-controlled vowels, short vowels, long vowels, and diphthongs. Despite the moderate ES for word recognition, the authors report a 3-year gain in reading level over the 3-month intervention period.

In summary, the present meta-analytic synthesis of single-subject research suggests that there are several effective interventions for improving the reading skills of students with learning disabilities. Overall, the intervention methods of phonics/direct instruction, whole word training, and oral reading practice improved the word recognition skills of children with reading disabilities in comparison to baseline levels.

SUMMARY

In summary, this chapter provides a comprehensive analysis of single-subject design studies. The results are not unlike those found earlier in Chapter 3. Similar to the findings in our group design studies, the primary findings were that methodological sophistication does influence the magnitude of outcomes. Additional findings were:(1) all domain areas (except handwriting) yield effect sizes at or above Cohen's .80 threshold for a substantial finding; (2) strategy instruction models better predicted ES estimates than direct instruction models when the results were qualified by the reported intellectual and reading level of the participants; (3) instructional components related to drill–repetition–practice–review, segmentation, small interactive groups, and the implementation of cues to use strategies contribute significant variance (15%) to estimates of ES; (4) the high IQ discrepancy groups yield lower ES when compared to the low IQ discrepancy groups in the domain of reading, whereas the reverse effect occurred when tasks were not reading measures; and (5) a Combined Model that includes components of direct and strategy instruction yields higher effect sizes for studies that include participants that (a) meet cutoff score criteria (IQ scores > 85 and reading scores < 90) or (b) meet IQ reading discrepancy score criteria but include participants in the low-average IQ range (85 to 92). As found earlier, the results are supportive of the pervasive influence of strategy instruction and direct instruction models across treatment domains and indicate that variations in sample definition are related to treatment outcomes.

Chapter 5

General Discussion

In this chapter we will review and then discuss the important findings reported in Chapters 3 and 4. Although we coded in excess of 300 variables in our synthesis related to the intervention research, for parsimony our discussions of the results are formulated around seven general findings. Unless otherwise specified, general conclusions from this synthesis are derived primarily from the group design studies.

THE MAGNITUDE OF CHANGE RELATED TO TREATMENT IS GREATER IN SOME ACADEMIC DOMAINS THAN IN OTHERS

The instructional areas we know most about in terms of treatment are in the domain of reading (e.g., word recognition, reading comprehension). The least researched domains are in the areas of intelligence, creativity (e.g., divergent and convergent thinking), and language. Based on Cohen's criteria of .80 as a substantive finding, only studies in the domains of reading comprehension, vocabulary, and creativity approached a threshold for a large effect when the confounds related to methodology were partialed from the analysis. The magnitude was .81 for reading comprehension, .73 for vocabulary, and .78 for creativity.

Studies that produced effect sizes in the moderate range (>.60 and <.70) were in the domains of cognitive processing (.69; e.g., metacognition, attribution, problem solving), word recognition (.65; real word recognition), memory (.66), writing (.66), intelligence (.61; performance on standardized tests), attitude/self-concept (.60; e.g., attitude scales), phonics/orthographic skills (.60; e.g., word skills such as reading pseudowords or recognizing correct spellings), and global achievement (.64; e.g., in terms of teacher grades, class ranking).

Those categories of dependent measures in which effect sizes were relatively weak (<.55) across intervention studies included spelling (.51), mathematics (.45), general reading (.46; these include measures in which word recognition and comprehension cannot be separated or are confounded on standardized tests), social skills (.47; e.g., behavior ratings), perceptual processes (.53; e.g., visual–motor skills, handwriting), and language processes (.50; e.g., listening comprehension).

For single-subject design studies, all domain areas except handwriting yield effect sizes at or above the .80 threshold. The most frequently investigated academic domains were word recognition, mathematics, and writing. Several domains of dependent measures, however, are not reflected in single-subject design research. These are in areas such as language (e.g., vocabulary), creativity, self-concept, and intelligence (e.g., memory).

NOT ALL TREATMENTS ARE EQUALLY EFFECTIVE

Before we isolate effective treatments, it is important to preface our conclusions with four observations. First, we assume that effective treatments (those studies that yield high effect sizes relative to other studies) that reflect diverse theoretical perspectives share some commonalities related to instructional components, tactics, and/or procedures. Our task was to identify those instructional and methodological ingredients that constitute an effective intervention for students with learning disabilities. Thus, we did not rely solely on the label of the independent variable provided by the authors themselves to characterize their treatments. Instead, we coded the methods and instructional components that made up the treatments. Therefore, based upon the occurrence or nonoccurrence of component information, studies were sorted into four general instructional models (Combined Model, DI Alone Model, SI Alone Model, NonDI + NonSI Model) and analyzed. We did not directly compare (although the data exists to be used), for example, effect size differences between peer tutoring (Jenkins & Jenkins, 1985), curriculum-based assessment (Deno, 1985), cooperative learning (Slavin, Karweit, & Madden, 1989), cognitive learning strategies (Deshler & Schumaker, 1988), adaptive educational strategies (Wang, 1992), and so forth. Instead, we focused on the overlapping (those components shared by all effect treatments) and nonoverlapping instructional (those components that independently contribute to outcomes) and methodological components that predict treatment outcomes.

Second, many of the intervention approaches used by public schools and/or clinics for children with learning disabilities have not been adequately researched. Thus, our findings may not match current instructional practices. Several popular interventions for children with learning disabilities were not included in our analysis either because of methodological flaws in published studies or because no data has been published. Some conspicuous interventions that were absent, that were rejected because of methodological flaws, and/or that yield generally weak outcomes were interventions related to medication in isolation of instruction, diet, whole language instruction, consulting teaching models, vision therapy (e.g., Irlen reading lenses), Reading Recovery programs, constructivist models, and so on.

Third, variations in methodology have a profound impact on treatment outcomes. As Table 3 indicates, if studies include control and treatment conditions that differ in (1) teachers, (2) setting, and/or (3) instructional loads (i.e., the steps and procedures of the treatment condition have minimal overlap with the control condition), and if studies fail to report psychometric data on the students with learning disabilities, then these studies yield high effect sizes no matter what the treatment imposed. Thus, we attempted to partial out the artifacts across studies prior to making judgments on potentially effective treatments.

Finally, what we know about treatment is biased by the publication of positive outcomes. The issue we confronted continually in our analysis is whether we could clearly differentiate instructional treatments that supersede others given that the literature is radically skewed toward publishing positive outcomes. This is a formidable task for individuals who conduct a meta-analysis because published manuscripts direct them to conclude that everything works. This conclusion, affectionately called the "the Dodo verdict" (i.e., "Everybody has won and all must have a prize"; see Parloff, 1984; Weisz et al., 1995) emanates from the landmark meta-analysis of Smith, Glass, and Miller (1980). In this synthesis, they found that therapy "is beneficial . . . consistently so and in may ways . . . different types of psychotherapy (verbal or behavioral, psychodynamic, client-centered, or systematic desensitization) do not produce different types or degrees of benefit. . . . It is clearly possible that all psychotherapies are equally effective" (pp. 184, 186).

Our results suggest that this picture is quite different in the area of learning disabilities. We find, generally, that when both published and nonpublished literatures (dissertations) are considered, a *Combined* Direct Instruction and Strategy Instruction Model is an effective procedure for remediating learning disabilities. The important instructional components that make up this treatment include attention to sequencing, drill–repetition–practice, segmenting information into parts or units for later synthesis, controlling task difficulty through prompts and cues, making use of technology, systematically modeling problem-solving steps, and making use of small interactive groups. We also found that regardless of the general model of instruction, only a few instructional components increase the predictive power of treatment effectiveness beyond what can be predicted by variations in methodology and age. These instructional components, the majority of which are reflected in the *Combined Model*, were:

1. *Sequencing*: breaking down the task, fading of prompts or cues, sequencing short activities, giving step-by-step prompts.
2. *Drill–repetition* and *practice–review*: daily testing of skills: for example, statements in the treatment description related to mastery criteria, distributed review and practice, using redundant materials or text, repeated practice, sequenced review, daily feedback, and/or weekly review.

3. *Segmentation*: breaking down a targeted skill into smaller units and then synthesizing the parts into a whole; for example, statements in the experimental condition included breaking down the task into short activities or step-by-step sequences, breaking down the targeted skill into smaller units, breaking the text or problem into component parts, segmenting and then synthesizing component parts.
4. *Directed questioning and responses*: the teacher asks "process-related" and/or "content-related" questions of students; for example, treatment may include dialectic questioning, students are directed by teacher to ask questions, teacher and student engage in dialogue, the teacher asks questions.
5. *Control difficulty or processing demands of a task*: tasks are sequenced from easy to difficult and only necessary hints and probes are provided to the child; for example, statements in the treatment reflect short activities with the level of difficulty controlled, the teacher provides necessary assistance, the teacher provides simplified demonstration, the task is sequenced from easy to difficult, discussion is given to a task analysis.
6. *Technology*: for example, use of a computer, a structured text, or flow charts to facilitate presentation; utilization of a structured curriculum, emphasis on pictorial representations, use of specific or structured material, use of media to facilitate presentation and feedback.
7. *Modeling of problem-solving steps by teacher*: teacher provides a demonstration of processes or steps to solve problem or explains how to do a task; for example, writing, comprehension, decoding words.
8. *Group instruction*: instruction occurs in a small group; students and/or teacher interact within the group.
9. *A supplement to teacher and peer involvement*: may include homework, or a parent or someone else who assists instruction.
10. *Strategy cues*: reminders to use strategies or multisteps; for example, the teacher verbalizes problem solving or procedures to solve, instruction makes use of "think-aloud" models, teacher presents benefits of strategy use or procedures.

We used a three-tier procedure to arrive at the above conclusions. In the first tier of our analysis we focused on two general (although not mutually exclusive) instructional models the literature considers as having a positive influence on treatment outcomes. We considered one approach (direct instruction) a bottom-up model and the other (strategy instruction) a top-down model. There has been lively debate over the years in the literature as to whether instruction should be top-down, emphasizing the knowledge base, heuristics, and explicit strategies, or bottom-up, emphasizing hierarchical instruction at the skill level (e.g., Adams, 1990; Palincsar & Brown, 1984; Vellutino & Scanlon, 1991). We considered both approaches viable for students with learning disabilities. Thus, in our analysis, we began by examining these two approaches as competing models.

The first approach we considered was direct instruction. Direct instruction studies were operationally defined in the following manner. In addition to looking for self-descriptive key words (e.g., the term *direct instruction* was assigned to the treatment approach) and looking at the instructional focus (e.g., a focus on skill) of the treatment, we labeled treatments as direct instruction if they included some of the following instructional components: (1) administering drills and probes, (2) administering feedback repeatedly, (3) rapid pacing of instruction, (4) allowing for individual instruction, (5) breaking the task into steps, (6) using a pictorial diagram, (7) instructing in a small group, and (8) having the teacher ask direct questions (e.g., "What sound does this letter make?"). With strategy instruction, we again looked for key words reflected in the description of the treatment (e.g., the term *strategy instruction*) and looked at the instructional focus (intervention focuses on processes, such as metacognition). We labeled treatments strategy instruction if they included some of the following methods: (1) systematic explanations and/or verbal elaborations of that direct task performance; (2) verbal modeling, questioning, and demonstration by the teacher of multiple steps and/or processes; (3) systematic reminders to use strategies, tactics, or procedures; and (4) verbal modeling and "think-aloud" models provided by the teacher to solve a problem.

Three findings emerged from this first tier of analysis: (1) strategy instruction produces larger effect sizes than those studies that do not use such procedures; (2) direct instruction models yield higher effect sizes than the nondirect instruction models; and (3) when strategy instruction and direct instruction presentation orders are varied in a regression model, strategy instruction bolsters outcomes (i.e., improves the R^2 of the ES estimate) independent of the contribution of direct instruction. Thus, the two models operate independent of each other.

Given that the two models were weakly correlated ($r = .17$), the results provide support for an independence model (i.e., both models make independent contributions to ES). However, we found that only 1% of the variance for direct instruction and 2% of the variance for strategy instruction was related to estimates of ES after the methodological composite score was entered in the analysis. Thus, the results of the first tier of analysis yield results of equivocal practical importance.

For the second tier of our analysis we divided the two general models into four models (Combined Direct Instruction and Strategy Instruction [Combined DI + SI], SI Alone, DI Alone, and NonSI + NonDI). We found that the Combined Model yields higher effect sizes than the three competing general models. Thus, for the second tier of the analysis, we found that although both strategy and direct instruction contribute independent variance to outcomes, the Combined Model was superior to the other three models across studies.

We also addressed the issue of whether the four models were actually reflective of distinct treatments (discriminant validity) by analyzing the instructional composition of each approach. Significant differences were found between the models in terms of the frequency of instructional components, as well as in terms of components significantly related to the magnitude of effect sizes. Three components of the Combined Model were distinct from the other models in predicting effect size. Those components were related to attributions about strategy, teacher modeling of problem-solving steps, and instruction occurring in the context of small interactive groups.

For the third tier of analysis, we ignored the four general models and attempted to isolate those components of instruction that predicted ES. Those components that optimally predicted ES estimates across all categories of dependent measures were sequencing, drill–repetition–practice, controlling task difficulty, segmentation of information, technology, small interactive groups, augmentation of teacher instruction (e.g., via homework), directed questioning/responding, and strategy cuing. The important findings were that only 9 of the 20 components significantly contributed to ES estimates. When the results from the comparisons of the four general models and the WLS regression models were collapsed, 10 instructional components were identified (listed above) as important components in predicting effect size. These findings coincided nicely with those of the single-subject design studies when the unit of analysis considered each dependent measure as independent of others. Those components in single-subject design studies that predicted effect sizes were drill–repetition–practice, segmentation, small interactive groups, and strategy cuing.

Thus, our general conclusion from this three-tier analysis is that not all treatments or instructional components are equally effective in predicting ES estimates. Interestingly, we did not find support for a common assumption that intense one-to-one instruction, no matter what the curriculum or combinations of methods, will prove effective (see Vellutino et al., 1996, for a discussion of this model). For example, our analysis suggests that one-to-one instruction also yields lower effect sizes than group instruction combined with one-to-one instruction.

SOME TREATMENT EFFECTS ARE SPECIFIC TO THE ACADEMIC PROBLEMS

Based on the previous discussion, the Combined Model (a model that includes the components of sequencing, drill–repetition–practice, segmentation, directed response/questioning, control of task difficulty, technology, small interactive groups, supplements to teacher instruction and strategy cuing) is a solid research-based approach towards the effective instruction of students with learning disabilities. As with any heuristic, however, the model reflects a general approach to remediation, and therefore needs modification, refinement, and/or elaboration when applied to isolated academic domains. Thus, there are instances in which various combinations of the Direct and Strategy Instruction Models (and by implication the instructional components that make up these models) interact with domains of instruction (e.g., reading, mathematics, writing). In the present synthesis, we found that the various combinations of the four models (Combined Model, DI Alone Model, SI Alone Model, and NonDI + NonSI Model [i.e., small group and individual instruction]) interacted across reading-related versus non-reading-related domains and within the reading-related domains (real word recognition vs. reading comprehension).

Before we summarize our findings related to the treatment × domain interactions, we must make three comments. First, we reconfigured the treatment domains in our regression analysis by collapsing the 17 general categories (see Table 3) into four general contrast variables. These contrast variables reflect a progression from general treatment domains to specific domains. This reconfiguration was carried out to control for obvious confounds (correlations) related to treatment and domain. That is, a common problem in synthesizing treatment research is that the independent variables (e.g., strategy training or phonics instruction) and dependent measures (e.g., metacognition or phonological awareness) are sometimes correlated. This occurs because the treatments use activities, probes, and/or materials. in their daily instruction that overlap considerably with the dependent measures. Thus, to partially control for this confound, we clustered the dependent measures into four general contrast variables. The first contrast variable compared high language domains (such as reading, writing, spelling) with areas that make fewer demands on language or reflect fewer specialized language skills (e.g., mathematics draws on visual–spatial processing skills, as well as language skills). The second contrast variable compared reading measures and nonreading measures. Reading is clearly the most researched domain in learning disabilities; therefore the outcomes of studies that include reading measures were compared to all other domains. The third contrast variable focused on the important transfer measures of reading real words and reading comprehension. That is, the purpose of reading intervention for students with learning disabilities is to increase their ability to read words and understand text. A final contrast variable focused on comparing low-order skills (the category of dependent measures related to word skills) with high-order processes (the category of dependent measures related to cognitive processing).

Second, the four general treatments (Combined DI + SI, DI Alone, SI Alone; NonDI + NonSI) were also reconfigured into various combinations. One contrast compares an undifferentiated model of strategy or direct instruction (a treatment with high overlapping and minimal overlapping instructional components) with a model void of the majority of DI and SI components (referred to as the NonDI + NonSI Model). This latter model primarily reflects the components of one-to-one and small group instruction. This comparison addressed the issue of whether intense one-to-one and/or group instruction is just as effective as the competing DI Alone and/or SI Alone Models. The second contrast variable compares a bottom-up model (DI Alone) with the top-down instructional model (SI Alone). This contrast considers the issue of whether instruction in a domain is best predicted by a bottom-up or a top-down model. The final contrast variable compares the Combined Model with all other models.

Finally, we did not investigate potential three-way interactions between domain × treatment and related variables (aptitude, setting of instruction) because of the limited number of studies that could actually fill the various cell sizes in such an analysis. Instead we partialed from the analysis setting and aptitude variables to better isolate treatment × domain interactions.

The important findings related to the WLS regression analysis of main and two-way interactions for domain and treatment were as follows:

1. The Combined Model is more effective on reading-related measures (e.g., word recognition and comprehension) than on non-reading-related measures (e.g., mathematics, social skills).
2. The effectiveness of the Combined Model is particularly pronounced on reading comprehension measures when compared to reading recognition measures.
3. Bottom-up instruction (DI Alone) yields higher effect sizes than top-down instruction (SI Alone) models on word recognition, but not reading comprehension measures.
4. Classifications of dependent measures into very broad domains of tasks highly embedded in language (e.g., reading, writing, spelling), less embedded in language domains (e.g., social skills, mathematics, attitude), or subskill or process domains of transfer measures (e.g., phonics and metacognition may underlie word recognition and reading comprehension, respectively) were not sensitive to the influence of the treatment model combinations.

Taken together, there are two important findings. First, our results support the notion that a certain level of treatment specificity emerges across academic domains. The comparison of outcome measures showed that the effectiveness of the Combined Model is most pronounced on reading-related domains. Second, the results indicate that the advantages of bottom-up instruction when compared to other models emerge primarily on word recognition measures.

Why is this second finding important? The conception of reading as a bottom up process, is firmly rooted in intervention for LD readers (e.g., see Gittelman & Feingold, 1983; Lovett et al., 1990). Researchers who support the bottom-up model reason that accurate word recognition is a necessary condition for comprehension, and therefore emphasize oral word recognition and decoding in reading instruction. Instruction in processing begins with letter features, which give rise to letter identification, which in turn lead to word recognition. Once readers learn to recognize words, they translate that ability into some sort of code, and derive meaning in much the same manner as when listening to spoken language (see Byrne et al., 1992, for a review). Although several instructional approaches emphasize bottom-up processes in which meaning is constructed from the sum of letters, words, and sentences on a page, skilled reading has also been viewed as an interactive process between low- and high-order processing components (Adams, 1990). Thus, sharp divisions exist about the most effective method of teaching reading (see Palincsar & Brown, 1984; Chall, 1967; Vellutino & Scanlon, 1991, for a review). Not surprisingly, divergent conceptions of the reading process have yielded a difference of opinions in how best to meet the needs of readers with learning disabilities. For example, in contrast to the bottom-up model, other models of reading assume that meaning construction proceeds from the reader's internal knowledge base rather than from the page (see Dole, Duffy, Roehler, & Pearson, 1991, for a review). In this top-down approach, reading success is viewed as dependent on the reader's cognitive and language abilities, including familiarity with the topic of discourse, perspective, and knowledge of syntax (e.g., Baker & Brown, 1984; Palincsar & Brown, 1984; Paris et al., 1984; and see Pressley et al., 1990, and Wong, 1991, for a review). These instructional approaches focus on (1) understanding the gist of topics, (2) summarizing information to differentiate important from unimportant ideas, and (3) deciding whether a question must be answered with prior knowledge alone or with a combination of prior knowledge and text information.

Given the different theoretical orientations of these approaches, the superiority of the Combined Model over others in the reading comprehension domain is an important finding. The results are consistent with the notion that an individual's lower-order and higher-order skills interact in order for her or him to gather meaning from text. Clearly, comprehension of text cannot occur without some critical threshold of word recognition skills. LD children vary in these skills. What was unclear from the literature, however, is how treatments that focus on high- or low-order skills vary in outcomes. It appears that the bottom-up model is only pronounced at the word recognition level, whereas both approaches (the DI Alone and SI Alone Models) are comparable for predicting ES in the reading comprehension domain.

A synthesis of single-subject design studies also supports the notion that a certain level of treatment specificity emerges, at least within the reading domain. However, the level of specificity differs considerably from the group design studies. For single-subject design studies, the Combined Model yields higher effect sizes on nonreading than on reading measures. Further, in contrast to group design studies, the Combined Model yields smaller effect sizes on reading comprehension than on word recognition and nonreading measures. For single-subject design studies, reading comprehension appears to yield higher effect sizes with the DI Alone or SI Alone Models relative to the other treatment approaches. The differences in findings between single-subject and group design studies may be because the single-subject design studies comprised a proportionately smaller number of subjects in reading comprehension studies, or it may be because of the proportionately larger number of studies in nonreading domain areas (e.g., mathematics). Consistent with the group design studies, however, treatment effects did not occur at the skill or process level.

Taken together, the results converge on the notion that intervention approaches are more effective in some domains than in others. The impact of instruction at specific domain levels must be qualified by the type of research design (single subject vs. group design) and focus of instruction. Regardless, an analyses of both types of designs support the presence of treatment × domain interactions.

FEW COMPONENTS ARE SALIENT IN PREDICTING EFFECT SIZES WITHIN DOMAINS

Our results support the notion that the shared variance among instructional components (i.e., the combination of certain instructional components) is more important than any one component in isolation in predicting ES estimates. This is because (1) instructional components do not appear in isolation within a treatment and (2) in many cases their importance as predictors is enhanced in the context of other components. For example, phonics instruction not only includes instructional components related to segmentation (breaking words into rhymes or isolated sounds), but also occurs in the context of drill–repetition–practice, small group instruction, technology (structured materials), and so forth. We were interested, however, in identifying those isolated components that may predict ES independent of the other components. On this issue our results indicated the following:

1. *Word Recognition.* None of the 20 instructional components in isolation predicted (met a critical alpha) the general category of real word recognition. For the experimental measures that included real words, however, there was a pattern ($ps < .05$) that components related to drill–repetition–practice, attributions, and segmentation influenced ES. The instructional component of segmentation is related to increases in ES for experimental measures that reflect phonological processing.
2. *Reading comprehension.* The teachers' (or experimenters') modeling of strategies is an instructional component that predicts ES.
3. *Spelling.* Sequencing of lessons and segmentation are components that predict ES.
4. *Mathematics.* None of the 20 instructional components in isolation predicted (met a critical alpha) the general category of mathematics. An emerging pattern was that small interactive groups (as in reciprocal teaching) are predictive of ES.
5. *Writing.* In a reduced regression model, orientation to task was predictive of ES.
6. *Cognitive processing.* Peer modeling, segmentation, small interactive groups, and strategy cuing are components predictive of ES.
7. *Single-subject design studies.* Regardless of the unit of analysis, one component that predicted ES estimates was the use of small interactive groups. When the effect sizes were not averaged within studies, the components that positively predicted effect size were drill–repetition–practice, small interactive groups, and strategy cuing.

In sum, only a few components in isolation predict ES estimates within a domain (e.g., segmentation predicts outcomes on phonological measures and strategy cuing predicts outcomes on processing measures). Thus, although we were able to isolate components that independently predict effect sizes, the largest amount of variance related to ES (approximately 17%) occurs when instruction reflects the variance shared across specific components.

LD CHILDREN ARE CLOSER IN PERFORMANCE TO NLD CHILDREN WHEN TREATMENT CONDITIONS INCLUDE STRATEGY INSTRUCTIONS

Regardless of the treatment, the general trends in the findings were that NLD students (age-related peers) outperform LD students. The few significant variables that positively moderated ES between LD and NLD (i.e., decreased the effect size differences in performance) occurred when (1) variations in the instructional components between treatment and control were minimal, and (2) there was substantial psychometric information on the LD children. More important, we found that when variables related to method, reported versus nonreported setting, type of setting, size of instructional group, direct instruction, strategy instruction, age, degree of discrepancy, intelligence, and severity of reading are entered in a predetermined order or in a nonhierarchical fashion in a regression analysis, the only significant effect to emerge is strategy instruction. The results indicated that the ES differences between LD and NLD were significantly smaller when LD children were exposed to treatments that included strategy conditions than when compared to the competing treatment conditions.

HOW THE LD SAMPLE IS DEFINED INFLUENCES OUTCOME

We addressed two common assumptions related to sample characteristics and intervention. The first assumption is that the sample characteristics are irrelevant to the effect of treatment approaches. Support for this assumption emerges when treatment effects are independent of the characteristics of the sample. This assumption is derived from behavioral treatments that focus on the functional relationships between contingencies in the classroom context and the intensity and reliability of treatment delivery. Such procedures place secondary importance on sample description.

Our results across group design studies suggest that variables related to gender and age were independent of treatment effects. Thus, no matter what the gender ratio for instruction or the age of the sample, the main effects of treatment across these variables are statistically comparable. We found in our regression modeling that younger children yield higher effect sizes when setting, methodological, and aptitude variables were partialed from the analysis. However, all age levels produced high effect sizes, suggesting that instructional procedures are effective across a broad age spectrum.

No support for the above assumption (treatment effects are independent of the characteristics of the sample) was found, however, when the aptitude variables of intelligence and reading severity were considered. The results related to the influence of psychometric scores on ES can be summarized as follows:

1. Studies that report less psychometric information yield larger effect sizes than studies that report more psychometric information.
2. Those studies that report no information on IQ reveal higher effect sizes than those studies that report some information on IQ.
3. Those studies that report no information on reading or report reading scores below a standard score of 85 yield higher effect sizes than those studies that report reading scores between the standard score of 84 and 91 or greater than 90.

The results related to the IQ × Reading severity interaction are:

1. Those studies that produced the highest effect sizes had no psychometric information on intelligence or reading *or* report the smallest discrepancy between intelligence and reading (intelligence scores between 84 and 91 and reading scores between 84 and 91) when compared to other studies that report higher IQ (intelligence scores >91) and reading scores between 84 and 91.
2. Those studies that yielded the lowest effect sizes reported reading scores that were higher than intelligence scores (i.e., reading scores are above a standard score of 90 and intelligence scores are in the standard score range of 84 to 90) *or* report reading scores between 84 and 90 with no information on intelligence.

Taken together, these studies suggest that there are some sample characteristic variables that influence treatment outcome. Perhaps the most important is that studies that report minimal information on the psychometric characteristics of the sample produce higher effect sizes (i.e., inflate effect sizes) than studies that report standardized scores related to intelligence, reading, and mathematics. Thus, we found that intelligence scores play a critical role in predicting ES when reading is severe or in the average range, but less of a role in the moderately deficient range.

The results also showed that some treatments interacted with subject characteristics. For example, in the single-subject design studies, larger effect sizes occur for strategy instruction than for nonstrategy instruction when the reported reading scores are severe (<85) or in the moderate (>84 and <90) range. Likewise, for group design studies that include reading measures, we found that the positive effects of direct instruction are most pronounced for studies that include children with severe reading problems or those studies that fail to report reading severity. Those studies that report reading scores in the moderate or average range yield lower effect sizes with direct instruction models when compared to studies that use competing models.

Another key assumption in the field we addressed is that different subtypes of LD children respond differently to treatment. Historically, in the LD literature, as well as in practice, interest has been expressed in the value of subgrouping ability groups on isolated psychological parameters (e.g., visual learners vs. auditory learners; reading-disabled learners vs. math-disabled learners; whole word readers vs. phonetic readers). Perhaps the main rationale for such practices was to reduce the heterogeneity within the sample and therefore better match different subtypes to various instructional approaches. Within our data set, we provide one of the most comprehensive reviews of the LD intervention research that includes subgroups. On this issue, the findings of our synthesis across treatment studies is clear: (1) there is no agreed-upon subtype in which to make comparison across studies, and (2) a minuscule number of studies investigate whether subgroups (subtypes) of LD students responded differently to treatments. Stated simply, our synthesis suggests that the relationship between typology (subgroup) and treatment outcomes has a weak database. Thus, we did not find support for a belief asserting that effective instruction for the learning disabled is based on an analysis of individual processing strengths and weaknesses.

Perhaps the most important findings related to treatment outcomes are that the sorting of studies into operational definitions and nonoperational definitions did influence treatment outcomes. Reading scores at or below the 25th percentile in reading recognition (see Stanovich & Siegel, 1994; Siegel & Ryan, 1989) and standardized intelligence performance above 84 have been considered as critical cutoff scores for defining learning disabilities. The treatment validity of such a cutoff score definition, however, has not been tested as a function of treatment outcomes. Three contrast variables related to the definition of learning disabilities were considered: one compares studies that report psychometric information (report reading and/or intelligence scores) versus those studies that fail to report psychometric information, another compares studies that meet a cutoff score in reading at or below the 25th percentile (i.e., the 25th percentile is a standard score of 90) and report intelligence scores >84, and a third compares relativity high-IQ-discrepancy-defined samples (IQ is above 90) and low-IQ-discrepancy-defined samples (IQ scores below 90 but above 84). Results related to the latter two contrasts are of more interest than those that contrast studies that report psychometric criteria and those that do not. Unfortunately, we were unable to make comparisons to nondiscrepancy-defined groups because many of these children were excluded from the synthesis (i.e., the majority of studies include previously identified LD samples and most are placed in special education on discrepancy criteria).

The important results related to definition suggest that cutoff scores and variations of IQ in discrepancy scores qualify treatment effects. Of primary interest is how these definitions interact with the Combined Model. For both group and single-subject and group design studies, the Combined Model yields higher effect sizes when cutoff scores can be computed than when cutoff scores cannot be computed. For single-subject design studies, the Combined Model yields higher effect sizes for the lower IQ discrepancy studies when compared to those studies that report discrepancies, but with relatively higher IQ scores.

METHODOLOGICAL VARIATIONS HAVE A SIGNIFICANT IMPACT ON TREATMENT OUTCOMES

The mean ES values generated by our current analysis suggest that the previous estimates of magnitude were inflated (Swanson et al., 1996). Our previous meta-analysis reported a .91 ES for direct instruction and a 1.07 ES for strategy instruction, whereas the current analysis reports .82 for direct instruction and .84 for strategy instruction. This is because the previous meta-analyses (1) used unweighted least squares to estimate ES estimates, and/or (2) failed to partial out the influence of variations in methodology, and therefore generated mean effect values at a higher range.

The results of the current synthesis show that there are a number of other key variables related to methodology that can influence treatment outcome. Although we took care to differentiate the ES for those studies that made comparisons between conditions from those studies that used repeated measures, a number of effects related to methodology still influenced outcomes. Before we indicate those variables, we will discuss those methodological variables that in isolation did not seem to have an influence on treatment outcomes.

One variable that did not significantly influence ES was the number (or intensity) of instructional sessions. Although studies with shorter instructional sessions were seen to have a trend toward larger effect sizes than those that had longer sessions (greater than 31 sessions), this trend was not significant. This finding implies that (1) most treatment effects emerge quickly (shorter number of sessions) and (2) sustained treatment over a long period of time does not yield high effect sizes. The issue of generalization, however, was not addressed in this analysis. Another variable that did not seem to be critical was variation in materials (commercial or experimentally developed) between the control and experimental condition. Specifically, although there was a trend that the use of different materials between treatment and control conditions yield slightly higher effect sizes, there were no significant differences in ES. Another methodological variable that did not appear to be important in isolation is the "focus" of the control condition. We reasoned that control conditions that focus on the very same domain as a treatment condition would yield smaller effect sizes than those control conditions (because some variation is controlled) that focus on a completely different domain (i.e., mathematics vs. reading). We found a trend that the same domain as treatment had a slightly higher effect sizes when compared to the other types of control conditions. However, this comparison was not significant.

Surprisingly, the variables related to treatment integrity and our internal validity rating scale did not separate the studies in terms of the magnitude of ES. These two variables, however, were included in our methodological composite score. Although not significant in isolation, another methodological variable added to the composite score was the type of treatment assignment (random vs. nonrandom). Although we found a slight trend that those studies that provided no information on how treatments were assigned to subjects yielded larger effect sizes, these conditions did not vary from studies that used a random assignment of treatment or those that used no random assignment of treatment. Again, this methodological variable was used in the composite score and its added effect had an influence on treatment outcomes.

The results clearly show that outcomes are influenced by variations in some methodological variables. Those isolated methodological variables that yield significant effects on the magnitude of ES estimates are summarized as follows:

1. Studies that used a different teacher between control and experimental groups yielded significantly larger effect sizes than those studies that used the same teacher.
2. Those studies in which control and experimental treatment occurred in a different setting (e.g., classroom vs. resource room) yielded significantly higher effect sizes than those that occurred in the same classroom setting.
3. Those studies that relied on experimental measures yielded significantly higher effect sizes than those studies that relied on standardized measures.
4. Those studies that were published in dissertations yielded significantly lower effect sizes than those published in journals.
5. Those studies that had a *low* overlap in terms of the number of instructional components between control and experimental conditions yield significantly higher effect sizes than those studies that have a high overlap in terms of instructional components (sequences, steps, methods, and procedures).
6. Those studies that did not report the setting in which the intervention occurred yielded significantly lower effect sizes than those that did report the setting.

In terms of setting characteristics, the results for group design studies (as stated above) are clear. Setting information was further divided into those studies that reported treatment occurring in the self-contained classroom, the resource room, and the regular classroom. Significant differences related to setting occurred for group design, but not single-subject design studies. For group design studies, the highest effect sizes occurred in the resource room when compared to other settings. No significant differences emerged between studies that took place in a self-contained, regular classroom, or that report no information on the setting.

A pessimistic conclusion from the above observations is that almost any intervention that varies from the control condition in terms of setting, teacher, and number of instructional steps (and whose results are published in journals) yields larger effect sizes than any study that fails to control for such variations. Thus, poor methodology must be taken into consideration when interpreting treatment effects. For example, of the four studies that included treatments in the regular classroom, two involved administering the experimental condition in one school and the control condition in another school. Thus, different teachers and settings confounded any meaningful interpretation of treatment effects.

We think probably the most serious threat to interpreting treatment effects is situations in which intervention studies "stack the treatment condition" with more steps and procedures than the control condition. This artifact alone guarantees that the experiential condition will unequivocally yield higher effect sizes than studies with minimal overlap across all designs and domains (single-subject and group design, LD vs. NLD, reading vs. nonreading.)

In sum, we found substantial support for the assumption that artifacts related to methodology have a profound influence on treatment outcomes. However, we also found that when we partialed out the weighted composite score related to methodology, significant effects related to the type of treatment emerged.

QUALIFICATIONS

Before we discuss the implications of our findings in the next chapter, we would like to qualify any conclusions we might make. First, very few state departments of education or research organizations provided us with technical reports. Therefore, we cannot generalize our findings beyond published articles and dissertations. Although data were readily available across categories of children placed in special education in unpublished reports or state department documents, no state department or research organization provided treatment data (i.e., means and standard deviations) that focused primarily on LD students.

Second, we placed only a few restrictive parameters on how the primary authors of the intervention studies defined learning disabilities. We initially relied on whether studies "reported" that LD students or students with similar labels (e.g., dyslexics, reading disabled, educationally handicapped) were in the sample and were provided with treatment above and beyond their classroom placement. Thus, our synthesis was clearly biased toward studies that use previously defined children or adults classified as learning disabled by the schools, clinics, and the like. Eventually we refined this too generous criterion in two ways. First, we removed studies ($N = 74$) that did not state that the sample was in the average IQ range. We noted that many of these studies (approximately 54) included subjects with intelligence scores below 80, and thus the sample was more appropriately classified as mildly retarded. Based on this preliminary analysis, we implemented the criterion that the studies must state that the sample is in the average range of intelligence. Therefore, a general stipulation in the studies we synthesized is that the Sample Description section of each study states that LD students were in the normal range of intelligence and experienced problems in an academic or behavioral domain.

Second, because of the bias toward identified samples, we also implemented a computer search of articles that emerged for the combined terms "high risk" and "treatment" or "intervention" or "instruction." We conducted a hand search of the top five journals over a 30-year period (see Table 2) to locate intervention studies that included samples of children considered at risk for learning disabilities who meet two psychometric standards. These studies of "nonidentified" LD students were included in our synthesis only if IQs were reported to be at or above 84 (or if it was reported that subjects were in the average range based on standardized scores) and a standardized achievement score was reported (or stated) to be at or below the 25th percentile. Thirty-four studies of this type were located. Eighteen of them were included in our synthesis and 16 were eliminated because of methodological flaws (e.g., inability to calculate effect sizes) and limited sample information.

Some may argue that our inclusion criteria for studies in the present synthesis were still not restrictive enough. We must argue in reply, however, that if we had been unduly restrictive in how studies defined learning disabilities, we would have eliminated approximately 50% of the studies in our data pool. For example, if we had insisted that only published group design studies with reported IQ and reading scores be included, only 17 studies in the reading recognition domain and 18 in the reading comprehension domain would have been included in the synthesis. Unfortunately, this narrowing of the studies would not have provided an accurate picture of the intervention research that exists within special education for these particular students.

Third, we did not direct our analysis of state or district policies on how LD samples are defined. The only variable we used to capture the influence of policy on the sampling procedures was whether studies stated that participants exhibited a discrepancy between potential (usually reflective of an IQ test) and achievement (usually reflected by scores on some standardized achievement measures). This variable was dummy coded (studies mention discrepancy or related term plus state that students are 1 or more years behind vs. other studies). According to Mercer, Jordan, Allsopp, and Mercer (1996), most states (34) attempt to operationalize learning disabilities by reporting a discrepancy between intelligence and achievement. Consistent with this finding, the most frequent basis for selecting LD subjects (>70% of the studies; however, only 16% of the studies explicitly stated that subjects were at least 1 year behind in achievement) stated by the primary authors of studies was that the participants exhibited a discrepancy between academic performance and intellectual performance. However, we found this variable problematic because most studies report discrepancies across all sorts of achievement domains. Unfortunately, we did *not* test whether broadly defined samples versus narrowly defined discrepancy-defined samples provide greater external validity for intervention effectiveness (although that data was available to us). We did find, however, those group design studies that included reading measures yielded higher effect sizes for studies that reported participants a year or more behind in achievement versus those that reported participants a year or less behind in achievement.

Thus, we sorted studies by a priori sample characteristics. Based on the literature, we imposed our own definitions of learning disabilities for comparisons between studies rather than relying on federal, state, or particular school district definitions. Although there should have been greater homogeneity in our sample selection in terms of matching subject characteristics to the specific treatments (e.g., LD children exhibit clear deficits in reading as opposed to mathematics performance when placed in a reading intervention program), we assume that those learning difficulties addressed in the present studies bear a logical relationship to the target intervention.

Fourth, it is important to note that many of the studies published prior to 1980 did not meet the methodological criteria for inclusion in our analysis. No doubt, methodological factors that we examined in the articles and dissertations may create a bias in what we analyzed. On the other hand, it is worth mentioning that we used a number of sensitivity analyses (e.g., weighted regression analyses of methodological variables, investigating the relationships between measures and year of publication) to analyze variables that best predicted overall treatment effects. If effect sizes were related to the unreliability of measurement, range restrictions, or incomplete information, and so forth, these were taken into account when explaining treatment effects.

Fifth, we made a fairly conservative conclusion about the efficacy of current instructional programs for students with learning disabilities. Our conservatism emerges for several reasons. For example, in only a few studies did we find a condition in which LD students "approximate" the performance of chronological age-matched peers. Although a cursory review of our tables (e.g., Table 1) would suggest that there are several intervention programs that work with LD children, it would be an incorrect conclusion to suggest that such children can be successfully remediated in the academic domains in which their deficits reside. Rather we would prefer to take the position that there are some credible studies within the LD field that do produce moderate effect sizes when the artifacts related to methodology are partialed out. These effect sizes are qualified when these studies are classified on such variables as the amount of psychometric information available on subjects, the degree to which the treatment varies from the control condition on instructional steps and materials, and whether the study uses standardized measures or experimental measures, and so on.

Finally, our synthesis indicated that the majority of studies published on intervention for students with learning disabilities are poorly designed, have poor internal validity, fail to indicate if the LD sample is in the normal range of intelligence, and/or fail to provide usable information. We found approximately 900 studies that actually reported data, but less than one-third of those studies met the criteria for inclusion in our synthesis. Thus, approximately *two-thirds* of the studies that report intervention outcomes for students with learning disabilities have flawed designs (e.g., no control condition). In addition, of those studies that were included in the synthesis, less than 5% actually would be considered credible studies according to the methodological criteria (i.e., high weighting on the methodological composite score; see Table 4) we have outlined. These criteria are cumulative scores related to internal validity, treatment integrity, adequacy of description of the control condition, breadth of sample description, adequacy of treatment sessions and sampling procedures, and use of reliable dependent measures. This is not meant to be a pessimistic conclusion on the state of intervention research in learning disabilities, but only to provide direction for future publications and funding needs for children with learning disabilities.

SUMMARY

In summary, this chapter has highlighted seven general findings from the synthesis. Although this text provides a synthesis of intervention research conducted in the last 30 years for students with learning disabilities, our discussion of the major findings certainly does not exhaust the database. However, we can address some basic questions that have eluded the field of learning disabilities for some time. For example, we can now answer questions about what is an effective approach to instructing students with learning disabilities. We can also highlight the components that make up that approach. Thus, the current findings, combined with an earlier meta-analysis (Swanson et al., 1996), provide evidence that educational intervention for students with learning disabilities produces positive effects of respectable magnitude. The magnitudes of these effects for a substantial proportion of the educational treatments are in a practical range of importance by most teaching standards. Of course, other questions can be addressed. For example, we are able to address the issue about the importance of how samples with learning disabilities are defined. We demonstrated how critical information on the sample (such as IQ and reading scores) plays an important role on prognosis to treatment. We also can address questions about the domains of instruction. For example, we know a lot more about some academic areas (reading) than others (mathematics). What we have not addressed are the implications of the synthesis. The next chapter considers the implications of the findings in the areas of theory, practice, and policy.

Chapter 6

Implications

In this chapter we will address the implications of our synthesis. The outline for discussion includes (1) methodological issues that emerged across the group versus single-subject design studies, (2) theory and intervention research, (3) principles of instruction, and (4) policy issues related to instruction.

METHODOLOGICAL ISSUES

As reviewed in Chapter 5, there is a clear relationship across studies between methodological procedures and ES. Methodological variables significantly predict effect sizes across all intervention domains. What has not been directly addressed is the relationship between group design and single-subject designs in terms of interpreting treatment outcomes.

Group-Design Studies

We found many flaws in the various group design studies in terms of their internal validity. The most serious threats to interpreting LD group design research were clearly related to (1) classroom by treatment confounds and (2) the unit of analysis (i.e., nonindependence for treatments administered in groups). The majority of group design studies in our synthesis suffer from a classroom by treatment confound, which occurs when the treatment is implemented in one classroom and the control occurs in another. Although some interesting information can be derived from a study of this design, such a design makes assessment of the impact of learning extremely difficult. To overcome this issue the study must treat each classroom as an experimental unit in which the classroom mean scores replace the individual scores. In addition, in most of the studies analyzed, treatment procedures were implemented in small groups. Thus, student scores are not independent because they are influenced by the dynamics unique to small group sessions. For example, during a small-group presentation some student's behavior might be disruptive and have a negative learning effect upon the other students in the small group. Given that the disruption can negatively impact the score, those scores cannot be considered independent. Unfortunately, few if any studies reported mean scores of instructional units.

Single-Subject Design Studies

In terms of interpreting effect sizes at the mean level, group design and single-subject design effect sizes are somewhat comparable. That is, when the last three variable sessions of baseline and treatment are used to calculate effect sizes in single-subject designs, and the intercorrelations between baseline and treatment are partialed out, effect sizes for single-subject designs are generally in line with those for group design studies. Further, there are similarities between the two types of design studies in terms of sample definition, reported IQs and chronological age, number of instructional sessions, length of instructional sessions, sample segmentation (gender, ethnicity), and number of experimental measures used in the study. However, this is not to say there were no differences in outcomes related to the two designs. We considered five.

First, single-subject studies yield higher effect sizes across all domains (except for handwriting) than do group design studies. This finding would have been even more pronounced had effect sizes for single-subject designs been computed using Cohen's *d* across all baseline and treatment sessions. Under these conditions, effect sizes were almost a standard deviation higher for single-subject studies than for group design studies. Thus, single-subject design studies generate an unusual form of variance (one based on intraparticipant variances), which may not be compatible with conventional variance statistics in group designs.

Second, fewer and, in some cases, different components of instruction predict effect sizes between the two designs. On the surface, it appears that any intervention that uses a single-subject design works. That is, few moderator variables predicted ES when compared to the group design studies. This is probably because the homogeneity of variance is easily satisfied in single-subject design studies, whereas it is seldom satisfied in group designs.

Third, some of the findings related to single-subject design studies reflect a greater focus on skills, such as word recognition and computation, than on high-order activities, such as reading comprehension and problem solving. Although both types of designs focused on word recognition to a high degree, single-subject designs frequently focus on low-order skills such as mathematical computation and spelling, whereas group designs focus frequently on high-order skills, such as reading comprehension. The domain of writing is a frequent area of investigation for both types of designs. However, single-subject designs focus more on the mechanics of writing, while group designs focus on such areas as writing coherence. Underrepresented areas of study in the single-subject designs are word skills, such as phonological coding and language processing. Also underrepresented in the single-subject designs are studies on vocabulary, attitude, and, surprisingly, social skills.

Fourth, the two types of designs vary on internal validity. Single-subject designs are more likely than group design studies to suffer from floor and ceiling effects in the dependent measures. However, the percentage of overlap between the control and treatment conditions in procedures and steps of instruction is substantially higher in the single-subject design than in the group designs.

Finally, we found that the instructional component that best predicted effect sizes in single-subject designs is paradoxical. For single-subject designs, the single best predictor, after methodological variables are partialed out, is small group instruction. As we mentioned earlier, when group instruction is a medium of treatment presentation, then the unit of analysis should be the composite scores of the groups rather than the scores of individual subjects.

There was some overlap, however, when the two designs attempted to identify those instructional components, that when combined, accounted for most of the variance in effect sizes. For single-subject design studies, the components of drill–repetition–practice, segmentation, small interactive groups, and strategy cuing are important predictors of ES. For group design studies, sequencing, drill–repetition–practice, segmentation, directed response/questioning, control of task difficulty, technology, small interactive groups, mediation or augmentation of instruction by someone other than peers or teachers, and strategy cues were important predictors of ES. Thus, there is overlap on four components between single-subject studies and group design studies. No doubt, the overlap between the two designs gives some validity to the importance of these variables. The group design studies add an additional five variables to the instructional model.

THEORY AND INTERVENTION RESEARCH

The findings of this synthesis pose two conceptual problems for the field of learning disabilities. The first problem relates to the common assumption that specific lower-order processing deficits (e.g., problems in word recognition, word skills, spelling) are the major contributors to academic problems in LD students. The second problem relates to the assumption that learning disabilities are not due to poor instruction, but instead reflect information processing constraints, primarily in the area of language. Both of these assumptions would predict that some domain areas are more amendable to intervention than others. Related to these issues, however, the LD participants in these intervention studies exhibited no deficit that would suggest that one process is more resistant to treatment than another. Because low-order processing deficits have been primarily tied to the reading domain, we would expect extremely low effect sizes in reading (of .10–.20 magnitude) when compared to other domains. This did not happen in the present synthesis. Interestingly, all domains of reading (comprehension, word recognition, word skills) showed moderate effect sizes. The lowest effect sizes occurred in the domain of mathematics (.45) and when reading comprehension and word recognition were confounded (.44).

How does one reconcile these outcomes of intervention research with current models of learning disabilities that suggest that academic problems are related to specific processing deficits? We suggest that the results of this synthesis are consistent with most information-processing models of individual differences (e.g., Kail & Bisanz, 1993). These models suggest that elementary processes are best understood in the context of their combination with other operations. Although it is important to identify elementary processes that underlie LD readers' performance, such an approach may not be sufficient for explaining how cognitive processes are organized and work in unison to remediate academic deficits.

Three possible explanations can be garnered to explain the lack of "specificity" (i.e., performance in one domain is more resistant to change than performance in another domain) in intervention effects. The first means of reconciling the conceptual problem of "specificity" is to suggest that academic difficulties reflect "bootstrapping effects" (see Stanovich, 1986, p. 364, for a discussion of this concept). For example, in the area of reading, Stanovich (1986) stated: "Many things that facilitate further growth in reading . . . [for example,] general knowledge, vocabulary . . . are developed by reading itself" (p. 364). Thus, due to the mutual facilitation between reading and cognitive processing, such interrelationships would be expected to increase with skill improvement. The implicit assumption, however, is that deficits in lower-order skills underlie such bootstrapping effects, and that the majority of domains investigated reflect secondary problems.

Our hesitation in accepting this assumption was that the effect sizes between LD and NLD students were minimized on strategy when compared to nonstrategy conditions. If there is a core problem at a low level of processing, then one would not expect interventions that primarily focus on higher-order processes (metacognition) to supersede interventions that focus on the core deficits. Such was not the case in this synthesis.

On the other hand, one may argue that because of specific processing deficits, LD students engage in compensatory processing to gain information across a wide array of domain areas. Strategy instruction facilitates such compensatory processing. That is, a weakness at one level of processing (e.g., the phonological level) is compensated for by a greater reliance on skills that are intact at other levels (Stanovich, 1980); strategy instruction facilitates such compensation. The most common example of this hypothesis is applied to word recognition. For example, because of LD readers' poor phonological coding ability, such children's word recognition is augmented by visual, semantic, nonverbal, and contextual clues (e.g., Stanovich, 1980). Support for a compensatory hypothesis can be tested several ways (also see Walczyk, 1993, for compensatory model predictions). Most directly, the relative differences across domains can be compared. Again, we find no indirect evidence across the intervention studies *within* the language domain that suggests that greater gains occur in one domain when compared to another.

The second explanation suggests that no one process in isolation dominates others. Although several studies indicate that deficiencies in LD readers are related to phonological processes (e.g., Stanovich & Siegel, 1994), additional studies indicate problems in orthographic (e.g., McBride-Chang et al., 1993), semantic (e.g., Zecker & Zinner, 1987; Waterman & Lewandowski, 1993), metacognitive (e.g., Wong, 1987), and working memory (e.g., Siegel & Ryan, 1989; Swanson & Alexander, 1997) processes.

Another means of reconciling the specificity issue is to suggest that higher-order cognitive processing problems can exist in LD children *independently* of their specific problems in lower-order processes, such as phonological coding. Thus, LD children may be viewed as having difficulty accessing higher-level information and/or lower-order skills (phonological codes), or as switching between the two levels of processing. Several studies have characterized LD children as having difficulties in executive processing that relate to checking, planning, testing, and evaluating their performance (e.g., see Wong, 1991, and Swanson, 1993, for a review). Difficulties in coordinating multiple pieces of information have been applied to LD children in various information-processing models (e.g., see Pressley's [1991] good information processor model) and strategy intervention programs (e.g., see Wong, 1991, for a review).

Regardless of these explanations, some would argue that our inability to find areas that show *a resistance to change in some domains* (low effect sizes related to other domains), especially in the area of reading, undermines the concept of specificity. This argument, however, falters for three reasons. The first is that the notion of specificity does not necessarily need to be isolated to a few deficient domains. Rather, a more appropriate conceptualization may be that a cognitive deficit is reflected in a specific *operation,* such as manipulating, representing, storing, or allocating resources. The second reason is that individual differences in higher order processes (e.g., metacognition) have been found to be independent of general intelligence. That is, individuals with lower and higher cognitive processing skills, but with average or above average intelligence, perform differently on reading tasks (Daneman & Carpenter, 1980). Thus, a multitude of lower- and higher-order processes may operate independently of intelligence (as measured on psychometric tests).

The third reason is that the concept of specificity is not dependent on establishing a direct link between deficient cognitive mechanisms and intervention outcomes. This is because reading, math, and other academic domains involve the concurrent execution of several subcomponent processes in an interactive, hierarchical, and/or opportunistic fashion (e.g., Frederiksen & Warren, 1987; Hayes-Roth & Hayes-Roth, 1979; Rumelhart, 1977). That is, reading is not necessarily unidirectional in terms of beginning at the lowest level with phonological processing and proceeding upward to higher-order processes. Thus, the attempt to reduce LD children's reading difficulties to an isolated mechanism is not sufficient if one is to have a complete picture of intervention outcomes. Although it is essential to identify deficient elementary processes in LD students, how these processes coalesce into general operations and "how" instruction may facilitate this coalescence may provide a more complete picture of the information-processing ability and treatment outcomes for students with learning disabilities.

In sum, we would argue that in the context of intervention, a focus on isolated skills or processes (e.g., word skills, metacognition) may not be an appropriate focus. Processing components seldom act independently of other processes when an individual is engaged in a meaningful cognitive activity (such as the domains reflected in the current synthesis). Our synthesis identified some instructional components that together influence performance across a broad array of domains. We also suggest that what appears to moderate outcomes are levels of severity related to intelligence and reading and not necessarily isolated processes. Based on our findings related to the Combined Model, effective instruction is neither a bottom-up nor a top-down approach in isolation. Lower-order and higher-order skills interact in order to influence treatment outcomes. Obviously, performance at complex levels (writing prose, inferring the meaning of text) cannot occur without some critical threshold of skills. Children with learning disabilities vary in these skills. What is clear, however, is that varying degrees of success across treatment domains interact with treatments that focus on high- and low-order instruction (i.e., strategy instruction and direct instruction).

We think that cognitive models of instruction (as reflected in strategy instruction) have made a significant contribution to the intervention literature on learning disabilities. It seems overly simplistic, however, to assert that all students with learning disabilities benefit from systematic cognitive instruction. Because direct instruction and strategy instruction are complex combinations of various components, we would not argue that strategy instruction has better support than direct instruction for treatment outcomes. Thus, there are many commonalities between strategy intervention programs and direct instruction programs. No doubt, there are clear differences in focus. Cognitive interventions focus on routines and planful action and/or general principles of handling information, whereas direct instruction focuses on isolated skill acquisition to support higher-order processing. However, much of the teaching in both approaches occurs in an explicit manner, relying on oral presentation by the teacher and oral responses by the students. Thus, although directive instruction has been associated with the behavioral paradigms, cognitive paradigms use some of the same procedures. This point is illustrated in an article by Swanson (1988) that suggests that in practice both cognitive and behavioral models use many of the same procedures (e.g., feedback, monitoring, repetition). Thus, unless studies are coded at the instructional component level, one cannot clearly differentiate instructional approaches.

Our results clearly show that combinations of these specific components that reflect both of these orientations enhance treatment outcomes. It is clear, however, that merely sequencing material, providing drill repetition and practice of skills, using peers as mediators, and employing reinforcement or probing provides an *incomplete* characterization of effective intervention models across various domains. Perhaps the only compelling evidence we have that instructional research supports a general framework about strategy differences in students with learning disabilities is that strategy studies contributed independent variance to effect sizes and this model and not direct instruction narrowed the gap between LD and NLD children. Based on the frequency of positive outcomes related to strategy models across studies, we can assume that the LD student may be viewed as having poor or inefficient strategies (i.e., is not a good information processor) for approaching the complex requirements of academic tasks, and so is unable to meet his or her academic potential. The LD student may be further characterized as an inefficient learner, one who either lacks certain strategies or chooses inappropriate strategies and/or generally fails to engage effectively in self-monitoring behavior.

Given these assumptions and the findings that emanate from the present synthesis, two questions emerge: What rationale can be provided to continue further instructional research from a cognitive orientation when compared to other treatment orientations? and What general principles of such instruction must be further tested before a cognitive approach becomes a viable and testable model?

In answer to the first question, two advantages to conceptualizing LD students' cognitive abilities in terms of strategy deficiencies for the present and future intervention research are considered (several advantages are discussed in Swanson, 1990):

1. *A focus is placed on what is modifiable.* We did not find any academic domain, cognitive process, or social skill that was not responsive to instruction. Perhaps learning disability is best conceptualized in terms of children who have cognitive processes that are highly susceptible or less susceptible to instruction, rather than in terms of fundamental or general differences in ability. Thus, rather than focusing on isolated elementary processing deficiencies, strategy research focuses on types of questions that are more educationally relevant. For example, a focus is placed on what LD students can do without instruction, what they can do with instruction, what can be done to modify existing instruction, and what can be done to modify existing classroom materials to improve instruction.

2. *It allows for theorizing and instructional development.* For example, materials can be developed to maximize strategy use. Effective instruction entails (a) information about a number of strategies, (b) how to control and implement those procedures, and (c) how to gain recognition of the importance of effort and personal causality in producing successful performance. Further, any of these components taught in isolation is likely to have rather diminished value in the classroom context.

Given the above rationale for strategy or cognitive models of instruction, the second question that must be addressed involves the major instructional principles that must be tested (see Rosenshine, 1995). The principles listed below have been tested in a laboratory setting (see Levin, 1986, and Swanson, 1989, for a review), but need to be addressed within the context of classroom settings (Swanson, 1984).

PRINCIPLES OF INSTRUCTION TO BE TESTED IN SUBSEQUENT INTERVENTION RESEARCH

Several articles from laboratory research have suggested principles for effective instruction. The ones discussed below are adapted from Levin (1986, 1988), Pressley (1994), and Swanson (1989). These guidelines, derived from experimental studies on cognition, learning, and memory, provide bases for evaluating the principles that can be derived from the intervention research. We will review each guideline and comment on how existing intervention research further informs (or does not inform) us about the validity of those principles.

Instruction Must Operate on the Law of Parsimony

This principle was directly addressed. The WLS regression model indicated that only 9 of the 20 possible components predicted ES estimates in group design studies and only 4 of the 20 possible in single-subject design studies. Thus, a high saturation of components (entering all 20 in the regression model) does not increase performance.

Components related to effective strategy instructional programs are reviewed by Pressley, Borkowski, and Schneider (1989). Some of these components include advance organizers (to provide students with a type of mental scaffolding upon which to build new understanding; i.e., organizers tap information already in the students' minds and give them new concepts to help them organize this information), organization (information questions directed at students to stop them from time to time to assess their understanding), elaboration (thinking about the material to be learned in a way that connects the material to information or ideas already in their mind), generative learning (learners must work to make sense out of what they are learning by summarizing the information), and general study strategies (e.g., underlining, note taking, summarizing, asking questions, outlining, and working in pairs to summarize sections of materials), think about and control one's thinking process (metacognition), and attributions (evaluating the effectiveness of a strategy). A number of the "multiple component packages" that are tested in the present synthesis (e.g., Chan et al., 1990; Englert et al., 1992; Graham & Harris, 1989a; Olsen, Wong, & Marx, 1983; Sawyer et al., 1992; Schunk & Rice, 1992; Wong et al., 1994) include some of these components. Other components that were encompassed in some of the studies include the following: skimming, imagining, drawing, elaborating, paraphrasing, mnemonics, accessing prior knowledge, reviewing, orienting to critical features, and so on. The best of these programs involve (1) teaching a few strategies well rather than superficially, (2) teaching students to monitor their own performance, (3) teaching students when and where to use a strategy in order to enhance generalization, (4) teaching strategies as an integrated part of an existing curriculum, and (5) teaching that includes a great deal of supervised student feedback and practice.

The problem with such intervention packages, however, at least in terms of instructional intervention, is that little is known about *which* components best predict student performance. Further, as we found in our synthesis, those studies that "load" the treatment condition with minimal overlap to the control condition, bias, as well as obscure, treatment outcomes. The multiple component approaches that are typically found in LD strategy intervention studies must be carefully contrasted with a component analysis approach that involves the systematic combination of instructional components known to have an additive effect on performance (see Graham & Harris, 1989b, and Sawyer, Graham, & Harris, 1992, for progress in this area). We assume that good instructional strategies are composed of the *sufficient* and *necessary* processes for accomplishing their intended goal, consuming as few intellectual processes as necessary to do so (Pressley et al., 1992; Pressley & Ghatala, 1990). The current synthesis addressed this issue. In the present synthesis, we were able to identify a few key instructional components that predict effect sizes. Thus, demonstrating change on a dependent measure did not appear to require extensive multicomponent intervention packages.

The Use of Effective Instructional Strategies Does Not Necessarily Eliminate Processing Differences

If LD children are presented an instructional strategy that allows for the efficient processing of information, then improvement in performance is assumed to affect the same processes as in NLD students. However, this assumption cannot be tested in the present synthesis. One means to test this assumption is to compare the effect sizes between LD versus NLD students in an academic domain (e.g., reading comprehension or word recognition) *and* the effect sizes in a domain assumed to underlie that domain (metacognition or phonics skills). Unfortunately, the small number of studies that included both academic and cognitive measures, as well as included both LD and NLD subjects, prevented our testing of this principle.

Instructional Strategies Serve Different Purposes

A test of this principle occurs by determining whether different instructional components can predict ES as a function of the academic domain. This principle can be tested by determining whether the instructional components that predict effect sizes across studies are the same components that predict effect sizes within domains. A review of Table 10 is relevant to this issue. As Tables 9 and 10 show, there were some components that emerged within domains in the prediction of ES that matched the components that emerged across studies. Further, some individual components played a greater role in predicting effect sizes in some domains than in others. This may have occurred for a number of reasons; but the most probable reason is the meager number of studies reflected in some domains.

As a number of intervention studies we review in the Appendices indicate, many intervention studies have looked at enhancing LD children's performance through the use of advance organizers, skimming, questioning, taking notes, summarizing, and so on (e.g., Borkowski, Weyhing, & Carr, 1988; Chan, 1991; Englert et al., 1992; Gajria & Salvia, 1992). But apart from the fact that LD students have been exposed to various types of strategies, the question of which intervention strategies are the most effective for a particular academic domain is unclear (or at least obscured in the present synthesis). We know in some laboratory situations, such as in remembering facts, that the key word approach appears to be more effective than direct instruction models (Scruggs & Mastropieri, 1989). However, it appears reasonable to assume that the rank ordering of different instructional strategies changes in reference to the different types of learning outcomes expected. Thus, it appears that certain instructional programs (e.g., decoding) are better suited to enhancing students' decoding of words or their understanding of what they previously read, while other strategies (e.g., summarization) are better suited to enhancing students' text comprehension (Gajria & Salvia, 1992). The point is that there are a number of ways that different and/or combinations of instructional strategies can affect different cognitive outcomes, but the current analysis was unable to dissect the subtle strategy differences on performance outcomes. For example, strategies for writing (e.g., Englert et al., 1992; Welch, 1992) had some of the same steps and procedures as strategies for reading comprehension (e.g., Chan, 1991), but different combinations of writing strategy versus reading comprehension strategy instruction components predicted effect sizes.

In sum, our synthesis supports the assumption that certain components play more of a role than others in predicting ES within domains. When the methodological variables were partialed out in the present analysis, the synthesis indicated that different components and different combinations of instructional components significantly predicted effect sizes. There was no one *combination* of instructional components that cut across all dependent measures in predicting effect sizes that also occurred within domains.

Comparable Performance Does Not Mean a Comparable Process to Instructional Strategies

This principle cannot be addressed by the current synthesis. That is, because of the limited number of effect sizes, we could not test whether instructional variables interact with aptitude variables in predicting effect sizes between LD and NLD children. Testing of the above principle in subsequent intervention studies is important, however, for two reasons. First, there have been recent studies (Swanson, 1993) that suggest that LD students use different strategies than NLD students on tasks in which they seem to have little difficulty; it is likely that these tasks will be overlooked by the teacher for possible intervention.

Second, it is commonly assumed that because LD children have isolated processing deficits and require instructional strategies to compensate for these processing deficits (e.g., using context to identify a previously unknown word), they process information comparable to their normal counterparts on those tasks with which they have little trouble. Yet several authors suggest that there are a number of alternative ways for achieving the correct response, and there is some indirect evidence that LD children may use qualitatively different mental operations and processing routes than their NLD counterparts (Shankweiler, Liberman, Mark, Fowler, & Fisher, 1979). Unfortunately, these assumptions cannot be assessed within the context of this synthesis of literature because there were few studies that included normal achieving children.

Strategies Must Be Considered in Relation to a Student's Knowledge Base and Capacity

In the present synthesis, we did find that variations in IQ play a significant role in predicting treatment outcomes. In fact, IQ scores interacted with direct instruction for group design studies that included reading measures and with single-subject design studies that included strategy models. However, few studies directly tested whether the students' domain-specific knowledge base (e.g., high and low knowledge of a domain) interacts with treatment outcome. Some support for this assumption, however, has been found in the experimental literature. Numerous authors (e.g., Borkowski & Turner, 1990; Harris & Pressley, 1991; Levin, 1986, 1988; Marks et al., 1993; Pressley et al., 1992) suggest that there must be a match between strategy and learner characteristics. One important variable that has been overlooked in the LD intervention literature is processing constraints (Swanson, 1984). Most LD instructional research has, either implicitly or explicitly, considered cognitive capacity (a hardware problem) to be a confounding variable, but researchers have made little attempt to measure its influence.

In sum, the principle related to capacity constraints could not be directly addressed in the present analysis. However, the relationship between general knowledge constraints (as reflected in IQ scores) and intervention outcomes was supported. Unfortunately, few studies from the present synthesis of literature addressed the notion of processing constraints. Thus, we cannot address issues about "how" or "what" processes related to "compensatory" instruction will improve academic performance.

Comparable Instructional Procedures May Not Eliminate Performance Differences

This principle was clearly supported. Several of the intervention studies reviewed indicated that residual differences remain between LD and NLD children even when the LD children are instructed in strategy use (Chan, 1991; Gelzheiser, 1984; Graham & Harris, 1989b). For example, in a study in the present synthesis by Gelzheiser (1984), LD and NLD children were compared on their ability to use organizational strategies. After instruction in organizational strategies, LD and NLD subjects were compared on their ability to recall information on a posttest. The results indicated that LD children were comparable in strategy use to the NLD children, but were deficient in overall performance. The results basically support the notion that groups of children with different learning histories may continue to learn differently, even when the groups are equated in terms of strategy use. Thus, while a learning disability may involve difficulties in learning to use a strategy, some of these LD students will require additional intervention to equate performance differences with their normal achieving counterparts.

Good Instructional Approaches for NLD Students Are Not Necessarily Good Approaches for LD Students

This principle could not be tested in this synthesis. In the present synthesis, it must be emphasized that we found no domains in which treatment results of the LD students exceeded those of the NLD students on posttest outcomes. Although some instructional programs (i.e., strategy instruction) may better bridge the gap between LD and NLD students, this is so because the NLD participants primarily served as a control condition and therefore were not exposed to the experimental condition. Thus, we were unable to test whether interactions would have emerged if both LD and NLD students were exposed to the same treatment. To address this principle we would have to determine whether an interaction occurs between LD and NLD students as a function of instructional condition. The majority of studies we reviewed did not directly compare LD and NLD students, and/or report interactions.

Instructional Strategies as Taught Do Not Necessarily Become Transformed into Efficient Generalization Strategies

We could not test this principle. In the current synthesis, very few studies actually tested transfer and generalization effects related to treatment. A nicely designed study by Lovett et al. (1994) that was included in our synthesis did evaluate the transfer of reading skill instruction on spelling measures. Lovett et al. found generalization to spelling on the word recognition decoding task that was coupled with a strategy component. Thus, there was some generalization between reading skills that required the ability to transform certain reading strategies and apply them to spell correctly. This study suggests a need to detail the mechanisms that allow children to take what they learn and generalize it to another activity.

One of the mechanisms that may help future research and generalization training is to teach children the transformation of strategies. This principle is based on the assumption that one mechanism that promotes expert performance is related to strategy transformation (Pressley, Brown, El-Dinary, & Allferbach, 1995). It often appears that children who become proficient at certain tasks have learned simple strategies, and that through practice they discover ways to modify the strategies into more efficient and powerful procedures. In particular, the proficient learner uses higher-order rules to eliminate unnecessary or redundant steps in order to hold on to increasing amounts of information. The LD child, in contrast, may learn most of the skills related to performing an academic task and may perform appropriately on that task by carefully and systematically following prescribed rules or strategies. Although LD children can be taught strategies, some evidence suggests that the difference between LD and NLD children (experts in this case) is that the latter have modified such strategies to become more efficient. It is plausible that the LD child remains a novice because he or she fails to transform simple strategies into more efficient forms.

POLICY ISSUES RELATED TO INTERVENTION RESEARCH

Next we will discuss four implications of the present syntheses related to policy and the funding of intervention research. These relate to funding practices, publication, definitional/classification issues, reading, and special education placement. We will attempt to generalize, as well as to qualify, from our synthesis findings related to each of these issues.

Funding and Publication

The results indicated that many of the methodologically sound studies cite no funding source. We also found a slight trend that some funding sources are isolated to some academic domains. Another interesting finding is that a large number of the studies that we rejected from our synthesis—because we could not calculate their ES (and other sorts of methodological variables that contaminated our interpretation)—do cite a funding source. We also found that a large number of these rejected studies were published in major special education journals. Thus, indirectly, there may be a relationship between studies we considered credible and funding/publication variables. For us, a particularly interesting finding was that few intervention studies build upon each other (as indicated by the citations, frequency of similar authors, institutional affiliation of studies). A further vexing situation is that minimal information is available regarding the fidelity (treatment integrity) and/or degree to which intervention studies actually carry out their announced treatment approach. Because intervention studies as a whole cannot as yet address some rather straightforward questions (e.g., what instruction works with a particular child with certain learning characteristics?), we conclude that more comprehensive and methodologically sound intervention research is needed.

One of many possible solutions to some of the above problems is to increase the *veracity* of the studies that show positive outcomes. Few studies provide measures of treatment integrity, and even fewer intervention studies do follow-ups or independent replications of their findings. Perhaps the lack of follow-up studies and independent replication is a "policy and/or researcher consensus problem." Intervention researchers are leery about their work being replicated, in much the same way that teachers don't like the idea of somebody verifying their claims that reading program *X* worked with student *A*, but not with student *B*. A common defense when outcomes differ from what is in the mainstream is that the replication was done poorly and that the particular version of the intervention created by the investigators did not represent well the intervention as studied previously. Sometimes this defense is appropriate, but at other times replication failure should be taken seriously (see Pressley & Harris, 1994, for a review of these issues). A change in the consensus of opinion about independent replication appears appropriate. The following four suggestions should be considered (also see Pressley & Harris, 1994, whole issue, for review):

Suggestion 1

We could learn more about what works with LD children if intervention studies were replicated by independent research groups. A simple reform of publication practices is called for: editors of research journals in the field of learning disabilities should publish *only* those intervention studies that include an independent replication. This would, of course, include studies that yield different conclusions.

Suggestion 2

Another simple reform could be instituted by funding agencies (e.g., U.S. Department of Education). They should insist that they will grant research intervention dollars *only* if applicants guarantee high internal validity and will assure independent replications. If this reform were carried out, the number of grant awards would surely decrease by some fraction. The positive outcome of this reform, however, would be some sort of truth in advertising about the importance of credible intervention studies with LD students. What is a credible study? *A credible empirical study, quite simply, is one that is methodologically sound. Credibility is a function of the study's internal validity characteristics, plain and simple* (see Pressley & Harris, 1994).

Suggestion 3

Another reform involves the consumers (teachers, administrators, and policymakers) of LD research. They should learn to value research that has passed the test of peer review and replication. We found many examples of research studies cited in the literature for students with learning disabilities even though these studies had not been tested scientifically. Part of the problem relates to the sophistication (actually, the supposed lack of sophistication) of the teacher as a consumer. There is a consistent trend to dummy-down research for teachers (and administrators, and policymakers). Thus, researchers fail to communicate and teachers fail to adequately identify a credible study.

Suggestion 4

Our fourth reform calls for placing emphasis on the technology of transfer *only* when an accumulation of credible intervention studies is replicated. A related problem is that some researchers believe that replicating complex cognitive and social interactive conditions is almost out of the question. It could be argued, however, that it might not be the replication of intervention research in various contexts that is at issue, but rather the research base behind the generalizability of effective procedures. The technology of transfer needs to be less interpretive and more explicit. This means that a rigorous approach should not be compromised because of the variability that emerges in various classroom settings, but rather that the technology of transfer must also include a high degree of rigor.

Definitional Issues and Intervention Outcomes

An important issue to consider when evaluating intervention research is the validity of how LD groups are defined and what role these definitions play in predicting treatment outcomes. In our synthesis we found that the detail to which a sample is defined (i.e., how much psychometric information is provided, whether cutoff scores can be calculated, and whether the discrepancy groups have IQs in the low average or average range) interacts with combinations of strategy and direct instructions approaches in predicting treatment outcomes.

Our synthesis only partially addressed the issue of whether discrepancy-defined groups responded differently than did groups who had achievement scores that were in the same range as their IQ scores. As Figure 4 (from Chapter 3) illustrates, those studies that include samples with IQs in the 85–90 range and reading scores in the 85–90 range yield higher effect sizes in treatment outcomes than studies that include samples with IQs in the 90+ range and reading scores in the 85–90 range. We say "partially addressed" because our sorting of studies into different definitional categories may not reflect variables that underlie how subjects were selected for intervention in the first place. For example, we relied on standard reading scores as a means of sorting studies for analysis, but some of the studies included groups with a broad array of academic difficulties, of which reading was only one of the problems.

Regardless, our synthesis clearly indicated that one of the most frequent identifiers of LD children provided by the primary authors, across all studies, is that some "sort of" discrepancy exists between the targeted sample's current grade placement and/or IQ and their current achievement. Perhaps the implicit assumption for the inclusion of discrepancy groups is that children who experience reading, writing, math, and/or other difficulties, unaccompanied by a low IQ, are distinct in processing from the general, "run-of-the-mill" poor, garden variety, slow, or mildly retarded learners. Yet the validity of this assumption has been seriously questioned. That is, when compared to nondiscrepancy-defined poor achievers, LD-defined groups are more similar in processing difficulties than different (e.g., Stanovich & Siegel, 1994; however, see Fuchs, Mather, Fuchs, & Lipsey, in press, for a different view).

How can intervention research address this conceptual issue? We will briefly review issues on the usefulness of operationally defined groups, which in turn will serve as a basis for introducing the concept of "definitional validity" as related to treatment intervention. To understand the challenges of discrepancy-based classification and treatment outcomes, however, we need to review briefly the important conceptual issues.

Discrepancy Definitions

Several studies have argued against the idea that generally backward and specific reading retardation groups are distinct (see reviews by Fletcher et al., 1994, Siegel, 1992, and Stanovich & Siegel, 1994). These studies indicate that children classified with learning disabilities (specifically in the area of reading) reflect a normal distribution of a multifactorial trait in reading characteristic of other poor readers (Fletcher et al., 1993; Stanovich & Siegel, 1994). In short, discrepancy-defined and nondiscrepancy-defined groups of poor achievers are more alike than different. (However, see Fuchs, Fuchs, & Mather, in press, for a comprehensive meta-analysis that challenges this assumption.)

The implication of these findings is that a major construct of the field has been ostensibly weakened (see Mercer et al., 1996, for a review). We say "weakened" because the impact and implications of such findings, to date, have not filtered down to actual diagnostic practices at the state or district level. In contrast, most of the discussion in practitioner-related journals focuses on the differences between objectively measured domains, such as reading, and general intelligence. This discussion focuses on the reliability (e.g., lack of stability related to the regression toward the mean) and/or methodology (formulas) for calculating discrepancy scores (e.g., Reynolds, 1981; Shepherd, Smith, & Vojir, 1983). Thus, discussion has been isolated to methodology (more conservative formulas that account for such issues as regression and overidentification), not necessarily to issues of construct validity (meaningful classification systems). In essence, the refinement of methodology (comparing formulas in terms of their ability to identify accurately) has operated independent of the construct validity issue (i.e., similar to an argument that a test may be reliable but not necessarily valid).

Several criticisms for the line of research that compares discrepancy and nondiscrepancy groups and that finds no differences in performance can be garnered. These criticisms are not powerful in and of themselves because they are limited to indicating problems in the depth of our knowledge, rather than to actually isolating serious conceptual flaws. We will briefly list these criticisms, then proceed to more substantive issues related to definition and intervention outcomes.

First, there is a mismatch between conventional wisdom and research outcomes. Most laypeople view learning disabilities as reflecting some sort of difference between what an individual really can do and what the individual actually does in certain situations (Swanson & Christie, 1994). While models of learning disabilities do not have to match a layperson's understanding, the notion of discrepancy is a frequently reported phenomena by parents of LD children and by LD adults themselves (Gerber & Reiff, 1991). (The weakness of this argument, of course, is that people who are generally slow in all academic areas may also operate with the notion that "I have more potential than I am showing.")

Second, there has been very little empirical evidence available on the validity of a discrep-

ancy score other than between intelligence and reading. A discrepancy in discriminating between groups may have validity in the deficient areas of mathematics, problem solving, writing, and so on.

Third, we don't know why a discrepancy emerges between IQ and achievement (e.g., reading) in a psychological sense (in contrast to statistical artifacts). Very little research has directly focused on understanding the determinants and consequences of a discrepancy.

Fourth, most research designed to test the discrepancy model is conceptualized in terms of searching for the association of deficits. Support for the null hypothesis provides a very insecure basis for theorizing. That is, findings that differences between poor readers and LD readers are statistically comparable or variations of a score on the same reading continuum are not theoretically compelling. More compelling is the possibly of dividing discrepancy groups into subgroups in terms of those who show disassociation in processes and those who do not (similar to Torgesen and Morgans [1990] rationally defined subgroups). In neuropsychology, for example, there has been a tendency to deemphasize associations and to place greater reliance on *disassociation* as a source of theoretical insight (Shallice, 1988).

Fifth, several important questions are not answered in this line of research. For example, "Is the discrepancy score merely an artifact or is there something that mediates this difference that has not been controlled in subsequent studies?" One could make the argument that the right questions haven't been asked or studied. That is, "Do the learning difficulties of children with learning disabilities stem from problems different from those characterized as poor learners without an IQ discrepancy?" is not the right question to ask. Rather, the right question is "Which processes that supersede reading, but are in the cognitive domain, mediate the emergence of discrepancies and nondiscrepancies in low achievers?"

Substantive Issues

Although the above arguments are serious, they are not compelling. It is our argument that attempts to validate the use of potential achievement discrepancies in the identification of LD children rests on some very key assumptions *of which some of those assumptions are related to intervention research.* In a nutshell, our argument is that current classification procedures merely reflect the artifacts of difference scores discussed in the literature of the 1950s. If we are to make progress in accurately classifying children as learning disabled from a discrepancy model, some key assumptions must be met. These assumptions are provided below.

1. *Construct integrity.* The beginning step in capturing the notion of a discrepancy is to define the measures and match those measures to the construct definition. A critical test of the construct validity of discrepancy groups as distinct from nondiscrepancy groups stands a greater chance of being assessed if the constructs included in the classification of groups are firmly grounded in theory. Most critically, there is little reason to believe, and certainly a lot of empirical support to disbelieve, the contention that some arbitrarily weighted function of

two variables (IQ and reading recognition) will properly define a construct (see Cronbach & Furby, 1970, p. 79).

Although several intervention studies in our syntheses relied on the WISC-R and standardized achievement tests to determine discrepancy scores, this is not an argument for conceptual integrity within a research study. Most studies use discrepancy scores as a basis for defining groups *as if* such scores were independent of construct validity concerns. Neither theoretical rationale nor any empirical evidence is available to substantiate the claim that IQ tests (e.g., WISC-III, WISC-R) capture the construct of "potential." Put quite simply, it is just not the case that individuals with comparable IQ have the same potential. For example, an accurate testing of a discrepancy versus a nondiscrepancy definition of LD is based on the assumption that IQ tests are related to processes of critical importance to potential and achievement. Unfortunately, a difference between an intelligence score on the Wechsler and a serious performance deficit on the Wide Range Achievement Test in the area of reading is not a valid test of the discrepancy model. Neither test fits into a theoretical framework of intelligence or reading.

2. *Independence of measures.* Discrepancy scores (or discrepancy-defined groups) are correlated with their component parts, and therefore the discrepancy measure will relate significantly to other variables correlated with the component parts (Cronbach & Furby, 1970). That is, when different scores are correlated with their component parts, there is a greater than chance tendency for them to be correlated with other variables that are also associated with those component parts. An example of this rule is as follows. We know that reading recognition (word skill accuracy) is highly correlated with measures of phonological awareness. Therefore, when (a) reading recognition is part of the discrepancy score, and (b) when groups are comparable on reading recognition performance, then performance is comparable on processes (phonological awareness) related to reading. Thus, the potential for a relationship between a discrepancy group and a nondiscrepancy group on a number of processes related to reading is high because the discrepancy group is little more than a surrogate for the poor reading group. This problem (called "circularity in findings") has been recognized in the literature for some time (Cronbach & Gleser, 1953). In fact, it can be demonstrated that systematic relationships between component (correlate scores) and difference scores exist even when the difference scores are generated randomly (Wall & Payne, 1973). For example, Wall and Payne (1973) demonstrated that when the components related to job satisfaction included the use of how the job *should be,* versus the way it *actually is,* the discrepancy scores were correlated with the component measures, even when component scores were assigned randomly to subjects.

More specifically, it is reasonable to assume that a spurious relationship exists when the observed relationship between two variables (e.g., intelligence and reading) is largely attributable to the relationship between both variables and a third variable. Thus, when discrepancy and nondiscrepancy groups are compared, it is imperative that the mediating variables shared between the two groups be partialed out before a clear test of differences can occur.

3. *Direction of outcomes.* The direction of the discrepancy must be consequential in performance outcomes. A critical assumption in testing the discrepancy model is that differences in the direction of the profiles are important. The fact that somebody has a high reading score in combination with a low intelligence score should reflect a different set or level of interrelations among processes than a student with a high IQ score but a low reading score. Interestingly, this basic assumption has not really been subjected to direct test in the literature. Consequently, a major assumption in variable selection for classification purposes, that the direction of the discrepancy is theoretically consequential (Cronbach & Furby, 1970), has not been proven. The field of learning disabilities, of course, assumes that the direction in which the discrepancy occurs is important. From the studies we synthesized, however, we found a few studies that reported *higher* reading than IQ scores. Further, these studies yielded higher effect sizes than studies that reported IQs above 90 and reading scores below 85.

Our point is that no study equating different uses of discrepancy scores has been done to determine if direction is consequential in treatment outcomes. It would appear to us that the information that goes into a discrepancy must have face validity in terms of the direction of outcomes. If the direction is unimportant, those measures used to determine a discrepancy should be removed from the classification criteria.

4. *Responsiveness to instruction.* The discrepancy model can only be validated if assessed on something above and beyond its components and its correlates. As we previously stated, we know that different scores are systematically related to their components. Thus one cannot test the construct validity of the discrepancy model with such scores. What needs to be tested, however, is whether the discrepancy scores accomplish something beyond their components. One obvious test is whether children defined by discrepancies are more likely to respond favorably (or unfavorably) to one treatment when compared to those poor achieving children without discrepancies. We found a significant interaction between discrepancies defined by variations in IQ and instruction for the single-subject design studies. *Responsiveness to instruction was mediated not by how discrepant the reported reading scores were from IQ, but rather by whether the discrepancies occurred at the lower end or the higher end of the IQ range.*

In sum, responsiveness to instruction seems to be a missing test in the majority of studies comparing discrepancy groups. We provide tentative support for the notion that the discrepancy model is a usable construct when it comes to intervention outcomes. Studies that report relatively high IQs and discrepancy are less responsive to some forms of instruction than those studies that report samples with discrepancy but with lower IQs.

Reading Instruction Issues

Reading is clearly the most investigated domain in our synthesis. We also found that several intervention studies published in the last 10 years have placed an emphasis on word recognition and word skills, primarily because of the high incidence of deficits related to phonological awareness in LD samples. "Phonological awareness" refers to one's sensitivity to the sound structure of speech. There have been consistent cases made that phonological awareness skills are a primary deficit in children with learning disabilities, particularly in the area of reading (Foorman, Francis, Fletcher, & Lynn, 1996; Stanovich & Siegel, 1994). The advantage of this emphasis is that it does give "specificity" to the field of learning disabilities. Further, it is obvious that reading performance is strongly related to decoding skill (Adams, 1990).

As we stated in the Introduction, however, there has been some debate about whether the emphasis of intervention in word reading should be directed at the whole word level, and/or at the analytic level (isolated sounds), and/or at the synthesis level (sound units). There are several negative outcomes in the debate over reading instruction for students with learning disabilities. The most important is that the teaching of whole language without due attention to decoding places LD children at greater risk than the use of more traditional programs. That is, children who cannot discover the alphabetic principal independently are denied explicit instruction on the regularity conventions of letter strings.

Our synthesis clearly shows that phonics instruction (and variations thereof) influences word skill measures. For example, the segmentation component of our possible 20 components was clearly related to word skill measures (see Table 9). However, on the important issues related to transfer measures (e.g., real word recognition, reading comprehension), the results are equivocal. We did not find unequivocal support for the notion that phonics instruction, in isolation from a number of other instructional components, significantly bolsters the reading of words (or, for that matter, the comprehension of text). This is a very important finding. To illustrate, several individual studies will be briefly reviewed. For example, Vellutino et al. (1996) suggested that after 15 weeks of 30-minute, daily, one-to-one tutoring in which phonological awareness was emphasized, the alphabetic principal and sight word vocabulary and comprehensive strategies were successful in remediating at-risk readers. However, when we analyzed this particular study, we were unable to calculate effect sizes (see tables of the original article). That is, the one-to-one intensive tutoring when compared to two other conditions (both traditional remedial programs in the schools) did not yield any effect sizes that were computable from the information presented. Indirectly, we could compute from the tables effect sizes on high and low readers among the three conditions, of which two were variations of the school approach of tutoring and classroom remediation when compared to the experimental treatment of intensive one-to-one instruction. The effect sizes were less than .10. In another study, Torgesen et al. (1997) suggested gains for reading disabled students (approximately 10 years old) who received one-to-one tutoring and synthetic and analytic phonics instruction with a skilled clinician for 2 hours daily over 8 weeks. However, when we calculated effect sizes for real word recognition measures, the magnitude of change was .19 (Word Identification subtest of the Woodcock Reading Mastery Test [WRMT]) when compared to the control conditions. In a study by Kennedy and Backman (1993) participants were instructed in a Lindamood Program that emphasized identification of speech sounds and orthographic symbols. The Lindamood Program was a supplement to regular private school LD instruction that included phonics. Control subjects also received private instruction that included phonics. With only 10 subjects in each condition, the effect size on the Slosson Oral Reading Test was .14 and on the Gray Oral Reading Test was .28. As in other studies, high effect sizes were found for the processes directly related to instruction (phonics), but meager effect sizes were found related to real word recognition.

Lovett et al. (1994) yield effect sizes between the strategy instruction and phonics instruction combination (the Benchmark Program; $N = 20$) of –.24 (in favor of the control condition) for word recognition on the Wide Range Achievement Test (WRAT) and –.67 (in favor of the control condition) on the WRMT word recognition subtest compared to the control condition, which included no reading instruction. When the phonics-direct instruction alone condition was compared to the control condition, the effect size was .60 on the WRAT and –.12 (in favor of the control) on the WRMT. Approximately 20 participants were in the three conditions, with participants ranging in age from 8 to 13 years. Thus, the control condition, which included no reading instruction, yielded higher effect sizes than the combined conditions (phonics + strategy instruction), and the direct instruction + phonics conditions were superior on one measure (WRAT), but inferior on a parallel measure (WRMT). These findings are difficult to interpret, especially given that different materials and age variations confound the results.

Brown and Felton (1990) argue that they found significant trends in their data supporting a structured phonics approach (using the Lippincott Basic Reading Program; 1991) over literature-based instruction or whole word instruction for 1st graders at risk for reading deficits due to poor phonological processing. Although we calculated the effect size after 2 years of instruction to be .52 on the word identification test of the WRMT (in favor of the phonics condition), it is important to realize that two different settings were used for comparisons (which means by inference that at least two different teachers were used). As we indicated in Chapter 3, whenever different settings or different teachers are used when comparing treatment to controls, effect sizes are highly inflated.

A study that overcomes some of these artifacts (which, unfortunately, we discovered too late to include in our synthesis) is reported by Foorman et al. (1997). They compared three interventions (synthetic phonics—Orton–Gillingham Approach; analytic phonics—focus on onsets and rimes—and sight word programs) in 2nd and 3rd graders identified with reading disabilities for 60 minutes a day for 1 school year. For word reading (an experimental measure of words selected from 1st and 2nd grade cumulative vocabulary lists in which half the words include predictable spelling patterns and half unpredictable or exceptional spelling patterns), no significant differences emerged between treatment conditions (see Table 8, pp. 106–107). The estimated effect sizes varied from 0 to .18 for the various comparisons.

In sum, the research does not seem to suggest unequivocally that phonics instruction is a sufficient condition for transfer to real words. There have been other reviews that suggest phonological awareness is an important, but not necessarily a sufficient, condition for learning to read (Adams, 1990; see Vellutino & Scanlon, 1991, for a review). We would not argue that phonological deficits, such as phonological awareness, cannot act as a critical precursor to reading problems in some LD children, but we would like to argue that its importance has been greatly exaggerated. The question that emerges is, Why have all the other language deficits in this population been overlooked in the last few years (i.e., compare the frequency of intervention studies in word recognition vs. language processing)?

One obvious reason is that certain neuropsychological models of reading have concentrated on reading as a bottom-up process in which words are first decoded and then meaning is assigned within the text. There is a good reason for this emphasis: those who have advocated a top-down model of reading acquisition have also overstated their case. One cannot deny that phonological segmentation plays a part in learning to read. However, we need to look at other sorts of variance in reading ability. *Perhaps more bothersome is the attempt to discount higher-order deficits as a possible basis for learning problems in students with learning disabilities.* This attempt is especially intriguing to us because the reading intervention studies we analyzed failed to provide unequivocal support for a bottom-up approach (i.e., strategy approaches were also effective).

Some would argue that there is a possible theoretical compromise: just call the general language problems (e.g., comprehension of text) in children with learning disabilities in the area of reading secondary manifestations of phonological processing. This compromise, however, when applied to children with learning disabilities in the early school grades, would lead to the dismissal of low verbal skills (e.g. phonological awareness) as a mere consequence of limited reading ability. A child who reads a lot will learn new words, and with them, new information; this new information is denied the LD reader who falls behind in a number of language areas. While we agree with this assumption, it is not necessarily the whole explanation. Some studies have shown substantial correlations between syntactic and semantic skills measured at 4 years of age, before children even start to receive reading instruction, and their reading performance at 8½ years of age (Bishop & Adams, 1990). We favor the view that some general language processes directly influence reading performance.

Another compromise is to view general language problems in children with learning disabilities (e.g., semantic and syntactic deficits) as underlying problems in phonological processes. For example, several studies (e.g., Shankweiler & Crain, 1986) argue that a deficient capacity to form phonetic representations limits the development of semantic and syntactic competence. However, there are extremes to this position. Apparently even nonlinguistic deficits may be interpreted as phonological disorders. For example, Jorm, Share, MacLean, and Mathews (1986) found "finger localization to be predictive of specific reading retardation and suggested that this may be a class of phonological processing disability" (p. 52). No doubt, with a sufficient imagination, any task that involves verbal stimulus or response can be deemed a reflection of phonological processing.

Although there has been a great deal of emphasis on the decoding skills of LD readers, there is another body of research that focuses on the metacognitive abilities of LD children and reading comprehension (see Wong, 1991, for a review). Unfortunately, not unlike word recognition intervention studies, this research has also suffered from several methodological flaws related to control group and systematic treatment comparisons. Some of the better designed studies are provided by Graves (1986), Graves and Levin (1989), and Wong and Jones (1982). Graves (1986) reported successful outcomes with LD students related to comprehension training. She contrasted two training conditions, one in which direct instruction and main idea identification were paired with self-monitoring training, and one in which only direct instruction and main idea identification were provided. These instructional conditions in turn were contrasted with a control or no training condition. Graves found that the training condition of combined direct instruction plus self-monitoring produced the best results in identifying main ideas. This finding was subsequently replicated by Graves and Levin (1989).

Wong and Jones (1982) also attempted to enhance reading comprehension of LD students through a metacognitive program. A total of six 8th and 9th graders with learning disabilities was compared with a reading-match control group of 6th graders. Half of the students in both the LD and 6th-grade reading-match groups were given self-questioning training procedures through which they learned to monitor their understanding of text. The other half served as a control group. In the experimental condition, the steps in comprehension monitoring included probing questions, such as "What are you studying this passage for?," "Find the main idea in the paragraph and underline it," "Think of a question about the main idea," and so on. Wong and Jones found that training increased the awareness of important textual units for adolescents with learning disabilities. Although these intervention results were positive, they primarily focused on older students who have, in some cases, already learned to compensate for their word recognition problems. In a study by Palincsar and Brown (1984), there was significant improvement in the reading comprehension skills of 7th graders who had good word recognition skills, but poor comprehension ability. Positive effects were obtained following 20 sessions of reciprocal teaching in which children were trained to adopt and practice the strategies of expert comprehenders through a process of interactive dialogue. In this study, however, successfully treated students were less skilled normal readers (not LD students), and therefore it is difficult to know whether this type of intervention will generalize to an LD sample.

Taken together, what can be concluded from the studies that have made comparisons among reading training treatment conditions? First, it is clear that cognitive treatment enhances reading comprehension. Second, in terms of treatment effects, the word decoding approach has an advantage only in the area of word processes. When real words are read in and out of context, the results are equivocal. Finally, given the abundance of poorly designed studies conducted in the past, it is clear why we do not have specific information regarding the efficacy of current remedial techniques for children who are LD readers.

In terms of suggested intervention practice, we think Marilyn Adams's 1990 synthesis of the literature captures our position. In her *Beginning to Read,* she states that "deep and thorough knowledge of letters, spelling, and words, and of phonological translations of all three, are of inescapable importance to both skillful reading and its acquisition. By extension, instruction designed to develop children's sensitivity to spellings and their relationship to pronunciation should be of paramount importance in the development of reading skills. This is, of course, precisely what is intended of good phonics instruction" (p. 416). She further states, however, that

> no good program succumbs to the simplistic hypotheses that letter sound relations are the most basic of reading skills. Rather, with respect to knowledge that is critical to reading, that which can be developed through phonics instruction represents neither the top nor the bottom, but only a realm in between. Before children learn to read, they must learn to recognize individual letters. They must become aware of the structure of language, from sentences and words to phonemes. And, most important, they must develop a basic understanding of the forms and functions of text and of its personal value to their own lives. Finally, none of the programs embodies the misguided hypothesis that reading skills are best developed from the bottom up. In a reading situation, as in any effective communication situation, the message or text does not rely on one critical source of information. The rest must come from the reader's own prior knowledge. Further, in a reading situation, as in any other learning situation, the learnability of a pattern depends critically on the prior knowledge in higher order relationships that it invokes. In both fluent reading and its acquisition, the reader's knowledge must be aroused interactively and in parallel. Neither understanding nor learning can proceed hierarchically from the bottom up. (pp. 421–422)

Full Inclusion

We narrowly define full inclusion in the context of our syntheses as students with learning disabilities who receive full-time education (with or without treatment) in a general (regular) education classroom. The settings of intervention and the effect sizes that emerge in these settings were directly coded in our analysis. Our results for group design studies indicated that those studies that do not report the setting ($N = 102$) in which the intervention occurred yield lower effect sizes than those that do report the setting (see Table 4). Setting information was further divided into those studies that report treatment occurring in the self-contained classroom, in the resource room, in the regular classroom, and where no information is provided about the type of classroom setting in which the treatment occurred. We found that larger effect sizes occurred in resource rooms than in other settings. As shown, however, only four studies, with a total sample size of 151 participants, provided information on effect sizes related to the regular classroom. Of these four studies, two were confounded by using different schools to represent treatment and control conditions.

Before discussing our observations, we must note some qualifications. Much has been written on the issue of full inclusion for students with learning disabilities (see Roberts & Mather, 1995, for a review), but little of this discussion involves a synthesis of outcomes related to intervention. Some authors suggest that special education has great things to offer, and then go on to argue that the real problem is that special education has been offering them in the wrong place (see Fuchs & Fuchs, 1994; and Kauffman & Hallahan, 1995, for a comprehensive review of various arguments). Their assumption is that special education as we now conceive it, that is, in terms of pull-out programs, is conceptually flawed and therefore what is unique about instruction for LD students needs to occur in the regular classroom. On this issue, our results show that interventions that took place in the pull-out classroom yielded larger effect sizes than interventions in other settings.

No doubt, there has been a trend, traceable to financial reasons, to leave LD students in the regular classroom (see Shanker, 1993, for a review of this issue). Much of this policy is also fueled by the lack of conclusive research on outcomes when such children are offered special instruction in pull-out programs (e.g., resource rooms) or the regular classroom (Fuchs & Fuchs, 1994a, 1994b). Our synthesis does indicate, however, at least in some cases, that the setting in which high effect sizes emerge is the special education setting. Of course, this conclusion calls for a qualification about how many intervention studies actually reported where treatment occurred. The more substantive issue, however, is whether teachers in the regular classroom can effectively accommodate such children. We have no data on this issue in our synthesis. We did not code whether treatment was better carried out by the regular classroom teacher than by the special education teacher.

Generalizations on treatment outcomes as a function of setting in our synthesis data are constrained by the lack of direct contrasts between special versus regular education settings *within* a study. Further, the research question "Which setting parameters of an instructional environment best maximize potential and productivity (however defined) in a general setting?" is not directly addressed in our synthesis. It is clear that many children with learning disabilities can be educated in full integration classrooms, and some cannot. Unfortunately, some school districts (and states, e.g., Colorado) are moving toward full inclusion models despite the lack of well-designed supportive research and sufficient information on individual differences in response to instruction (e.g., severe vs. moderate learning disabilities).

In addition to the above issues, it is also quite evident that regular classroom teachers are responsible for teaching growing numbers of diverse learners. This increase results largely from the growth in the number of children living in poverty and those who come from non-English-speaking backgrounds. The full inclusion model (or models) places increasing numbers of special students in the general education classrooms and also imposes more demands on these regular classroom teachers. Thus, diverse learners, such as students with learning disabilities and children from limited English-speaking backgrounds, are reported to have a variety of problems in the areas of memory, language, strategies, vocabulary, and so on. In addition, there are demands (or at least expectations) that these students perform to some particular standard. Although few regular classroom teachers would deny the tremendous diversity within their classrooms, especially in the area of achievement, within the field of learning disabilities we may be amplifying the impact of such diversity.

A conservative interpretation of our intervention studies supports a full continuum of services (high effect sizes were found in both placements). This is a generous interpretation on two accounts: (1) the trend in the data support pull-out programs, and (2) there are few studies on intervention that occur in the regular classroom setting. Unless it can be shown that all children with learning disabilities don't benefit from pull-out programs (our synthesis suggests that they do) when compared to integrated-classroom programs, special education placements should be left in place.

SUMMARY

Our synthesis has characterized intervention research within the field of learning disabilities over the last 30 years. We identified studies that yield high effect sizes and those that are methodologically sound. In spite of the limitations in subject descriptions, we were also able to identify some aptitude variables (intellectual range and severity of reading deficiency) that played an important role in predicting treatment outcomes. One aptitude variable, whether groups are defined by cutoff scores or variations in discrepancy as a function of low and high IQ, influenced treatment outcomes. We also provide information on the controversial issue of reading and conclude that both whole word and phonics approaches do make a significant contribution to treatment outcome and that neither clearly supersedes the other in terms of transfer measures (reading real words and comprehending text).

A proper research agenda for the next decade of intervention research would include the investigation of which treatment approaches are most effective, the causal processes by which they work, and the characteristics of LD children, teachers, and settings that most influence these particular results. Because most of the studies that we analyzed were only crude comparisons between undifferentiated treatment packages and control conditions, not enough attention was paid to potential interactions of instruction and LD characteristics. Such a research agenda is justified by basic assumptions in special education. Thus, the question is not whether a particular intervention works, but how it works and how it can be retooled to work much better.

References

Aaron, P. G., Frantz, S. S., & Manges, A. R. (1990). Dissociation between comprehension and pronunciation in dyslexic and hyperlexic children. *Reading and Writing, 2*(3), 243–264.

Adams, M. J. (1990). *Beginning to read.* Cambridge, MA: MIT Press.

Arter, J. A., & Jenkins, J. R. (1979). Differential diagnosis-prescriptive teaching: A critical appraisal. *Review of Educational Research, 49*, 517–555.

Baker, L., & Brown, A. L. (1984). Metacognitive skills of reading. In D. L. Forrest-Pressley, G. E. MacKinnon, & T. G. Waller (Eds.), *Metacognition, cognition, and human performance* (Vol. 1, pp. 155–205). San Diego, CA: Academic Press.

Bandura, A. (1989). Regulation of cognitive processes through perceived self-efficacy. *Developmental Psychology, 25*, 729–735.

Bateman, B. (1992). Learning disabilities: The changing landscape. *Journal of Learning Disabilities, 25*, 29–39.

Becker, W., & Carnine, D. (1980). Direct instruction: An effective approach for educational intervention with the disadvantaged and low performers. In B. Lahey & A. Kazdin (Eds.), *Advances in child clinical psychology*. New York: Plenum Press.

Bishop, D. V. M., & Adams, C. (1990). A prospective study of the relationship between specific language impairment, phonological disorder, and reading retardation. *Journal of Child Psychology and Psychiatry, 31*, 1027–1050.

Boder, E. (1973). Developmental dyslexia: A diagnostic approach based on three atypical reading-spelling patterns. *Developmental Medicine and Child Neurology, 15*, 663–687.

Bollen, K. A. (1989). *Structural equations with latent variables*. New York: Wiley-Interscience.

Borkowski, J. G., Estrada, M. T., Milstead, M., & Hale, C. A. (1989). General problem-solving skills: Relations between metacognition and strategic processing. *Learning Disability Quarterly, 12*, 57–70.

Borkowski, J. G., & Turner, L. A. (1990). Transsituational characteristics of metacognition. In W. Schneider & F. E. Weinert (Eds.), *Interactions among aptitudes, strategies, and knowledge in cognitive performance* (pp. 159–176). New York: Springer-Verlag.

Borkowski, J. G., Weyhing, R. S., & Carr, M. (1988). Effects of attributional retraining on strategy-based reading comprehension in learning-disabled students. *Journal of Educational Psychology, 80*, 46–53.

Bos, C. S., & Anders, P. L. (1990). Effects of interactive vocabulary instruction on the vocabulary learning and reading comprehension of junior-high learning disabled students. *Learning Disability Quarterly, 12*(1), 31–42.

Bos, C. S., Anders, P. L., Filip, D., & Jaffe, L. E. (1985). Semantic feature analysis and long-term learning. *National Reading Conference Yearbook, 34*, 42–47.

Brailsford, A., Smart, F., & Das, J. P. (1984). Strategy training and reading comprehension. *Journal of Learning Disabilities, 17*(5), 287–293.

Branwhite, A. B., (1983). Boosting reading skills by direct instruction. *British Journal of Educational Psychology, 53*(3), 291–298.

Brinker, R. P. (1990). In search of the foundation of special education: Who are the individuals and what are the differences? *Journal of Special Education, 24*, 174–184.

Brophy, J. E. (1986). Research linking teacher behavior to student achievement: Potential implications for instruction of Chapter 1 students. In B. I. Williams, P. A. Richmond, & B. J. Mason (Eds.), *Designs for compensatory education: Conference proceedings and papers* (Vol. 4, pp. 122–179). Washington, DC: Research and Evaluation Associations.

Brophy, J. E., & Good, T. (1986). Teacher-effects results. In M. C. Wittrock (Ed.), *Handbook of research on teaching* (3rd ed.). New York: Macmillan.

Brown, F. S., & Felton, R. C. (1990). Effects of instruction on beginning reading skills in children at risk for reading disability. *Reading and Writing: An Interdisciplinary Journal, 2*, 223–241.

Bryk, A. S., & Raudenbush, S. W. (1992). *Hierarchical linear models: Applications and data analysis methods*. Newbury Park, CA: Sage.

Busk, P. L., & Serlin, R. C. (1992). Meta-analysis for single-case research. In T. R. Kratochwill & J. R. Levin (Eds.), *Single-case research design and analysis: New directions for psychology and education* (pp. 187–212). Hillsdale, NJ: Erlbaum.

Byrne, B., Freebody, P., & Gates, A. (1992). Longitudinal data on relations of word-reading strategies to comprehension, reading time, and phonemic awareness. *Reading Research Quarterly, 27*, 140–151.

Campbell, D. T., & Stanley, J. C. (1963). Experimental and quasi-experimental designs for research on teaching. In N. L. Gage (Ed.), *Handbook of research on teaching* (pp. 171–246). Chicago: Rand McNally.

Chabot, R. J., Petros, T. V., & McCord, G. (1983). Developmental and reading ability differences in accessing information from semantic memory. *Journal of Experimental Child Psychology, 35*, 128–142.

Chalfant, J. C., & Scheffelin, M. A. (1969). *Central processing dysfunctions in children: A review of research. Phase three of a three-phase project* (NINDS Monograph). Bethesda, MD: U.S. Department of Health, Education and Welfare.

Chall, J. (1967). *Learning to read: The great debate*. New York: McGraw-Hill.

Chan, L. K. S. (1991). Promoting strategy generalization through self-instructional training in students with reading disabilities. *Journal of Learning Disabilities, 24*(7), 427–433.

Chan, L. K. S., Cole, P. G., & Morris, J. N. (1990). Effects of instruction in the use of a visual-imagery strategy on the reading-comprehension competence of disabled and average readers. *Learning Disability Quarterly, 13*(1), 2–11.

Chiang, B., Thorpe, H. W., & Darch, C. B. (1980). Effects of cross-age tutoring on word-recognition performance of learning disabled students. *Learning Disability Quarterly, 3*(4), 11–19.

Cohen, J. (1970). Approximate power and sample size determination for common one-sample and two-sample hypothesis tests. *Educational and Psychological Measurement, 30*(4), 811–831.

Cohen, J. (1988). *Statistical power analysis for the behavioral sciences* (2nd ed.) New York: Academic Press.

Cohen, J., & Cohen, P. (1983). *Applied multiple regression/correlation analysis for the behavioral sciences*. Hillsdale, NJ: Erlbaum.

Coltheart, V., Avons, S. E., Masterson, J., & Laxon, V. J. (1991). The role of assembled phonology in reading comprehension. *Memory and Cognition, 19*(4), 387–400.

Cooney, J., & Swanson, H. L. (1987). Overview of research on learning disabled children's memory development. In H. L. Swanson (Ed.), *Memory and learning disabilities* (pp. 2–40). Greenwich, CT: JAI Press.

Cooper, H. (1989). *Integrating research: A guide for literature reviews*. New York: Russell Sage Foundation.

Cooper, H., & Hedges, L. V. (1994). *The handbook of research synthesis*. New York: Russell Sage Foundation.

Cooper, H., Nye, B., Charlton, K., Lindsey, J., & Greathouse, S. (1996). The effects of summer vacation on achievement scores: A narrative and meta-analysis review. *Review of Educational Research, 66*, 227–268.

Cosden, M. A., & English, J. P. (1987). The effects of grouping, self esteem, and locus of control on microcomputer performance and help seeking by mildly handicapped students. *Journal of Educational Computing Research, 3*(4), 443–459.

Cronbach, L. J., & Furby, L. (1970). How we should measure "change" or should we? *Psychological Bulletin, 74*, 68–80.

Cronbach, L. J., & Gleser, G. C. (1953). Assessing similarity between profiles. *Psychological Bulletin, 74*, 68–80.

Cronbach, L. J., & Snow, R. E. (1977). *Aptitudes and instructional methods: A handbook for research on interactions*. New York: Irvington.

Cruickshank, W. M., Bentzen, F. A., Ratzeburg, F. H., & Tannhauser, M. T. (1961). *A teaching method for brain-injured and hyperactive children*. Syracuse, NY: Syracuse University Press.

Daneman, M., & Carpenter, P. A. (1980). Individual differences in working memory and reading. *Journal of Verbal Learning and Verbal Behavior, 19*, 450–466.

Darch, C., & Gersten, R. (1985). The effects of teacher presentation rate and praise on LD students' oral reading performance. *British Journal of Educational Psychology, 55*(3), 295–303.

Darch, C., & Kameenui, E. J. (1987). Teaching LD students critical reading skills: A systematic replication. *Learning Disability Quarterly, 10*(2), 82–90.

Das, J. P., Kirby, J. R., & Jarman, R. F. (1979). *Simultaneous and successive cognitive processes*. New York: Academic Press.

Deno, S. L. (1985). Curriculum-based measurement: The emerging alternative. *Exceptional Children, 52*, 219–232.

Deshler, D. D., & Schumaker, J. B. (1988). An instructional model for teaching students how to learn. In J. Graden, J. Zins, & M. Curtis (Eds.), *Alternative educational delivery systems: Enhancing instructional options for all students* (pp. 391–411). Washington, DC: National Association of School Psychologists.

Deshler, D. D., Schumaker, J. B., & Lenz, B. K. (1984a). Academic and cognitive interventions for LD adolescents: Part 1. *Journal of Learning Disabilities, 17*, 108–117.

Deshler, D. D., Schumaker, J. B., Lenz, B. K., & Ellis, E. (1984b). Academic and cognitive interventions for LD adolescents: Part 2. *Journal of Learning Disabilities, 17*, 170–187.

Dixon, P., LeFevre, J., & Twilley, L. C. (1988). Word knowledge and working memory as predictors of reading skill. *Journal of Educational Psychology, 80*, 465–472.

Dole, J. A., Duffy, G. G., Roehler, L. R., & Pearson, P. D. (1991). Moving from the old to the new: Research on reading comprehension instruction. *Review of Educational Research, 61*(2), 239–264.

Eagly, A. H., & Wood, W. (1994). Using research synthesis for future research. In H. Cooper & L. V. Hedges (Eds.), *The handbook of research synthesis* (pp. 458–500). New York: Russell Sage Foundation.

Engelmann, S., & Carnine, D. W. (1982). *Theory of instruction: Principles and applications*. New York: Irvington.

Englert, C. S., Raphael, T. E., & Anderson, L. M. (1992). Socially mediated instruction: Improving students' knowledge about talk and writing. *Elementary School Journal, 92*(4), 411–449.

Faith, M. S., Allison, D. B., & Gorman, B. S. (1997). Meta-analysis of single-case research. In R. D. Franklin, D. B. Allison, & B. S. Gorman (Eds.), *Design and analysis of single-case research* (pp. 245–277). Mahwah, NJ: Erlbaum.

Farmer, M. E., Klein, R., & Bryson, S. E. (1992). Computer-assisted reading: Effects of whole word feedback on fluency and comprehension in readers with severe disabilities. *Remedial and Special Education, 13*, 50–60.

Federal Register. (1977). *The rules regulating implementing of P. L. 94–142*. Washington, DC : U.S. Government Printing Office.

Fiedorowicz, C.A.M. (1986). Training of component reading skills. *Annals of Dyslexia, 36*, 318–334.

Fletcher, J., Shaywitz, S. E., Shankweiler, D. P., Katz, L., Liberman, I., Stuebing, K., Francis, D., Fowler, A., & Shaywitz, B. A. (1994). Cognitive profiles of reading disability: Comparisons of discrepancy and low achievement definitions. *Journal of Educational Psychology, 86*, 6–23.

Foorman, B. R., Francis, D. J., Fletcher, J. M., & Lynn, A. (1996). Relation of phonological and orthographic processing to early reading: Comparing two approaches to regression-based, reading-level-match design. *Journal of Educational Psychology, 88*, 639–652.

Foorman, B. R., Francis, D. J., Winikates, D., Mehta, P., Schatschneider, C., & Fletcher, J. M. (1997). Early interventions for children with reading disabilities. *Scientific Studies of Reading, 1*(3), 255–276.

Forness, S. R., Kavale, K. A., Blum, I. M., & Lloyd, J. W. (1997). Mega-analysis of meta-analyses: What works in special education and related services. *Teaching Exceptional Children, 29*(6), 4–9.

Francis, D. J., Shaywitz, S. E., Stuebing, K. K., Shaywitz, B. A., & Fletcher, J. M. (1996). Developmental lag versus deficit models of reading disability: A longitudinal, individual growth curves analysis. *Journal of Educational Psychology, 88*, 3–17.

Franklin, R. D., Allison, D. B., & Gorman, B. S. (Eds.). (1996). *Design and analysis of single-case research*. Mahwah, NJ: Erlbaum.

Franklin, R. D., Gorman, B. S., Beasley, T. M., & Allison, D. B. (1996). Graphical display and visual analysis. In R. D. Franklin, D. B. Allison, & B. S. Gorman (Eds.), *Design and analysis of single-case research* (pp. 119–158). Mahwah, NJ: Erlbaum.

Frederiksen, J. R. (1981). Sources of process interaction in reading. In A. M. Lesgold & C. A. Perfetti (Eds.), *Interactive process in reading* (pp. 367–386). Hillsdale, NJ: Erlbaum.

Frederiksen, J. R., & Warren, B. M. (1987). A cognitive framework for developing expertise in reading. In R. Glaser (Ed.), *Advances in instructional psychology* (Vol. 3, pp. 1–39) Hillsdale, NJ: Erlbaum.

Freeman, T. J., & McLaughlin, T. F. (1984). Effects of a taped-words treatment on learning-disabled students' sight-word oral reading. *Learning Disabilities Quarterly, 7,* 49–54.

Frostig, M., Lefever, D. W., & Whittlesey, J. R. B. (1964). *The Marianne Frostig Developmental Test of Visual Perception.* Palo Alto, CA: Consulting Psychology Press.

Fuchs, D., & Fuchs, L. S. (1994a). Classwide curriculum-based measurement: Helping general educators meet the challenge of student diversity. *Exceptional Children, 60,* 518–537.

Fuchs, D., & Fuchs, L. S. (1994b). Inclusive school movement and the radicalization of special education reform. *Exceptional Children, 60,* 294–309.

Fuchs, D., Mathes, P., Fuchs, L., & Lipsey, M. (in press). *Is LD just a fancy term for underachievers?* To be submitted as a final report to the U.S. Department of Education.

Fuchs, D. (in press). *U.S. Department of Education: A comparison between discrepancy and nondiscrepancy groups.*

Gajria, M., & Salvia, J. (1992). The effects of summarization instruction on text comprehension of students with learning disabilities. *Exceptional Children, 58*(6), 508–516.

Gelzheiser, L. M. (1984). Generalization from categorical memory tasks to prose by learning disabled adolescents. *Journal of Educational Psychology, 76*(6), 1128–1138.

Gettinger, M., Bryant, N. D., & Fayne, H. R. (1982). Designing spelling instruction for learning disabled children: An emphasis on unit size, distributed practice, and training for transfer. *Journal of Special Education, 16*(4), 439–448.

Gittelman, R., & Feingold, I. (1983). Children with reading disorders, Part 1: Efficacy of reading remediation. *Journal of Child Psychology and Psychiatry, 24*(2), 167–191.

Gerber, P. I., & Reiff, H. B. (1991). *Speaking for themselves: Ethnographic interviews with adults with learning disabilities.* Ann Arbor: University of Michigan Press.

Glass, G. V., McGraw, B., & Smith, M. L. (1981). *Meta-analysis in social research.* Beverly Hills, CA: Sage.

Gleser, L. J., & Olkin, I. (1994). Stochastically dependent effect sizes. In H. Cooper & L. V. Hedges (Eds.), *The handbook of research synthesis* (pp. 339–355). New York: Russell Sage Foundation.

Graham, S., & Harris, K. R. (1989). Components analysis of cognitive strategy instruction: Effects on learning disabled students' compositions and self-efficacy. *Journal of Educational Psychology, 81*(3), 353–361.

Graham, S., & Harris, K. R. (1989a). Cognitive training: Implications for written language. In J. Hughes & R. Hall (Eds.), *Cognitive behavioral psychology in the schools: A comprehensive handbook* (pp. 247–279). New York: Guilford Press.

Graham, S., & Harris, K. R. (1989b). A components analysis of cognitive strategy instruction: Effects on learning disabled students' compositions and self-efficacy. *Journal of Educational Psychology, 81,* 353–361.

Graham, S., & Harris, K. R. (1993). Cognitive strategy instruction: Methodological issues and guidelines in conducting research. In S. Vaughn & C. Bos (Eds.), *Research issues in learning disabilities* (pp. 146–158). New York: Springer-Verlag.

Graham, S., & Harris, K. R. (1996). Self-regulation and strategy instruction for students who find writing and learning challenging. In C. M. Levy & S. Ransdell (Eds.), *The science of writing: Theories, methods, individual differences, and applications* (pp. 347–360). Mahwah, NJ: Erlbaum.

Graves, A. W. (1986). Effects of direct instruction and metacomprehension on finding main ideas. *Learning Disability Research, 1,* 90–100.

Graves, A. W., & Levin, J. R. (1989). Comparison of monitoring and mnemonic text-processing strategies in learning disabled students. *Learning Disability Quarterly, 12*(3), 212–236.

Guthrie, J. T., VanMeter, P., McCann, A. D., & Wigfield, A. (1996). Growth of literacy engagement: Changes in motivations and strategies. *Reading Research Quarterly, 31*(3), 306–332.

Hallahan, D. (1992). Some thoughts on why the prevalence of learning disabilities has increased. *Journal of Learning Disabilities, 25*, 523–528.

Hallahan, D. P., & Cruickshank, W. M. (1973). *Psychoeducational foundations of learning disabilities*. Englewood Cliffs, NJ: Prentice-Hall.

Harris, K. R., & Graham, S. (1985). Improve learning disabled students' composition skills: Self-control strategy training. *Learning Disability Quarterly, 8*, 27–36.

Harris, K. R., & Pressley, M. (1991). The nature of cognitive strategy instruction: Interactive strategy construction. *Exceptional Children, 57*, 392–404.

Harwell, M. R. (1992). Summarizing monte carlo results in methodological research. *Journal of Educational Statistics, 17*, 297–313.

Hayes-Roth, B., & Hayes-Roth, F. (1979). A cognitive model of planning. *Cognitive Sciences, 3*, 275–310.

Hedges, L. V. (1982a). Estimation of the effect size from a series of independent experiments. *Psychological Bulletin, 92*, 490–499.

Hedges, L. V. (1982b). Fitting categorical models to effect sizes from a series of experiments. *Journal of Educational Statistics, 7*, 119–137.

Hedges, L. V. (1982c). Fitting continuous models to effect size data. *Journal of Educational Statistics, 7*, 245–270.

Hedges, L. V. (1994a). Fixed effects models. In H. Cooper & L. V. Hedges (Eds.), *The handbook of research synthesis* (pp. 285–299). New York: Russell Sage Foundation.

Hedges, L. V. (1994b). Statistical considerations. In H. Cooper & L. V. Hedges (Eds.), *The handbook of research synthesis* (pp. 29–38). New York: Russell Sage Foundation.

Hedges, L. V., & Olkin, I. (1985). *Statistical methods for meta-analysis*. San Diego, CA: Academic Press.

Herdman, C., & LeFevre, J. (1992). Individual differences in the efficiency of word recognition. *Journal of Educational Psychology, 84*, 95–105.

Hunter, J. E., & Schmidt, F. L. (1990). *Methods of meta-analysis: Correcting error and bias in research findings*. Newbury Park, CA: Sage.

Hunter, J. E., & Schmidt, F. L. (1994). Correcting for sources of artificial variation across studies. In H. Cooper & L. V. Hedges (Eds.), *The handbook of research synthesis* (pp. 323–336). New York: Russell Sage Foundation.

Hurford, D. P. (1990). Training phonemic segmentation ability with a phonemic discrimination intervention in second- and third-grade children with reading disabilities. *Journal of Learning Disabilities, 23*, 564–569.

Jenkins, J. R., & Jenkins, L. M. (1985). Peer tutoring in elementary and secondary programs. *Focus on Exceptional Children, 17*(6), 1–12.

Johnson, L., Graham, S., & Harris, K. R. (1997). The effects of goal setting and self-instruction on learning a reading comprehension strategy: A study of students with learning disabilities. *Journal of Learning Disabilities, 30*(1), 80–91.

Jorm, A. F. (1979). The cognitive and neurological basis of developmental dyslexia: A theoretical framework and review. *Cognition, 7*, 19–33.

Jorm, A. F., Share, D., Maclean, R., & Matthews, R. (1986). Cognitive factors at school entry predictive of specific reading retardation and general reading awkwardness: A research note. *Journal of Child Psychology and Psychiatry, 27*, 45–54.

Just, M. A., & Carpenter, P. A. (1992). A capacity theory of comprehension: Individual differences in working memory. *Psychological Review, 99*, 122–149.

Kail, R., & Bisanz, J. (1993). The information processing perspective on cognitive/development in childhood and adolescence. In R. Sternberg & C. A. Berg (Eds.), *Intellectual development* (Vol 1, pp. 229–260). New York: Cambridge University Press.

Kameenui, E. J. (1991). Toward a scientific pedagogy of learning disabilities: A sameness in the message. *Journal of Learning Disabilities, 24*, 364–372.

Kameenui, E. J., Jitendra, A. K., & Darch, C. B. (1995). Direct instruction reading as contronym and eonomine. *Reading and Writing Quarterly: Overcoming Learning Difficulties, 11*(1), 3–17.

Kass, C. E. (1970). *Final report: Advanced institute for Leadership Personnel in Learning Disabilities.* Tucson: Department of Health, Education, and Welfare, University of Arizona.

Kauffman, J. M., & Hallahan, D. P. (Eds.). (1995). *The illusion of full inclusion: A comprehensive critique of a current special education bandwagon.* Austin, TX: PRO-ED.

Kendall, J. R., & Hood, J. (1979). Investigating the relationship between comprehension and word recognition: Oral reading analysis of children with comprehension or word recognition disabilities. *Journal of Reading Behavior, 11*(1), 41–48.

Kennedy, K. M., & Backman, J. (1993). Effectiveness of the Lindamood Auditory Discrimination in Depth Program with students with learning disabilities. *Learning Disabilities Research and Practice, 8*(4), 253–259.

Keogh, B. K., Major-Kingsley, S., Omori-Gordon, H., & Reid, H. (1982). A system of marker variables for the field of learning disabilities. *Alexander R. Luria Research Monograph Series on Learning Disabilities, 1,* 1–95.

Kerstholt, M. T., Van Bon, W. H. J., & Schreuder, R. (1994). Training in phonemic segmentation: The effects of visual support. *Reading and Writing: An Interdisciplinary Journal, 6*(4), 361–385.

Kirk, S. A. (1963). Behavioral diagnosis and remediation of learning disabilities. *Proceedings from the Conference on the Exploration on Problem for Perpetually Handicapped Children, 1,* 1–23.

Kirk, S. A., & Kirk, W. D. (1971). *Psycholinguistic learning disabilities: Diagnosis and remediation.* Chicago: University of Illinois Press.

Leinhardt, G., & Greeno, J. G. (1986). The cognitive skill of teaching. *Journal of Educational Psychology, 78*(2), 75–95.

Lessen, E., Dudzinski, M., Karsh, K., & Van Acker, R. (1989). A survey of ten years of academic intervention research with learning disabled students: Implications for research and practice. *Learning Disabilities Focus, 4,* 106–122.

Levin, J. R. (1986). Four cognitive principles of learning strategy instruction. *Educational Psychologist, 21,* 3–17.

Levin, J. R. (1988). Elaboration-based learning strategies: Powerful theory = powerful application. *Contemporary Educational Psychology, 13,* 191–205.

Lindsley, O. R. (1964). Direct measurement and prosthesis of retarded behavior. *Journal of Education, 147,* 62–81.

Lipsey, M. W., & Wilson, D. B. (1993). The efficacy of psychological, educational, and behavioral treatment: Confirmation from meta-analysis. *American Psychologist, 48*(12), 1181–1209.

Lomax, R. G. (1983). Applying structural modeling to some component processing of reading comprehension development. *Journal of Experimental Education, 52,* 33–40.

Lovegrove, W., Martin, F., & Slaghuis, W. (1986). A theoretical and experimental case for a visual deficit in specific reading disability. *Cognitive Neuropsychology, 3,* 225–267.

Lovett, M. W., Borden, S. L., DeLuca, T., Lacerenza, L., Benson, N. J., & Brackstone, D.

(1994). Treating the core deficits of developmental dyslexia: Evidence of transfer of learning after phonologically- and strategy-based reading training programs. *Developmental Psychology, 30*, 805–822.

Lovett, M. W., Ransby, M. J., Hardwick, N., Johns, M. S., & Donaldson, S. A. (1989). Can dyslexia be treated? Treatment-specific and generalized treatment effects in dyslexic children's response to remediation. *Brain and Language, 37*(1), 90–121.

Lovett, M. W., Warren-Chaplin, P. M., Ransby, M. J., & Borden, S. L. (1990). Training the word recognition skills of reading disabled children: Treatment and transfer effects. *Journal of Educational Psychology, 82*(4), 769–780.

Lucangeli, D., Galderisi, D., & Cornoldi, C. (1995). Specific and general transfer effects following metamemory training. *Learning Disabilities Research and Practice, 10*(1), 11–21.

MacArthur, C. A., Schwartz, S. S., & Graham, S. (1991). Effects of a reciprocal peer revision strategy in special education classrooms. *Learning Disabilities Research, 6*(4), 201–210.

Manis, F., Custodio, R., & Szeszulski, P. A. (1993). Development of phonological and orthographic skill: A two-year longitudinal study of dyslexic children. *Journal of Experimental Child Psychology, 56*, 64–86.

Marks, M., Pressley, M., Coley, J. D., Craig, S., Gardner, R., Rose, W., & DePinto, T. (1993). Teachers' adaptations of reciprocal teaching: Progress toward a classroom-compatible version of reciprocal teaching. *Elementary School Journal, 94*, 267–283.

Martin, E. (1988). Response to: Intervention research in learning disabilities. In S. Vaughn & C. Bos (Eds.), *Research in learning disabilities* (pp. 173–184). San Diego, CA: Little, Brown, and Company.

Matyas, T. A., & Greenwood, K. M. (1997). Serial dependency in single-case time series. In R. D. Franklin, D. B. Allison, & B. S. Gorman (Eds.), *Design and analysis of single-case research* (pp. 215–243). Mahwah, NJ: Erlbaum.

McBride-Chang, C., Manis, F. R., Seidenberg, M. S., Custodio, R., & Doi, L. M. (1993). Print exposure as a predictor of word reading and reading comprehension in disabled and nondisabled readers. *Journal of Educational Psychology, 85*, 230–238.

McCarthy, J. J., & Kirk, S. A. (1961). *Illinois Test of Psycholinguistic Abilities: Experimental version*. Urbana: University of Illinois Press.

Meichenbaum, D. (1977). *Cognitive behavior modification*. New York: Plenum Press.

Mercer, C. D., Jordan, L., Allsopp, D. H., & Mercer, A. R. (1996). Learning disabilities definitions and criteria used by stated education departments. *Learning Disability Quarterly, 19*, 217–232.

Mercer, C. D., & Mercer, A. R. (1981). *Teaching students with learning problems*. Columbus, OH: Merrill.

Miller, N., & Pollock, V. E. (1994). Meta-analytic synthesis for theory development. In H. Cooper & L. Hedges (Eds.), *The handbook of research synthesis* (pp. 457–484). New York: Russell Sage Foundation.

Moats, L. C., & Lyon, G. R. (1993). Learning disabilities in the United States: Advocacy, science, and the future of the field. *Journal of Learning Disabilities, 26*(5), 282–294.

Morrison, S. R., & Siegel, L. S. (1991). Learning disabilities: A critical review of definitional and assessment issues. In J. E. Obrzut & G. W. Hynd (Eds.), *Neurological foundations of learning disabilities* (pp. 79–97). San Diego, CA: Academic Press.

Myers, P., & Hammill, D. D. (1990). *Learning disabilities: Basic concepts, argument practices, and instructional strategies*. Austin, TX: PRO-ED.

Naylor, J. G., & Pumfrey, P. D. (1983). The alleviation of psycholinguistic deficits and some effects on the reading attainments of poor readers: A sequel. *Journal of Research in Reading, 6*(2), 129–153.

Newcomer, P. L., & Hammill, D. D. (1975). ITPA and academic achievement. *Teacher, 28,* 731–741.

Olofsson, A. (1992). Synthetic speech and computer aided reading for reading disabled children. *Reading and Writing, 4*(2), 165–178.

Olsen, J. L., Wong, B. Y. L., & Marx, R. W. (1983). Linguistic and metacognitive aspects of normally achieving and learning disabled children's communication process. *Learning Disability Quarterly, 6*(3), 289–304.

Olson, R., Kliegl, R., Davidson, B., & Foltz, G., (1985). Individual and developmental differences in reading disability. In G. E. MacKinnon & T. Waller (Eds.), *Reading research: Advances in theory and practice* (Vol. 4, pp. 1–64). San Diego, CA: Academic Press.

Olson, R. K., Wise, B., Conners, F., & Rack, J. P. (1990). Organization, heritability, and remediation of component word recognition and language skills in disabled readers. In T. H. Carr & B. A. Levy (Eds.), *Reading and its development: Component skills approaches* (pp. 261–322). San Diego, CA: Academic Press.

Palincsar, A. S. (1986a). Metacognitive strategy instruction. *Exceptional Children, 53,* 118–124.

Palincsar, A. S. (1986b). The role of dialogue in providing scaffolded instruction. *Educational Psychologist, 21*(1–2), 73–98.

Palincsar, A. S., & Brown, A. L. (1984). Reciprocal teaching of comprehension-fostering and comprehension-monitoring activities. *Cognition and Instruction, 1,* 117–175.

Palincsar, A. S., & Brown, A. L. (1988). Teaching and practicing thinking skills to promote comprehension in the context of group problem solving. *RASE: Remedial and Special Education, 9,* 53–59. (Special Issue: The challenge of reading with understanding in the intermediate grades.)

Paris, S. G., Cross, D. R., & Lipson, M. Y. (1984). Informed strategies for learning: A program to improve children's reading awareness and comprehension. *Journal of Educational Psychology, 76,* 1239–1252.

Parloff, M. B. (1984). Psychotherapy research and its incredible credibility crisis. *Clinical Psychology Review, 4,* 95–109.

Perfetti, C. A. (1985). *Reading ability.* New York: Oxford University Press.

Pflaum, S. W. (1980). The predictability of oral reading behaviors on comprehension in learning disabled and normal readers. *Journal of Reading Behavior, 12,* 231–236.

Pressley, M. (1991). Can learning disabled children become good information processors? How can we find out? In L. Feagans, E. Short, & L. Meltzer (Eds.), *Subtypes of learning disabilities* (pp. 137–162). Hillsdale, NJ: Erlbaum.

Pressley, M. (1994). Embracing the complexity of individual differences in cognition: Studying good information processing and how it might develop. *Learning and Individual Differences, 6*(3), 259–284.

Pressley, M., Borkowski, J. G., & Schneider, W. (1989). Good information processing: What it is and how education can promote it. *International Journal of Educational Research, 13,* 857–867.

Pressley, M., Brown, R., El-Dinary, P. B., & Allferbach, P. (1995). The comprehension instruction that students need: Instruction fostering constructively responsive reading. *Learning Disabilities Research and Practice, 10*(4), 215–224.

Pressley, M., Burkell, J., Cariglia-Bull, T., Lysynchuk, L., McGoldrick, J. A., Schneider, B., Symons, S., & Woloshyn, V. (1990). *Cognitive strategy instruction.* Cambridge, MA: Brookline Books.

Pressley, M., El-Dinary, P. B., Gaskins, I., Schuder, T., Berrgman, J. L., Almasi, J., & Brown, R. (1992). Beyond direct explanation: Transactional instruction of reading comprehension strategies. *Elementary School Journal, 92*, 513–556.

Pressley, M., & Ghatala, E. S. (1990). Self-regulated learning: Monitoring learning from text. *Educational Psychologist, 25*, 19–34.

Pressley, M., & Harris, K. R. (1994). Increasing the quality of educational intervention research. *Educational Psychology Review, 6*, 191–208.

Prior, M., Frye, S., & Fletcher, C. (1987). Remediation for subgroups of retarded readers using a modified oral spelling procedure. *Developmental Medicine and Child Neurology, 29*(1), 64–71.

Rack, J. P., Snowling, M. J., & Olson, R. K. (1992). The nonword reading deficit in developmental dyslexia: A review. *Reading Research Quarterly, 27*, 28–53.

Resnick, L. B. (1987). Constructing knowledge in school. In L. S. Liben (Ed.), *Development and learning: Conflict or congruence?* (pp. 19–50). Hillsdale, NJ: Erlbaum.

Reynolds, C. R. (1981). The fallacy of "two years below grade level for age" as a diagnostic criterion for reading disorders. *Journal of School Psychology, 11*, 250–258.

Roberts, R., & Mather, N. (1995). Legal protections for individuals with learning disabilities: The IDEA, Section 504, and the ADA. *Learning Disabilities Research and Practice, 10*, 160–168.

Rose, T. L., & Sherry, L. (1984). Relative effects of two previewing procedures on LD adolescents' oral reading performance. *Learning Disability Quarterly*, *7*, 39–44.

Rosenshine, B. (1982, April). *The master teacher and the master developer*. Paper presented at the annual convention of the American Educational Research Association, New York.

Rosenshine, B. (1995). Advances in research on instruction. *Journal of Educational Research, 88*(5), 262–268.

Rosenshine, B., & Stevens, R. (1986). Teaching functions. In M. C. Wittrock (Ed.), *Handbook of research on teaching* (3rd ed.). New York: Macmillan.

Rosenthal, R. (1994). Parametric measures of effect size. In H. Cooper & L. V. Hedges (Eds.), *The handbook of research synthesis* (pp. 231–244). New York: Russell Sage Foundation.

Rumelhart, D. E. (1977). Toward an interactive model of reading. In S. Dornic (Ed.), *Attention and performance* (Vol. 6, pp. 573–603). Hillsdale, NJ: Erlbaum.

SAS Institute. (1992a). *SAS/Stat users guide: Version 6*. Cary, NC: Author.

SAS Institute. (1992b). *SAS technical report P-229*. Cary, NC: Author.

Sawyer, R. J., Graham, S., & Harris, K. R. (1992). Direct teaching, strategy instruction, and strategy instruction with explicit self-regulation: Effects on the composition skills and self-efficacy of students with learning disabilities. *Journal of Educational Psychology*, *84*(3), 340–352.

Schmidt, F. L. (1992). What do data really mean? Research findings, meta-analysis, and cumulative knowledge in psychology. *American Psychologist, 47*, 1173–1181.

Schunk, D. H. (1985). Participation in goal setting: Effects on self-efficacy and skills of learning-disabled children. *Journal of Special Education, 19*(3), 305–317.

Schunk, D. H., & Rice, J. M. (1992). Influence of reading-comprehension strategy information on children's achievement outcomes. *Learning Disabilities Quarterly, 15*(1), 51–64.

Scruggs, T. E., & Mastropieri, M. A. (1989). Mnemonic instruction of LD students: A field-based evaluation. *Learning Disability Quarterly, 12*(2), 119–125.

Scruggs, T. E., & Mastropieri, M. A. (1993). Issues in conduction intervention research: Secondary students. In S. Vaughn & C. Bos (Eds.), *Research issues in learning disabilities* (pp. 130–145). New York: Springer-Verlag.

Scruggs, T. E., & Mastropieri, M. A. (in press). Summarizing single subject research: Issues and applications. *Behavior Modification.*

Seidenberg, M. S., & McClelland, J. L. (1989). A distributed, developmental model of word recognition and naming. *Psychological Review, 96,* 523–568.

Shallice, T. (1988). *From neuropsychology to mental structures.* Cambridge, UK: Cambridge University Press.

Shanker, A. (1993, September 19). Where we stand: A rush to inclusion. *New York Times,* Week in Review Section, p. 9.

Shankweiler, D., & Crain, S. (1986). Language mechanisms and reading disorder: A modular approach. *Cognition, 24,* 139–168.

Shankweiler, D., Liberman, I., Mark, L., Fowler, C., & Fisher, F. (1979). The speech code and learning to read. *Journal of Experimental Psychology: Human Learning and Memory, 5,* 531–545.

Share, D. L., & Stanovich, K. E. (1995). Cognitive processes in early reading development: Accommodating individual differences into a model of acquisition. *Issues in Education, 1,* 1–58.

Shepherd, L. A., Smith, M. L., & Vojir, C. P. (1983). Characteristics of pupils identified as learning disabled. *American Educational Research Journal, 20,* 309–331.

Siegel, L. S. (1985). Psycholinguistic aspects of reading disabilities. In L. S. Siegel & F. Morrison (Eds.), *Cognitive development in atypical children* (pp. 45–66). New York: Springer-Verlag.

Siegel, L. S. (1992). An evaluation of the discrepancy definition of dyslexic. *Journal of Learning Disabilities, 25,* 618–629.

Siegel, L. S. (1993). The cognitive basis of dyslexia. In M. Howe & R. Pasnak (Eds.), *Emerging themes in cognitive development* (pp. 33–52). New York: Springer-Verlag.

Siegel, L. S., & Linder, A. (1984). Short-term memory processes in children with reading and arithmetic disabilities. *Developmental Psychology, 20,* 200–207.

Siegel, L. S., & Ryan, E. B. (1989). The development of working memory in normally achieving and subtypes of learning disabled children. *Child Development, 60,* 973–980.

Simmons, D. C., & Kameenui, E. J. (1996). A focus on curriculum design: When children fail. *Focus on Exceptional Children, 28*(7), 1–16.

Slavin, R. E. (1986). Best evidence synthesis: An alternative to meta-analytic and traditional reviews. *Educational Researcher, 15,* 5–11.

Slavin, R. E. (1987). Grouping for instruction in the elementary school. *Educational Psychologist, 22,* 109–127.

Slavin, R. E., Karweit, N. L., & Madden, N. A. (1989). *Effective programs for students at risk.* Needham Heights, MA: Allyn & Bacon.

Slavin, R. E., Stevens, R. J., & Madden, N. A. (1988). Accommodating student diversity in reading and writing instruction: A cooperative learning approach. *RASE: Remedial and Special Education, 9*(1), 60–66. (Special Issue: The challenge of reading with understanding in the intermediate grades.)

Smith, M. L., Glass, G. V., & Miller, T. L. (1980). *The benefits of psychotherapy.* Baltimore: Johns Hopkins University Press.

Snow, R. E. (1994). Abilities in academic tasks. In R. J. Sternberg & R. K. Wagner (Eds.), *Mind in context: Interactionist perspective on human intelligence* (pp. 3–37). New York: Cambridge University Press.

Snow, R. E., & Swanson, J. (1992). Instructional psychology: Aptitude, adaptation, and assessment. *Annual Review of Psychology, 43,* 583–626.

Snowling, M. J. (1981). Phonemic deficits in developmental dyslexia. *Psychological Research, 43,* 219–234.

Spear-Swerling, L., & Sternberg, R. J. (1994). The road not taken: An integrative theoretical model of reading disability. *Journal of Learning Disabilities, 27*(2), 91–103, 122.

Spector, J. E. (1995). Phonemic awareness training: Application of principles of direct instruction. *Reading and Writing Quarterly: Overcoming Learning Difficulties, 11*(1), 37–51.

Stanovich, K. E. (1980). Toward an interactive-compensatory model of individual differences in the development of reading fluency. *Reading Research Quarterly, 16*, 32–65.

Stanovich, K. E. (1986). Matthew effects in reading: Some consequences of individual differences in the acquisition of literacy. *Reading Research Quarterly, 21*, 360–406.

Stanovich, K. E., & Siegel, L. S. (1994). Phenotypic performance profile of children with reading disabilities: A regression-based test of the phonological-core difference model. *Journal of Educational Psychology, 86*, 24–53.

Stephens, T. M. (1977). *Teaching skills to children with learning and behavior disorders*. Columbus, OH: Merrill.

Strauss, A. A., & Kephart, N. C. (1955). *Psychopathology and education of the brain-injured child, Vol. 2: Progress in theory and clinic.* New York: Grune & Stratton.

Sullivan, J. (1972). The effects of Kephart's Perceptual Motor Training on a reading clinic sample. *Journal of Learning Disabilities, 5*, 32–38.

Swanson, H. L. (1982). Conceptual processes as a function of age and enforced attention in learning disabled children: Evidence for deficient rule learning. *Contemporary Educational Psychology, 7*, 152–160.

Swanson, H. L. (1984). Does theory guide practice? *Remedial and Special Education, 5*(5), 7–16.

Swanson, H. L. (1987). Verbal coding deficits in the recall of pictorial information by learning disabled readers: The influence of a lexical system. *American Educational Research Journal, 24*, 143–170.

Swanson, H. L. (1988). Toward a metatheory of learning disabilities. *Journal of Learning Disabilities, 21*, 196–209.

Swanson, H. L. (1989). Central processing strategy difference in gifted, normal achieving, learning disabled, and mentally retarded children. *Journal of Experimental Child Psychology, 47*, 378–397.

Swanson, H. L. (1990). Instruction derived from the strategy deficit model: Overview of principles and procedures. In T. E. Scruggs & B. Y. L. Wong (Eds.), *Intervention research in learning disabilities* (pp. 34–65). New York: Springer-Verlag.

Swanson, H. L. (1991). Operational definitions of learning disabilities. *Learning Disability Quarterly, 14*, 242–254.

Swanson, H. L. (1992). Generality and modifiability of working memory among skilled and less skilled readers. *Journal of Educational Psychology, 64*(4), 473–488.

Swanson, H. L. (1993). Working memory in learning disability subgroups. *Journal of Experimental Child Psychology, 56*, 87–114.

Swanson, H. L., & Alexander, J. E. (1997). Cognitive processes as predictors of word recognition and reading comprehension in learning-disabled and skilled readers: Revisiting the specificity hypothesis. *Journal of Educational Psychology, 89*(1), 128–158.

Swanson, H. L., Carson, C., & Sachse-Lee, C. M. (1996). A selective synthesis of intervention research for students with learning disabilities. *School Psychology Review, 25*(3), 370–391.

Swanson, H. L., Carson, C., & Sachse-Lee, C. (1996). Intervention research in learning disabilities: Is there support for a deficit model? In T. Scruggs & M. Mastropieri (Eds.), *Advances in learning and behavioral disabilities* (pp. 51–179). Greenwich, CT: JAI Press.

Swanson, H. L., & Christie, L. (1994). Implicit notions about learning disabilities: Some directions for definitions. *Learning Disabilities Research and Practice, 9*, 242–252.

Swanson, H. L., O'Shaughnessy, T., McMahon, C., Hoskyn, M., & Sache-Lee, C. (1998). A selective synthesis of single subject intervention research on students wiht learning disabilities. In T. Scruggs & M. Mastropieri (Eds.), *Advances in learning and behavioral disabilities* (pp. 79–125). Greenwich, CT: JAI Press.

Thorpe, H. W., Lampe, S., Nash, R. T., & Chiang, B. (1981). The effects of the kinesthetic–tactile component of the VAKT procedure on secondary LD students' reading performance. *Psychology in the Schools, 18*(3), 334–340.

Tobias, S. (1981). Adaptation to individual differences. In F. H. Farley & N. J. Gordon, (Eds.), *Psychology and education: The state of the union* (pp. 40–81). Berkeley, CA: McCutchan.

Torgesen, J. K., & Morgan, S. (1990). Phonological synthesis tasks: A developmental, functional, and componential analysis. In H. L. Swanson & B. Keogh (Eds.), *Learning disabilities: Theoretical and research issues* (pp. 263–276). Hillsdale, NJ: Erlbaum.

Torgesen, J. K., Wagner, R. K., Rashotte, C. A., Alexander, A. W., & Conway, T. (1997). Preventive and remedial intervention for children with severe reading disabilities. *Learning Disabilities: A Multi-Disciplinary Journal, 8*, 51–61.

Turner, M. L., & Engle, R. W. (1989). Is working memory capacity task dependent? *Journal of Memory and Language, 28*, 127–154.

U.S. Department of Education. (1994). *Sixteenth annual report to Congress on the implementation of Individuals with Disabilities Education Act.* Washington, DC: U.S. Government Printing Office.

VanStrien, J. W., Stolk, B. D., & Zuiker, S. (1995). Hemisphere-specific treatment of dyslexia subtypes: Better reading with anxiety-laden words? *Journal of Learning Disabilities, 28*(1), 30–34.

Vellutino, F., & Scanlon, D. M. (1991). The effects of instructional bias on word identification. In I. L. Rieben & C. A. Perfetti (Eds.), *Learning to read: Basic research and its implications* (pp. 189–204). Hillsdale, NJ: Erlbaum.

Vellutino, F., Scanlon, D. M., Sipay, E., Small, S., Pratt, A., Chen, R., & Denckla, M. (1996). Cognitive profiles of difficult-to-remediate and readily remediated poor readers: Early intervention as a vehicle for distinguishing between cognitive and experiential deficits as basic causes of specific reading disability. *Journal of Educational Psychology, 88*, 601–638.

Vellutino, F., Scanlon, D. M., & Spearing, D. (1995). Semantic and phonological coding in poor and normal readers. *Journal of Experimental Child Psychology, 59*, 76–123.

Walczyk, J. J. (1993). Are general resource notions still viable in reading research? *Journal of Educational Psychology, 85*, 127–135.

Wall, T. D., & Payne, D. (1973). Are deficiency scores deficient? *Journal of Applied Psychology, 58*, 322–326.

Wang, M. C. (1992). *Adaptive education strategies: Building on diversity*. Baltimore: Brookes.

Waterman, B., & Lewandowski, L. (1993). Phonological and semantic processing in reading disabled and nondisabled males at two age-levels. *Journal of Experimental Child Psychology, 55*, 87–103.

Waters, G. S., Caplan, D., & Leonard, C. (1992). The role of phonology in reading comprehension: Implications of the effects of homophones on processing sentences with referentially dependent categories. *Quarterly Journal of Experimental Psychology: Human Experimental Psychology, 44*, 343–372.

Weisz, J. R., Weiss, B., Han, S. S., Granger, D. A., & Morton, T. (1995). Effects of psychotherapy with children and adolescents revisited: A meta-analysis of treatment outcome studies. *Psychological Bulletin, 117*(3), 450–468.

Welch, M. (1992). The PLEASE strategy: A meta-cognitive learning strategy for improving the paragraph writing of students with learning disabilities. *Learning Disability Quarterly, 15*(2), 119–128.

Wiederholt, J. L. (1974). Historical perspectives on the education of the learning disabled. In L. Mann & D. A. Sabatino (Eds.), *The second review of special education* (pp. 103–152). Austin, TX: PRO-ED.

Wiederholt, J. L., & Hammill, D. D. (1971). Use of the Frostig-Horne Visual Perceptual Program in the urban school. *Psychology in Schools, 8*, 268–274.

Wiederholt, J. L., Hammill, D. D., & Brown, V. (1978). *The resource teacher: A guide to effective practices.* Boston: Allyn & Bacon.

Williams, J. P. (1979). Reading instruction today. *American Psychologist, 34*, 917–922.

Wong, B. Y. L. (1986). Metacognition and special education: A review of a view. *Journal of Special Education, 20*(1), 9–29.

Wong, B. Y. L. (1987). How do the results of metacognitive research impact on the learning disabled individual? *Learning Disability Quarterly, 10*, 189–195.

Wong, B. Y. L. (1991). Assessment of metacognitive research in learning disabilities: Theory, research, and practice. In H. L. Swanson (Ed.), *Handbook on the assessment of learning disabilities* (pp. 265–284). Austin, TX: PRO-ED.

Wong, B. Y. L., Butler, D. L., Ficzere, S. A., Kuperis, S., Corden, M., & Zelmer, J. (1994). Teaching problem learners revision skills and sensitivity to audience through two instructional modes: Student–teacher versus student–student interactive dialogues. *Learning Disabilities Research and Practice, 9*(2), 78–90.

Wong, B. Y. L., & Jones, W. (1982). Increasing metacomprehension in learning disabled and normally-achieving students through self-questioning training. *Learning Disability Quarterly, 5*, 228–240.

Wong, B. Y. L., & Wong, R. (1986). Study behavior as a function of metacognitive knowledge about critical task variables: An investigation of above average, average, and learning disabled readers. *Learning Disability Research, 1*, 101–111.

Woodcock, R. W., & Johnson, M. B. (1989). *Woodcock–Johnson Psycho-Educational Battery—Revised.* Allen, TX: DLM Teaching Resources.

Zecker, S. G., & Zinner, T. E. (1987). Semantic code deficit for reading disabled children on an auditory lexical decision task. *Journal of Reading Behavior, 19*, 177–189.

Appendix A

Studies Selected for General Synthesis

1. Amerikaner, M., & Summerlin, M. L. (1982). Group counseling with learning disabled children: Effects of social skills and relaxation training on self-concept and classroom behavior. *Journal of Learning Disabilities, 15*(6), 340–343.
2. Argulewicz, E. N. (1982). Effects of an instructional program designed to improve attending behaviors of learning disabled students. *Journal of Learning Disabilities, 15*(1), 23–27.
3. Ault, M. J., Wolery, M., Gast, D. L., Doyle, P. M., & Martin, C. P. (1990). Comparison of predictable and unpredictable trial sequences during small-group instruction. *Learning Disability Quarterly, 13*(1), 12–29.
4. Ayllon, T., Layman, D., & Kandel, H. J. (1975). A behavioral educational alternative to drug control of hyperactive children. *Journal of Applied Behavior Analysis, 8*(2), 137–146.
5. Ayres, A. J. (1972). Improving academic scores through sensory integration. *Journal of Learning Disabilities, 5*(6), 338–343.
6. Bakker, D. J., Bouma, A., & Gardien, C. J. (1990). Hemisphere-specific treatment of dyslexia subtypes: A field experiment. *Journal of Learning Disabilities, 23*(7), 433–438.
7. Balcerzak, J. P. (1986). The effects of an aptitude treatment interaction approach with intermediate aged learning disabled students based on emphasizing the individual's strength in simultaneous or sequential processing in the areas of mathematics, reading, and self-concept (Ph.D. diss., State University of New York, 1985). *Dissertation Abstracts International, 47*(3-A), 630.
8. Barbetta, P. M., & Heward, W. L. (1993). Effects of active student response during error correction on the acquisition and maintenance of geography facts by elementary students with learning disabilities. *Journal of Behavioral Education, 3*(3), 217–233.
9. Bay, M., Staver, J. R., Bryan, T., & Hale, J. B. (1992). Science instruction for the mildly handicapped: Direct instruction versus discovery teaching. *Journal of Research in Science Teaching, 29*(6), 555–570.
10. Beals, V. L. (1985). The effects of large group instruction on the acquisition of spe-

cific learning disabled adolescents (Ph.D. diss., University of Kansas, 1984). *Dissertation Abstracts International, 45*(9-A), 2478.
11. Bell, K. E., Young, K. R., Salzberg, C. L., & West, R. P. (1991). High school driver education using peer tutors, direction instruction, and precision teaching. *Journal of Applied Behavior Analysis, 24*(1), 45–51.
12. Belmont, I., & Birch, H. G. (1974). The effect of supplemental intervention on children with low reading-readiness scores. *Journal of Special Education, 8*(1), 81–89.
13. Berninger, V. W., Lester, K., Sohlberg, M. M., & Mateer, C. (1991). Interventions based on the multiple connections model of reading for developmental dyslexia and acquired deep dyslexia. *Archives of Clinical Neuropsychology, 6*(4), 375–391.
14. Billingsley, F. F. (1977). The effects of self- and externally-imposed schedules of reinforcement on oral reading performance. *Journal of Learning Disabilities, 10,* 549–558.
15. Blandford, B. J., & Lloyd, J. W. (1987). Effects of a self-instructional procedure on handwriting. *Journal of Learning Disabilities, 20*(6), 342–346.
16. Blick, D. W., & Test, D. W. (1987). Effects of self-recording on high school students' on-task behavior. *Learning Disability Quarterly, 10*(3), 203–213.
17. Bos, C. S., & Anders, P. L. (1990). Effects of interactive vocabulary instruction on the vocabulary learning and reading comprehension of junior-high learning disabled students. *Learning Disability Quarterly, 13*(1), 31–42.
18. Bos, C. S., & Anders, P. L. (1992). Using interactive teaching and learning strategies to promote text comprehension and content learning for students with learning disabilities. *International Journal of Disability, Development and Education, 39*(3), 225–238.
19. Bos, C. S., Anders, P. L., Filip, D., & Jaffe, L. E. (1985). Semantic feature analysis and long-term learning. *National Reading Conference Yearbook, 34,* 42–47.
20. Bos, C. S., Anders, P. L., Filip, D., & Jaffe, L. E. (1989). The effects of an interactive instructional strategy for enhancing reading comprehension and content area learning for students with learning disabilities. *Journal of Learning Disabilities, 22,* 384–390.
21. Boyer, A. W. (1991). Improving the expository paragraph writing of learning disabled elementary school students using small group strategies instruction and word processing (Ph.D. diss., University of Kentucky, 1990). *Dissertation Abstracts International, 52*(1-A), 129–130.
22. Brailsford, A., Snart, F., & Das, J. P. (1984). Strategy training and reading comprehension. *Journal of Learning Disabilities, 17*(5), 287–293.
23. Branwhite, A. B. (1983). Boosting reading skills by direct instruction. *British Journal of Educational Psychology, 53*(3), 291–298.
24. Brigham, F. J., Scruggs, T. E., & Mastropieri, M. A. (1992). Teacher enthusiasm in learning disabilities classrooms: Effects on learning and behavior. *Learning Disabilities Research and Practice, 7*(1), 68–73.
25. Brown, I. S., & Felton, R. C. (1990). Effects of instruction on beginning reading skills in children at risk for reading disability. *Reading and Writing: An Interdiscriplanary Journal, 2,* 223–241.
26. Brown, R. T., & Alford, N. (1984). Ameliorating attentional deficits and concomitant academic deficiencies in learning disabled children through cognitive training. *Journal of Learning Disabilities, 17,* 20–26.
27. Bryant, N. D., Drabin, I. R., & Gettinger, M. (1981). Effects of varying unit size on spelling achievement in learning disabled children. *Journal of Learning Disabilities, 14*(4), 200–203.
28. Bryant, N. D., Fayne, H. R., & Gettinger, M. (1982). Applying the mastery learning model to sight word instruction for disabled readers. *Journal of Experimental Education, 50*(3), 116–121.

29. Bryant, S. T. (1979). Relative effectiveness of visual–auditory versus visual–auditory–kinesthetic–tactile procedures for teaching sight words and letter sounds to young, disabled readers (Ph.D. diss., Columbia University, 1979). *Dissertation Abstracts International, 40*(5-A), 2588–2589.
30. Bulgren, J. A., Hock, M. F., Schumaker, J. B., & Deshler, D. D. (1995). The effects of instruction in a paired associates strategy on the information mastery performance of students with learning disabilities. *Learning Disabilities Research and Practice, 10*(1), 22–37.
31. Bulgren, J. A., Schumaker, J. B., & Deshler, D. D. (1988). Effectiveness of a concept teaching routine in enhancing the performance of LD students in secondary-level mainstream classes. *Learning Disability Quarterly, 11*(1), 3–17.
32. Burkwist, B. J., Mabee, W. S., & McLaughlin, T. F. (1987). The effect of a daily report card system on inappropriate classroom verbalizations with a junior high school learning-disabled student. *Techniques, 3*(4), 265–272.
33. Campbell, B. J., Brady, M. P., & Linehan, S. (1991). Effects of peer-mediated instruction on the acquisition and generalization of written capitalization skills. *Journal of Learning Disabilities, 24,* 6–14.
34. Carte, E., Morrison, D., Sublett, J., Uemura, A., & Setrakian, W. (1984). Sensory integration therapy: A trial of a specific neurodevelopmental therapy for the remediation of learning disabilities. *Developmental and Behavioral Pediatrics, 5*(4), 189–194.
35. Cartelli, L. M. (1978). Paradigmatic language training for learning disabled children. *Journal of Learning Disabilities, 11*(5), 54–59.
36. Carter, B. G. (1985). For the learning disabled: Semantic mapping or SQ3R? (Ph.D. diss., University of Nevada–Reno, 1984). *Dissertation Abstracts International, 46*(3-A), 674.
37. Case, L. P., Harris, K. R., & Graham, S. (1992). Improving the mathematic problem-solving skills of students with learning disabilities: Self-regulated strategy development. *Journal of Special Education, 26*(1), 1–19.
38. Chan, L. K. S. (1991). Promoting strategy generalization through self-instructional training in students with reading disabilities. *Journal of Learning Disabilities, 24*(7), 427–433.
39. Chan, L. K. S., & Cole, P. G. (1986). The effects of comprehension monitoring training on the reading competence of learning disabled and regular class students. *Remedial and Special Education, 7*(4), 33–40.
40. Chan, L. K. S., Cole, P. G., & Morris, J. N. (1990). Effects of instruction in the use of a visual-imagery strategy on the reading-comprehension competence of disabled and average readers. *Learning Disability Quarterly, 13*(1), 2–11.
41. Chase, C. H., Schmitt, R. L., Russell, G., & Tallal, P. (1984). A new chemotherapeutic investigation: Piracetum effects on dyslexia. *Annals of Dyslexia, 34,* 29–48.
42. Chiang, B. (1986). Initial learning and transfer effects of microcomputer drills on LD students' multiplication skills. *Learning Disability Quarterly, 9*(2), 118–123.
43. Chiang, B., Thorpe, H. W., & Darch, C. B. (1980). Effects of cross-age tutoring on word-recognition performance of learning disabled students. *Learning Disability Quarterly, 3*(4), 11–19.
44. Cochrane, M., & Ballard, K. D. (1986). Teaching five special needs children in a regular primary classroom using a consultation–collaboration model. *Exceptional Child, 33*(2), 91–102.
45. Cole, K. B. (1993). Efficacy and generalization of instruction in sequential expository writing for students with learning disabilities (Ph.D. diss., Northern Illinois University, 1992). *Dissertation Abstracts International, 53*(7-A), 2326

46. Collins, M., & Carnine, D. (1988). Evaluating the field test revision process by comparing two versions of a reasoning skills CAI Program. *Journal of Learning Disabilities, 21*(6), 375–379.
47. Commeyras, M. (1992). Dialogical-thinking reading lessons: Promoting critical thinking among "learning-disabled" students (Ph.D. diss., University of Illinois, 1991). *Dissertation Abstracts International, 52*(7-A), 2480–2481.
48. Cornelius, P. L., & Semmel, M. I. (1982). Effects of summer instruction on reading achievement regression of learning disabled students. *Journal of Learning Disabilities, 15*(7), 409–413.
49. Cosden, M. A., & English, J. P. (1987). The effects of grouping, self esteem, and locus of control on microcomputer performance and help seeking by mildly handicapped students. *Journal of Educational Computing Research, 3*(4), 443–459.
50. Cuvo, A. J., Ashley, K. M., Marso, K. J., Zhang, B. L., & Fry, T. A. (1995). Effect of response practice variables on learning spelling and sight vocabulary. *Journal of Applied Behavior Analysis, 28*, 155–173.
51. Daly, E. J., & Martens, B. K. (1994). A comparison of three interventions for increasing oral reading performance: Application of the instructional hierarchy. *Journal of Applied Behavior Analysis, 27*(3), 459–469.
52. Danoff, B., Harris, K. R., & Graham, S. (1993). Incorporating strategy instruction with the writing process in the regular classroom: Effects on the writing of students with and without learning disabilities. *Journal of Reading Behavior, 25*(3), 295–322.
53. Darch, C., & Carnine, D. (1986). Teaching content area material to learning disabled students. *Exceptional Children, 53*(3), 240–246.
54. Darch, C., & Eaves, R. C. (1986). Visual displays to increase comprehension of high school learning-disabled students. *Journal of Special Education, 20*(3), 309–318.
55. Darch, C., & Gersten, R. (1985). The effects of teacher presentation rate and praise on LD students' oral reading performance. *British Journal of Educational Psychology, 55*(3), 295–303.
56. Darch, C., & Gersten, R. (1986). Direction-setting activities in reading comprehension: A comparison of two approaches. *Learning Disability Quarterly, 9*(3), 235–243.
57. Darch, C., & Kameenui, E. J. (1987). Teaching LD students critical reading skills: A systematic replication. *Learning Disability Quarterly, 10*(2), 82–90.
58. Das, J. P., Mishra, R. K., & Pool, J. E. (1995). An experiment on cognitive remediation of word-reading difficulty. *Journal of Learning Disabilities, 28*(2), 66–79.
59. DeBoskey, D. S. (1982). An investigation of the remediation of learning disabilities based on brain-related tasks as measured by the Halstead–Reitan Neuropsychological test battery (Ph.D. diss., University of Tennessee, 1982). *Dissertation Abstracts International, 43*(6-B), 2032.
60. DeLaPaz, S. (1995). *An analysis of the effects of dictation and planning instruction on the writing of students with learning disabilities* (unpublished Ph.D. diss., University of Maryland).
61. DeLaPaz, S. (in press). Strategy instruction in planning: Teaching students with learning and writing disabilities to compose persuasive and expository essays. *Learning Disability Quarterly*.
62. Deno, S. L., & Chiang, B. (1979). An experimental analysis of the nature of reversal errors in children with severe learning disabilities. *Learning Disability Quarterly, 2*, 40–50

63. DiGangi, S. A., Maag, J. W., & Rutherford, R. B. (1991). Self-graphing of on-task behavior: Enhancing the reactive effects of self-monitoring on on-task behavior and academic performance. *Learning Disability Quarterly, 14*, 221–230.
64. DiVeta, S. K., & Speece, D. L. (1990). The effects of blending and spelling training on the decoding skills of young poor readers. *Journal of Learning Disabilities, 23*(9), 579–582.
65. Dixon, M. E. (1984). Questioning strategy instruction participation and reading comprehension of learning disabled students (Ph.D. diss., University of Arizona, 1983). *Dissertation Abstracts International, 44*(11-A), 3349.
66. Dowis, C. L., & Schloss, P. (1992). The impact of mini-lessons on writing skills. *Remedial and Special Education, 13*(5), 34–42.
67. DuPaul, G. J., & Henningson, P. N. (1993). Peer tutoring effects on the classroom performance of children with attention deficit hyperactivity disorder. *School Psychology Review, 22*(1), 134–143.
68. Duvall, S. F., Delquadri, J. C., Elliott, M., & Hall, R. V. (1992). Parent-tutoring procedures: Experimental analysis and validation of generalization in oral reading across passages, settings, and time. *Journal of Behavioral Education, 2*, 281–303.
69. Ellis, E. S., Deshler, D. D., & Schumaker, J. B. (1989). Teaching adolescents with learning disabilities to generate and use task-specific strategies. *Journal of Learning Disabilities, 22*(2), 108–130.
70. Ellis, E. S., & Graves, A. W. (1990). Teaching rural students with learning disabilities: A paraphrasing strategy to increase comprehension of main ideas. *Rural Special Education Quarterly, 10*, 2–10.
71. Englert, C. S., Hiebert, E. H., & Stewart, S. R. (1985). Spelling unfamiliar words by an analogy strategy. *Journal of Special Education, 19*(3), 291–306.
72. Englert, C. S., & Mariage, T. V. (1991). Making students partners in the comprehension process: Organizing the reading "posse." *Learning Disability Quarterly, 14*(2), 123–138.
73. Englert, C. S., Raphael, T. E., & Anderson, L. M. (1992). Socially mediated instruction: Improving students' knowledge about talk and writing. *Elementary School Journal, 92*(4), 411–449.
74. Englert, C. S., Raphael, T. E., Anderson, L. M., Anthony, H. M., & Stevens, D. D. (1991). Making strategies and self talk visible: Writing instruction in regular and special education classrooms. *American Educational Research Journal, 28*(2), 337–372.
75. Fantasia, K. L. (1982). An investigation of formal analysis as an intervention to improve word problem computation for learning disabled children (Ph.D. diss., University of Washington, 1981). *Dissertation Abstracts International, 42*(12-A), 5085.
76. Farmer, M. E., Klein, R., & Bryson, S. E. (1992). Computer-assisted reading: Effects of whole word feedback on fluency and comprehension in readers with severe disabilities. *Remedial and Special Education, 13*, 50–60.
77. Fawcett, A. J., Nicolson, R. I., & Morris, S. (1993). Computer-based spelling remediation for dyslexic children. *Journal of Computer Assisted Learning, 9*(3), 171–183.
78. Fiedorowicz, C. A. M. (1986). Training of component reading skills. *Annals of Dyslexia, 36*, 318–334.
79. Fiedorowicz, C. A. M., & Trites, R. L. (1987). *An evaluation of the effectiveness of computer-assisted component reading subskills training.* Ontario, Canada: Queen's Printer.
80. Fletcher, C. M., & Prior, M. R. (1990). The rule learning behavior of reading disabled and normal children as a function of task characteristics and instruction. *Journal of Experimental Child Psychology, 50*(1), 39–58.

81. Fortner, V. L. (1986). Generalization of creative productive-thinking training to LD students' written expression. *Learning Disability Quarterly*, *9*(4), 274–284.

82. Foster, K. (1983). The influence of computer-assisted instruction and workbook of the learning of multiplication facts by learning disabled and normal students (Ph.D. diss., Florida State University, 1983). *Dissertation Abstracts International*, *42*(9-A), 3953.

83. Fuchs, L. S., Fuchs, D., Hamlett, C. L., Phillips, N. B., & Bentz, J. (1994). Classwide curriculum-based measurement: Helping general educators meet the challenge of student diversity. *Exceptional Children*, *60*(6), 518–537.

84. Gajria, M., & Salvia, J. (1992). The effects of summarization instruction on text comprehension of students with learning disabilities. *Exceptional Children*, *58*(6), 508–516.

85. Gelzheiser, L. M. (1984). Generalization from categorical memory tasks to prose by learning disabled adolescents. *Journal of Educational Psychology*, *76*(6), 1128–1138.

86. Gettinger, M., Bryant, N. D., & Fayne, H. R. (1982). Designing spelling instruction for learning disabled children: An emphasis on unit size, distributed practice, and training for transfer. *Journal of Special Education*, *16*(4), 439–448.

87. Gittelman, R., & Feingold, I. (1983). Children with reading disorders, Part 1: Efficacy of reading remediation. *Journal of Child Psychology and Psychiatry*, *24*(2), 167–191.

88. Glaman, G. M. V. (1975). Use of ability measures to predict the most appropriate method or sequence of mathematics instruction for learning disabled junior high students (Ph.D. diss., University of Minnesota, 1974). *Dissertation Abstracts International*, *35*(11-A), 7154.

89. Graham, S. (1990). The role of production factors in learning disabled students' compositions. *Journal of Educational Psychology*, *82*(4), 781–791.

90. Graham, S., & Harris, K. R. (1989). Components analysis of cognitive strategy instruction: Effects on learning disabled students' compositions and self-efficacy. *Journal of Educational Psychology*, *81*(3), 353–361.

91. Graham, S., MacArthur, C., Schwartz, S., & Page-Voth, V. (1992). Improving the compositions of students with learning disabilities: Using a strategy involving product and process goal setting. *Exceptional Children*, *58*(4), 322–334.

92. Graves, A. W. (1986). Effects of direct instruction and metacomprehension training on finding main ideas. *Learning Disabilities Research*, *1*(2), 90–100.

93. Graybill, D., Jamison, M., & Swerdlik, M. E. (1984). Remediation of impulsivity in learning disabled children by special education resource teachers using verbal self-instruction. *Psychology in the Schools*, *21*(2), 252–254.

94. Griffin, C. C., Simmons, D. C., & Kameeenui, E. J. (1991). Investigating the effectiveness of graphic organizer instruction on the comprehension and recall of science content by students with learning disabilities. *Reading, Writing, and Learning Disabilities*, *7*(4), 355–376.

95. Guyer, B. P., & Sabatino, D. (1989). The effectiveness of a multisensory alphabetic phonetic approach with college students who are learning disabled. *Journal of Learning Disabilities*, *22*(7), 430–434.

96. Hallahan, D. P., Lloyd, J., Kosiewicz, M. M., Kauffman, J. M., & Graves, A. W. (1979). Self-monitoring of attention as a treatment for a leaning disabled boy's off-task behavior. *Learning Disability Quarterly*, *2*, 24–32

97. Hallahan, D. P., Marshall, K. J., & Lloyd, J. W. (1981). Self-recording during group instruction: Effects on attention to task. *Learning Disability Quarterly*, *4*(4), 407–413.

98. Harper, J. A. (1986). A comparison of the effectiveness of microcomputer and workbook instruction on reading comprehension performance of high incidence handi-

capped students (Ph.D. diss., Southern Illinois University–Carbondale, 1985). *Dissertation Abstracts International, 46*(11A), 3318–3319.

99. Harris, K. R. (1986). Self-monitoring of attentional behavior versus self-monitoring of productivity: Effects on on-task behavior and academic response rate among learning disabled children. *Journal of Applied Behavior Analysis, 19*(4), 417–423.
100. Harris, K. R., & Graham, S. (1985). Improving learning disabled students' composition skills: Self-control strategy training. *Learning Disability Quarterly, 8*, 27–36.
101. Harris, K. R., Graham, S., Reid, R., McElroy, K., & Hamby, R. S. (1994). Self-monitoring of performance: Replication and cross-task comparison studies. *Learning Disability Quarterly, 17*(2), 121–139.
102. Hazel, J. S., Schumaker, J. B., Sherman, J. A., & Sheldon, J. (1982). Application of a group training program in social skills and problem solving to learning disabled and non-learning disabled youth. *Learning Disability Quarterly, 5*, 398–408.
103. Helper, M. M., Farber, E. D., & Feldgaier, S. (1982). Alternative thinking and classroom behavior of learning impaired children. *Psychological Reports, 50*(2), 415–420.
104. Hine, M. S., Goldman, S. R., & Cosden, M. A. (1990). Error monitoring by learning handicapped students engaged in collaborative microcomputer-based writing. *Journal of Special Education, 23*(4), 407–422.
105. Hollingsworth, M., & Woodward, J. (1993). Integrated learning: Explicit strategies and their role in problem-solving instruction for students with learning disabilities. *Exceptional Children, 59*(5), 444–455.
106. Howell, R., Sidorenko, E., & Jurica, J. (1987). The effects of computer use on the acquisition of multiplication facts by a student with learning disabilities. *Journal of Learning Disabilities, 20*, 336–341.
107. Hughes, C. A., & Schumaker, J. B. (1991). Test-taking strategy instruction for adolescents with learning disabilities. *Exceptionality, 2*(4), 205–221.
108. Humphries, T. W., Wright, M., Snider, L., & McDougall, B. (1992). A comparison of the effectiveness of sensory integrative therapy and perceptual–motor training in treating children with learning disabilities. *Developmental and Behavioral Pediatrics, 13*(1), 31–40.
109. Hurford, D. P. (1990). Training phonemic segmentation ability with a phonemic discrimination intervention in second- and third-grade children with reading disabilities. *Journal of Learning Disabilities, 23*, 564–569.
110. Hurford, D. P., & Sanders, R. E. (1990). Assessment and remediation of a phonemic discrimination deficit in reading disabled second and fourth graders. *Journal of Experimental Child Psychology, 50*(3), 396–415.
111. Hutchinson, N. L. (1993). Effects of cognitive strategy instruction on algebra problem solving of adolescents with learning disabilities. *Learning Disability Quarterly, 16*(1), 34–63.
112. Hutchinson, N. L., Freeman, J. G., Downey, K. H., & Kilbreath, L. (1992). Development and evaluation of an instructional module to promote career maturity for youth with learning disabilities. *Canadian Journal of Counselling, 26*(4), 290–299.
113. Idol, L., & Croll, V. J. (1987). Story-mapping training as a means of improving reading comprehension. *Learning Disability Quarterly, 10*, 214–229.
114. Idol-Maestas, L. (1981). Increasing the oral reading performance of a learning disabled adult. *Learning Disability Quarterly, 4*(3), 294–301.
115. Jaben, T. H. (1983). The effects of creativity training on learning disabled student's creative written expression. *Journal of Learning Disabilities, 16*(5), 264–265.

116. Jaben, T. H. (1985). Effect of instruction for creativity on learning disabled students' drawings. *Perceptual and Motor Skills, 61*(3, pt. 1), 895–898.
117. Jaben, T. H. (1986). Impact of instruction on behavior disordered and learning disabled students' creative behavior. *Psychology in the Schools, 23*(4), 401–405.
118. Jaben, T. H. (1987). Effects of training on learning disabled students' creative written expression. *Psychological Reports, 60*(1), 23–26.
119. Jaben, T. H., Treffinger, D. J., Whelan, R. J., Hudson, F. G., Stainback, S. B., & Stainback, W. (1982). Impact of instruction on learning disabled students' creative thinking. *Psychology in the Schools, 19*(3), 371–373.
120. Johnson, L., Graham, S., & Harris, K. R. (1997). The effects of goal setting and self-instructions on learning a reading comprehension strategy: A study with students with learning disabilities. *Journal of Learning Disabilities, 30*, 88–91.
121. Jones, K. M., Torgesen, J. K., & Sexton, M. A. (1987). Using computer guided practice to increase decoding fluency in learning disabled children: A study using the Hint and Hunt I Program. *Journal of Learning Disabilities, 20*(2), 122–128.
122. Kane, B. J., & Alley, G. R. (1980). Tutored, instructional management program in computational mathematics for program in incarcerated learning disabled juvenile delinquents. *Journal of Learning Disabilities, 13*(3), 148–151.
123. Kendall, P. C., & Braswell, L. (1982). Cognitive-behavioral self-control therapy for children: A components analysis. *Journal of Consulting and Clinical Psychology, 50*(5), 672–689.
124. Kennedy, K. M., & Backman, J. (1993). Effectiveness of the Lindamood Auditory Discrimination in Depth Program with students with learning disabilities. *Learning Disabilities Research and Practice, 8*(4), 253–259.
125. Kershner, J. R., Cummings, R. L., Clarke, K. A., Hadfield, A. J., & Kershner, B. A. (1990). Two-year evaluation of the Tomatis Listening Training Program with learning disabled children. *Learning Disability Quarterly, 13*, 43–53.
126. Kerstholt, M. T., Van Bon, W. H. J., & Schreuder, R. (1994). Training in phonemic segmentation: The effects of visual support. *Reading and Writing: An Interdisciplinary Journal, 6*(4), 361–385.
127. Kim, Y. O. (1992). The effect of teaching a test-taking strategy to high school students with learning disabilities (Ph.D. diss., West Virginia University, 1991). *Dissertation Abstracts International, 53*(1-A), 121.
128. King-Sears, M. E., Mercer, C. D., & Sindelar, P. T. (1992). Toward independence with keyword mnemonics: A strategy for science vocabulary instruction. *Remedial and Special Education, 13*(3), 22–33.
129. Kitterman, J. F. (1984). Error verification and microcomputer mediation of a spelling task with learning disabled students (Ph.D. diss., Ball State University, 1984). *Dissertation Abstracts International, 45*(2-A), 491–492.
130. Klingner, J. K., & Vaughn, S. (1996). Reciprocal teaching of reading comprehension strategies for students with learning disabilities who use English as a second language. *Elementary School Journal, 96*, 275–293.
131. Kosiewicz, M. M., Hallahan, D. P., & Lloyd, J. (1981). The effects of an LD student's treatment choice on handwriting performance. *Learning Disability Quarterly, 4*, 281–286.
132. Kosiewicz, M. M., Hallahan, D. P., Lloyd, J., & Graves, A. W. (1982). Effects of self-instruction and self-correction procedures on handwriting performance. *Learning Disability Quarterly, 5*(1), 71–78.
133. Kraetsch, G. A. (1981). The effects of oral instructions and training on the expansion of written language. *Learning Disability Quarterly, 4*, 82–90.

134. Kunka, A. S. K. (1984). A modality–instruction interaction study of elementary learning disabled students using two types of electronic learning aids for math instruction (Ph.D. diss., University of Pittsburgh, 1983). *Dissertation Abstracts International, 45*(2-A), 387.
135. Lahey, B. B., Busemeyer, M. K., Ohara, C., & Beggs, V. E. (1977). Treatment of severe perceptual–motor disorders in children diagnosed as learning disabled. *Behavior Modification, 1*(1), 123–140.
136. Lalli, E. P., & Shapiro, E. S. (1990). The effects of self-monitoring and contingent reward on sight word acquisition. *Education and Treatment of Children, 13*, 129–141.
137. Larson, K. A., & Gerber, M. M. (1987). Effects of social metacognitive training for enhancing overt behavior in learning disabled and low achieving delinquents. *Exceptional Children, 54*(3), 201–211.
138. Lenkowsky, R. S., Barwosky, E. I., Dayboch, M., Puccio, L., & Lenkowsky, B. E. (1987). Effects of bibliotherapy on the self-concept of learning disabled, emotionally handicapped adolescents in a classroom setting. *Psychological Reports, 61*(2), 483–488.
139. Lenz, B. K., Ehren, B. J., & Smiley, L. R. (1991). A goal attainment approach to improve completion of project-type assignments by adolescents with learning disabilities. *Learning Disabilities Research and Practice, 6*(3), 166–176.
140. Leong, C. K., Simmons, D. R., & Izatt-Gambell, M. A. (1990). The effect of systematic training in elaboration on word meaning and prose comprehension in poor readers. *Annals of Dyslexia, 40*, 192–215.
141. Lerner, C. H. (1978). The comparative effectiveness of a language experience approach and a basal-type approach to remedial reading instruction for severely disabled readers in a senior high school (Ph.D. diss., Temple University 1978). *Dissertation Abstracts International, 39*(2-A), 779–780.
142. Lloyd, J., Cullinan, D., Heins, E. D., & Epstein, M. H. (1980). Direct instruction: Effects on oral and written language comprehension. *Learning Disability Quarterly, 3*(4), 70–76.
143. Lloyd, J. W., Hallahan, D. P., Kosiewicz, M. M., & Kneedler, R. D. (1982). Reactive effects of self-assessment and self-recording on attention to task and academic productivity. *Learning Disability Quarterly, 5*, 216–227.
144. Lorenz, L., & Vockell, E. (1979). Using the neurological impress method with learning disabled readers. *Journal of Learning Disabilities, 12*(6), 420–422.
145. Losh, M. A. (1991). The effect of the strategies intervention model on the academic achievement of junior high learning-disabled students (Ph.D. diss., University of Nebraska, 1991). *Dissertation Abstracts International, 52*(3-A), 880.
146. Lovett, M. W., Borden, S. L., DeLuca, T., Lacerenza, L., Benson, N. J., & Brackstone, D. (1994). Treating the core deficits of developmental dyslexia: Evidence of transfer of learning after phonologically- and strategy-based reading training programs. *Developmental Psychology, 30*(6), 805–822.
147. Lovett, M. W., Ransby, M. J., & Barron, R. W., (1988). Treatment, subtype, and word type effects on dyslexic children's response to remediation. *Brain and Language, 34*(2), 328–349.
148. Lovett, M. W., Ransby, M. J., Hardwick, N., Johns, M. S., & Donaldson, S. A. (1989). Can dyslexia be treated? Treatment-specific and generalized treatment effects in dyslexic children's response to remediation. *Brain and Language, 37*(1), 90–121.
149. Lovett, M. W., & Steinbach, K. A. (in press). The effectiveness of remedial programs for reading disabled children of different ages: Is there decreased benefit for older children? *Learning Disability Quarterly*.

150. Lovett, M. W., Warren-Chaplin, P. M., Ransby, M. J., & Borden, S. L. (1990). Training the word recognition skills of reading disabled children: Treatment and transfer effects. *Journal of Educational Psychology, 82*(4), 769–780.
151. Lovitt, T., Rudsit, J., Jenkins, J., Pious, C., & Benedetti, D. (1986). Adapting science materials for regular and learning disabled seventh graders. *Remedial and Special Education, 7*, 31–39.
152. Lucangeli, D., Galderisi, D., & Cornoldi, C. (1995). Specific and general transfer effects following metamemory training. *Learning Disabilities Research and Practice, 10*(1), 11–21.
153. Lundberg, I., & Olofsson, A. (1993). Can computer speech support reading comprehension? *Computers in Human Behavior, 9*(2–3), 283–293.
154. Maag, J. W., Reid, R., & DiGangi, S. A. (1993). Differential effects of self-monitoring attention, accuracy, and productivity. *Journal of Applied Behavior Analysis, 26*(3), 329–344.
155. MacArthur, C. A., & Haynes, J. B. (1995). Student assistant for learning from text (SALT): A hypermedia reading aid. *Journal of Learning Disabilities, 28*(3), 150–159.
156. MacArthur, C. A., Haynes, J. A., Malouf, D. B., Harris, K., & Owings, M. (1990). Computer assisted instruction with learning disabled students: Achievement, engagement, and other factors that influence achievement. *Journal of Educational Computing Research, 6*(3), 311–328.
157. MacArthur, C. A., Schwartz, S. S., & Graham, S. (1991). Effects of a reciprocal peer revision strategy in special education classrooms. *Learning Disabilities Research, 6*(4), 201–210.
158. Manning, B. H. (1984). Problem-solving instruction as an oral comprehension aid for reading disabled third graders. *Journal of Learning Disabilities, 17*(8), 457–461.
159. Maron, L. R. (1993). A comparison study of the effects of explicit versus implicit training of test-taking skills for learning-disabled fourth-grade students (Ph.D. diss., University of Wisconsin-Madison, 1992). *Dissertation Abstracts International, 53*(9-B), 4613.
160. Marsh, L. G., & Cooke, N. L. (1996). The effects of using manipulatives in teaching math problem solving to students with learning disabilities. *Learning Disabilities Research and Practice, 11*, 58–65.
161. Martin, K. F., & Manno, C. (1995). Use of a check-off system to improve middle school students' story compositions. *Journal of Learning Disabilities, 28*(3), 139–149.
162. Mathes, P. G., & Fuchs, L. S. (1993). Peer-mediated reading instruction in special education resource rooms. *Learning Disabilities Research and Practice, 8*(4), 233–243.
163. Mathews, R. M., & Fawcett, S. B. (1984). Building the capacities of job candidates through behavioral instruction. *Journal of Community Psychology, 12*(2), 123–129.
164. McCollum, P. S., & Anderson, R. P. (1974). Group counseling with reading disabled children. *Journal of Counseling Psychology, 21*(2), 150–155.
165. McCurdy, B. L., Cundari, L., & Lentz, F. E. (1990). Enhancing instructional efficiency: An examination of time delay and the opportunity to observe instruction. *Education and Treatment of Children, 13*(3), 226–238.
166. McIntyre, S. B., Test, D. W., Cooke, N. L., & Beattie, J. (1991). Using count-bys to increase multiplication facts fluency. *Learning Disability Quarterly, 14,* 82–88.
167. McNaughton, D., Hughes, C., & Ofiesh, N. (1997). Proofreading for students with learning disabilities: Integrating computer and strategy use. *Learning Disabilities Research and Practice, 12*(1), 16–28.
168. Meyer, L. A. (1982). The relative effects of word-analysis and word-supply correc-

tion procedures with poor readers during word-attack training. *Reading Research Quarterly, 17*(4), 544–555.

169. Miller, S. P., & Mercer, C. D. (1993). Using data to learn about concrete-semiconcrete-abstract instruction for students with math disabilities. *Learning Disabilities Research and Practice, 8*(2), 89–96.
170. Montague, M. (1992). The effects of cognitive and metacognitive strategy instruction on the mathematical problem solving of middle school students with learning disabilities. *Journal of Learning Disabilities, 25*(4), 230–248.
171. Montague, M., Applegate, B., & Marquard, K. (1993). Cognitive strategy instruction and mathematical problem-solving performance of students with learning disabilities. *Learning Disabilities Research and Practice, 8*(4), 223–232.
172. Montague, M., & Bos, C. S. (1986). The effect of cognitive strategy training on verbal math problem solving performance of learning disabled adolescents. *Journal of Learning Disabilities, 19*(1), 26–33.
173. Montague, M., & Leavell, A. G. (1994). Improving the narrative writing of students with learning disabilities. *Remedial and Special Education, 15*(1), 21–33.
174. Moore, L., Carnine, D., Stepnoski, M., & Woodward, J. (1987). Research on the efficiency of low-cost networking. *Learning Disability Quarterly, 20*(9), 574–576.
175. Morgan, A. V. (1991). A study of the effects of attribution retraining and cognitive self-instruction upon the academic and attentional skills, and cognitive–behavioral trends of elementary-age children served in self-contained learning disabilities programs (Ph.D. diss. College of William and Mary, 1990). *Dissertation Abstracts International, 51*(8-B), 4035.
176. Naylor, J. G., & Pumfrey, P. D. (1983). The alleviation of psycholinguistic deficits and some effects on the reading attainments of poor readers: A sequel. *Journal of Research in Reading, 6*(2), 129–153.
177. Nelson, S. L. (1985). Modifying impulsivity in learning disabled boys on matching, maze, and WISC-R performance scales (Ph.D. diss., University of Southern California, 1984). *Dissertation Abstracts International, 45*(7-B), 2316–2317.
178. Newby, R. F., Caldwell, J., & Recht, D. R. (1989). Improving the reading comprehension of children with dysphonetic and dyseidetic dyslexia using story grammar. *Journal of Learning Disabilities, 22*, 373–380.
179. O'Connor, P. D., Stuck, G. B., & Wyne, M. D. (1979). Effects of a short-term intervention resource-room program on task orientation and achievement. *Journal of Special Education, 13*(4), 375–385.
180. Olofsson, A. (1992). Synthetic speech and computer aided reading for reading disabled children. *Reading and Writing, 4*(2), 165–178.
181. Olsen, J. L., Wong, B. Y. L., & Marx, R. W. (1983). Linguistic and metacognitive aspects of normally achieving and learning disabled children's communication process. *Learning Disability Quarterly, 6*(3), 289–304.
182. Olson, R. K., & Wise, B. W. (1992). Reading on the computer with orthographic and speech feedback. *Reading and Writing: An Interdisciplinary Journal, 4*(2), 107–144.
183. Omizo, M. M., Cubberly, W. E., & Omizo, S. A. (1985). The effects of rational–emotive education groups on self-concept and locus of control among learning disabled children. *Exceptional Child, 32*(1), 13–19.
184. Omizo, M. M., Lo, F. G., & Williams, R. E. (1986). Rational–emotive education, self-concept, and locus of control among learning-disabled students. *Journal of Humanistic Education, 25*(2), 58–69.
185. Omizo, M. M., & Williams, R. E. (1982). Biofeedback-induced relaxation training as

an alternative for the elementary school learning-disabled child. *Biofeedback and Self-Regulation, 7*(2), 139–148.

186. Pany, D., & Jenkins, J. R. (1978). Learning word meanings: A comparison of instructional procedures. *Learning Disability Quarterly, 1*(2), 21–32.
187. Pany, D., Jenkins, J. R., & Schreck, J. (1982). Vocabulary instruction: Effects on word knowledge and reading comprehension. *Learning Disability Quarterly, 5*(3), 202–215.
188. Pihl, R. O., Parkes, M., Drake, H., & Vrana, F. (1980). The intervention of a modulator with learning disabled children. *Journal of Clinical Psychology, 36*(4), 972–976.
189. Porinchak, P. M. (1984). Computer-assisted instruction in secondary school reading: Interaction of cognitive and affective factors (Ph.D. diss., Hofstra University, 1983). *Dissertation Abstracts International, 45*(2-A), 478.
190. Prater, M. A., Joy, R., Chilman, B., Temple, J., & Miller, S. R. (1991). Self-monitoring of on-task behavior by adolescents with learning disabilities. *Learning Disability Quarterly, 14*, 165–177.
191. Prior, M., Frye, S., & Fletcher, C. (1987). Remediation for subgroups of retarded readers using a modified oral spelling procedure. *Developmental Medicine and Child Neurology, 29*(1), 64–71.
192. Ratekin, N. (1979). Reading achievement of disabled learners. *Exceptional Children, 45*(6), 454–458.
193. Reid, R., & Harris, K. R. (1993). Self-monitoring of attention versus self-monitoring of performance: Effects on attention and academic performance. *Exceptional Children, 60*(1), 29–40.
194. Reilly, J. P. (1991). Effects of a cognitive–behavioral program designed to increase the reading comprehension skills of learning-disabled students (Ph.D. diss., College of William and Mary, 1991). *Dissertation Abstracts International, 52*(3-A), 865.
195. Reynolds, C. J. (1986). The effects of instruction in cognitive revision strategies on the writing skills of secondary learning disabled students (Ph.D. diss. Ohio State University, 1985). *Dissertation Abstracts International, 46*(9-A), 2662.
196. Rivera, D., & Smith, D. D. (1988). Using a demonstration strategy to teach mid-school students with learning disabilities how to compute long division. *Journal of Learning Disabilities, 21*, 77–81.
197. Roberts, M., & Smith, D. D. (1980). The relationship among correct and error oral reading rates and comprehension. *Learning Disability Quarterly, 3*(1), 54–64.
198. Rose, T. L., McEntire, E., & Dowdy, C. (1982). Effects of two error-correction procedures on oral reading. *Learning Disability Quarterly, 5*(2), 100–105.
199. Rose, T. L., & Sherry, L. (1984). Relative effects of two previewing procedures on LD adolescents' oral reading performance. *Learning Disability Quarterly, 7*, 39–44.
200. Rosenberg, M. S. (1986). Error-correction during oral reading: A comparison of three techniques. *Learning Disability Quarterly, 9*, 182–192.
201. Rosenberg, M. S. (1989). The effects of daily homework assignments on the acquisition of basic skills by students with learning disabilities. *Journal of Learning Disabilities, 2*, 314–323.
202. Ross, P. A., & Braden, J. P., (1991). The effects of token reinforcement versus cognitive behavior modification on learning-disabled students' math skills. *Psychology in the Schools, 28*(3), 247–256.
203. Rudel, R. G., & Helfgott, E. (1984). Effect of piracetam on verbal memory of dyslexic boys. *American Academy of Child Psychiatry, 23*(6), 695–699.
204. Ruhl, K. L., Hughes, C. A., & Gajar, A. H. (1990). Efficacy of the pause procedure

for enhancing learning disabled and nondisabled college students' long-and short-term recall of facts presented through lecture. *Learning Disability Quarterly, 13*(1), 55–64.
205. Salend, S. J., & Lamb, E. A. (1986). Effectiveness of a group-managed interdependent contingency system. *Learning Disability Quarterly, 9*, 268–273.
206. Salend, S. J., & Meddaugh, D. (1985). Using a peer-mediated extinction procedure to decrease obscene language. *The Pointer, 30*(1), 8–11.
207. Salend, S. J., & Nowak, M. R. (1988). Effects of peer-previewing on LD students' oral reading skills. *Learning Disability Quarterly, 11*, 47–52.
208. Salend, S. J., Reeder, E., Katz, N., & Russell, T. (1992). The effects of a dependent group evaluation system. *Education and Treatment of Children, 15*(1), 32–42.
209. Sawyer, R. J., Graham, S., & Harris, K. R. (1992). Direct teaching, strategy instruction, and strategy instruction with explicit self-regulation: Effects on the composition skills and self-efficacy of students with learning disabilities. *Journal of Educational Psychology, 84*(3), 340–352.
210. Scanlon, D., Deshler, D. D., & Schumaker, J. B. (1996). Can a strategy be taught and learned in secondary inclusive classrooms? *Learning Disabilities Research and Practice, 11*, 41–57.
211. Scheerer-Neumann, G. (1981). The utilization of intraword structure in poor readers: Experimental evidence and a training program. *Psychological Research, 43*(2), 155–178.
212. Schiemek, N., (1983). Errorless discrimination training of digraphs with a learning disabled student. *School Psychology Review, 12*, 101–105.
213. Schulte, A. C., Osborne, S. S., & McKinney, J. D. (1991). Academic outcomes for students with learning disabilities in consultation and resource programs. *Exceptional Children, 57*(2), 162–172.
214. Schumaker, J. B., Deshler, D. D., Alley, G. R., Warner, M. M., Clark, F. L., & Nolan, S. (1982). Error monitoring: A learning strategy for improving adolescent academic performance. In M. W. Cruickshank & J. W. Lerner (Eds.), *Coming of age* (Vol 3, pp. 170–183). Syracuse, NY: Syracuse University Press.
215. Schunk, D. H. (1985). Participation in goal setting: Effects on self-efficacy and skills of learning-disabled children. *Journal of Special Education, 19*(3), 305–317.
216. Schunk, D. H., & Cox, P. D. (1986). Strategy training and attributional feedback with learning disabled students. *Journal of Educational Psychology, 78*(3), 201–209.
217. Scruggs, T. E., & Mastropieri, M. A. (1989). Mnemonic instruction of LD students: A field-based evaluation. *Learning Disability Quarterly, 12*, 119–125.
218. Scruggs, T. E., & Mastropieri, M. A. (1992). Classroom applications of mnemonic instruction: Acquisition, maintenance, and generalization. *Exceptional Children, 58*(3), 219–229.
219. Scruggs, T. E., Mastropieri, M. A., & Tolfa-Veit, D. (1986). The effects of coaching on the standardized test performance of learning disabled and behaviorally disordered students. *Remedial and Special Education, 7*(5), 37–41.
220. Scruggs, T. E., & Tolfa, D. (1985). Improving the test-taking skills of learning-disabled students. *Perceptual and Motor Skills, 60*(3), 847–850.
221. Seabaugh, G. O., & Schumaker, J. B. (1994). The effects of self-regulation training on the academic productivity of secondary students with learning problems. *Journal of Behavioral Education, 4*(1), 109–133.
222. Sheare, J. B. (1978). The impact of resource programs upon the self-concept and

peer acceptance of learning disabled children. *Psychology in the Schools, 15*(3), 406–412.

223. Simmonds, E. P. M. (1990). The effectiveness of two methods for teaching a constraint-seeking questioning strategy to students with learning disabilities. *Journal of Learning Disabilities, 23*(4), 229–232.
224. Simmonds, E. P. M. (1992). The effects of teacher training and implementation of two methods for improving the comprehension skills of students with learning disabilities. *Learning Disabilities Research and Practice, 7*(4), 194–198.
225. Simpson, S. B., Swanson, J. M., & Kunkel, K. (1992). The impact of an intensive multisensory reading program on a population of learning-disabled delinquents. *Annals of Dyslexia, 42*, 54–66.
226. Sinatra, R. C., Stahl-Gemake, J., & Berg, D. N. (1984). Improving reading comprehension of disabled readers through semantic mapping. *Reading Teacher, 38*(1), 22–29.
227. Sindelar, P. T., Honsaker, M. S., & Jenkins, J. R. (1982). Response cost and reinforcement contingencies of managing the behavior of distractible children in tutorial settings. *Learning Disability Quarterly, 5*, 3–13.
228. Smith, M. A. (1989). The efficacy of mnemonics for teaching recognition of letter clusters to reading disabled students (Ph.D. diss., University of Oregon, 1989). *Dissertation Abstracts International, 50*(5-A), 1259–1260.
229. Smith, P. L., & Friend, M. (1986). Training learning disabled adolescents in a strategy for using text structure to aid recall of instructional prose. *Learning Disabilities Research, 2*(1), 38–44.
230. Snider, V. E. (1989). Reading comprehension performance of adolescents with learning disabilities. *Learning Disability Quarterly, 12*(2), 87–96.
231. Somerville, D. E., & Leach, D. J. (1988). Direct or indirect instruction?: An evaluation of three types of intervention programme for assisting students with specific reading difficulties. *Educational Research, 30*(1), 46–53.
232. Sowell, V., Parker, R., Poplin, M., & Larsen, S. (1979). The effects of psycholinguistic training on improving psycholinguistic skills. *Learning Disability Quarterly, 2*(3), 69–78.
233. Straub, R. B., & Roberts, D. M. (1983). Effects of nonverbal-oriented social awareness training program on social interaction ability of learning disabled children. *Journal of Nonverbal Behavior, 7*(4), 195–201.
234. Sullivan, J. (1972). The effects of Kephart's perceptual motor-training on a reading clinic sample. *Journal of Learning Disabilities, 5*(10), 545–551.
235. Swanson, L. (1981). Modification of comprehension deficits in learning disabled children. *Learning Disability Quarterly, 4*, 189–202.
236. Swanson, H. L. (1985). Effects of cognitive–behavioral training on emotionally disturbed children's academic performance. *Cognitive Therapy and Research, 9*(2), 201–216.
237. Swanson, H. L., Kozleski, E., & Stegink, P. (1987). Disabled readers' processing of prose: Do any processes change because of intervention? *Psychology in the Schools, 24*(4), 378–384.
238. Swanson, H. L., & Scarpati, S. (1984). Self-instruction training to increase academic performance of educationally handicapped children. *Child and Family Behavior Therapy, 6*(4), 23–39.
239. Swanson, H. L., & Trahan, M. F. (1992). Learning disabled readers' comprehension of computer mediated text: The influence of working memory, metacognition and attribution. *Learning Disabilities Research and Practice, 7*(2), 74–86.

240. Tansey, M. A. (1985). Brainwave signatures—an index reflective of the brain's functional neuroanatomy: Further findings on the effect of EEG sensorimotor rhythm biofeedback training on the neurologic precursors of learning disabilities. *International Journal of Psychophysiology, 3*(2), 85–99.

241. Thorpe, H. W., Lampe, S., Nash, R. T., & Chiang, B. (1981). The effects of the kinesthetic–tactile component of the VAKT procedure on secondary LD students' reading performance. *Psychology in the Schools, 18*(3), 334–340.

242. Tollefson, N., Tracy, D. B., Johnsen, E. P., Farmer, A. W., & Buenning, M. (1984). Goal setting and personal responsibility training for LD adolescents. *Psychology in the Schools, 21*(2), 224–233.

243. Torgesen, J. K., Wagner, R. K., Rashotte, C. A., Alexander, A. W., & Conway, T. (1997). Preventive and remedial interventions for children with severe reading disabilities. *Learning Disabilities, 8*(1), 51–61.

244. Trapani, C., & Gettinger, M. (1989). Effects of social skills training and cross-age tutoring on academic achievement and social behaviors of boys with learning disabilities. *Journal of Research and Development in Education, 23*(1), 1–9.

245. VanDaal, V. H. P., & Reitsma, P. (1990). Effects of independent word practice with segmented and whole-word sound feedback in disabled readers. *Journal of Research in Reading, 13*(2), 133–148.

246. VanDaal, V. H. P., & Reitsma, P. (1993). The use of speech feedback by normal and disabled readers in computer-based reading practice. *Reading and Writing: An Interdisciplinary Journal, 5*(3), 243–259.

247. VanDaal, V. H. P., & Van Der Leij, D. (1992). Computer-based reading and spelling practice for children with learning disabilities. *Journal of Learning Disabilities, 25*(3), 186–195.

248. VanDen Meiracker, M. (1987). Effectiveness of teacher-based versus computer-based instruction on reading comprehension of subtypes of learning disabled children (Ph.D. diss., University of North Carolina Chapel Hill, 1986). *Dissertation Abstracts International, 47*(9-A), 3398–3399.

249. VanReusen, A. K., & Bos, C. S. (1994). Facilitating student participation in individualized education programs through motivation strategy instruction. *Exceptional Children, 60*(5), 466–475.

250. VanStrien, J. W., Stolk, B. D., & Zuiker, S. (1995). Hemisphere-specific treatment of dyslexia subtypes: Better reading with anxiety-laden words? *Journal of Learning Disabilities, 28*(1), 30–34.

251. Vaughn, S., Schumm, J. S., & Gordon, J. (1993). Which motoric condition is most effective for teaching spelling to students with and without learning disabilities? *Journal of Learning Disabilities, 26*(3), 193–198.

252. Vivion, H. K. (1985). Using a modified cloze procedure to effect an improvement in reading comprehension in reading disabled children with good oral language (Ph.D. diss., Vanderbilt University, 1984). *Dissertation Abstracts International, 46*(3-A), 663.

253. Wade, J. F. (1979). The effects of component deficit remediation and academic deficit remediation on improving reading achievement of learning disabled children (Ph.D. diss. University of Arizona, 1979). *Dissertation Abstracts International, 40*(3-A), 1412.

254. Wade, J. F., & Kass, C. E. (1987). Component deficit and academic remediation of learning disabilities. *Journal of Learning Disabilities, 20*(7), 441–447.

255. Wallace, G. W., & Bott, D. A. (1989). Statement-pie: A strategy to improve the paragraph writing skills of adolescents with learning disabilities. *Journal of Learning Disabilities, 22*, 541–545.

256. Wanat, P. E. (1983). Social skills: An awareness program with learning disabled adolescents. *Journal of Learning Disabilities, 16*(1), 35–38.
257. Warner, J. M. R. (1973). The effects of two treatment modes upon children diagnosed as having learning disabilities (Ph.D. diss., University of Illinois, 1973). *Dissertation Abstracts International, 34*(3-A), 1142–1143.
258. Waterman, D. E. (1974). Remediation of word attack skills in slow readers by total body movement learning games (Ph.D. diss., University of Tulsa, 1973). *Dissertation Abstracts International, 34*(7-A), 4049.
259. Weidler, S. D. (1986). The remediation of disabled readers' metacognitive strategies via cognitive self-instruction (Ph.D. diss., Pennsylvania State University, 1985). *Dissertation Abstracts International, 46*(9-A), 2645–2646.
260. Weinstein, G., & Cooke, N. L. (1992). The effects of two repeated reading interventions on generalization of fluency. *Learning Disability Quarterly, 15*, 21–28.
261. Welch, M. (1992). The PLEASE strategy: A meta-cognitive learning strategy for improving the paragraph writing of students with learning disabilities. *Learning Disability Quarterly, 15*(2), 119–128.
262. Whang, P. L., Fawcett, S. B., & Mathews, R. M. (1984). Teaching job-related social skills to learning disabled adolescents. *Analysis and Intervention in Developmental Disabilities, 4*(1), 29–38.
263. White, C. V., Pascarella, E. T., & Pflaum, S. W. (1981). Effects of training in sentence construction on the comprehension of learning disabled children. *Journal of Educational Psychology, 71*(5), 697–704.
264. Whitman, D. M. (1986). The effects of computer-assisted instruction on mathematics achievement of mildly handicapped students (Ph.D. diss., University of South Carolina, 1985). *Dissertation Abstracts International, 46*(10A), 3000–3001.
265. Williams, J. P., Brown, L. G., Silverstein, A. K., & deCani, J. S. (1994). An instructional program in comprehension of narrative themes for adolescents with learning disabilities. *Learning Disability Quarterly, 17*, 205–221.
266. Wilsher, C., Atkins, G., & Manfield, P. (1985). Effect of piracetam on dyslexic's reading ability. *Journal of Learning Disabilities, 18*, 19–25.
267. Wilson, C. L. (1989). An analysis of a direct instruction procedure in teaching word problem-solving to learning disabled students (Ph.D. diss., Florida State University, 1988). *Dissertation Abstracts International, 50*(2-A), 416.
268. Wilson, C., & Sindelar, P. T. (1991). Direct instruction in math word problems: Students with learning disabilities. *Exceptional Children, 57*(6), 512–519.
269. Wise, B. W., Ring, J., Sessions, L., & Olson, R. K. (in press). Phonological awareness with and without articulation: A preliminary study. *Learning Disability Quarterly.*
270. Wong, B. Y. L., Butler, D. L, Ficzere, S. A., & Kuperis, S. (1996). Teaching low achievers and students with learning disabilities to plan, write, and revise opinion essays. *Journal of Learning Disabilities, 29*, 197–212.
271. Wong, B. Y. L., Butler, D. L., Ficzere, S. A., Kuperis, S., Corden, M., & Zelmer, J. (1994). Teaching problem learners revision skills and sensitivity to audience through two instructional modes: Student–teacher versus student–student interactive dialogues. *Learning Disabilities Research and Practice, 9*(2), 78–90.
272. Wong, B. Y. L., & Jones, W. (1982). Increasing metacomprehension in learning disabled and normally achieving students through self-questioning training. *Learning Disability Quarterly, 5*(3), 228–240.
273. Wood, D. A., Rosenberg, M. S., & Carran, D. T. (1993). The effects of tape-record-

ed self-instruction cues on the mathematics performance of students with learning disabilities. *Journal of Learning Disabilities, 26*(4), 250–258.

274. Zieffle, T. H., & Romney, D. M. (1985). Comparison of self-instruction and relaxation training in reducing impulsive and inattentive behavior of learning disabled children on cognitive tasks. *Psychological Reports, 57*(1), 271–274.

275. Zipprich, M. A. (1995). Teaching web making as a guided planning tool to improve student narrative writing. *Remedial and Special Education, 16*(1), 3–15, 52.

Appendix B

Sample of Studies Disqualified from Synthesis

REASONS FOR STUDIES NOT BEING INCLUDED IN SYNTHESIS (N = 467)

Several other studies (N = 155) were disqualified simply from information reported in the abstract. Primary reasons for articles not included in our synthesis include the following: **(1)** Can't calculate effect sizes; **(2)** Missing critical data (e.g., sample size); **(3)** IQ below average or not reported; **(4)** Can't separate LD effect size from other sample; **(5)** Not an LD sample or sample description unclear; **(6)** Not enough intervention sessions; **(7)** No data on LD subjects; **(8)** No instructional control group; **(9)** Not original data or duplicate data; **(10)** No manipulation, not an intervention study; **(11)** No data on LD students; **(12)** No information on achievement and/or behavior problems; **(13)** No data; and **(14)** Experimental design issues.

1. Abbott, S. P., Reed, E., Abbott, R. D., & Berninger, V. W. (in press). Year-long, balanced reading/writing tutorial: A design experiment used for dynamic assessment. *Learning Disability Quarterly*. **(8)**
2. Abegglen, S. R. (1985). The efficacy of computer-assisted instruction with educationally handicapped high school students (Ph.D. diss., Memphis State University, 1984). *Dissertation Abstracts International, 45*(10-A), 3109. **(8)**
3. Abikoff, H., Ganales, D., Reiter, G., Blum, C., Foley, C., & Klein, R. G. (1988). Cog-

Note. The purpose of citing these studies is to illustrate how exhaustive our research was. A number of studies in these references reflect high internal validity. However, these studies did not meet *all* the criteria for inclusion.

nitive training in academically deficient ADDH boys receiving stimulant medication. *Journal of Abnormal Child Psychology, 16*(4), 411–432. **(1)**

4. Abramson, E. E., & Crocker, R. W. (1978). Rapid elimination of out-of-seat behavior by the use of response cost and reinforcement. *Behavioral Engineering, 4*, 103–105. **(5)**
5. Abroms, K. I., & Meeker, M. (1980). Learning disabilities: A diagnostic and educational challenge. *Journal of Learning Disabilities, 9*, 28–35. **(10)**
6. Ackerman, P. T., Anhalt, J. M., & Dykman, R. A. (1986). Inferential word-decoding weakness in reading disabled children. *Learning Disability Quarterly, 9*, 315–324. **(6)**
7. Adams, M. J., & Bruck, M. (1993). Word recognition: The interface of educational policies and scientific research. *Reading and Writing: An Interdisciplinary Journal, 5*, 113–139. **(10)**
8. Alexander, A. W., Andersen, H. G., Heilman, P. C., Voeller, K. K. S., & Torgesen, J. K. (1991). Phonological awareness training and remediation of analytic decoding deficits in a group of severe dyslexics. *Annals of Dyslexia, 41*, 193–206. **(8)**
9. Algozzine, K. M., Morsink, C. V., & Algozzine, B. (1986). Classroom ecology in categorical special education classrooms: And so, they counted the teeth in the horse! *Journal of Special Education, 20*, 209–217. **(7)**
10. Anderson, V., & Roit, M. (1993). Planning and implementing collaborative strategy instruction for delayed readers in grades 6–10. *Elementary School Journal, 94*, 121–137. **(9)**
11. Armstrong, S. W. (1983). The effects of material difficulty upon learning disabled children's oral reading and reading comprehension. *Learning Disability Quarterly, 6*, 339–348. **(1)**
12. Arnold, L. E., Barneby, N., McManus, J., Smeltzer, D. J., Conrad, A., Winer, G., & Desgranges, L. (1977). Prevention by specific perceptual remediation for vulnerable first-graders. *Archives of General Psychiatry, 34*, 1279–1294. **(1)**
13. Atkins, M., & Rohrbeck, C. A. (1993). Gender effects in self-management training: Individual versus cooperative interventions. *Psychology in the Schools, 30*, 362–368. **(5)**
14. Baarstad, D. L. (1972). The early identification of children with perception problems and subsequent implementation of intervention techniques (Ph.D. diss., Brigham Young University, 1972). *Dissertation Abstracts International, 33*(6-A), 2786. **(5)**
15. Baber, G., & Bacon, E. H. (1995). Effect of instructional cues on memory for new words by poor readers. *Education and Treatment of Children, 18*, 117–127. **(2)**
16. Bailet, L. L., & Lyon, G. R. (1985). Deficient linguistic rule application in a learning disabled speller: A case study. *Journal of Learning Disabilities, 18*, 162–165. **(1)**
17. Barbeito, C. L. (1973). A comparison of two methods for teaching prepositions to language handicapped pre-school children (Ph.D. diss., University of Denver, 1972). *Dissertation Abstracts International, 45*(10-B), 3367. **(5)**
18. Barbetta, P. M., Heron, T. E., & Heward, W. L. (1993). Effects of active student response during error correction on the acquisition, maintenance, and generalization of sight words by students with developmental disabilities. *Journal of Applied Behavior Analysis, 26*(1), 111–119. **(5)**
19. Barbetta, P. M., Heward, W. L., & Bradley, D. M. C. (1993). Relative effects of whole-word and phonetic-prompt error correction on the acquisition and maintenance of sight words by students with developmental disabilities. *Journal of Applied Behavior Analysis, 26*(1), 99–110. **(5)**
20. Barbetta, P. M., Heward, W. L., Bradley, D. M., & Miller, A. D. (1994). Effects of immediate and delayed error correction on the acquisition and maintenance of sight

words by students with developmental disabilities. *Journal of Applied Behavior Analysis, 27*, 177–178. **(4)**

21. Barker, T. A., & Torgesen, J. (1995). An evaluation of computer-assisted instruction in phonological awareness with below average readers. *Journal of Educational Computing Research, 13*, 89–103. **(3)**
22. Barone, C., Trickett, E. J., Schmid, K. D., & Leone, P. E. (1993). Transition tasks and resources: An ecological approach to life after high school. *Prevention and School Transitions, 10*, 179–204. **(4)**
23. Bendell, D., Tollefson, N., & Fine, M. (1980). Interaction of locus-of-control orientation and the performance of learning disabled adolescents. *Journal of Learning Disabilities, 13*, 32–35. **(6)**
24.. Bender, W. N. (1986). Instructional grouping and individualization for mainstreamed learning disabled children and adolescents. *Child Study Journal, 16*, 207–215. **(10)**
25. Bergerud, D., Lovitt, T. C., & Horton, S. (1988). The effectiveness of textbook adaptations in life science for high school students with learning disabilities. *Journal of Learning Disabilities, 21*, 70–76. **(4)**
26. Berninger, V. W., Abbott, R. D., Whitaker, D., Sylvester, L., & Nolen S. B. (in press). Integrating low-level and high-level skills in instructional protocols for writing disabilities. *Learning Disability Quarterly*. **(3)**
27. Berrol, C. F. (1979). The effects of two movement remediation programs on selected measures of perceptual–motor ability, academic achievement, and behavior on first grade children manifesting learning and perceptual–motor problems (Ph.D. diss., University of California–Berkeley, 1978). *Dissertation Abstracts International, 39*(9A), 5443–5444. **(5)**
28. Blackbourn, J. M. (1989). Acquisition and generalization of social skills in elementary-aged children with learning disabilities. *Journal of Learning Disabilities, 22*, 28–34. **(8)**
29. Blake, R., Field, B., Foster, C., Platt, F., & Wertz, P. (1991). Effect of FM auditory trainers on attending behaviors of learning-disabled children. *Language, Speech, and Hearing Services in Schools, 22*(3), 111–114. **(3)**
30. Blankenship, C. S. (1978). Remediating systematic inversion errors in subtraction through the use of demonstration and feedback. *Learning Disability Quarterly, 1*, 12–22. **(1)**
31. Blau, H., Schwalb, E., Zanger, E., & Blau, H. (1969). Developmental dyslexia and its remediation. *Reading Teacher, 22*, 649–653, 669. **(5)**
32. Blechman, E. A., Kotanchik, N. L., & Taylor, C. J. (1981). Families and schools together: Early behavioral intervention with high risk children. *Behavior Therapy, 12*, 308–319. **(7)**
33. Bluechardt, M. H., & Shephard, R. J. (1995). Using an extracurricular physical activity program to enhance social skills. *Journal of Learning Disabilities, 26*, 160–169. **(1)**
34. Boettcher, J. V. (1973). Computer-based education: Classroom application and benefits for the learning-disabled student. *Annals of Dyslexia, 33*, 203–219. **(8)**
35. Borkowski, J. G., Weyhing, R. S., & Carr, M. (1988). Effects of attributional retraining on strategy-based reading comprehension in learning-disabled students. *Journal of Educational Psychology, 80*(1), 46–53. **(3)**
36. Bos, C. S., & Allen, A. (1989). Vocabulary instruction and reading comprehension with bilingual learning disabled students. *National Reading Conference Yearbook, 38*, 173–179. **(9)**

37. Bos, C. S., & Filip, D. (1984). Comprehension monitoring in learning disabled and average students. *Learning Disability Quarterly*, *17*, 229–233. **(6)**
38.. Bowman, J. E., & Davey, B. (1986). Effects of presentation mode on the comprehension-monitoring behaviors of LD adolescents. *Learning Disability Quarterly*, *9*, 250–257. **(6)**
39. Bradley, P. E., Battin, R. R., & Sutter, E. G. (1979). Effects of individual diagnosis and remediation for the treatment of learning disabilities. *Clinical Neuropsychology*, *1*(2), 25–32. **(1)**
40. Braggins, J. M. (1976). The efficacy of perceptual motor, language, and distinctive features training with first graders (Ph.D. diss., Syracuse University, 1975). *Dissertation Abstracts International*, *37(4-A)*, 2070. **(5)**
41. Brier, N. (1994). Targeted treatment for adjudicated youth with learning disabilities: Effects on recidivism. *Journal of Learning Disabilities*, *27*(4), 215–222. **(1)**
42. Brigham, F. J., Scruggs, T. E., & Mastropieri, M. A. (1995). Elaborative maps for enhanced learning of historical information: Uniting spatial, verbal, and imaginal information. *Journal of Special Education*, *28*, 440–460. **(6)**
43. Brignac, B. (1984). A comparison of four intervention strategies on the acquisition of sight words with the learning disabled (Ph.D. diss., Georgia State University, 1983). *Dissertation Abstracts International*, *45*(2-A), 487. **(14)**
44. Broski, D. C. (1975). Comprehension of rate-altered discourse by primary school children with identified auditory or visual strengths (Ph.D. diss., Michigan State University, 1974). *Dissertation Abstracts International*, *35*(9-A), 5962. **(8)**
45. Brown, A. L., & Palincsar, A. S. (1982). Inducing strategic learning from texts by means of informed, self-control training. *Topics In Learning and Learning Disabilities*, *2*(1), 1–17. **(1)**
46. Brown, R. I. (1966). A remedial reading program for the adolescent illiterate. *Journal of Special Education*, *1*(4), 409–417. **(8)**
47. Brownell, M. T., Mellard, D. F., & Deshler, D. D. (1993). Differences in the learning and transfer performance between students with learning disabilities and other low-achieving students on problem-solving tasks. *Learning Disability Quarterly*, *16*, 138–156. **(6)**
48. Bryan, T., Cosden, M., & Pearl, R. (1982). The effects of cooperative goal structures and cooperative models on LD and NLD students. *Learning Disability Quarterly*, *5*, 415–421. **(6)**
49. Buerger, T. A. (1968). A follow-up of remedial reading instruction. *Reading Teacher*, *21*, 329–334. **(5)**
50. Bugental, D. B., Whalen, C. K., & Henker, B. (1977). Causal attributions of hyperactive children and motivational assumptions of two behavior-change approaches: Evidence for an interactionist position. *Child Development*, *48*, 874–884. **(2)**
51. Bulgren, J., Schumaker, J. B., & Deshler, D. D. (1994). The effects of a recall enhancement routine of the test performance of secondary students with and without learning disabilities. *Learning Disabilities Research and Practice*, *9*, 2–11. **(6)**
52. Bursuck, W. D., & Lessen, E. (1987). A classroom-based model for assessing students with learning disabilities. *Learning Disabilities Focus*, *3*, 17–29. **(10)**
53. Butler, D. L. (1995). Promoting strategic learning by postsecondary students with learning disabilities. *Journal of Learning Disabilities*, *28*, 170–190. **(8)**
54. Cancelli, A. S., Harris, A. M., Friedman, D. L., & Yoshida, R. K. (1993). Type of instruction and the relationship of classroom behavior to achievement among learning disabled children. *Journal of Classroom Interaction*, *28*, 13–19. **(1)**

55. Carr, S. C., & Punzo, R. P. (1993). The effects of self-monitoring of academic accuracy and productivity on the performance of students with behavioral disorders. *Behavioral Disorders, 18*, 241–250. **(5)**
56. Case, L. P., Mamlin, N., Harris, K. R., & Graham, S. (in press). Self-regulated strategy development: A theoretical and practical perspective. In T. E. Scruggs & M. A. Mastropieri (Eds.), *Advances in learning and behavioral disabilities* (Vol. 9). Greenwich, CT: JAI Press. **(10)**
57. Cavallaro, C. C., & Poulson, C. L. (1985). Teaching language to handicapped children in natural settings. *Education and Treatment of Children, 8*, 1–24. **(5)**
58. Chan, L. K. S., Cole, P. G., & Barfett, S. (1987). Comprehension monitoring: Detection and identification of text inconsistencies by LD and normal students. *Learning Disability Quarterly, 10*, 114–124. **(6)**
59. Cipani, E., Hayes, E., & Swope, R. (1981). The effects of a behavioral "package program" on deficit skills in emotionally handicapped students. *Corrective and Social Psychiatry and Journal of Behavior Technology Methods and Therapy, 27*, 48–61. **(5)**
60. Clark, F. L., Deshler, D. D., Schumaker, J. B., Alley, G. R., & Warner, M. M. (1984). Visual imagery and self-questioning: Strategies to improve comprehension of written material. *Journal of Learning Disabilities, 17*, 145–149. **(6)**
61. Clark, L. W. (1991). A descriptive study of transition programs available to learning-disabled and behaviorally disordered student, grades K–12, in the state of Kansas (Ph.D. diss., Kansas State University, 1990). *Dissertation Abstracts International, 51*(8-A), 2705. **(3)**
62. Clements, S. D., & Barnes, S. M. (1978). The three Rs and central processing training. *Academic Therapy, 13*, 535–547. **(10)**
63. Cohen, A. L., Torgesen, J. K., & Torgesen, J. L. (1988). Improving speed and accuracy of word recognition in reading disabled children: An evaluation of two computer program variations. *Learning Disability Quarterly, 11*, 333–341. **(1)**
64. Cohen, M., Krawiecki, N., & DuRant, R. H. (1987). The neuropsychological approach to the remediation of dyslexia. *Archives of Clinical Neuropsychology, 2*, 163–173. **(1)**
65. Cole, K. S., Dale, P. S., Mills, P. E., & Jenkins, J. R. (1993). Interaction between early intervention curricula and student characteristics. *Exceptional Children, 60*(1), 17–28. **(4)**
66. Collette-Harris, M., & Minke, K. A. (1978). A behavioral experimental analysis of dyslexia. *Behaviour Research and Therapy, 16*(4), 291–295. **(1)**
67. Collins, M., Carnine, D., & Gersten, R. (1987). Elaborated corrective feedback and the acquisition of reasoning skills: A study of computer-assisted instruction. *Exceptional Children, 54*, 254–262. **(4)**
68. Condus, M. M., Marshall, K. J., & Miller, S. R. (1986). Effects of the keyword mnemonic strategy on vocabulary acquisition and maintenance by learning disabled children. *Journal of Learning Disabilities, 19*, 609–613. **(1)**
69. Conrad, W. G., Dworkin, E. S., Shai, A., & Toblessen, J. E. (1971). Effects of amphetamine therapy and prescriptive tutoring on the behavior and achievement of lower class hyperactive children. *Journal of Learning Disabilities, 4*, 45–53. **(3)**
70. Cook, J. E., Nolan, G. A., & Zanotti, R. J. (1980). Treating auditory perception problems: The NIM helps. *Academic Therapy, 15*(4), 473–481. **(3)**
71. Cook, S. B., Scruggs, T. E., Mastropieri, M. A., & Casto, G. C. (1985–1986). Handicapped students as tutors. *Journal of Special Education, 19*, 483–492. **(9)**
72. Cosden, M. A., Gerber, M. M., Semmel, D. S., Goldman, S. R., & Semmel, M. I.

(1987). Microcomputer use within micro-educational environments. *Exceptional Children, 53*, 399–409. **(10)**

73. Cowin, P., & Graff, V. (1969). Comprehensive treatment of the older disabled reader. *Bulletin of the Orton Society, 19*, 100–112. **(1)**
74. Crawford, D. B., & Carnine, D. (1995). *Promoting and assessing higher order thinking in history: Using performance assessment to evaluate effects of instruction* (unpublished manuscript). **(5)**
75. Cunningham, M. M. (1978). Perceptual ability and associational learning in normal and learning disabled children. *Perceptual and Motor Skills, 47*, 1200. **(1)**
76. Curley, J. F., & Reilly, L. J. (1983). Sensory process instruction with learning disabled children. *Perceptual and Motor Skills, 57*, 1219–1226. **(6)**
77. Curtis, M. E., & Chmelka, M. B. (1994). Modifying the Laubach Way to Reading Program for use with adolescents with LDs. *Learning Disabilities Research and Practice, 9*(1), 38–43. **(8)**
78. Dally, A. (1978). Language remediation with primary school-age children. *Language, Speech, and Hearing Services in School, 9*, 85–90. **(1)**
79. Davidson, M. S. (1985). Computer assisted instruction in arithmetic for specific learning disabilities students in the elementary school (Ph.D. diss., University of South Florida, 1985). *Dissertation Abstracts International, 46*(3-A), 674. **(5)**
80. Day, J. D., & Zajakowski, A. (1991). Comparisons of learning ease and transfer propensity in poor and average readers. *Journal of Learning Disabilities, 24*, 421–426, 433. **(8)**
81. Densem, J. F., Nuthall, G. A., Bushnell, J., & Horn, J. (1989). Effectiveness of a sensory integrative therapy program for children with perceptual–motor deficits. *Journal of Learning Disabilities, 22*, 221–229. **(4)**
82. Dowell, H. A., Storey, K., & Gleason, M. (1994). A comparison of programs designed to improve the descriptive writing of students labeled learning disabled. *Developmental Disabilities Bulletin, 22*(1), 73–91. **(3)**
83. Driscoll, M. C., & Abetson, C. (1972). Programmed instruction versus therapist instruction. *American Journal of Occupational Therapy, 26*, 78–80. **(1)**
84. Duffy, F. H., & McAnulty, G. (1990). Neurophysiological heterogeneity and the definition of dyslexia: Preliminary evidence for plasticity. *Neuropsychologia, 28*, 555–571. **(10)**
85. Duran, G. Z. (1992). Language of instruction, reading achievement, and language proficiency for learning-disabled and non-learning-disabled Hispanic limited-English proficient students (Ph.D. diss., University of Arizona, 1991). *Dissertation Abstracts International, 52*(7-A), 2499–2500. **(8)**
86. Durand, V. M., & Carr, E. G. (1991). Functional communication training to reduce challenging behavior: Maintenance and application in new settings. *Journal of Applied Behavior Analysis, 24*, 251–264. **(5)**
87. Eiserman, W. D. (1988). Three types of peer tutoring: Effects on the attitudes of students with learning disabilities and their regular class peers. *Learning Disability Quarterly, 21*, 249–252. **(1)**
88. Elkind, J., Cohen, K., & Murray, C. (1993). Using computer-based readers to improve reading comprehension of students with dyslexia. *Annals of Dyslexia, 43*, 238–259. **(3)**
89. Englert, C. S. (1984). Effective direct instruction practices in special education settings. *Remedial and Special Education, 5*, 38–47. **(7)**
90. Englert, C. S., Garmon, A., Mariage, T., Rozendal, M., Tarrant, K., & Urba, J.

(1995). The Early Literacy Project: Connecting across the literacy curriculum. *Learning Disability Quarterly*, *18*(4), 253–275 **(1)**

91. English, J. P., Gerber, M. M., & Semmel, M. I. (1985). Microcomputer administered spelling tests: Effects on learning handicapped and normally achieving students. *Journal of Reading, Writing, and Learning Disabilities*, *1*(2), 165–176. **(3)**
92. Eucher, J. N. (1985). Self-instructional training as a treatment for impulsivity in learning disabled children with cognitive differences (Ph.D. diss., University of Iowa, 1984). *Dissertation Abstracts International*, *45*(9-A), 2803. **(6)**
93. Faulkner, H. J., & Levy. B. A. (1994). How text difficulty and reader skill interact to produce differential reliance on word and content overlap in reading transfer. *Journal of Experimental Child Psychology*, *58*, 1–24. **(3, 6)**
94. Fawcett, A. J., & Nicolson, R. I. (1991). Vocabulary training for children with dyslexia. *Journal of Learning Disabilities*, *24*(6), 379–383. **(1)**
95. Fayne, H. R., & Gettinger, M. (1980). Narrowing the gap between research and practice in sight word reading instruction. *Psychology in the School*, *18*(2), 240–245. **(3)**
96. Feldman, S. C., Schmidt, D. E., & Deutsch, C. P. (1968). Effect of auditory training on reading skills of retarded readers. *Perceptual and Motor Skills*, *26*, 467–480. **(5)**
97. Felton, R. H. (1993). Effects of instruction on the decoding skills of children with phonological-processing problems. *Journal of Learning Disabilities*, *26*(9), 583–589. **(10)**
98. Fiedorowicz, C. A. M., & Trites, R. L. (1991). From theory to practice with subtypes of reading disabilities. In B. P. Rourke (Ed.), *Neuropsychological validation of learning disability subtypes* (pp. 243–266). New York: Guilford Press. **(8)**
99. Fisher, D. F. (1981). Compensatory training for disabled readers: Implementing and refining. *Journal of Learning Disabilities*, *14*, 451–454. **(3)**
100. Fisher, G. L., Jenkins, S. J., Meyers, F. D., & Bullis, C. K. (1986). The use of remedial teacher-counselors with disabled readers. *Techniques*, *2*, 60–66. **(8)**
101. Fitzgerald, G., Flick, L., & Milich, R. (1986). Computer-assisted instruction for students with attentional difficulties. *Journal of Learning Disabilities*, *19*, 376–379. **(1)**
102. Fleisher, L. S., & Jenkins, J. R. (1978). Effects of contextualized and decontextualized practice conditions on word recognition. *Learning Disability Quarterly*, *1*, 39–47. **(1)**
103. Fleisher, L. S., & Jenkins, J. R. (1983). The effect of word-and comprehension-emphasis on reading performance. *Learning Disability Quarterly*, *6*(2), 146–154. **(5)**
104. Foorman, B. R., Francis, D. J., Beeler, T., Winikates, D., & Fletcher, J. M. (1997). Early interventions for children with reading problems: Study designs and preliminary findings. *Learning Disabilities*, *8*(1), 63–71. **(1)**
105. Foorman, B. R., Francis, D. J., Novy, D. M., & Liberman, D. (1991). How letter-sound instruction mediates progress in first-grade reading and spelling. *Journal of Educational Psychology*, *83*(4), 456–469. **(5)**
106. Foorman, B. R., Jenkins, L., & Francis, D. J. (1993). Links among segmenting, spelling, and reading words in first and second grades. *Reading and Writing: An Interdisciplinary Journal*, *5*, 1–15. **(3)**
107. Foster, K., & Torgesen, J. K. (1983). The effects of directed study on the spelling performance of two subgroups of learning disabled students. *Learning Disability Quarterly*, *6*, 252–257. **(6)**
108. Frankel, F., Forness, S. R., Rowe, S. L., & Westlake, J. (1979). Individualizing schedules of instruction for school children with learning and behavior problems. *Psychology in the Schools*, *16*, 270–279. **(8)**

109. Freeman, T. J., & McLaughlin, T. F. (1984). Effects of a taped-words treatment procedure on learning disabled students' sight-word oral reading. *Learning Disability Quarterly, 7*, 49–54. **(3)**
110. Freides, D., & Messina, C. A. (1986). Memory improvement via motor encoding in learning disabled children. *Learning Disability Quarterly, 19*, 113–115. **(6)**
111. Friedman, S. G., & Hofmeister, A. M. (1984). Matching technology to content and learners: A case study. *Exceptional Children, 51*, 130–134. **(8)**
112. Fuchs, D., Fuchs, L. S., & Fernstromm, P. (1992). Case-by-base reintegration of students with learning disabilities. *Elementary School Journal, 92*(3), 263–281. **(3)**
113. Fuchs, L. S. (1988). Effects of computer-managed instruction on teachers' implementation of systematic monitoring programs and student achievement. *Journal of Educational Research, 81*, 294–304. **(4)**
114. Fuchs, L. S., Bahr, C. M., & Reith, H. J. (1989). Effects of goal structures and performance contingencies on the math performance of adolescents with learning disabilities. *Journal of Learning Disabilities, 22*, 554–560. **(3)**
115. Fuchs, L. S., Fuchs, D., & Bishop, N. (1992). Teacher planning for students with learning disabilities: Differences between general and special educators. *Learning Disabilities Research and Practice, 7*, 120–128. **(4)**
116. Fuchs, L. S., & Maxwell, L. (1988). Interactive effects of reading mode, production format, and structural importance of text among LD pupils. *Learning Disability Quarterly, 11*, 97–105. **(6)**
117. Fuller, P. W. (1978). Attention and the EEG alpha rhythm in learning disabled children. *Journal of Learning Disabilities, 11*, 303–312. **(10)**
118. Ganschow, L., (1985). Diagnosing and remediating writing problems of gifted students with language learning disabilities. *Journal for the Education of the Gifted, 9*, 25–43. **(8)**
119. Gatejen, J. (1979). The effects of individual educational planning on the perceptual capacities and processes of "at-risk" preschool and kindergarten children (Ph.D. diss., University of San Francisco, 1979). *Dissertation Abstracts International, 40*(3-A), 1355–1356. **(5)**
120. Geary, D. C. (1990). A componential analysis of an early learning deficit in mathematics. *Journal of Experimental Child Psychology, 49*, 363–383. **(3)**
121. Gelzheiser, L. M., Cort, R., & Shepherd, M. J. (1987). Is minimal strategy instruction sufficient for LD children? Testing the production deficiency hypothesis. *Learning Disability Quarterly, 10*, 267–275. **(6)**
122. Gelzheiser, L. M., Shepherd, M. J., & Wozniak, R. H. (1986). The development of instruction to induce skill transfer. *Exceptional Children, 53*, 125–129. **(6)**
123. Gerard, J. A. (1978). An investigation into the efficacy of a task analysis model for the diagnosis and remediation of handwriting problems of the learning disabled (Ph.D. diss., Boston College, 1978). *Dissertation Abstracts International, 39*(3-A), 1474–1475. **(3)**
124. Gerber, M. M. (1984). Orthographic problem-solving ability of learning disabled and normally achieving students. *Learning Disability Quarterly, 7*, 157–164. **(1)**
125. Gerber, M. M. (1986). Generalization of spelling strategies by LD students as a result of contingent imitation/modeling and mastery criteria. *Learning Disability Quarterly, 19*, 530–537. **(4)**
126. Getman, D. G. (1986). Fernald instruction with emotionally handicapped nonreaders (Ph.D. diss., Yeshiva University, 1985). *Dissertation Abstracts International, 46* (11-A), 3303. **(5)**

127. Gettinger, M. (1993). Effects of invented spelling and direct instruction on spelling performance of second-grade boys. *Journal of Applied Behavior Analysis, 26*(3), 281–291. **(3)**
128. Giannotti, T. J., & Doyle, R. E. (1982). The effectiveness of parental training on learning disabled children and their parents. *Elementary School Guidance and Counseling, 17*, 131–136. **(1)**
129. Gleason, M., Carnine, D., & Vala, N. (1991). Cumulative versus rapid introduction of new information. *Exceptional Children, 57*, 353–358. **(6)**
130. Good, C. E., Eller, B. F., Spanger, R. S., & Stone, J. E. (1981). The effect of an operant intervention program on attending and other academic behavior with emotionally disturbed children. *Journal of Instructional Psychology, 9*, 25–33. **(3)**
131. Gottesman, R. L., Croen, L. G., Cerullo, F. M., & Nathan, R. G. (1983). Diagnostic intervention for inner-city primary graders with learning difficulties. *Elementary School Journal, 83*(3), 239–249. **(3)**
132. Gottlieb, B. W. (1984). Effects of relative competence on learning disabled children's oral reading performance. *Learning Disability Quarterly, 7*, 108–112. **(3)**
133. Graham, S., & Freeman, S. (1985). Strategy training and teacher- vs. student-controlled study conditions: Effects on LD students' spelling performance. *Learning Disability Quarterly, 8*, 267–274. **(6)**
134. Graham, S., Harris, K. R., & Reid, R. (1992). Developing self-regulated learners. *Focus on Exceptional Children, 24*, 1–16. **(10)**
135. Graham, S., MacArthur, C., & Schwartz, S. (1995). The effects of goal setting and procedural facilitation on the revising behavior and writing performance of students with writing and learning problems. *Journal of Educational Psychology, 87*(2), 230–240. **(1)**
136. Graves, A., Montague, M., & Wong, Y. L. (1990). The effects of procedural facilitation on the story composition of learning disabled students. *Learning Disabilities Research, 5*, 88–93. **(3)**
137. Gray, S. R. (1992). The effects of modified discipline-based art instruction on mainstreamed students' attitudes, achievement and classroom performance in a public school system (Ph.D. diss., Brigham Young University, 1992). *Dissertation Abstracts International, 53*(6-A), 1770. **(8)**
138. Grayson, P. M. (1986). Evaluation of a television-based social problem solving curriculum for learning disabled children (Ph.D. diss., State University of New York-Stony Brook, 1986). *Dissertation Abstracts International, 47*(4-A), 1245. **(3)**
139. Greenwood, C. R., Arrega-Mayer, C., & Carta, J. J. (1994). Identification and translation of effective teacher-developed instructional procedures for general practice. *Remedial and Special Education, 15*, 140–151. **(10)**
140. Griffin, C. C., & Tulbert, B. L. (1995). The effect of graphic organizers on students' comprehension and recall of expository text: A review of the research and implications for practice. *Reading and Writing Quarterly, 11*, 73–89. **(10)**
141. Grossen, B. J. (1989). A study of the effect of response form in computer assisted instruction of class reasoning skills (Ph.D. diss., University of Oregon, 1988). *Dissertation Abstracts International, 50*(2A), 410. **(3)**
142. Gruneberg, M. M., Sykes, R. N., & Hammond, V. (1991). Face–name association in learning-disabled adults: The use of a visual associative strategy. *Neuropsychological Rehabilitation, 1*, 113–116. **(6)**
143. Gurney, D., Gersten, R., Dimino, J., & Carnine, D. (1990). Story grammar: Effective literature instruction for high school students with learning disabilities. *Journal of Learning Disabilities, 23*, 335–342, 348. **(1)**

144. Guthrie, J. T., & Seifert, M. (1977). Letter–sound complexity in learning to identify words. *Journal of Educational Psychology, 69,* 686–696. **(5)**
145. Guyer, B. P., Banks, S. R., & Guyer, K. E. (1993). Spelling improvement for college students who are dyslexic. *Annals of Dyslexia, 43,* 186–193. **(1)**
146. Hagin, R. A. (1973). Models of intervention with learning disabilities: Ephemeral and otherwise. *School Psychology Monograph, 1,* 1–24. **(10)**
147. Haight, S. L., & Fachting, D. D. (1986). Materials for teaching sexuality, love, and maturity to high school students with learning disabilities. *Journal of Learning Disabilities, 19,* 344–350. **(8)**
148. Haines, D. J., & Torgesen, J. K. (1979). The effects of incentives on rehearsal and short-term memory in children with reading problems. *Learning Disability Quarterly, 2,* 48–55. **(6)**
149. Hall, E. A. (1991). An ethnographic and sociolinguistic examination of the mainstreaming of learning-disabled second and third graders (Ph.D. diss., University of California, Los Angeles, 1991). *Dissertation Abstracts International, 52*(1-A), 203. **(10)**
150. Hallenbeck, M. J. (1996). The cognitive strategy in writing: Welcome relief for adolescents with learning disabilities. *Learning Disabilities Research and Practice, 11,* 107–119. **(1)**
151. Hallett, M. (1985). The effectiveness of microcomputer assisted instruction for fourth, fifth, and sixth grade students in spelling, language skill development, and math (Ph.D. diss., University of Idaho, 1984). *Dissertation Abstracts International, 46*(6-A), 1511. **(4)**
152. Hansen, C. L., & Lovitt, T. C. (1976). The relationship between question type and mode of reading on the ability to comprehend. *Journal of Special Education, 10,* 53–60. **(1)**
153. Harber, J. R. (1983). The effects of illustrations on the reading performance of learning disabled and normal children. *Learning Disability Quarterly, 6,* 55–60. **(1)**
154. Hargis, C. H., Gickling, E. E., & Mahmoud, C. C. (1975). The effectiveness of TV in teaching sight words to students with learning disabilities. *Journal of Learning Disabilities, 8,* 44–46. **(8)**
155. Haring, N. G., & Hauck, M. A. (1969). Improved learning conditions in the establishment of reading skills with disabled readers. *Exceptional Children, 35,* 341–352. **(1)**
156. Harris, K. R. (1986). The effects of cognitive-behavior modification on private speech and task performance during problem solving among learning-disabled and normally achieving children. *Journal of Abnormal Child Psychology, 14*(1), 63–67. **(6)**
157. Harris, K. R. (1990). Developing self-regulated learners: The role of private speech and self-instructions. *Educational Psychologist, 25,* 35–49. **(10)**
158. Harris, K. R., & Graham, S. (1992). Self-regulated strategy development: A part of the writing process. In M. Pressley, K. R. Harris, & J. Guthrie (Eds.), *Promoting academic competence and literacy: Cognitive research and instructional innovation* (pp. 207–309). New York: Academic Press. **(10)**
159. Harris, K. R., Graham, S., & Freeman, S. (1988). Effects of strategy training on metamemory among learning disabled students. *Exceptional Children, 54,* 332–338. **(6)**
160. Hashimoto, H. (1978). Some effects of task analysis assessment versus diagnostic-remedial assessment on the behavior of children during reading instruction (Ph.D. diss., University of California–Berkeley with San Francisco State University, 1977). *Dissertation Abstracts International, 39*(2-A), 811. **(3)**
161. Havertape, J. F., & Kass, C. E. (1978). Examination of problem solving in learning

disabled adolescents through verbalized self-instructions. *Learning Disability Quarterly*, *1*, 94–104. **(6)**

162. Hawkins, S. (1985). Early intervention in preventing reading problems. *Academic Therapy*, *21*, 193–197. **(1)**
163. Haynes, J. A., Kapinus, B. A., Malouf, D., & MacArthur, C. (1985). Effects of computer-assisted instruction on disabled readers' metacognition and learning of new words. *National Reading Conference Yearbook*, *34*, 205–212. **(3)**
164. Haynes, M. C., & Jenkins, J. R. (1986). Reading instruction in special education resource rooms. *American Educational Research Journal*, *23*, 161–190. **(10)**
165. Heckerl, J. R., & Sansbury, R. J. (1968). A study of severe reading retardation. *Reading Teacher*, *21*, 724–729. **(8)**
166. Heckerl, J. R., & Webb, S. M. (1969). An educational approach to the treatment of children with learning disabilities. *Journal of Learning Disabilities*, *2*, 199–204. **(10)**
167. Heider, J. P. (1979). Time with the psychologist as a reinforcement for work completion. *School Psychology Digest*, *8*, 335–338. **(1)**
168. Henderson, A. J., & Shores, R. E. (1982). How learning disabled student's failure to attend to suffixes affects their oral reading performance. *Journal of Learning Disabilities*, *15*, 178–182. **(3)**
169. Hess, A. M., Rosenberg, M. S., & Levy, G. K. (1990). Reducing truancy in students with mild handicaps. *Research and Special Education*, *11*, 14–19. **(4)**
170. Hess, L. J., Wagner, M., DeWald, B., & Conn, P. (1993). Conversation skill intervention programme for adolescents with learning disabilities. *Child Language Teaching and Therapy*, *9*, 13–31. **(1)**
171. Higgins, K., & Boone, R. (1990). Hypertext computer study guides and the social studies achievement of students with learning disabilities, remedial students, and regular education students. *Journal of Learning Disabilities*, *23*(9), 529–540. **(3)**
172. Hinton, G. C., & Knights, R. M. (1971). Children with learning problems: Academic history, academic prediction, and adjustment three years after assessment. *Exceptional Children*, *37*, 513–519. **(14)**
173. Hofmeister, A. M., Engelmann, S., & Carnine, D. (1989). Developing and validating science education video discs. *Journal of Research in Science Teaching*, *26*, 665–677. **(8)**
174. Holborow, P., Elkins, J., & Berry, P. (1981). The effect of the Feingold diet on "normal" school children. *Journal of Learning Disabilities*, *14*, 143–147. **(1)**
175. Holmes, B. C. (1985). The effects of a strategy and sequenced materials on the inferential comprehension of disabled readers. *Learning Disability Quarterly*, *18*, 542–546. **(3)**
176. Horner, R. H. (1994). Functional assessment: Contributions and future directions. *Journal of Applied Behavior Analysis*, *27*, 401–404. **(10)**
177. Horton, S. V., & Lovitt, T. C. (1989). Using study guides with three classifications of secondary students. *Journal of Special Education*, *22*, 447–462. **(6)**
178. Horton, S. V., Lovitt, T. C., & Bergerud, D. (1990). The effectiveness of graphic organizers for three classifications of secondary students in content area classes. *Journal of Learning Disabilities*, *23*, 12–22, 29. **(6)**
179. Horton, S. V., Lovitt, T. C., Givens, A., & Nelson, R. (1989). Teaching social studies to high school students with academic handicaps in a mainstreamed setting: Effects of a computerized study guide. *Journal of Learning Disabilities*, *22*, 102–107. **(6)**
180. Horton, S. V., Lovitt, T. C., & Slocum, T. (1988). Teaching geography to high school students with academic deficits: Effects of a computerized MAP tutorial. *Learning Disability Quarterly*, *11*, 371–379. **(6)**

181. Hosek, G. A. (1985). A comparison of the learning disabilities resource room and regular classroom activities during time allocated for reading instruction (Ph.D. diss., University of Florida, 1984). *Dissertation Abstracts International, 46*(3-A), 675–676. **(10)**
182. Howard-Rose, D., & Rose, C. (1994). Students' adaptation to task environments in resource room and regular class settings. *Journal of Special Education, 28*(1), 3–26. **(8)**
183. Hui, E. K. P. (1991). Using Data Pac for Hong Kong Chinese children with reading difficulties. *Educational Psychology in Practice, 7*, 180–186. **(8)**
184. Humphries, T. W., Snider, L., & McDougall, B. (1993). Clinical evaluation of the effectiveness of sensory integrative and perceptual motor therapy in improving sensory integrative function in children with learning disabilities. *Occupational Therapy Journal of Research, 13*, 163–182. **(8)**
185. Hurford, D. P., Johnston, M., Nepote, P., Hampton, S., Moore, S., Neal, J., Mueller, A., McGeorge, K., Huff, L., Awad, A., Tatro, C., Juliano, C., & Huffman, D. (1994). Early identification and remediation of phonological-processing deficits in first-grade children at risk for reading disabilities. *Journal of Learning Disabilities, 10*, 647–659. **(1)**
186. Hurford, D. P., & Shedelbower, A. (1993). The relationship between discrimination and memory ability in children with reading disabilities. *Contemporary Educational Psychology, 18*, 101–113. **(6)**
187. Hutcheson, L., Selig, H., & Young, N. (1990). A success story: A large urban district offers a working model for implementing multisensory teaching into the resource and regular classroom. *Annals of Dyslexia, 40*, 79–96. **(8)**
188. Hutton, J. B., & Polo, L. (1976). A sociometric study of learning disability children and type of teaching strategy. *Group Psycho-Therapy, Psycho-Drama and Sociometry, 29*, 113–120. **(8)**
189. Idol, L. (1987). Group story mapping: A comprehension strategy for both skilled and unskilled readers. *Journal of Learning Disabilities, 20*(4), 196–205. **(3)**
190. Idol-Maestas, L. (1985). Getting ready to read: Guided probing for poor comprehenders. *Learning Disability Quarterly, 8*, 243–254. **(3)**
191. Illovsky, J., & Fredman, N. (1976). Group suggestion in learning disabilities of primary grade children: A feasibility study. *International Journal of Clinical and Experimental Hypnosis, 24*, 87–97. **(12)**
192. Ito, H. R. (1980). Long-term effects of resource room programs on learning disabled children's reading. *Journal of Learning Disabilities, 13*(6), 322–326. **(8)**
193. Jaben, T. H. (1985). Effects of instruction on elementary-age students' productive thinking. *Psychological Reports, 57*(3, Pt.1), 900–902. **(1)**
194. Jaben, T. H. (1986). Impact of creativity instruction on learning disabled students' divergent thinking. *Journal of Learning Disabilities, 19*(6), 342–343. **(1)**
195. Jason, L. A., Christensen, H., & Carl, K. (1982). Programmed versus naturalistic approaches in enhancing study-related behavior. *Journal of Clinical Child Psychology, 11*(3), 249–254. **(3)**
196. Jenkins, J. R., Barksdale, A., & Clinton, L. (1978). Improving reading comprehension and oral reading: Generalization across behaviors, settings, and time. *Journal of Learning Disabilities, 11*, 607–617. **(5)**
197. Jenkins, J. R., Heliotis, J. D., Stein, M. L., & Haynes, M. C. (1987). Improving reading comprehension by using paragraph restatements. *Exceptional Children, 54*(10), 54–59. **(3)**
198. Jenkins, J. R., Larson, K., & Fleisher, L. (1983). Effects of error correction on word recognition and reading comprehension. *Learning Disability Quarterly, 6*, 139–145. **(3)**

199. Johns, J. L. (1977). Children's conceptions of a spoken word: A developmental study. *Reading World, 16*, 248–257. **(8)**
200. Johnson, G., Gersten, R., & Carnine, D. (1987). Effects of instructional design variables on vocabulary acquisition of LD students: A study of computer-assisted instruction. *Journal of Learning Disabilities, 20*, 206–213. **(3)**
201. Johnson, R. T., & Johnson, D. W. (1983). Effects of cooperative, competitive, and individualistic learning experiences on social development. *Exceptional Children, 49*(4), 323–329. **(4)**
202. Johnson, R. T., Johnson, D. W., Scott, L. E., & Ramolae, B. A. (1985). Effects of single-sex and mixed-sex cooperative interaction on science achievement and attitudes and cross-handicap and cross-sex relationships. *Journal of Research in Science Teaching, 22*, 207–220. **(4)**
203. Jones, J. (1969). Dyslexia: Identification and remediation in a public school setting. *Journal of Learning Disabilities, 2*, 533–538. **(8)**
204. Kamann, M. P., & Wong, B. Y. L. (1993). Inducing adaptive coping self-statements in children with learning disabilities through self-instruction training. *Journal of Learning Disabilities, 26*, 630–638. **(8)**
205. Kameenui, E. J., Simmons, D. C., & Darch, C. B. (1987). LD children's comprehension of selected textual features: Effects of proximity of information. *Learning Disability Quarterly, 10*, 237–248. **(6)**
206. Kapadia, E. S., & Fantuzzo, J. W. (1988). Effects of teacher- and self-administered procedures on the spelling performance of learning-handicapped children. *Journal of School Psychology, 26*(1), 49–58. **(3)**
207. Kaplan, B. J., Polatajko, H. J., Wilson, B. N., & Faris, P. D. (1993). Reexamination of sensory integration treatment: A combination of two efficacy studies. *Journal of Learning Disabilities, 26*, 342–347. **(1)**
208. Karraker, R. J. (1977). Self versus teacher selected reinforcers in a token economy. *Exceptional Children, 43*, 454–455. **(5)**
209. Kavale, K. A. (1984). A meta-analytic evaluation of the Frostig Test and Training Program. *Exceptional Child, 31*, 134–141. **(10)**
210. Kearney, C. A., & Drabman, R. S. (1993). The write–say method for improving spelling accuracy in children with learning disabilities. *Journal of Learning Disabilities, 26*, 52–56. **(1)**
211. Keel, M. C., & Gast, D. L. (1992). Small-group instruction for students with learning disabilities: Observational and incidental learning. *Exceptional Children, 58*(4), 357–368. **(8)**
212. Keene, S., & Davey, B. (1987). Effects of computer-presented text on LD adolescents' reading behaviors. *Learning Disability Quarterly, 10*, 283–290. **(6)**
213. Kerchner, L. B., & Kistinger, B. J. (1984). Language processing/word processing: Written expression, computers and learning disabled students. *Learning Disability Quarterly, 7*(4), 329–334. **(3)**
214. Keresztenyi, S. B. (1986). Uses of computer technology in education programs for mentally retarded, learning disabled, and emotionally disturbed students in New York State (Ph.D. diss., Columbia University Teachers College, 1986). *Dissertation Abstracts International, 47*(6-A), 2120. **(10)**
215. Kezele, G. L. (1985). Psychoeducational intervention with learned helplessness: An analysis of attributional factors of learning disabled adolescents in conjunction with composing written language tasks in the academic setting (Ph.D. diss., Marquette University, 1985). *Dissertation Abstracts International, 46*(6-A), 1564. **(3)**

216. Kinder, D., & Carnine, D. (1991). Direct instruction: What it is and what it is becoming. *Journal of Behavioral Education, 1*, 193–213. **(10)**
217. Kirchner, D. M. (1991). Using verbal scaffolding to facilitate conversational participation and language acquisition in children with pervasive developmental disorders. *Journal of Childhood Communication Disorders, 14*, 81–98. **(9)**
218. Kitz, W. R., & Nash, R. T. (1992). Testing the effectiveness of the project success summer program for adult dyslexics. *Annals of Dyslexia, 42*, 3–24. **(8)**
219. Kline, F. M., Schumaker, J. B., & Deshler, D. D. (1991). Development and validation of feedback routines for instructing students with learning disabilities. *Learning Disability Quarterly, 14*, 191–206. **(6)**
220. Klingner, J. K., Vaughn, S., & Schumm, J. S. (in press). Collaborative strategic reading during social studies in heterogeneous fourth-grade classrooms. *Elementary School Journal.* **(3)**
221. Konopak, B. C., Williams, N. L., & Jampole, E. S. (1991). Use of mnemonic imagery for content learning. *Reading, Writing, and Learning Disabilities, 7*, 309–319. **(10)**
222. Kos, R. (1991). Persistence of reading disabilities: The voices of four middle school students. *American Educational Research Journal, 28*, 875–895. **(8)**
223. Koscinski, S. T., & Gast, D. L. (1993). Computer-assisted instruction with constant time delay to teach multiplication facts to students with learning disabilities. *Learning Disabilities Research and Practice, 8*, 157–168. **(3)**
224. Koskinen, P. S., Wilson, R. M., Gambrell, L. B., & Jensema, C. J. (1986). Using closed captioned television to enhance reading skills of learning disabled students. *Thirty-Fifth Yearbook of the National Reading Conference, 35*, 61–65. **(3)**
225. Kuder, S. J. (1990). Effectiveness of the DISTAR reading program for children with learning disabilities. *Journal of Learning Disabilities, 23*, 69–71. **(1)**
226. Kuder, S. J. (1991). Language abilities and progress in a direct instruction reading program for students with learning disabilities. *Journal of Learning Disabilities, 24*, 124–127. **(8)**
227. Laconte, M., Shaw, D., & Dunn, I. (1993). The effects of a rational–emotive affective education program for high-risk middle school students. *Psychology in the Schools, 30*, 274–281. **(5)**
228. LaCroix, K. J. O. (1987). The effect of instruction in a metacognitive strategy on functional reading of learning disabled students (Ph.D. diss., Louisiana State University and Agricultural and Mechanical College, 1986). *Dissertation Abstracts International, 47*(8-A), 2973. **(3)**
229. Landis, B. C. (1986). Training secondary LD students in the use of semantic maps: Effects on prose recall (Ph.D. diss., Ball State University, 1985). *Dissertation Abstracts International, 46*(9-A), 2661. **(3)**
230. Lane, P. R. (1970). Educational therapy for adolescent nonreaders. *Academic Therapy, 6*(2), 155–159. **(10)**
231. Larson, B. L., & Roberts, B. B. (1986). The computer as a catalyst for mutual support and empowerment among learning disabled students. *Journal of Learning Disabilities, 19*(1), 52–55. **(1)**
232. Larson, K. A. (1989). Task-related and interpersonal problem-solving training for increasing school success in high-risk young adolescents. *Research and Special Education, 10*, 32–42. **(4)**
233. Lazerson, D. B., Foster, H. L., Brown, S. I., & Hummel, J. W. (1988). The effectiveness of cross-age tutoring with truant, junior high school students with learning disabilities. *Learning Disability Quarterly, 21*, 253–255. **(1)**

234. Leinhardt, G., Zigmond, N., & Cooley, W. W. (1981). Reading instruction and its effects. *American Educational Research Journal, 18*(3), 343–361. **(8)**

235. Leon, J. A., & Pepe, H. J. (1983). Self-instructional training: Cognitive behavior modification for remediating arithmetic deficits. *Exceptional Children, 50*(1), 54–60. **(3)**

236. Leshowitz, B., Jenkens, K., Heaton, S., & Bough, T. L. (1993). Fostering critical thinking skills in students with learning disabilities: An instructional program. *Journal of Learning Disabilities, 26*, 483–490. **(4)**

237. Levy, B. A., Abello, B., & Lysynchuk, L. (1997). Transfer form word training to reading in context: Gains in reading fluency and comprehension. *Learning Disability Quarterly, 20*, 173–188. **(3)**

238. Lew, M., & Bryant, R. (1984). The effect of cooperative groups on regular class spelling achievement of special needs learners. *Educational Psychology, 4*(4), 275–283. **(3)**

239. Lieber, J., & Semmel, M. I. (1987). The relationship group size and performance on a microcomputer problem-solving task for learning handicapped and nonhandicapped students. *Journal of Educational Computing Research, 3*(2), 171–187. **(1)**

240. Lindsey, J. D., & Frith, G. H. (1981). Effects of exceptionality status and art instruction on Good enough-Harris standard IQs. *American Journal of Mental Deficiency, 85*(6), 658–660. **(6)**

241. Lloyd, J., Saltzman, N. J., & Kauffman, J. M. (1981). Predictable generalization in academic learning as a result of preskills and strategy training. *Learning Disability Quarterly, 4*, 203–216. **(6)**

242. Locher, P. J. (1985). Use of haptic training to modify impulse and attention control deficits of learning disabled children. *Learning Disability Quarterly, 18*, 89–93. **(3)**

243. Logan, R., & Colarusso, R. (1978). The effectiveness of the MWM and GOAL programs in developing general language abilities. *Learning Disability Quarterly, 1*, 32–38. **(5)**

244. Lovett, M. W. (1991). Reading, writing, and remediation: Perspectives on the dyslexic learning disability from remedial outcome data. *Learning and Individual Differences, 3*, 295–305. **(10)**

245. Lovett, M. W., Barron, R. W., Forbes, J. E., Cuksts, B., & Steinbach, K. A. (1994). Computer speech-based training of literacy skills in neurologically impaired children: A controlled evaluation. *Brain and Language, 47*, 117–154. **(1)**

246. Lovett, M. W., Benson, N. J., & Olds, J. (1990). Individual difference predictors of treatment outcome in the remediation of specific reading disability. *Learning and Individual Differences, 2*, 287–314. **(9)**

247. Lovitt, T. C., & DeMier, D. M. (1984). An evaluation of the Slingerland Method with LD youngsters. *Learning Disability Quarterly, 17*, 267–272. **(1)**

248. Lovitt, T. C., & Hurlburt, M. (1974). Using behavior analysis techniques to assess the relationship between phonics instruction and oral reading. *Journal of Special Education, 8*, 57–72. **(5)**

249. Lovitt, T., Rudsit, J., Jenkins, J., Pious, C., & Benedetti, D. (1985). Two methods of adapting science materials for learning disabled and regular seventh graders. *Learning Disability Quarterly, 8*, 275–285. **(4)**

250. Luchow, J. P., & Shepherd, M. J. (1981). Effects of multisensory training in perceptual learning. *Learning Disability Quarterly, 4*, 38–43. **(6)**

251. Luiselli, J. K., Helfen, C. S., & Colozzi, G. (1977). Teachers' use of reinforcement and time-out procedures to modify disruptive classroom behavior of special education students. *School Applications of Learning Theory, 9*, 49–64. **(5)**

252. MacArthur, C. A., Graham, S., & Schwartz, S. (1991). Knowledge of revision and

revising behavior among students with learning disabilities. *Learning Disability Quarterly, 14*, 61–73. **(8)**

253. MacArthur, C. A., Graham, S., Schwartz, S. S., & Schafer, W. D. *Evaluation of a writing instruction model that integrated a process approach, strategy instruction, and word processing* (unpublished manuscript). **(8)**
254. MacArthur, C. A., Haynes, J. A., & Malouf, D. B. (1986). Learning disabled students' engaged time and classroom interaction: The impact of computer assisted instruction. *Journal of Educational Computing Research, 2*(2), 189–198. **(10)**
255. MacArthur, C. A., & Shneiderman, B. (1986). Learning disabled students' difficulties in learning to use a word processor: Implications for instruction and software evaluation. *Journal of Learning Disabilities, 19*, 248–253. **(8)**
256. Macklem, G. L. (1987). No one wants to play with me. *Academic Therapy, 22*(5), 477–484. **(10)**
257. Madden, N. A., & Slavin, R. E. (1982). Effects of cooperative learning on the social acceptance of mainstreamed academically handicapped students. *Center for Social Organization of Schools Report, The Johns Hopkins University, 321*, 23. **(4)**
258. Maheady, L., Harper, G. F., Mallette, B., & Winstanley, N. (1991). Training and implementation requirements associated with the use of a classwide peer tutoring system. *Education and Treatment of Children, 14*, 177–198. **(4)**
259. Maheady, L., Sacca, M. K., & Harper, G. F. (1987). Classwide student tutoring teams: The effects of peer-mediated instruction on the academic performance of secondary mainstreamed students. *Journal of Special Education, 21*(3), 107–121. **(4)**
260. Maher, C. A. (1985). Procedure for mainstreaming handicapped adolescents into regular education classrooms. *Techniques, 1*, 380–388. **(4)**
261. Malec, J. (1985). Personality factors associated with severe traumatic disability. *Rehabilitation Psychology, 30*, 165–172. **(5)**
262. Malone, L. D., & Mastropieri, M. A. (1992). Reading comprehension instruction: Summarization and self-monitoring training for students with learning disabilities. *Exceptional Children, 58*, 270–279. **(6)**
263. Malouf, D. B. (1987). The effect of instructional computer games on continuing student motivation. *Journal of Special Education, 21*(4), 27–38. **(6)**
264. Malouf, D. B., MacArthur, C. A., & Radin, S. (1986). Using interactive videotape-based instruction to teach on-the-job social skills to handicapped adolescents. *Journal of Computer-Based Instruction, 13*, 130–133. **(4)**
265. Mandoli, M., Mandoli, P., & McLaughlin, T. F. (1982). Effects of same-age peer tutoring on the spelling performance of a mainstreamed elementary LD student. *Learning Disability Quarterly, 5*, 185–190. **(14)**
266. Marandola, P., & Imber, S. C. (1979). Glasser's classroom meeting: A humanistic approach to behavior change with preadolescent inner-city learning disabled children. *Journal of Learning Disabilities, 12*, 383–387. **(3)**
267. Marble, J. M. (1974). An analysis of the effectiveness of individualized reading instruction upon self-concept of disadvantaged students with reading disabilities (Ph.D. diss., Mississippi State University, 1973). *Dissertation Abstracts International, 34*(8-A), 4571–4572. **(5)**
268. Margalit, M., & Caspi, M. (1985). A change in teacher–child interaction through paradoxical intervention. *Exceptional Child, 32*, 41–45. **(1)**
269. Margalit, M., Weisel, A., & Shulman, S. (1987). The facilitation of information processing in learning disabled children using computer games. *Educational Psychology, 7*, 47–54. **(6)**
270. Marston, D. (1987). The effectiveness of special education: A time series analysis of

reading performance in regular and special education settings. *Journal of Special Education, 21*(4), 13–26. **(4)**

271. Martin, F., Mackenzie, B., Lovegrove, W., & McNicol, D. (1993). Irlen lenses in the treatment of specific reading disability: An evaluation of outcomes and processes. *Australian Journal of Psychology, 45*, 141–150. **(1)**
272. Martino, L., & Johnson, D. W. (1979). Cooperative and individualistic experiences among disabled and normal children. *Journal of Social Psychology, 107*(2), 177–183. **(3)**
273. Mastropieri, M. A., Scruggs, T. E., & Levin, J. R. (1985). Mnemonic strategy instruction with learning disabled adolescents. *Journal of Learning Disabilities, 18*, 94–100. **(6)**
274. Mastropieri, M. A., Scruggs, T. E., Levin, J. R., Gaffney, J., & McLoone, B. (1985). Mnemonic vocabulary instruction for learning disabled students. *Learning Disability Quarterly, 8*, 57–63. **(6)**
275. Mastropieri, M., Scruggs, T. E., McLoone, B., & Levin, J. R. (1985). Facilitating learning disabled students' acquisition of science classifications. *Learning Disability Quarterly, 8*, 299–309. **(6)**
276. Mastropieri, M. A., Scruggs, T. E., Whittaker, M. E. S., & Bakken, J. P. (1994). Applications of mnemonic strategies with students with mild mental disabilities. *Remedial and Special Education, 15*(1), 34–43. **(5)**
277. Matefy, R. E. (1978). Evaluation of a remediation program using senior citizens as psychoeducational agents. *Community Mental Health Journal, 14*, 327–336. **(4)**
278. Mather, N., & Healey, W. C. (1984). The efficacy of a memory strategy for eliminating reversal behavior. *Journal of Learning Disabilities, 17*(2), 84–88. **(14)**
279. Matthews, C. (1991). Serial processing and the "phonetic route": Lessons learned in the functional reorganization of deep dyslexia. *Journal of Communication Disorders, 24*, 21–39. **(5)**
280. Mayhall, W. F., Jenkins, J. R., Chestnut, N. J., Rose, M. A., Schroeder, K. L., & Jordan, B. (1975). Supervision and site of instruction as factors in tutorial programs. *Exceptional Children, 42*(3), 151–154. **(3)**
281. McCloskey, M. L., & Quay, L. C. (1987). Effects of coaching on handicapped children's social behavior and teachers' attitudes in mainstreamed classrooms. *Elementary School Journal, 87*, 425–435. **(4)**
282. McCormick, S., & Hill, D. S. (1984). An analysis of the effects of two procedures for increasing disabled readers' inferencing skills. *Journal of Educational Research, 77*, 219–226. **(5)**
283. McCoy, K. M., & Pany, D. (1986). Summary and analysis of oral reading corrective feedback research. *Reading Teacher, 39*, 548–554. **(10)**
284. McLaughlin, T. F., Swain, J. C., Brown, M., & Fielding L (1986). The effects of academic consequences on inappropriate social behavior of special education middle school students. *Techniques, 2*, 310–316. **(4)**
285. McLoone, B. B., Scruggs, T. E., Mastropieri, M. A., & Zucker, S. F. (1986). Memory strategy instruction and training with learning disabled adolescents. *Learning Disabilities Research, 2*, 45–53. **(6)**
286. Meadows, N. B. W. (1989). The effects of individual, teacher-directed, and cooperative learning instructional methods on the comprehension of expository text (Ph.D. diss., University of Washington, 1988). *Dissertation Abstracts International, 50*(2-A), 406. **(3)**
287. Mehring, T. A. (1982). The interaction of selected aptitude and cognitive style mea-

sures with a learning strategies intervention used to teach self-questioning to junior high school learning disabled adolescents (Ph.D. diss., University of Kansas, 1981). *Dissertation Abstracts International, 42*(7-A), 3109. **(8)**

288. Mesibov, G. B., Schroeder, C. S., & Wesson, L. (1977). Parental concerns about their children. *Journal of Pediatric Psychology, 2*, 13–17. **(5)**
289. Meyers, M. J. (1980). The significance of learning modalities, modes of instruction, and verbal feedback for learning to recognize written words. *Learning Disability Quarterly, 3*(3), 62–69. **(6)**
290. Miller, S. R., Sabatino, D. A., & Miller, T. L. (1977). Influence of training in visual perceptual discrimination on drawings by children. *Perceptual and Motor Skills, 44*(2), 479–487. **(4)**
291. Miller, T. L., & Sabatino, D. A. (1978). An evaluation of the teacher consultant model as an approach to mainstreaming. *Exceptional Children, 45*(2), 86–91. **(1)**
292. Millman, P. G. (1985). The effects of computer-assisted instruction on attention deficits, achievement, and attitudes of learning disabled children (Ph.D. diss., University of Virginia, 1984). *Dissertation Abstracts International, 45*(10-A), 3114. **(3)**
293. Minuchin, S., Chamberlain, P., & Graubard, P. (1967). A project to teach learning skills to disturbed, delinquent children. *American Journal of Ortho-Psychiatry, 37*, 558–567. **(5)**
294. Miramontes, O., Cheng, L., & Trueba, H. T. (1984). Teacher perceptions and observed outcomes: An ethnographic study of classroom interactions. *Learning Disability Quarterly, 7*, 349–357. **(8)**
295. Montali, J., & Lewandowski, L. (1996). Bimodal reading: Benefits of a talking computer for average and less skilled readers. *Journal of Learning Disabilities, 29*, 271–279. **(8)**
296. Moore, D. K. (1986). Modality preference: Prediction via the visual aural digit span text? *Journal of Psychoeducational Assessment, 4*, 263–272. **(6)**
297. Morgan, R. T. T. (1976). "Paired reading" tuition: A preliminary report on a technique for cases of reading deficit. *Child Care, Health and Development, 2*, 13–28. **(1, 8)**
298. Morgan, R., & Lyon, E. (1979). "Paired reading": A preliminary report on a technique for parental tuition of reading-retarded children. *Journal of Child Psychology and Psychiatry and Allied Disciplines, 20*, 151–160. **(1)**
299. Morocco, C. C., Dalton, B., & Tivnan, T. (1992). The impact of computer-supported writing instruction on fourth-grade students with and without learning disabilities. *Reading and Writing Quarterly: Overcoming Learning Difficulties, 8*(1), 87–113. **(4)**
300. Morrison, J. A. (1984). An evaluation of the perceptual deficit hypothesis and verbal processing theory in a sample of 114 second-grade Spanish readers (Ph.D. diss., University of Southern California, 1984). *Dissertation Abstracts International, 44*(12-A), 3639–3640. **(4)**
301. Mosby, R. J. (1979). A bypass program of supportive instruction for secondary students with learning disabilities. *Journal of Learning Disabilities, 12*(3), 187–190. **(1)**
302. Mulcahy, R. F. (1991). Developing autonomous learners. *Alberta Journal of Educational Research, 37*, 385–397. **(1)**
303. Nelson, J. R., Smith, D. J., & Dodd, J. M. (1994). The effects of learning strategy instruction on the completion of job applications by students with learning disabilities. *Journal of Learning Disabilities, 27*, 104–110, 122. **(6)**
304. Neuman, D. (1991). Learning disabled students' interactions with commercial courseware: A naturalistic study. *Educational Technology Research and Development, 39*(1), 31–49. **(8)**

305. Newcomer, P. L., & Magee, P. (1977). The performance of learning (reading) disabled children on a test of spoken language. *Reading Teacher, 30*, 896–900. **(10)**
306. Nulman, J. H., & Gerber, M. M. (1984). Improving spelling performance by imitating a child's errors. *Journal of Learning Disabilities, 17*, 328–333. **(8)**
307. Nutter, R. E., McDavis, R. J., & Boone, R. (1985). Counseling interventions used with exceptional students: A statewide assessment. *School Counselor, 32*, 224–230. **(10)**
308. O'Connor, P. D., Sofo, F., Kendall, L., & Olsen, G. (1990). Reading disabilities and the effects of colored filters. *Journal of Learning Disabilities, 23*, 597–603, 620. **(1)**
309. O'Connor, R. E., Jenkins, J. R., Cole, K. N., & Mills, P. E. (1993). Two approaches to reading instruction with children with disabilities: Does program design make a difference? *Exceptional Children, 59*, 312–323. **(4)**
310. Odom, S. L., Jenkins, J. R., Speltz, M. L., & DeKlyen, M. (1982). Promoting social integration of young children at risk for learning disabilities. *Learning Disability Quarterly, 5*, 379–387. **(4)**
311. Okolo, C. M. (1992). The effects of computer-based attribution retraining on the attributions, persistence, and mathematics computation of students with learning disabilities. *Journal of Learning Disabilities, 25*(5), 327–334. **(3)**
312. Olson, R., Foltz, G., & Wise, B. (1986). Reading instruction and remediation with the aid of computer speech. *Behavior Research Methods, Instruments and Computers, 18*, 93–99. **(3)**
313. Omizo, M. M., & Cubberly, W. E. (1983). The effects of reality therapy classroom meetings on self-concept and locus of control among learning disabled children. *Exceptional Child, 30*(3), 201–209. **(3)**
314. Omizo, M. M., & Omizo, S. A. (1987). The effects of eliminating self-defeating behavior of learning-disabled children through group counseling. *School Counselor, 34*(4), 282–288. **(3)**
315. Omizo, M. M., Omizo, S. A., & Suzuki, L. A. (1987). Intervention strategies. *Academic Therapy, 22*(4), 427–432. **(10)**
316. Omizo, M. M., Williams, R. E., & Omizo, S. A. (1986). The effects of participation in parent group sessions on child-rearing attitudes among parents of learning disabled children. *Exceptional Child, 33*, 134–139. **(5)**
317. O'Neill, M. J. (1978). An evaluation of a method for developing learning strategies in kindergarten children with potential learning disabilities (Ph.D. diss., University of Toronto, Canada, 1975). *Dissertation Abstracts International, 39*(3-A), 1504. **(5)**
318. Outhred, L. (1989). Word processing: Its impact on children's writing. *Learning Disability Quarterly, 22*, 262–264. **(8)**
319. Palmeri, J. J. (1980). Relaxation and cognitive coping statements as supplemental remedial interventions for learning problems in children (Ph.D. diss., Hofstra University, 1980). *Dissertation Abstracts International, 40*(12-B), 5796–5797. **(5)**
320. Pany, D., & McCoy, K. M. (1988). Effects of corrective feedback on word accuracy and reading comprehension of readers with learning disabilities. *Journal of Learning Disabilities, 21*, 546–550. **(6)**
321. Paquin, M. J. (1978). The effects of pupil self-graphing on academic performance. *Education and Treatment of Children, 1*, 5–16. **(1)**
322. Parmar, R. S., Cawley, J. F., & Miller, J. H. (1994). Differences in mathematics performance between students with learning disabilities and students with mild retardation. *Exceptional Children, 60*(6), 549–563. **(13)**
323. Parmar, R. S., DeLuca, C. B., & Janczak, T. M. (1994). Investigations into the rela-

tionship between science and language abilities of students with mild disabilities. *Remedial and Special Education, 15*(2), 117–126. **(13)**

324. Pascarella, E. T., Pflaum, S. W., Bryan, T. H., & Pearl, R. A. (1983). Interaction of internal attribution for effort and teacher response mode in reading instruction: A replication note. *American Educational Research Journal, 20*(2), 269–276. **(10)**
325. Perkins, V. L. (1988). Feedback effects on oral reading errors of children with learning disabilities. *Learning Disability Quarterly, 21*, 244–248. **(6)**
326. Pflaum, S. W., & Pascarella, E. T. (1980). Interactive effects of prior reading achievement and training in context on the reading of learning-disabled children. *Reading Research Quarterly, 16*(1), 138–158. **(1)**
327. Pflaum, S. W., Pascarella, E. T., Auer, C., Augustyn, L., & Boswick, M. (1982). Differential effects of four comprehension-facilitating conditions on LD and normal elementary-school readers. *Learning Disability Quarterly, 5*, 106–116. **(6)**
328. Phillips, N. B., Hamlett, C. L., Fuchs, L. S., & Fuchs, D. (1993). Combining classwide curriculum-based measurement and peer tutoring to help general educators provide adaptive education. *Learning Disabilities Research and Practice, 83*(3), 148–156. **(5)**
329. Pollack, H. A. (1985). The effects of two types of feedback in microcomputer instruction for teaching a visual discrimination task to learning disabled students (Ph.D. diss., Boston University, 1984). *Dissertation Abstracts International, 46*(2-A), 406–407. **(6)**
330. Portsmouth, R., Wilkins, J., & Airey, W. J. (1985). Home based reading for special school pupils. *Educational Psychology in Practice, 1*(2), 52–58. **(3)**
331. Quist, S. (1995). The effects of using graphic organizers with LD students to increase comprehension. (M. A. project, Kean College of New Jersey ; 41 pages). **(3)**
332. Ragland, E. U., Kerr, M. M., & Strain, P. S. (1981). Social play of withdrawn children: A study of the effects of teacher-mediated peer feedback. *Behavior Modification, 5*, 347–359. **(5)**
333. Ragland, G. G., & Wright, E. (1986). The influence of an academic skills resource lab on the competency test performance of mildly handicapped students. *High School Journal, 70*, 25–32. **(10)**
334. Ransby, M. J., & Melonari, S. A. *Can reading disabled young adolescents profit from exposure to taped books? A pilot outcome study* (unpublished manuscript). **(1)**
335. Rawson, H. E. (1992). Effects of intensive short-term remediation on academic intrinsic motivation of "at-risk" children. *Journal of Instructional Psychology, 19*, 274–285. **(8)**
336. Reid, R., & Harris, K. R. (1989). Self-monitoring of performance. *LD Forum, 15*, 39–42. **(10)**
337. Reid, R., Maag, J. W., Vasa, S. F., & Wright, G. (1994). Who are the children with attention deficit-hyperactivity disorder? A school-based survey. *Journal of Special Education, 28*, 117–137. **(5)**
338. Reilly, L. J. (1982). The role of sensory processes in remedial academic instruction with the learning disabled (Ph.D. diss., St. John's University, 1982). *Dissertation Abstracts International, 42*(12-B), 4920. **(6)**
339. Reilly, S. S., & Barber-Smith, D. (1982). Expanded use of captioned films for learning disabled students. *Exceptional Children, 48*(4), 361–363. **(6)**
340. Reiter, S. M., Mabee, W. S., & McLaughlin, T. F. (1985). Self-monitoring: Effects for on-task and time to complete assignments. *Remedial and Special Education, 6*, 50–51. **(1)**

341. Reynolds, C. J., Hill, D. S., Swassing, R. H., & Ward, M. E. (1988). The effects of revision strategy instruction on the writing performance of students with learning disabilities. *Journal of Learning Disabilities, 21*, 540–545. **(6)**
342. Reynolds, M. C., Heistad, D., Peterson, J., & Dehli, R. (1992). A study of days to learn. *Remedial and Special Education, 13*, 20–26. **(4)**
343. Richardson, E. (1984). The impact of phonemic processing instruction on the reading achievement of reading-disabled children. *Annals of the New York Academy of Sciences, 433*, 97–118. **(10)**
344. Richardson, E., Ostereicher, M. H., Bialer, I., & Winsberg, B. G. (1975). Teaching beginning reading skills to retarded children in community classrooms: A programmatic case study. *Mental Retardation, 13*, 11–15. **(3)**
345. Rickard, H. C., Clements, C. B., & Willis, J. W. (1970). Effects of contingent and noncontingent token reinforcement upon classroom performance. *Psychological Reports, 27*, 903–908. **(4)**
346. Ritter, D. R. (1978). Surviving in the regular classroom: A follow-up of mainstreamed children with learning disabilities. *Journal of School Psychology, 16*, 253–256. **(8)**
347. Rivera, D. M., & Smith, D. D. (1987). Influence of modeling on acquisition and generalization of computation skills: A summary of research findings from three sites. *Learning Disability Quarterly, 10*(1), 69–80. **(14)**
348. Robinson, C. A. (1986). Effects of confluent education on high school students identified as learning disabled. *Exceptional Child, 33*(3), 193–197. **(8)**
349. Robinson, G. L. W., & Conway, R. N. F. (1990). The effects of Irlen colored lenses on students' specific reading skills and their perception of ability: A 12-month validity study. *Journal of Learning Disabilities, 23*(10), 589–596. **(8)**
350. Robinson, P. W., Newby, T. J., & Ganzell, S. L. (1981). A token system for a class of underachieving hyperactive children. *Journal of Applied Behavior Analysis, 14*, 307–315. **(3)**
351. Roessler, R. T., & Johnson, V. A. (1987). Developing job maintenance skills in learning disabled youth. *Journal of Learning Disabilities, 20*, 428–432. **(3)**
352. Rooney, K. J., Hallahan, D. P., & Lloyd, J. W. (1984). Self-recording of attention by learning disabled students in the regular classroom. *Journal of Learning Disabilities, 17*, 360–364. **(3)**
353. Rose, M. C., Cundick, B. P., & Higbee, K. L. (1983). Verbal rehearsal and visual imagery: Mnemonic aids for learning-disabled children. *Learning Disability Quarterly, 16*, 352–354. **(6)**
354. Rose, T. L. (1986). Effects of illustrations on reading comprehension of learning disabled students. *Journal of Learning Disabilities, 19*(9), 542–544. **(6)**
355. Rose, T. L., & Beattie, J. R. (1986). Relative effects of teacher-directed and taped previewing on oral reading. *Learning Disability Quarterly, 9*, 193–199. **(1)**
356. Rose, T. L., & Furr, P. M. (1984). Negative effects of illustrations as word cues. *Journal of Learning Disabilities, 17*, 334–337. **(3)**
357. Rose, T. L., & Robinson, H. H. (1984). Effects of illustration on learning disabled students' reading performance. *Learning Disability Quarterly, 3*(1), 165–171. **(3)**
358. Rubin, J. M. (1986). Evaluation of the self-contained elementary school program for the learning disabled child in the city school district of the city of Newburgh (Ph.D. diss., Columbia University Teacher's College, 1986). *Dissertation Abstracts International, 47*(6-A), 2123. **(10)**
359. Rubino, C. A., & Minden, H. A. (1973). An analysis of eye-movements in children with a reading disability. *Cortex, 9*, 217–220. **(6)**

360. Ruhl, K. L., & Suritsky, S. (1995). The pause procedure and/or an outline: Effect on immediate free recall and lecture notes taken by college students with learning disabilities. *Learning Disability Quarterly*, *18*, 2–11. **(6)**

361. Ryan, G. (1990). Computer literacy instruction for learning disabled students with reading disabilities (Ph.D. diss., Boston College, 1988). *Dissertation Abstracts International*, *50*(9-A), 2862. **(8)**

362. Sachs, A. (1984). Accessing scripts before reading the story. *Learning Disability Quarterly*, *7*, 226–228. **(6)**

363. Sawyer, D. J. (1992). Language abilities, reading acquisition, and developmental dyslexia: A discussion of hypothetical and observed relationships. *Journal of Learning Disabilities*, *25*, 82–95. **(10)**

364. Schell, R. M., Pelham, W. E., Bender, M. E., Andree, J. A., Law, T., & Robbins, F. R. (1986). *Behavioral Assessment*, *8*, 373–384. **(3)**

365. Schmidt, M., Weinstein, T., Niemic, R., & Walberg, H. J. (1985–1986). Computer-assisted instruction with exceptional children. *Journal of Special Education*, *4*, 493–501. **(13)**

366. Schmidt, M. W. (1989). Method of questioning and placement of questions: Effects on LD students' comprehension. *Learning Disability Quarterly*, *12*, 192–198. **(6)**

367. Schumaker, J. B., & Deshler, D. D. (1992). Validation of learning strategy interventions for students with learning disabilities: Results of a programmatic research effort. In B. Y. L. Wong (Ed.), *Contemporary intervention research in learning disabilities* (pp. 22–46). New York: Springer-Verlag. **(10)**

368. Schumaker, J. B., Deshler, D. D., Alley, G. R., Warner, M. M., & Denton, P. H. (1982). Multipass: A learning strategy for improving reading comprehension. *Learning Disability Quarterly*, *5*, 295–304. **(1)**

369. Schumaker, J. B., & Ellis, E. S. (1982). Social skills training of LD adolescents: A generalization study. *Learning Disability Quarterly*, *5*, 409–414. **(1)**

370. Schunk, D. H., & Rice, J. M. (1992). Influence of reading-comprehension strategy information on children's achievement outcomes. *Learning Disability Quarterly*, *15*(1), 51–64. **(3)**

371. Schworm, R. W. (1979). The effects of selective attention on the decoding skills of children with learning disabilities. *Journal of Learning Disabilities*, *12*, 639–644. **(1)**

372. Scruggs, T. E., & Mastropieri, M. A. (1986). Improving the test-taking skills of behaviorally disordered and learning disabled children. *Exceptional Children*, *53*(1), 63–68. **(4)**

373. Scruggs, T. E., Mastropieri, M. A., Brigham, F. J., & Sullivan, G. S. (1992). Effects of mnemonic reconstructions on the spatial learning of adolescents with learning disabilities. *Learning Disability Quarterly*, *15*, 154–162. **(6)**

374. Scruggs, T. E., Mastropieri, M. A., Levin, J. R., & Gaffney, J. S. (1985). Facilitating the acquisition of science facts in learning disabled students. *American Educational Research Journal*, *22*, 575–586 **(6)**

375. Scruggs, T. E., Mastropieri, M. A., Sullivan, G. S., & Hesser, L. S. (1993). Improving reasoning and recall: The differential effects of elaborative interrogation and mnemonic elaboration. *Learning Disability Quarterly*, *16*, 233–240. **(6)**

376. Scruggs, T. E., & Osguthorpe, R. T. (1986). Tutoring interventions within special education settings: A comparison of cross-age and peer tutoring. *Psychology in the Schools*, *23*, 187–193. **(4)**

377. Searcy, J. B. (1984). A comparative study of reading instruction programs in a multicultural school system based on word recognition and reading comprehension errors

(Ph.D. diss., University of Alabama, 1983). *Dissertation Abstracts International, 44*(8-A), 2444. **(4)**

378. Serwer, B. L., Shapiro, B. J., & Shapiro, P. P. (1973). The comparative effectiveness of four methods of instruction on the achievement of children with specific learning disabilities. *Journal of Special Education, 7*(5), 37–41. **(3)**
379. Shafto, F., & Sulzbacher, S. (1977). Comparing treatment tactics with a hyperactive preschool child: Stimulant medication and programmed teacher intervention. *Journal of Applied Behavior Analysis, 10*, 13–20. **(5)**
380. Shapiro, E. S. (1989). Teaching self-management skills to learning disabled adolescents. *Learning Disability Quarterly, 12*, 275–287. **(1)**
381. Sharpe, L. W. (1976). The effects of a creative thinking skills program on intermediate grade educationally handicapped children. *Journal of Creative Behavior, 10*, 138–145. **(1)**
382. Shelfbine, J. (1990). A syllabic-unit approach to teaching decoding of polysyllabic words to fourth- and sixth-grade disabled readers. *Yearbook of the National Reading Conference, 39*, 223–229. **(5)**
383. Shipe, D., & Miezitis, S. (1969). A pilot study in the diagnosis and remediation of special learning disabilities in preschool children. *Journal of Learning Disabilities, 2*, 579–592. **(5)**
384. Siddle, B. G. (1980). Interpersonal problem-solving training with adolescents: A cognitive behavior modification approach (Ph.D. diss., Arizona State University, 1980). *Dissertation Abstracts International, 41*(2-B), 701. **(4)**
385. Simmons, D. C., Kameenui, E. J., & Darch, C. B. (1988). The effect of textual proximity on fourth- and fifth-grade LD students' metacognitive awareness and strategic comprehension behavior. *Learning Disability Quarterly, 11*, 380–395. **(6)**
386. Sinatra, R., & Venezia, J. F. (1986). A visual approach to improved literacy skills for special education adolescents: An exploratory study. *Exceptional Child, 33*(3), 187–192. **(8)**
387. Sindelar, P. T. (1982). The effects of cross-aged tutoring on the comprehension skills of remedial reading students. *Journal of Special Education, 16*(2), 199–206. **(3)**
388. Sindelar, P. T., Bursuck, W. D., & Halle, J. W. (1986). The effects of two variations of teacher questioning on student performance. *Education and Treatment of Children, 9*, 56–66. **(4)**
389. Sindelar, P. T., Smith, M. A., Harriman, N. E., Hale, R. L., & Wilson, R. J. (1986). Teacher effectiveness in special education programs. *Journal of Special Education, 20*, 195–207. **(10)**
390. Singh, T. (1993). The deficit approach to dyslexia: An appraisal. *Psycho-Lingua, 23*(1), 1–10. **(10)**
391. Skinner, C. H., Adamson, K. L., Woodward, J. R., Jackson, R. R., Atchison, L. A., & Mims, J. W. (1993). A comparison of fast-rate, slow-rate, and silent previewing interventions on reading performance. *Journal of Learning Disabilities, 26*(10), 674–681. **(1)**
392. Skinner, C. H., Ford, J. M., & Yunker, B. D. (1991). A comparison of instructional response requirements on the multiplication performance of behaviorally disordered students. *Behavioral Disorders, 17*, 56–65. **(3)**
393. Skinner, C. H., Smith, E. S., & Mclean, J. E. (1994). The effects of intertrial interval duration on sight-word learning rates in children with behavioral disorders. *Behavioral Disorders, 19*(2), 98–107. **(3)**
394. Skorina, J. K. (1974). A study of the effects of ritalin intervention upon the percep-

tual competencies of children diagnosed as giving evidence of psychoneurological learning disabilities (Ph.D. diss., Wayne State University, 1973). *Dissertation Abstracts International, 34* (11-A), 7055–7056. **(3)**

395. Slavin, R. E., Madden, N. A., & Leavey, M. (1984). Effects of team assisted individualization on the mathematics achievement of academically handicapped and nonhandicapped students. *Journal of Educational Psychology, 76*, 813–819. **(3)**
396. Smith, D. D. (1979). The improvement of children's oral reading through the use of teacher modeling. *Journal of Learning Disabilities, 12*(3), 172–175. **(3)**
397. Smith, D. D., & Lovitt, T. C. (1973). The educational diagnosis and remediation of written b and d reversal problems: A case study. *Journal of Learning Disabilities, 6*(6), 356–363. **(3)**
398. Smith, D. D., & Lovitt, T. C. (1976). The differential effects of reinforcement contingencies on arithmetic performance. *Journal of Learning Disabilities, 9*(1), 21–29. **(3)**
399. Smith, K. N. (1985). A study of parent locus of control and attitudes as related to intervention for learning disabled children (Ph.D. diss., Kansas State University, 1984). *Dissertation Abstracts International, 45*(9-A), 2813. **(7)**
400. Snart, F. (1979). Strategy training for children with learning difficulties. *Mental Retardation Bulletin, 7*(2), 61–73. **(8)**
401. Snow, J. H., Barnett, L., Cunningham, K., & Ernst, M. (1988). Cross-modal development with normal and learning disabled children. *International Journal of Clinical Neuropsychology, 10*, 74–80. **(6)**
402. Sovik, N. (1977). Individual instruction in Norwegian (The PODIN Project). *Scandinavian Journal of Educational Research, 21*, 197–232. **(5)**
403. Sparks, S. S. (1982). The relation of off-task behavior to performance among educable mentally retarded, learning disabled, and normal middle school students. (Ph.D. diss., The University of Florida, 1981). *Dissertation Abstracts International, 42*(9-A), 3953. **(10)**
404. Speltz, M. L. (1982). The effects of standardized and three types of group contingencies on the academic and social behaviors of learning disabled children (Ph.D. diss., University of Missouri, 1980). *Dissertation Abstracts International, 42*(8-B), 3245. **(3)**
405. Sprafkin, J., Watkins, L. T., & Gadow, K. D. (1990). Efficacy of a television literacy curriculum for emotionally disturbed and learning disabled children. *Journal of Applied Developmental Psychology, 11*(2), 225–244. **(1)**
406. Stapleton, L. E. (1973). A long-range diagnostic-prescriptive reading intervention program employing the Frostic Test of Visual Perceptual development and the Illinois Test of Psycholinguistic Abilities with low socioeconomic, semi-urban, elementary students of the Okaloosa County Florida Public School (Ph.D. diss., Florida State University, 1973). *Dissertation Abstracts International, 34*(6-A), 3161–3162. **(5)**
407. Steele, K., & Barling, J. (1982). Self-instruction and learning disabilities: Maintenance, generalization, and subject characteristics. *Journal of General Psychology, 106*, 141–154. **(3)**
408. Stevens, K. B., Blackhurst, A. E., & Slaton, D. B. (1991). Teaching memorized spelling with a microcomputer: Time delay and computer-assisted instruction. *Journal of Applied Behavior Analysis, 24*(1), 153–160. **(4)**
409. Stevens, R. J., & Slavin, R. E. (1995). The cooperative elementary school: Effects on students' achievement, attitudes, and social relations. *American Educational Research Journal, 32*, 321–351. **(3)**
410. Stowitschek, C. E., Lewis, B. L., Shores, R. E., & Ezzell, D. L. (1980). Procedures for

analyzing student performance data to generate hypotheses for the purpose of educational decision making. *Behavioral Disorders*, *5*, 136–150. **(3)**

411. Stricker, A. G. (1989). Application of an intelligent CAI tutoring system to spelling instruction for learning disabled students (Ph.D. diss., Texas A & M University, 1988). *Dissertation Abstracts International*, *50*(4-A), 909. **(3)**
412. Stromer, R. (1977). Remediating academic deficiencies in learning disabled children. *Exceptional Children*, *43*, 432–440. **(3)**
413. Stump, C. S., Lovitt, T. C., Fister, S., Kemp, K., Moore, R., & Schroeder, B. (1992). Vocabulary intervention for secondary-level youth. *Learning Disability Quarterly*, *15*(3), 207–222. **(3)**
414. Sugai, G., & Smith, P. (1986). The equal additions method of subtraction taught with a modeling technique. *Remedial and Special Education*, *7*, 40–48. **(3)**
415. Sutaria, S. (1979). A summer program for children with learning disabilities. *Journal of Learning Disabilities*, *12*, 191–193. **(1)**
416. Talbot, E., Pepin, M., & Loranger, M. (1992). Computerized cognitive training with learning disabled students: A pilot study. *Psychological Reports*, *71*(3, Pt. 2), 1347–1356. **(5)**
417. Tansey, M. A. (1984). EEG sensorimotor rhythm biofeedback training: Some effects on the neurologic precursors of learning disabilities. *International Journal of Psychophysiology*, *1*, 163–177. **(1)**
418. Taves, R. A. H., Hutchinson, N. L., & Freeman, J. G. (1992). The effect of cognitive instruction in the development of employment interview skills in adolescents with learning disabilities. *Canadian Journal of Counselling*, *26*(2), 87–95. **(1)**
419. Taylor, L., Adelman, H. S., & Kaser-Boyd, N. (1985). Minors' attitudes and competence toward participation in psychoeducational decisions. *Professional Psychology: Research and Practice*, *16*, 226–235. **(10)**
420. Tenney, R. A., & Osguthorpe, R. T. (1990). Elementary age special education students using self-directed or tutor-assisted computer-aided instruction to develop keyboarding skills. *Journal of Educational Computing Research*, *6*,(2), 215–229. **(4)**
421. Thomas, A., & Pashley, B. (1982). Effects of classroom training on LD students' task persistence and attributions. *Learning Disability Quarterly*, *5*, 133–144. **(1)**
422. Thorkildsen, R. (1985a). Using an interactive video disc program to teach social skills to handicapped children. *American Annals of the Deaf*, *130*, 383–385. **(13)**
423. Thorkildsen, R. (1985b). Microelectronic technology and the hearing impaired: The future. *American Academy of the Deaf*, *130*, 324–331. **(1)**
424. Thornhill, C. H. (1989). A study of the effectiveness of preventative interventions for children at risk in a Florida school district (Ph.D. diss., University of Central Florida, 1989). *Dissertation Abstracts International*, *50*(5-A), 1174. **(5)**
425. Thorpe, H. W., Chiang, B., & Darch, C. B. (1981). Individual and group feedback systems for improving oral reading accuracy in learning disabled and regular class children. *Journal of Learning Disabilities*, *14*, 332–334, 367. **(3)**
426. Thurlow, M. L., Ysseldyke, J. E., Wotruba, J. W., & Algozzine, B. (1993). Instruction in special education classrooms under varying student–teacher ratios. *Elementary School Journal*, *93*, 305–320. **(10)**
427. Tindal, G., & Hasbrouck, J. (1991). Analyzing student writing to develop instructional strategies. *Learning Disabilities Research and Practice*, *6*, 237–245. **(10)**
428. Top, B. L., & Osguthorpe, R. T. (1987). Reverse-role tutoring: The effects of handicapped students tutoring regular class students. *Elementary School Journal*, *87*, 413–423. **(4)**

429. Torgesen, J. K., Dahlem, W. E., & Greenstein, J. (1987). Using verbatim text recordings to enhance reading comprehension in learning disabled adolescents. *Learning Disabilities Focus, 3,* 30–38. **(4)**

430. Torgesen, J. K., Waters, M. D., Cohen, A. L., & Torgesen, J. L. (1988). Improving sight-word recognition skills in LD children: An evaluation of three computer program variations. *Learning Disability Quarterly, 11,* 125–132. **(1)**

431. Torneus, M. (1984). Phonological awareness and reading: A chicken and egg problem? *Journal of Educational Psychology, 76,* 1346–1358. **(5)**

432. Traynelis-Yurek, E. (1985). Preferred versus non-preferred hand: A comparative study. *Academic Therapy, 21,* 29-36. **(1)**

433. Trifiletti, J. J., Frith, G. H., & Armstrong, S. (1984). Microcomputers versus resource rooms for LD students: A preliminary investigation of the effects on math skills. *Learning Disability Quarterly, 7*(1), 69–76. **(3)**

434. Trovato, J., Harris, J., Pryor, C. W., & Wilkinson, S. C. (1992). Teachers in regular classrooms: An applied setting for successful behavior programming. *Psychology in the Schools, 29,* 52–60. **(5)**

435. Uhry, J. K., Shepherd, M. J. (1997). Teaching phonological recoding to young children with phonological processing deficits: The effect on sight vocabulary acquisition. *Learning Disability Quarterly, 20,* 104–125. **(8)**

436. Vadasy, P. F., Jenkins, J. R., Antil, L. R., Wayne, S. K., & O'Connor, R. E. (1997). Community-based early reading intervention for at-risk first graders. *Learning Disabilities Research and Practice, 12*(1), 29–39. **(8)**

437. Vadasy, P. F., Jenkins, J. R., Antil, L. R., Wayne, S. K., & O'Connor, R. E. (in press). The effectiveness of one-to-one tutoring by community tutors for at-risk beginning readers. *Learning Disability Quarterly.* **(3)**

438. Vallecorsa, A. L., & deBettencourt, L. U. (1992). Teaching composing skills to learning disabled adolescents using a process-oriented strategy. *Journal of Developmental and Physical Disabilities, 4*(4), 277–297. **(1)**

439. VanBon, W. H. J., Boksebeld, L. M., Tonneke, A. M., Freide, F., & VandenHurk, A. J. M. (1991). A comparison of three methods of reading-while-listening. *Journal of Learning Disabilities, 24,* 471–476. **(1)**

440. Varnhagen, S. (1983). Learning disabled adults and the use of microcomputer programs. *Mental Retardation and Learning Disability Bulletin, 11,* 122–127. **(1)**

441. Vaughn, S., McIntosh, R., & Spencer-Rowe, J. (1991). Peer rejection is a stubborn thing: Increasing peer acceptance of rejected students with learning disabilities. *Learning Disabilities Research and Practice, 6*(2), 83–88. **(8)**

442. Vaughn, S., Schumm, J. S., & Gordon, J. (1992). Early spelling acquisition: Does writing really beat the computer? *Learning Disability Quarterly, 15,* 223–228. **(6)**

443. Vaughn, S., Schumm, J. S., & Kouzekanani, K. (1993). What do students with learning disabilities think when their general education teachers make adaptations? *Journal of Learning Disabilities, 26,* 545–555. **(10)**

444. Vellutino, F. R. (1991). Introduction to three studies on reading acquisition: Convergent findings on theoretical foundations of code-oriented versus whole-language approaches to reading instruction. *Journal of Education Psychology, 83,* 437–443. **(1)**

445. Vellutino, F. R., Scanlon, D. M., Sipay, E. R., Small, S. G., Pratt, A., Cheven, R., & Denckla, M. B. (1997). Cognitive profiles of difficult-to-remediate and readily remediated poor readers: Early intervention as a vehicle for distinguishing between cognitive and experiential deficits as basic causes of specific reading disability. *Journal of Educational Psychology, 88*(4), 601–638. **(1)**

446. Voss, C. A. (1985). Cognitive–behavioral training in teaching reading to children with learning disabilities (Ph.D. diss., Hofstra University, 1984). *Dissertation Abstracts International, 45*(8-A), 2706–2707. **(1)**

447. Welch, M., & Jensen, J. B. (1990). Write, P.L.E.A.S.E.: A video-assisted strategic intervention to improve written expression of inefficient learners. *Remedial and Special Education, 12*, 37–47. **(5)**

448. Whyte, L. A. (1984). Characteristics of learning disabilities persisting into adolescence. *Alberta Journal of Educational Research, 30*, 14–25. **(10)**

449. Wiig, E. H., & Semel, E. M. (1973). Comprehension of linguistic concepts requiring logical operations by learning-disabled children. *Journal of Speech and Hearing Research, 16*(4), 627–636. **(1)**

450. Williams, M. C., Lecluyse, K., & Rock-Faucheux, A. (1992). Effective interventions for reading disability. *Journal American Optometry Association, 63*, 411–417. **(6)**

451. Wilson, R., & Wesson, C. (1991). Increasing achievement of learning disabled students by measuring and controlling task difficulty. *Learning Disabilities, Research and Practice, 6*, 34–39. **(10)**

452. Wise, B. W., & Olson, R. K. (1992). How poor readers and spellers use interactive speech in a computerized spelling program. *Reading and Writing: An Interdisciplinary Journal, 4*, 145–163. **(3)**

453. Wise, B. W., Olson, R. K., & Treiman, R. (1990). Subsyllabic units in computerized reading instruction: Onset-rime vs. postvowel segmentation. *Journal of Experimental Child Psychology, 49*, 1–19. **(3)**

454. Wolff, D. E., Desberg, P., & Marsh, G. (1985). Analogy strategies for improving word recognition in competent and learning disabled readers. *Reading Teacher, 38*, 412–416. **(6)**

455. Wong, B. Y. L. (1979). Increasing retention of main ideas through questioning strategies. *Learning Disability Quarterly, 2*(2), 42–47. **(6)**

456. Wong, B. Y. L. (1980). Activating the inactive learner: Use of questions/ prompts to enhance comprehension and retention of implied information in learning disabled children. *Learning Disability Quarterly, 3*(1), 29–37. **(6)**

457. Wong, B. Y. L. (1997). Research on genre-specific strategies in enhancing writing in adolescents with learning disabilities. *Learning Disability Quarterly, 20*, 110–159. **(8)**

458. Wong, B. Y. L., Butler, D. L., Ficzere, S. A., & Kuperis, S. (1996). Teaching adolescents with learning disabilities and low achievers to plan, write, and revise opinion compare-and-contrast essays. *Learning Disabilities Research and Practice, 12*(1), 2–15. **(8)**

459. Wong, B. Y. L., & Wilson, M. (1984). Investigating awareness of and teaching passage organization in learning disabled children. *Journal of Learning Disabilities, 17*, 477–482. **(6)**

460.. Wong, B. Y. L., Wong, R., & Blenkinsop, J. (1989). Cognitive and metacognitive aspects of learning disabled adolescents' composing problems. *Learning Disability Quarterly, 12*, 300–322. **(8)**

461. Woodward, J. (1994). The role of models in secondary science instruction. *Remedial and Special Education, 15*, 94–104. **(10)**

462. Wright, J., & Cashdan, A. (1991). Training metacognitive skills in backward readers: A pilot study. *Educational Psychology in Practice, 7*, 153–162. **(1)**

463. Yanok, J. (1993). College students with learning disabilities enrolled in developmental education programs. *College Student Journal, 27*(1), 166–174. **(3)**

464. Zaragoza, N., & Vaughn, S. (1992). The effects of process writing instruction on

three 2nd-grade students with different achievement profiles. *Learning Disabilities Research and Practice*, *7*, 184–193. **(8)**

465. Zawaiza, T. W., & Gerber, M. M. (1993). Effects of explicit instruction on math word-problem solving by community college students with learning disabilities. *Learning Disability Quarterly*, *16*, 64–79. **(6)**
466. Zentall, S. S., & Ferkis, M. A. (1993). Mathematic problem solving for youth with ADHD, with and without learning disabilities. *Learning Disability Quarterly*, *16*, 6–18. **(10)**
467. Zinar, E. H. (1976). Intervention procedures for classroom management using the guided inquiry mode and programmed materials: A consultant model (Ph.D. diss., University of California-Los Angeles, 1975). *Dissertation Abstracts International*, *36*(11-A), 7225. **(8)**

DISSERTATIONS WE WERE UNABLE TO OBTAIN FROM HOME CAMPUS ($N = 16$)

1. Bott, D. A. (1984). Math performance across six modality combinations: A study of children with learning problems (Ph.D. diss., University of Florida, 1983). *Dissertation Abstracts International*, *45*(4-A), 1091.
2. Bucher, A. K. (1978). The effect of supplementary phonics training on the transfer skills taught by a linguistic approach to reading instruction (Ph.D. diss., Catholic University of America, 1977). *Dissertation Abstracts International*, *38*(11-A), 6489–6490.
3. Campbell, E. F. (1978). The effects of learning disabilities remediation, attention training, and the Hawthorne effect on learning disabled children (Ph.D. diss., Hofstra University, 1977). *Dissertation Abstracts International*, *38*(9-B), 4423–4424.
4. Childs, S. A. (1987). A comparison of indoor versus outdoor teaching interventions upon the academic skill acquisition and interaction behaviors of selected students with learning disabilities (Ph.D. diss., Ohio State University, 1986). *Dissertation Abstracts International*, *47*(7-A), 2449.
5. Cottom, B. G. (1991). The effects of the Multisensory Authoring Computer System (MACS) with and without voice accompaniment on the word recognition of students with learning disabilities (Ph.D. diss., Johns Hopkins University, 1991). *Dissertation Abstracts International*, *52*(6-A), 2086.
6. Freund, L. A. (1986). The influence of instruction on the interrogative strategies of learning disabled children (Ph.D. diss., Columbia University Teachers College, 1986). *Dissertation Abstracts International*, *47*(6-A), 2118.
7. Gartland, D. (1987). The effects of varying amounts of teacher directed instruction and monitored independent seatwork on the acquisition of syllabication rules by severely disabled children (Ph.D. diss., Pennsylvania State University, 1986). *Dissertation Abstracts International*, *47*(11-A), 4055.
8. Gisondo, J. (1978). Learning disabilities remediation using individual or group techniques in clinic and school settings (Ph.D. diss., Hofstra University, 1978). *Dissertation Abstracts International*, *39*(5-A), 2830.
9. Keddy, B. A. S. (1991). Computer keyboarding instruction for students with learning disabilities: Computer-assisted versus traditional versus mnemonic methods (Ph.D. diss., Columbia University Teachers College, 1990). *Dissertation Abstracts International*, *51*(10-A), 3392.

10. Klein, R. W. (1990). Social skills training and parent intervention with learning-disabled children (Ph.D. diss., University of Florida, 1989). *Dissertation Abstracts International, 51*(6-A), 1911.
11. Klosterman, D. G. (1974). A comparison of self-instructional techniques and a guided-learning approach in instructing learning-disabled children in a one-to-one tutorial situation (Ph.D. diss., University of Cincinnati, 1972). *Dissertation Abstracts International, 34*(8-B), 4021.
12. Mullins, N. J. (1989). An analysis of the effects of three procedures for increasing word knowledge of older disabled readers (Ph.D. diss., Ohio State University, 1989). *Dissertation Abstracts International, 50*(4-A), 911.
13. Ruppert, E. T. (1976). The effect of the synthetic-multisensory method of language instruction upon psycholinguistic abilities and reading achievement (Ph.D. diss., American University, 1976). *Dissertation Abstracts International, 37*(2-A), 920–921.
14. Rusalem, H. J. (1972). Effect of group training in short-term memory on children enrolled in classes for the learning disabled (Ph.D. diss., Columbia University, 1972). *Dissertation Abstracts International, 33*(5-A), 2202.
15. Shapero, S. (1978). The effects of parents' use of direct and supplemental reading instruction on the oral reading performance of their learning disabled children (Ph.D. diss., University of Washington, 1978). *Dissertation Abstracts International, 39*(6-A), 3519.
16. Simmonds, E. P. M. D. (1986). The effects of two methods of intervention in the use of an efficient questioning strategy on the performance of learning disabled children (Ph.D. diss., Columbia University Teachers College, 1986). *Dissertation Abstracts International, 47*(6-A), 4913.

Appendix C

Meta-Analysis Project

CODING SHEET

Article Analysis

1. Complete citation of article (APA style) ____________________
____
____
____
2. Institutional affiliation of first or corresponding author (school, university, etc.) ____________________
____
3. Institutional affiliation of editor of journal (check journal cover) __________
____
4. Department or program affiliation of first or corresponding author ____________________ (*Note:* If work was done as a doctoral student, give credit to training university.)
5. Number of coauthors __________
6. Funding source(s) ____________________ (e.g., Office of Special Education and Rehabilitation Services—field initiated research, National Institute of Mental Health, university—faculty grant, etc.)
7. Gender of first author F _1_ M _2_
8. Subject area discussed or focused upon in the article on intervention (refer to key term in title or abstract, e.g., reading, math) ____________________

9. Frequency of citations (refer to Social Science Citation Index 2 years after publication date) ______________

10. Number of references in article ____________ *and* number of references different from journal ___________

Name of Researcher ______________________________
Name of Interrater ______________________________
%Interrater Agreement ___________________________

Design and Methodological Analysis

11. Who is the most frequent author cited in reference sections—*other than* the author of article (if a bimodel score emerges, list both authors)? _________

    ____

12. Hypothesis is directional (specific outcomes predicted) 1 , or nondirectional (null) 2 , none given 3 (hypotheses usually occur in paragraph before Methods section) (circle one)

13. Sampling procedure (circle appropriate boxes)
    - 1 Randomly selected from school district (includes schools or students)
    - 2 Randomly selected within schools
    - 3 Randomly assigned to treatment condition
    - 4 Stratified sampling (subgroups are selected and randomly assigned to treatment)
    - 5 Stratified sampling *but not* randomly assigned to treatment
    - 6 *Intact sample *but no* random assignment to treatment
    - 7 Intact sample *but* random assignment to treatment
    - 8 Table of random numbers mentioned
    - 9 Volunteer sampling
    - 10 Other (specify) ______________________________
    - 11 No information

    Note. *Intact (the word "random" is not provided—if the word "random" or "stratified" is not used at all in the study, then most likely #6)

14. Geographic region from where sample selected (United States) (stated in the article Methods section)
    - 1 ___ Midwest
    - 2 ___ Northeast
    - 3 ___ Northwest
    - 4 ___ Southeast
    - 5 ___ Southwest
    - 6 ___ East North Central
    - 7 ___ West North Central
    - 8 ___ East South Central
    - 9 ___ Mountain

10 ___ Pacific
11 ___ South
12 ___ West
13 ___ North Central
14 ___ No information
15 ___ Other ______________________________(e.g., Canada, England)

Descriptive Data on LD Subjects

15. Psychometric and behavioral data (includes all testing data usually found in Subjects section of article standardized and nonstandardized related to sample description)

	Experimental		Control[a]		Mixed	
Name of Measure						
WAIS						
WAIS-R						
WISC						
WISC-R						
WISC III						
WRAT						
Reading						
Arithmetic						
Spelling						
WRAT-R						
Reading						
Arithmetic						
Spelling						

Note. If not broken down into control versus experimental, enter in mixed column.

[a]Descriptive data on control sample (circle one)

Type of control group (1 = LD control, 2 = NLD-CA matched control, 3 = younger ability [e.g., reading matched], 4 = other—please define)

If type of control = 1, 2, and 3, make additional copy of form to record.

16. Psychometric and behavioral data (includes all testing data usually found in Subjects section of article standardized and nonstandardized related to sample description; include *complete* title of test)

	Experimental		Control[a]		Mixed	
Name of Measure	*M*	*SD*	*M*	*SD*	*M*	*SD*

Note. If not broken down into control versus experimental, enter in mixed column.

[a]Descriptive data on control sample (circle one)

Type of control group (1 = LD control, 2 = NLD-CA matched control, 3 = younger ability [e.g., reading matched], 4 = other—please define)

If type of control = 1, 2, and 3, make additional copy of form to record.

17. Type of research design and methodology used to assess intervention
 - _1_ Survey
 - _2_ Case study
 - _3_ Time-series analysis*
 - _4_ Reversal design (or variation)
 - _5_ Multiple baseline (or variation)
 - _6_ Criterion changing (or variation)
 - _7_ Multielement (or variation of alternating treatment design)

_8_ One group pretest–posttest design
_9_ Pretest–posttest design with control and experimental group
_10_ Posttest-only design with control and experimental group randomly assigned to treatment and only a posttest is given
_11_ Observational or naturalistic study—Ethnographic
_12_ Single-factor design—compare two or more groups on a single factor, for example, word recognition
_13_ Static group comparison design—a group of subjects are administered treatment and posttested while another group is only posttested
_14_ Solomon design or Latin square design
_15_ Factorial design—determines the effect of two or more independent variables
_16_ Correlational design
_17_ Factor analysis
_18_ Regression
_19_ Path analysis
_20_ Other: list
_21_ Longitudinal study

**Note*. If #3, 4, 5, 6, or 7 selected, then study is single subject. If #11, then study is narrative.

18. Statistical analysis (may circle more than one response)
_1_ No statistical analysis
_2_ Descriptive (frequency, percentages, central tendency, and variability)
_3_ Percent nonoverlapping data
_4_ Chi-square
_5_ Independent and dependent *t*-test (test of separate random sample)
_6_ Planned orthogonal comparisons (e.g., Dunn, Dunnett, planned orthogonal contrasts—e.g., *t*-test)
_7_ Post-hoc multiple comparison (e.g., Tukey, Newman–Keuls, Scheffe)
_8_ One-way ANOVA
_9_ Factorial ANOVA
_10_ Trend analysis
_11_ One-way ANCOVA
_12_ Factorial ANCOVA
_13_ Part/partial correlation
_14_ Multiple regression
_15_ Discriminant analysis
_16_ Path analysis
_17_ Canonical correlation
_18_ Factor analysis
_19_ Cluster analysis
_20_ One way MANOVA/MANCOVA
_21_ Factorial MANOVA/MANCOVA
_22_ Meta-analysis

23 Other correlational (list the type) ____________________
24 Other nonparametric (list the type) ____________________
25 Other (list the type) ____________________

19. Study contains information on the validity and reliability of dependent measures used to assess treatment effects?
___ a. Study uses standardized tests to assess treatment effects?
yes 1 or no 2 (circle)
___ Number of standardized measures?
___ b. Study includes reliability coefficient on experimental measures?
yes 1 or no 2 (circle)
___ Number of experimental measures reliability indicated
___ Total number of experimental measures
___ c. Type of reliability measure on experimental measure (check)
___ Interobserver
___ Internal reliability (e.g., coefficient alpha, KR20)
___ Test–retest
___ Parallel forms
___ d. Study includes rationale for experimental measures (cites previous study) yes 1 or no 2 (circle)
___ Study includes coefficient on validity of experimental measures
___ Number of experimental measures in which validity coefficient reported
___ Total number of experimental measures

20. For single-subject design studies (#3 through #7 on item 17)
Interrater reliability _____ (yes 1 or no 2)
Cohen's kappa _____ (yes 1 or no 2)
Range __________ to __________
Mean ________
How often assessed ______________
Total # of sessions in total study ____________

Type of recording (check)
1___ Duration
2___ Time sampling
3___ Interval
4___ Frequency
5___ Permanent product
6___ Other (specify)____________________

21. How many experiments does the study include? ____

22. Does information on LD group *state* the following or use the following concepts (found in sample description) (check the appropriate boxes)?
___ 1. PL 94-142
___ 2. Specific disability in reading, math, writing, process, etc.
___ 3. General, weak achievement (no particular deficits are specified)

___ 4. Discrepancy
___ 5. State definition or state law
___ 6. IQ and achievement score
___ 7. Children already placed in special education class
___ 8. Referred by:
 ___ 8a. teacher
 ___ 8b. district
 ___ 8c. parent
 ___ 8d. school
 ___ 8e. clinic
 ___ 8f. other (specify) ______________________________
___ 9. Discrepancy formula or equation
___ 10. Exclusion
___ 11. Cutoff scores
 Type of cutoff scores
 ___ 11a. grade equivalent
 ___ b. percentile
 ___ c. standard score
 ___ d. raw score
 ___ e. other (specify) ______________________________
___ 12. Age scores
___ 13. Grade scores
___ 14. NJCLD (National Joint Committee for Learning Disabilities)
___ 15. DSM-III-R (DSM-III)
___ 16. Previous school identification
___ 17. Length of time in special education
___ 18. Responsiveness to previous instruction
___ 19. Potential
___ 20. Family history
___ 21. Underachievement
___ 22. CNS or neurological dysfunction
___ 23. Process problem
___ 24. Indicates sample has specific deficit in
 a ___ reading b ___ writing c ___ arithmetic/mathematics
 d ___ language e ___ memory f ___ receptive
 g ___ expressive h ___ other (specify)_______________
___ 25. Comorbidity
 a ___ ADHD
 b ___ MR
 c ___ emotional/behavioral disorders
 d ___ social skills
 e ___ other (specify) _____________
___ 26. Gifted
___ 27. Absence of other handicapping conditions
___ 28. School study team

___ 29. Students to be included in study must meet a level of proficiency in _______ performance.

a ___ reading b ___ writing c ___ arithmetic/mathematics
d ___ language e ___ memory f ___ receptive
g ___ expressive h ___ other (specify)______________

23. Check the concept terms (synonyms) or words used in the Introduction or Sample Description section (may include multiple checks)

1 ___ Academic skills
2 ___ Agraphia
3 ___ Aphasia
4 ___ Applied behavior analysis
5 ___ Asymmetry difference between right and left hemisphere
6 ___ Attention
7 ___ Attention deficit/ADHD
8 ___ Attribution
9 ___ Auditory memory
10 ___ Auditory perception/processing
11 ___ Auditory discrimination
12 ___ Behavior modification
13 ___ Behavioral/emotional adjustment
14 ___ Behavioral
15 ___ Cognition
16 ___ Cognitive
17 ___ Cognitive behavioral modification
18 ___ Cognitive skills
19 ___ Cooperative learning
20 ___ Direct instruction
21 ___ Directionality
22 ___ Dyscalculia/math disability
23 ___ Dysgraphia/writing disability/visual–motor
24 ___ Dyslexia/reading disability
25 ___ Educational achievement
26 ___ Functional assessment
27 ___ Generalization
28 ___ Goal setting
29 ___ Hemispheric dominance
30 ___ Integration
31 ___ Intellectual ability
32 ___ Language
33 ___ Lateralization
34 ___ Learning disabled
35 ___ Long-term memory
36 ___ Maintenance
37 ___ Memory
38 ___ Metacognition
39 ___ Minimal brain dysfunction
40 ___ Modeling
41 ___ Neurological deficit
42 ___ Organization
43 ___ Piagetian
44 ___ Planning
45 ___ Problem solving
46 ___ Recall
47 ___ Retention
48 ___ Self-efficacy
49 ___ Self-monitoring
50 ___ Self-regulation
51 ___ Sequencing
52 ___ Short-term memory
53 ___ Skill development
54 ___ Social learning
55 ___ Social perception
56 ___ Social skills
57 ___ Spatial perception
58 ___ Strategy
59 ___ Strategy instruction
60 ___ Transfer
61 ___ Verbal oral expression
62 ___ Verbalization
63 ___ Visual
64 ___ Visual discrimination
65 ___ Visual memory
66 ___ Visual motor
67 ___ Visual perception
68 ___ Visual spatial
69 ___ Working memory

Added terms

Academic remediation (125)
Academic behavior (119)
Balance (99)
Bypass (or modification) (75)
Checklists (76)
Classroom survival skills (130)
Coaching test-taking skills (86)
Cognitive-processing strategies (117)
Comprehension (122)
Computer-assisted instruction (87)
Cooperative learning (79)
Creative writing (124)
Creative thinking (88)
Creativity training (106)
Cross-age tutoring (84)
Decoding skills program (131)
DISTAR reading method (70)
Divergent thinking (89)
Educational intervention (105)
Equal addition method (120)
Friendly and hostile interaction between NLD and LD (80)
Gross motor skills deficit (74)
Group counseling (93)
Hyperactivity (100)
Individual differences (121)
Kephart's perceptual motor training (97)
Linguistic stucture (92)
Locus of control (104)
Logicogrammatical (94)
Mainstreaming (72)
Metacomprehension (85)
Naturally available consequence (77)
Nonverbal communication (107)
On-task behavior (118)
One-to-one tutoring (96)
Oral and written language stimulation (132)
Orthographic structure (114)
Overload (91)
Parental involvement (112)
Peer tutoring (95)
Phonetic segmentation ability (134)
Phonetic discrimination training (133)
Phonics (129)
Private speech (115)
Psycholinguistic skills training (78)
Rehearsal (116)
Reinforcement (123)
Scoptic sensitivity (135)
Selective attention (73)
Self-correction (82)
Self-concept (103)
Self-instruction (verbal) (110)
Sensory motor integration (98)
Social affect training (108)
Spatial relations (109)
Spelling (90)
Spelling deficit (102)
Stigmatization of LD pupils (81)
Teacher- and self-administered procedures (128)
Test-taking skills (113)
Training in context (83)
Viewing prompts (111)
Visual figure ground (126)
Visual closure (127)
Word reading mastery (101)
Writing reversal problem (71)

General Background Markers

General Background Markers identify study-relevant information that provides a context for interpreting LD sample data and intervention effects. These markers refer to control/comparison groups as well as to LD samples.

24. Year of study (check)
    Month and year data collection began ___________
    Month and year data collection completed ___________
    Not indicated___________

25. *Exclusionary criteria used for selection of LD subjects (check)

1 ___	Other than normal intelligence	9 ___	Physical disabilities
2 ___	Achievement consistent with general ability	10 ___	Sex
3 ___	Sensory or sensorimotor deficits	11 ___	Race/ethnicity
4 ___	Neurological problems	12 ___	Language
5 ___	Emotional problems	13 ___	Socioeconomic status
6 ___	Behavioral problems	14 ___	School or classroom placement
7 ___	Hyperactivity	15 ___	Reading
8 ___	Medication	16 ___	Math
		17 ___	Other (specify) ___________

*(children who were excluded from sample)

b. Sample in experimental condition differs from the control condition in the following ways (check)

1 ___ Sample size
2 ___ Proportion of males to females
3 ___ Age
4 ___ Socioeconomic status
5 ___ Ethnicity
6 ___ Intelligence
7 ___ Achievement
8 ___ Materials
9 ___ Person administering treatments
10 ___ Setting
11 ___ Other (specify) ___________________________

c. Internal validity (1 = yes, 2 = no, 3 = not stated, 4 = not applicable)

___ Subject mortality was equal in control and experimental condition
___ Control subjects believed they were receiving a treatment
___ Controls were exposed to same materials as trained subjects
___ Controls were exposed to the same amount of time as experimental conditions

___ Same experimenter(s) provide treatment for all conditions
___ There were checks to determine if students did as they were instructed
___ Alternate forms were used if a dependent measure was repeated
___ There were no ceiling or floor effects (ceiling—mean scores between 90% or .90)
(floor effect—mean score between 0 and 10% or .10)
___ Interrater reliabilities reported
___ Regression to the mean ruled out as an alternative explanation of treatment effects
___ Correlations were computed within groups

d. External validity (1 = yes, 2 = no, 3 = not stated)
___ Standardization sample for measures used in study was similar to sample included in experiment
___ There was a measure of transfer to school subjects or behaviors other than the one in which training occurred
___ There was a measure of transfer to tasks or behaviors other than the one in which training occurred
___ There was a measure of transfer to settings or behaviors other than the one in which training occurred

26. Geographic location of study (must be stated directly in article)
   a. State ____________________
   b. City ____________________
   c. School district ____________________
   d. School(s) ____________________

27. Provide information on all dependent measures administered to assess treatment effects.

Dependent Measure**		Treatment (e.g., 1, 2, 3, etc.)						Control ( )*											
	N	Pre			Post			Pre			Post								
		M	*SD*	*n*	*M*	*SD*	*n*	*M*	*SD*	*n*	*M*	*SD*	*n*	*t*	χ^2	*r*	*F*	*p*	*df*
1.																			
2.																			
3.																			
4.																			
5.																			
6.																			
7.																			
8.																			
9.																			
10.																			
11.																			
12.																			
13.																			
14.																			
15.																			

*( ) refers to treatment or control 1, 2, 3, etc. (if more than one treatment and control, circle the appropriate number). Label the number below the table (e.g., treatment = 1, phonics; trt = 2, language experience; trt = 3, whole language).

** Indicate if dependent measure by experimenter made, report reliability next to experimental measure if available (e.g., pseudoword lists, $r = .63$).

28. Provide information on all dependent measures administered to assess treatment.

Dependent Measure**		Treatment (e.g., 1, 2, 3, etc.)						Control ( )*											
	N	Pre			Post			Pre			Post								
		M	*SD*	*n*	*M*	*SD*	*n*	*M*	*SD*	*n*	*M*	*SD*	*n*	*t*	χ^2	*r*	*F*	*p*	*df*
1.																			
2.																			
3.																			
4.																			
5.																			
6.																			
7.																			
8.																			
9.																			
10.																			
11.																			
12.																			
13.																			
14.																			
15.																			

*( ) refers to treatment or control 1, 2, 3, etc. (if more than one treatment and control, circle the appropriate number). Label the number below the table (e.g., treatment = 1, phonics; trt =2, language experience; trt = 3, whole language).

** Indicate if dependent measure by experimenter made, report reliability next to experimental measure if available (e.g., pseudoword lists, $r = .63$).

29. Provide information on all dependent measures administered to assess treatment effects.

Dependent Measure**		Treatment (e.g., 1, 2, 3, etc.)						Control ( )*											
	N	Pre			Post			Pre			Post								
		M	SD	n	M	SD	n	M	SD	n	M	SD	n	t	χ^2	r	F	p	df
1.																			
2.																			
3.																			
4.																			
5.																			
6.																			
7.																			
8.																			
9.																			
10.																			
11.																			
12.																			
13.																			
14.																			
15.																			

*( ) refers to treatment or control 1, 2, 3, etc. (if more than one treatment and control, circle the appropriate number). Label the number below the table (e.g., treatment = 1, phonics; trt = 2, language experience; trt = 3, whole language).

** Indicate if dependent measure by experimenter made, report reliability next to experimental measure if available (e.g., pseudoword lists, $r = .63$).

30. Age range in each intervention (check and then circle 1 or 2)
    ___ Elementary = K–6th grade or 5–12 years of age (code 1 or 2, respectively)
    ___ Secondary = 7th–12th grade or 13–21 years of age (code 1 or 2, respectively)

31. Need for academic intervention (check one)
    ___ Specified = preintervention test scores indicating the subject(s) was significantly below grade level or statements made that the subject(s) was deficient in the target skill(s)
    ___ Implied = no specified reasons provided for changing or teaching the target academic skill
    ___ No information

32. New versus retaught skill (check one)
    ___ New skill = author states information indicating that the target skill *had not* been previously taught to the subject(s)
    ___ Retaught skill = author states that there was an examination of the effects of an intervention on a skill that had been previously taught to, but was not part of, the subject's current repertoire of skills
    ___ No information*
    *use more lines if necessary

33. List independent variables (names of treatments) (use names given in articles)
    1 ______________________________ (e.g., phonemic)
    2 ______________________________ (e.g., language experience)
    3 ______________________________ (e.g., control)
    4 ______________________________
    5 ______________________________

34. ___ Treatment integrity (fidelity) was assessed yes 1 or no 2

35. Information related to treatment integrity (i.e., steps used to ensure that treatment was implement as planned) (type of measures)
    1 ___ Independent observers
    2 ___ Videotape
    3 ___ Audiotape
    4 ___ No information
    5 ___ Checklist
    6 ___ Stopwatch
    7 ___ Computer-assessed daily

36. Integrity (check)
    1 ___ Randomly done
    2 ___ Predetermined
    3 ___ No information

37. Number of sessions in which integrity of treatment implementation assessed? ______________

38. List material (experimental made and commercial name materials and publishers) used in experimental and control condition

Experimental	Control
1.	1.
2.	2.
3.	3.
4.	4.
5.	5
6.	6.

39. Social validation on success/failure of treatment (1 = yes, 2 = no, 3 = not available)
   ___ Social comparison = test scores of students with learning disabilities compared to test scores of regular education peers after treatment completed
   ___ Subject evaluation = professionals' (e.g., classroom teacher's) suggested criterion level or rate of accomplishment at which subjects should progress

40. Descriptive information on intervention
   a. *Antecedents to intervention*: List instructional methods, curriculum, and/or material (e.g., verbal vs. written directions, structured materials, training students in the use of mnemonic devices) to change the academic skill of interest *prior* to intervention (e.g., basal readers, first-grade level, Houghton-Mifflin instructional method was phonics instruction).

   b. Consequent intervention: Briefly describe teaching method or material introduced; as well as reinforcement contingencies, corrective feedback, strategies, etc., used to change an academic skill.

   c. Antecedent and consequent intervention: List if a combination of both types of interventions were to change performance (e.g., basal material already in use in the regular classroom was supplemented with corrective feedback).

d. The intervention includes the following components (place a ✓ beside component if stated or directly implied by author—the rater must look for key words; if an inference is required on the rater's part, leave blank).

1 ___ Breaking down task by skills**
2 ___ Child is asked to look over material prior to instruction
3 ___ Children are directed to focus on material presented
4 ___ Conduct probes of learning (intermittent test)**
5 ___ Diagram or pictorial presentation**
6 ___ Elaborate explanations*
7 ___ Fading of prompts or cues
8 ___ Homework
9 ___ Independent practice (e.g., complete worksheet on own)
10 ___ Individually paced**
11 ___ Information is provided before student discussion
12 ___ Instruction broken down into steps**
13 ___ Instruction individually**
14 ___ Instruction small group (2 to 5)**
15 ___ Instruction large group (>5)
16 ___ Level of difficulty applied to each student
17 ___ Mastery criteria
18 ___ Modeling—from peers
19 ___ Modeling—of skill by teachers**
20 ___ New curriculum
21 ___ Parent provides instruction
22 ___ Peer provides daily feedback on student performance
23 ___ Provide distributed practice (pacing) and review (weekly and monthly reviews)**
24 ___ Redundant text or materials
25 ___ Reminders to use certain strategies or procedures*
26 ___ Repeated practice (e.g., drill and repetition)
27 ___ Review of material on each session
28 ___ Reward and reinforcers
29 ___ Short activities sequenced by teacher
30 ___ Simplified demonstration
31 ___ Specialized film or video tape/audio tape
32 ___ Step-by-step prompts, multistep directions, or multistep processes*
33 ___ Student asks questions
34 ___ Task analysis
35 ___ Teacher and student talk back and forth*
36 ___ Teacher asks questions*
37 ___ Teacher demonstrates
38 ___ Teacher (or experimenter) presents new material**
39 ___ Teacher (or experimenter) provides daily feedback on student performance**

40 ___ Teacher (or experimenter) states learning objectives
41 ___ Teacher presents benefits of instruction
42 ___ Teacher provides only necessary assistance*
43 ___ Think-aloud models (modeling aloud by teacher)*
44 ___ Using media (e.g., computer) for elaboration or repetition
45 ___ Weekly review

*Reflects component related to strategy instruction
**Reflects component related to direct instruction

e. Student response includes:
1 ___ Analysis—Students make inferences, for example, identify reasons
2 ___ Application—using information to solve a problem, for example, apply the rules
3 ___ Comprehension—demonstrating understanding, for example, explain in their own words
4 ___ Evaluation—judging merits of responses
5 ___ Goal setting
6 ___ Organizing content
7 ___ Recognition— recalling or recognizing information as learned, for example, "What is the capital of ________?"
8 ___ Self-correction or self-monitoring
9 ___ Self-recording
10 ___ Self-statements
11 ___ Student is asked to focus attention
12 ___ Student is asked to make predictions
13 ___ Student is asked to reflect or slow down response
14 ___ Student is asked to summarize information
15 ___ Synthesis—planning

41. Group versus individual instruction
Circle whether the intervention was conducted with (1) groups of subjects or (2) with individual subjects regardless of the number of subjects reported in the study

42. Circle whether individual subject scores are the unit of analysis (1—means are averaged across subjects) or instruction group (2—means include instructional units)

43. Length of intervention
Code duration of the intervention as indicated by: (a) the total number of sessions, (b) the length of each session, (c) the number of sessions per week.
__________________(a) __________________(b) __________________(c)

43a. Environmental setting in which intervention occurred
1 ___ Regular classroom
2 ___ Resource room

3 ___ Pullout (different from resource room)
4 ___ Clinic
5 ___ Home
6 ___ After school
7 ___ Other (specify) ________________________________
8 ___ No information

43b. Time intervention took place (check appropriate box)
1 ___ After school
2 ___ Before school
3 ___ Morning
4 ___ Afternoon
5 ___ During regular instruction
6 ___ During study time
7 ___ As an addition to regular instruction
ADDED CODING
8 ___ No information
9 ___ All day

44. Generalization/transfer of training (check)
(A) Transfer of skill(s) occurred under the following conditions
1 ___ (a) the same skill under different instructional conditions
2 ___ (b) a similar skill under the same instructional conditions
3 ___ (c) the same skill in a different setting
4 ___ (d) the same skill with a different teacher
ADDED CODING
5 ___ (E) MORE THAN TWO

(B) How generalization was a ssessed? (check)
1 ___ To a different or more complex skill
2 ___ Across several skills
3 ___ No information
4 ___ Same skills on a bigger scale

(C) When was generalization assessed? (check)
1 ___ Pre-/postintervention
2 ___ Probed throughout intervention
3 ___ Postanalysis only
4 ___ Anecdotal information provided
5 ___ Halfway test

45. Instructional Materials (check)
___ (Yes) = materials that would normally be found in classrooms or would be available to regular or special classes (e.g., commercially available materials, investigator made materials but described in sufficient detail to allow for replication, can write to author for materials).
___ (No) = materials would not normally be available in classrooms or materials not described sufficiently to allow for replication.

46. Follow-up or maintenance data collected
Code how often and when the effects of the intervention were measured *after* the termination of the intervention itself.
Schedule of when maintenance data collected (check appropriate box) (2 answers needed): 1 = A, 2 = B

(A)			(B)			
1 ___	Once		4___	<2 months	7___	1 year
2 ___	2–4 sessions		5___	2 months–6 months	8___	>1 year
3 ___	Over 4 sessions		6___	>6 months	9___	>5 years

47. Detail on procedures for replication in classroom for teacher (check one)
1 ___ Sufficient detail. Suggested operationalization
(a) More than 3 or more paragraphs are provided in Methods section on implementation
(b) more than one paragraph in Discussion Section on instructional procedures.
2 ___ Adequate detail. Provides more than 3 paragraphs on treatment procedures in Methods section
3 ___ Marginal detail. Provides one complete paragraph in Methods section.
4 ___ Minimal detail. Provides information in Methods section but less than 4 sentences
5 ___ Not replicable from description. (none of the above)

48. Did author provide any indication that the intervention would be adopted by school(s)/teacher(s)?
1 ___ Yes
2 ___ No

49. Teaching implications and recommendations (limit evaluation to Discussion section of article)
(*Note.* Italics refer to key word or synonym.) Rating: yes 1 or no 2
Did the author make a recommendation for
___ *Teacher's* (the word "teacher" is stated) use of procedures in classroom
___ Type of *LD student* who would benefit from treatment
___ Type of *instructional materials* or procedures that could be used in resource or regular classroom

APPENDIX (MARKER VARIABLES 50–52)[a]

50. Descriptive markers refer to both the LD and control (NLD) sample. *Note.* If more than one experimental control, enter column for each and label. For single-subject design, just use experimental column—that is, subject is in both control and experimental condition.
If various control groups, the rater may need additional copies of pages 340 to 352.
If single-subject or repeated measure design, not necessary to complete the control group section of the matrix below.

[a]This appendix (pp. 340–350) is based on the seminal work of Keogh, Major-Kingley, Omori-Gordon, and Reid (1982).

	Experimental					Control (circle one LD, NLD-CA, NLD-A)				
		1	2	3	4		1	2	3	4
D1	**Total Sample Size**					**Total Sample Size**				
	Males					Males				
	Females					Females				
	Total					Total				
D2	**Chronological Age (Months)**					**Chronological Age (Months)**				
	Mean					Mean				
	Standard deviation					Standard deviation				
	Range					Range				
D3	**Grade Level(s) of LD Sample**					**Grade Level(s) of LD Sample**				
	Range reported (yes or no) **Indicate Range:**					Range reported (yes or no) **Indicate Range:**				
	A) Primary (Gr K–3) Specify grade level(s)					A) Primary (Gr K–3) Specify grade level(s)				
	B) Upper Elementary (Gr 4–6) Specify grade level(s)					B) Upper Elementary (Gr 4–6) Specify grade level(s)				
	C) Middle School (Gr 6–8) Specify grade level(s)					C) Middle School (Gr 6–8) Specify grade level(s)				
	D) High School (Gr 9–12) Specify grade level(s)					D) High School (Gr 9–12) Specify grade level(s)				
	E) College/University Specify year					E) College/University Specify year				
	Ungraded classrooms					Ungraded classrooms				
	No information					No information				
	Note. When the number is asked for, write it in; leave blank if not reported. Some articles do not provide number, but mention information—provide a check (✓) if mentioned.									
D4	**Locale (# in sample)**					**Locale (# in sample)**				
1	Rural (sparsely settled, largely agricultural)					Rural (sparsely settled, largely agricultural)				
2	Small town (population center, not a city)					Small town (population center, not a city)				
3	Suburban (residential area outlying a city)					Suburban (residential area outlying a city)				
4	Urban (densely settled, nonagricultural)					Urban (densely settled, nonagricultural)				
5	University community (university and surrounding locale; takes precedence over other categories)					University community (university and surrounding locale; takes precedence over other categories)				
6	Other **(indicate):**					Other **(indicate):**				
D5	**Race/ethnicity (# in sample)**					**Race/ethnicity (# in sample)**				
	Asian American					Asian American				
	Black/African American					Black/African American				

	Caucasian (not Hispanic)					Caucasian (not Hispanic)				
	Hispanic American					Hispanic American				
	Native American Indian					Native American Indian				
	Other (specify)					Other (specify)				
	Not given					Not given				
D6	**Sample Source (# in sample)**					**Sample Source (# in sample)**				
	Public school—day program					Public school—day program				
	Public school—residential program					Public school—residential program				
	Private school—day program					Private school—day program				
	Private school—residential program					Private school—residential program				
	Residential facilities (e.g., state hospital)					Residential facilities (e.g., state hospital)				
	University					University				
	Clinic/hospital					Clinic/hospital				
	Other sources					Other sources				
	Unspecified					Unspecified				
D7	**Socioeconomic (SES) Data**					**Socioeconomic (SES) Data**				
a)	**Socioeconomic Status (# in sample)**					**Socioeconomic Status (# in sample)**				
	Upper					Upper				
	Upper middle					Upper middle				
	Middle					Middle				
	Lower middle					Lower middle				
	Lower					Lower				
	Not available					Not available				
b)	**Methods used to derive SES**					**Methods used to derive SES**				
	U.S. Census Bureau Tract ratings					U.S. Census Bureau Tract ratings				
	Hollingshead Scale					Hollingshead Scale				
	School personnel estimates					School personnel estimates				
	Type of school (private, Title I, etc.)					Type of school (private, Title I, etc.)				
	Location of school					Location of school				
	Parental education					Parental education				
	Parental income					Parental income				
	Author stated					Author stated				
	Other					Other				
D8	**Language (# in sample)**					**Language (# in sample)**				
	English-speaking home					English-speaking home				
	Bilingual home (specify language)					Bilingual home (specify language)				
	Non-English-speaking home (specify language)					Non-English-speaking home (specify language)				

D9	**Educational History (# in sample)**					**Educational History (# in sample)**				
	In age-appropriate grade placement					In age-appropriate grade placement				
	Retained in grade					Retained in grade				
	Changed schools often					Changed schools often				
	Never classified LD prior to this study					Never classified LD prior to this study				
	Spent most of educational career in special classes					Spent most of educational career in special classes				
D10	**Educational Placement (# in sample)**					**Educational Placement (# in sample)**				
	Regular class with **NO** special educational services					Regular class with **NO** special educational services				
	Regular class **WITH** special educational services					Regular class **WITH** special educational services				
	Resource room					Resource room				
	Self-contained special education class					Self-contained special education class				
	Other **(specify):**					Other **(specify):**				
D11	**Physical and Health Status (# in sample)**					**Physical and Health Status (# in sample)**				
	Sensory deficits					Sensory deficits				
	Physical disabilities					Physical disabilities				
	On medication					On medication				
	Medically diagnosed neurological impairment					Medically diagnosed neurological impairment				
	Chronic illness					Chronic illness				
	Other (specify):					Other (specify):				
	Not specified					Not specified				

51. Substantive markers

Substantive markers are closely tied to most definitions of LD. They include intellectual ability, educational achievement, behavioral and emotional adjustment, etc. Substantive markers refer to the LD and control sample.

Rate all articles on intelligence and reading information, *then* based on focus of article, for example, social skills, math, language. Fill in appropriate information related to sample description.

S1	**General Intellectual Ability**					**General Intellectual Ability**				
a)	**Categories (# of sample)**					**Categories (# of sample)**				
	Superior or gifted ($M > 130$)					Superior or gifted ($M > 130$)				
	High Average ($M > 115$)					High Average ($M > 115$)				
	Average ($M > 95$ and < 115)					Average ($M > 95$ and < 115)				
	Low average ($M < 96$ and > 85)					Low average ($M < 96$ and > 85)				
	Below average ($M < 85$)					Below average ($M < 85$)				

b)	**Techniques used to determine intellectual ability**					**Techniques used to determine intellectual ability**				
	Standardized individual tests					Standardized individual tests				
	Standardized group tests					Standardized group tests				
	Teacher estimate					Teacher estimate				
	Other school personnel estimate					Other school personnel estimate				
	Researcher/research staff estimate					Researcher/research staff estimate				
	Other (specify):					Other (specify):				
	Criterion referenced					Criterion referenced				
c)	**Intellectual ability assessed by:**					**Intellectual ability assessed by:**				
	Clinic personnel					Clinic personnel				
	Researcher/research staff					Researcher/research staff				
	School psychologist					School psychologist				
	Special education teacher					Special education teacher				
	Regular education teacher					Regular education teacher				
	Speech pathologist (school)					Speech pathologist (school)				
	Other school support staff					Other school support staff				
	List:					**List:**				
d)	**Currency of intellectual ability information assessed:**					**Currency of intellectual ability information assessed:**				
	At time of study					At time of study				
	Less than 1 year prior to study					Less than 1 year prior to study				
	1 to 2 years prior to study					1 to 2 years prior to study				
	More than 2 years prior to study					More than 2 years prior to study				
	No information					No information				
e)	**Summary values of intellectual ability**					**Summary values of intellectual ability**				
	Means					Means				
	Standard deviation					Standard deviation				
	Range					Range				
S2	**Reading Achievement**					**Reading Achievement**				
a)	**Achievement estimate (# of sample)**					**Achievement estimate (# of sample)**				
	Above grade level					Above grade level				
	At grade level					At grade level				
	Less than 1 year below grade level					Less than 1 year below grade level				
	1.0–1.9 years below grade level					1.0–1.9 years below grade level				
	2.0–2.9 years below grade level					2.0–2.9 years below grade level				
	More than 2.9 years below grade level					More than 2.9 years below grade level				

b)	**Techniques used to determine reading level**					**Techniques used to determine reading level**				
	Standardized individual tests					Standardized individual tests				
	Standardized group tests					Standardized group tests				
	Teacher estimate					Teacher estimate				
	Other school personnel estimate					Other school personnel estimate				
	Researcher/research staff estimate					Researcher/research staff estimate				
	Other (specify):					Other (specify):				
	Criterion referenced					Criterion referenced				
c)	**Reading achievement assessed by (check)**					**Reading achievement assessed by (check)**				
	Clinic personnel					Clinic personnel				
	Researcher/research staff					Researcher/research staff				
	School psychologist					School psychologist				
	Special education teacher					Special education teacher				
	Regular education teacher					Regular education teacher				
	Speech pathologist (school)					Speech pathologist (school)				
	Other school support staff					Other school support staff				
	List:					**List:**				
d)	**When reading achievement was assessed (check)**					**When reading achievement was assessed (check)**				
	At time of study					At time of study				
	Less than 1 year prior to study					Less than 1 year prior to study				
	1 to 2 years prior to study					1 to 2 years prior to study				
	More than 2 years prior to study					More than 2 years prior to study				
	No information					No information				
e)	**Summary values of reading achievement**					**Summary values of reading achievement**				
	Mean					Mean				
	Standard deviation					Standard deviation				
	Range					Range				
S3	**Arithmetic Achievement**					**Arithmetic Achievement**				
a)	**Achievement estimate (# of sample)**					**Achievement estimate (# of sample)**				
	Above grade level					Above grade level				
	At grade level					At grade level				
	Less than 1 year below grade level					Less than 1 year below grade level				
	1.0–1.9 years below grade level					1.0–1.9 years below grade level				
	2.0–2.9 years below grade level					2.0–2.9 years below grade level				
	More than 2.9 years below grade level					More than 2.9 years below grade level				

b)	**Techniques used to determine arithmetic level**					**Techniques used to determine arithmetic level**				
	Standardized individual tests					Standardized individual tests				
	Standardized group tests					Standardized group tests				
	Teacher estimate					Teacher estimate				
	Other school personnel estimate					Other school personnel estimate				
	Researcher/research staff estimate					Researcher/research staff estimate				
	Other (specify):					Other (specify):				
	Criterion referenced					Criterion referenced				
c)	**Arithmetic achievement assessed by (check)**					**Arithmetic achievement assessed by (check)**				
	Clinic personnel					Clinic personnel				
	Researcher/research staff					Researcher/research staff				
	School psychologist					School psychologist				
	Special education teacher					Special education teacher				
	Regular education teacher					Regular education teacher				
	Speech pathologist (school)					Speech pathologist (school)				
	Other school support staff					Other school support staff				
	List:					**List:**				
d)	**When arithmetic achievement was assessed:**					**When arithmetic achievement was assessed:**				
	At time of study					At time of study				
	Less than 1 year prior to study					Less than 1 year prior to study				
	1 to 2 years prior to study					1 to 2 years prior to study				
	More than 2 years prior to study					More than 2 years prior to study				
	No information					No information				
e)	**Summary values of arithmetic achievement:**					**Summary values of arithmetic achievement:**				
	Mean					Mean				
	Standard deviation					Standard deviation				
	Range					Range				
S4	**Language Achievement**					**Language Achievement**				
a)	**Achievement estimate (# of sample)**					**Achievement estimate (# of sample)**				
	Above grade level					Above grade level				
	At grade level					At grade level				
	Less than 1 year below grade level					Less than 1 year below grade level				
	1.0–1.9 years below grade level					1.0–1.9 years below grade level				
	2.0–2.9 years below grade level					2.0–2.9 years below grade level				
	More than 2.9 years below grade level					More than 2.9 years below grade level				

b)	**Techniques used to determine language level**					**Techniques used to determine language level**					
	Standardized individual tests					Standardized individual tests					
	Standardized group tests					Standardized group tests					
	Teacher estimate					Teacher estimate					
	Other school personnel estimate					Other school personnel estimate					
	Researcher/research staff estimate					Researcher/research staff estimate					
	Other (specify):					Other (specify):					
	Criterion referenced					Criterion referenced					
c)	**Language achievement assessed by (check)**					**Language achievement assessed by (check)**					
	Clinic personnel					Clinic personnel					
	Researcher/research staff					Researcher/research staff					
	School psychologist					School psychologist					
	Special education teacher					Special education teacher					
	Regular education teacher					Regular education teacher					
	Speech pathologist (school)					Speech pathologist (school)					
	Other school support staff					Other school support staff					
	List:					**List:**					
d)	**When Language achievement was assessed:**					**When Language achievement was assessed:**					
	At time of study					At time of study					
	Less than 1 year prior to study					Less than 1 year prior to study					
	1 to 2 years prior to study					1 to 2 years prior to study					
	More than 2 years prior to study					More than 2 years prior to study					
	No information					No information					
e)	**Summary values of language achievement:**					**Summary values of language achievement:**					
	Mean					Mean					
	Standard deviation					Standard deviation					
	Range					Range					
S5	**_______Achievement**					**_______Achievement**					
a)	**Achievement estimate (# of sample)**					**Achievement estimate (# of sample)**					
	Above grade level					Above grade level					
	At grade level					At grade level					
	Less than 1 year below grade level					Less than 1 year below grade level					
	1.0–1.9 years below grade level					1.0–1.9 years below grade level					
	2.0–2.9 years below grade level					2.0–2.9 years below grade level					
	More than 2.9 years below grade level					More than 2.9 years below grade level					

b)	**Techniques used to determine _________ level**					**Techniques used to determine _________ level**				
	Standardized individual tests					Standardized individual tests				
	Standardized group tests					Standardized group tests				
	Teacher estimate					Teacher estimate				
	Other school personnel estimate					Other school personnel estimate				
	Researcher/research staff estimate					Researcher/research staff estimate				
	Other (specify):					Other (specify):				
	Criterion referenced					Criterion referenced				
c)	**________ Achievement assessed by (check)**					**________ Achievement assessed by (check)**				
	Clinic personnel					Clinic personnel				
	Researcher/research staff					Researcher/research staff				
	School psychologist					School psychologist				
	Special education teacher					Special education teacher				
	Regular education teacher					Regular education teacher				
	Speech pathologist (school)					Speech pathologist (school)				
	Other school support staff					Other school support staff				
	List:					**List:**				
d)	**When _______ achievement was assessed:**					**When _______ achievement was assessed:**				
	At time of study					At time of study				
	Less than 1 year prior to study					Less than 1 year prior to study				
	1 to 2 years prior to study					1 to 2 years prior to study				
	More than 2 years prior to study					More than 2 years prior to study				
	No information					No information				
e)	**Summary values of __________ achievement**					**Summary values of __________ achievement**				
	Mean					Mean				
	Standard deviation					Standard deviation				
	Range					Range				
S6	**Behavioral/social and emotional adjustment**					**Behavioral/social and emotional adjustment**				
a)	Characteristics (# in sample)					Characteristics (# in sample)				
	LD with minimal behavior/emotion problems					LD with minimal behavior/emotion problems				
	Primarily LD with secondary behavioral/emotional problems					Primarily LD with secondary behavioral/emotional problems				
	Primarily behaviorally/emotionally disturbed with secondary learning problems					Primarily behaviorally/emotionally disturbed with secondary learning problems				

b)	**Adjustment estimate (# in sample)**					**Adjustment estimate (# in sample)**				
	Adequate behavioral/emotional adjustment					Adequate behavioral/emotional adjustment				
	Mild behavioral/emotional problems					Mild behavioral/emotional problems				
	Moderate behavioral/emotional problems					Moderate behavioral/emotional problems				
	Severe behavioral/emotional problems					Severe behavioral/emotional problems				
c)	**Techniques used to determine behavioral/emotional adjustment (check)**					**Techniques used to determine behavioral/emotional adjustment (check)**				
	Clinical judgment					Clinical judgment				
	Standardized tests					Standardized tests				
	Behavior rating scales					Behavior rating scales				
	Teacher estimate					Teacher estimate				
	Researcher/research staff estimate					Researcher/research staff estimate				
	Other (specify):					Other (specify):				
d)	**Behavioral/emotional adjustment assessed by**					**Behavioral/emotional adjustment assessed by**				
	Clinic personnel					Clinic personnel				
	Parent					Parent				
	Researcher/research staff					Researcher/research staff				
	School psychologist					School psychologist				
	Special education teacher					Special education teacher				
	Regular education teacher					Regular education teacher				
	Speech pathologist (school)					Speech pathologist (school)				
	Other school support staff					Other school support staff				
	List					**List**				
e)	**Currency of behavioral/emotional adjustment was assumed (check)**					**Currency of behavioral/emotional adjustment was assumed (check)**				
	At time of study					At time of study				
	Less than 1 year prior to study					Less than 1 year prior to study				
	1 to 2 years prior to study					1 to 2 years prior to study				
	More than 2 years prior to study					More than 2 years prior to study				
	No information					No information				
f)	**Summary values of behavioral/emotional adjustment**					**Summary values of behavioral/emotional adjustment**				
	Mean					Mean				
	Standard deviation					Standard deviation				
	Range					Range				

52. Topical marker, report the following items:
    a. *Primary* domain focus of intervention (e.g., reading, spelling, writing, mathematics, problem solving, cognitive motivation, language/vocabulary, other). (write in if not on checklist below)

PRIMARY

1___READING
- a ___ Oral reading
- b ___ Reading comprehension
- c ___ Decoding
- d ___ Reading fluency
- e ___ Sight word vocabulary
- f ___ Letter identification reversal
- g ___ Word recognition
- h ___ Mat reading
- i ___ Main Idea
- j ___ General reading ability
- k ___ Critical reading skills
- l ___ Functional reading
- m___ Letter sounds
- n ___ Phonemic segmentation

2___MATH
- a ___ Computation skills
- b ___ Problem solving
- c ___ Developmental skills (e.g., counting skills)
- d ___ Word problems
- e ___ Number reversal
- f ___ Multiplication skills
- d ___ Peer interactions/peer perceptions

3___WRITTEN LANGUAGE
- a ___ Spelling
- b ___ Story writing
- c ___ Sentence structure
- d ___ Thematic content
- e ___ Grammar
- f ___ Creative writing
- g ___ Composition

4___LANGUAGE
- a ___ Pragmatics/social language
- b ___ Vocabulary
- c ___ Receptive language
- d ___ Expressive language
- e ___ Oral comprehension
- f ___ Discourse composition

5___BEHAVIOR
- a ___ On-task behavior/ academic engaged time
- b ___ Study skills
- c ___ Active participation in class/question asking
- d ___ Task completion
- e ___ Impulsivity
- f ___ Homework completion
- g ___ Social skills

6___PROBLEM SOLVING
- a ___ Math
- b ___ Social
- c ___ Other

7___VISUAL–MOTOR
- a ___ Writing skills
- b ___ Fine motor skills
- c ___ Gross motor skills
- d ___ Visual–perceptual discrimination

8___ PROCESSING ABILITIES
a ___ Language Processing
b ___ Memory
c ___ Attention
d ___ Psycholinguistic abilities
e ___ Planning
f ___ Transfer
g ___ Self-monitoring

9___Other
a ___ Achievement motivation
b ___ Self-concept/ self-esteem
c ___ Parent involvement
e ___ Alphabet reversal
f ___ Number reversal
g ___ Peer acceptance
h ___ Social studies achievement
i ___ Work completion
j ___ Test taking
k ___ Self efficacy
l ___ Locus of control
m___ Self-monitoring
n ___ Self-correction

b. Specific areas studied *within* subject or domain area (e.g., *Reading*: non-word recognition, text comprehension; *Arithmetic:* word problems, single digit computation)

____

____

c. Intervention used (intervention [steps] and control condition in 6 or fewer phrases) (steps are derived from Methods section on procedures and materials)

Intervention	Control
1. ______________	1. ______________
2. ______________	2. ______________
3. ______________	3. ______________
4. ______________	4. ______________
5. ______________	5. ______________
6. ______________	6. ______________

d. Data on dependent measures to assess treatment collected by (check)
1 ___ Clinic personnel
2 ___ Researcher/research staff
3 ___ School psychologist
4 ___ Special education teacher
5 ___ Regular education teacher
6 ___ Speech pathologist (school)
7 ___ Other school support staff (list:______________________)
8 ___ Other (specify) ______________________
9 ___ No information

e. When data were collected (check)
1 ___ At time of study
2 ___ Less than 1 year prior to study
3 ___ 1 to 2 years prior to study
4 ___ Over 2 years prior to study
5 ___ No information

0 = no information
1 = information available but inference required
2 = information clearly identified intervention

Note. Numbers 24 through 27 rated no matter what type of study.

		Rating
(33)	24. Documents statements on treatment outcomes by parents.	0 1 2
(34)	25. Documents statements on treatment outcomes by teachers.	0 1 2
(35)	26. Documents statements on treatment outcomes by. administration	0 1 2
(36)	27. Documents statements on treatment outcomes by groups or individuals in community.	0 1 2

*Analysis of Narrative Articles on Treatment
(Studies that are primarily qualitative in their analysis, e.g., interviews, survey, anecdotal logs)

		Rating
(10)	1. Provides information on previous uses of intervention.	0 1 2
(11)	2. Provides data that bears on topic.	0 1 2
(12)	3. Presents hypotheses and questions after analysis of data.	0 1 2
(13)	4. Based on data, states new questions and hypotheses.	0 1 2
(14)	5. States previous reviews' methodological inadequacies of intervention.	0 1 2
(15)	6. Lists pattern of results in present study to previous studies.	0 1 2
(16)	7. States the findings from intervention in terms of frequency and/or percentages.	0 1 2
(17)	8. Lists the independent and dependent variables of intervention.	0 1 2
(18)	9. Author states sampling errors.	0 1 2
(19)	10. Author states factors that influence the internal validity intervention (e.g., statistical regression, mortality, previous testing, history, maturation, bias selection of subjects).	0 1 2
(20)	11. Author states factors that influence the external validity intervention (e.g., reactivity to pretest, nonrandom subject selection, restricted defining of variables, Hawthorne novelty, or John Henry effect, treatment interference, experimenter bias or contamination).	0 1 2

			Rating	
(21) 12.	Descriptive analyses (e.g., discussion section) are used to explain differing outcomes of the present study.	0	1	2

* Narrative article includes intervention that is greater than equal to three teaching sessions on control condition but does not include means, *SD*, inferential statistic that can be used in meta-analysis.

			Rating	
(22) 13.	Provides a —new intervention	0	1	2
	—confirmation of old intervention	0	1	2
	—refinement of old intervention	0	1	2
	—disapproval of old intervention	0	1	2
(23) 14.	Provides recommendation for practice.	0	1	2
(24) 15.	Makes suggestions for future study.	0	1	2
(25) 16.	Reports information in the area of:			
	a. Sampling (e.g., random, stratified)	0	1	2
	b. Measurement (e.g., instrument)	0	1	2
	c. Findings	0	1	2
(26) 17.	Indicates outcomes of intervention positive.	0	1	2
(27) 18.	Indicates outcome of intervention negative.	0	1	2
(28) 19.	States the magnitude of the findings.	0	1	2
(29) 20.	Reports how intervention procedure was selected (e.g., computer search based on literature).	0	1	2
(30) 21.	States types of constructs or traits investigated in the intervention.	0	1	2
(31) 22.	Provides crude estimation of when research was begun on the given intervention.	0	1	2
(32) 23.	Classified intervention in terms of qualitative research (e.g., naturalistic ethnographic, etc.)	0	1	2

Appendix D

Mean Effect for Each Study Sorted by General Category of Dependent Measures Used in the Regression Analysis

GROUP DESIGN (EFFECT SIZE BASED ON POSTTEST SCORES ONLY)

Author	Year	k^a	Mean
Cognitive Processing			
Brown	1984	1	.97
Chase	1984	4	.15
Collins	1988	5	1.48
DeBoskey	1982	4	.32
Englert	1991	1	.85
Englert	1992	3	1.20
Gittelman	1983	4	.13
Graybill	1984	1	.89
Griffin	1991	3	.40
Hine	1990	3	.92
Humphries	1992	5	.13
Hutchinson	1993	1	2.78

Author	Year	K^a	Mean
Cognitive Processing (cont.)			
Kendall	1982	6	.50
Kim	1992	2	1.10
Klingner	1996	1	.57
Larson	1987	5	1.94
Leong	1990	3	1.12
Lovett	1989	5	.30
Lovett	1994	3	1.29
Lucangeli	1995	2	.85
MacArthur	1990	2	1.11
MacArthur	1991	9	.28
Morgan	1991	3	.33
Nelson	1984	2	.80
O'Connor	1979	2	2.44
Olsen	1983	1	2.40
Omizo	1982	3	.61
Omizo	1985	1	1.23
Omizo	1986	1	1.38
Reid	1993	2	.58
Reilly	1991	1	.27
Rudel	1984	3	.15
Schunk	1985	1	1.22
Schunk	1986	6	.40
Schunk	1992	4	1.49
Simmonds	1990	1	.26
Swanson	1992	2	.52
Tollefson	1984	4	.29
Wong	1994	2	.75
Wong	1996	2	.67
Zieffle	1985	1	.62
Word Recognition			
Ayres	1972	2	1.09
Bakker	1990	5	1.97
Balcerzak	1985	1	.59
Branwhite	1983	1	2.32
Brown	1984	1	.06
Brown	1990	3	.59
Bryant	1979	6	.31
Bryant	1982	1	1.59
Carte	1984	1	.43
Cartelli	1978	4	1.22
Cornelius	1982	2	.60

Author	Year	k^a	Mean
Word Recognition (cont.)			
Das	1995	4	.24
DeBoskey	1982	1	.67
Englert	1985	2	.32
Farmer	1992	5	.12
Fiedorowicz	1986	5	1.87
Fiedorowicz	1987	7	.30
Gettinger	1982	2	.90
Gittelman	1983	11	.64
Helper	1982	1	.50
Humphries	1992	1	.54
Jones	1987	5	1.95
Kendall	1982	2	.25
Kennedy	1993	1	.13
Kershner	1990	1	.03
Lorenz	1979	1	.27
Lovett	1994	7	.54
Lovett	1988	2	.62
Lovett	1989	12	.43
Lovett	1990	10	.66
Lovett	1998	4	.56
Lovett-1	1998	3	1.31
Lovett-2	1998	4	.31
Lucangeli	1995	1	.11
Lundberg	1993	2	.51
Maron	1993	2	.63
Mathes	1993	1	.46
Meyer	1982	1	.78
Morgan	1991	1	.21
Naylor	1983	1	2.12
Olofsson	1992	8	1.42
Olson	1992	1	.74
Porinchak	1984	1	.62
Prior	1987	5	1.32
Ratekin	1979	3	.74
Scruggs	1986	1	.54
Sullivan	1972	2	.49
Swanson	1992	2	.57
Torgesen	1997	1	.19
VanDaal	1990	1	1.57
VanDaal	1992	1	.61
VanDaal	1993	2	.09
Warner	1973	1	.68

Author	Year	k^a	Mean
Word Recognition (cont.)			
Waterman	1974	1	.95
Wise	1998	2	.00
Reading Comprehension			
Bos	1992	4	.70
Bos	1985	1	1.63
Bos	1992	7	1.16
Bos	1990	3	.97
Cartelli	1978	2	1.96
Chan	1990	4	.39
Chan	1986	3	1.44
Chan	1991	6	.80
Chase	1984	4	.49
Darch	1987	4	1.22
Darch	1986	4	1.12
Darch	1986	2	1.24
Darch	1986	6	1.10
DeBoskey	1982	1	.86
Dixon	1983	4	.58
Englert	1991	1	1.09
Farmer	1992	1	.07
Fiedorowicz	1987	16	.33
Gajria	1992	1	2.76
Gittelman	1983	9	.34
Graves	1986	1	2.70
Helper	1982	1	.46
Humphries	1992	1	1.10
Johnson	in press	5	.50
Klingner	1996	2	.21
Leong	1990	1	1.12
Lerner	1978	2	.07
Lovett	1989	7	.41
Lovett	1994	1	.33
Lovitt	1986	1	.78
Lucangeli	1995	1	1.24
Lundberg	1993	2	.36
MacArthur	1995	1	.52
Manning	1984	2	1.08
Mathes	1993	2	.51
Meadows	1989	8	.49
Meyer	1982	1	.46
Morgan	1991	2	.40

Author	Year	k^a	Mean
Reading Comprehension (cont.)			
Olofsson	1992	3	.80
Olsen	1983	1	2.07
Pany	1982	9	1.00
Ratekin	1979	1	.72
Reilly	1991	1	.36
Schulte	1991	1	.59
Scruggs	1985	1	.04
Scruggs	1986	1	.39
Simmonds	1992	2	1.53
Sinatra	1984	3	.21
Smith	1986	5	1.74
Snider	1989	1	1.57
Stevens	1995	1	.65
Sullivan	1972	6	.49
Swanson	1992	1	.28
Torgesen	1997	1	.26
Wade	1987	1	.38
Wade	1979	2	.12
White	1981	2	.63
Williams	1994	8	.92
Wong	1982	1	.56
Spelling			
Ayres	1972	2	.59
Brown	1984	1	.33
Brown	1990	2	.38
Bryant	1981	1	.83
Carte	1984	1	.34
Chase	1984	2	.40
Englert	1985	4	1.21
Fawcett	1993	1	.97
Gittelman	1983	8	.48
Humphries	1992	1	.17
Kendall	1982	2	.45
Kennedy	1993	1	.08
Kershner	1990	1	.03
Kerstholt	1994	2	.35
Lerner	1978	1	.03
Lovett	1994	3	.42
Lovett	1990	4	.84
Lovett	1989	6	.34
MacArthur	1990	4	.42

Author	Year	k^a	Mean
Spelling (cont.)			
MacArthur	1991	1	.70
Reid	1993	2	.32
Trapani	1989	1	.11
Vaughn	1993	2	.53
Wise	1997	1	2.66
Memory Recall			
Argulewicz	1982	2	.43
Brailsford	1984	4	1.31
Carter	1985	12	.55
Chan	1986	1	.86
Chase	1984	5	.27
DeBoskey	1982	2	1.04
Englert	1991	1	1.85
Gelzheiser	1984	2	.52
Pany	1978	1	.34
Ruhl	1990	1	1.17
Swanson	1992	1	.88
Zieffle	1985	1	.50
Mathematics			
Ayres	1972	2	.31
Brown	1984	1	.18
Carte	1984	1	.72
DeBoskey	1982	1	1.64
Foster	1983	1	.75
Fuchs	1994	3	.47
Gittelman	1983	12	.24
Glaman	1975	3	.23
Hutchinson	1993	2	1.15
Hutchinson	1992	1	.58
Kane	1980	1	.26
Kendall	1982	2	.71
Kershner	1990	1	.03
Kunka	1984	3	.23
Lovett	1994	1	.43
Lucangeli	1995	4	.34
Montague	1993	6	.36
Morgan	1991	2	.51
O'Connor	1979	6	1.77
Ross	1991	2	.25
Schulte	1991	1	.46

Author	Year	k^a	Mean
Mathematics			
Schunk	1985	1	1.46
Schunk	1986	1	.57
Scruggs	1986	3	.06
Stevens	1995	2	.50
Whitman	1986	4	.08
Wilson	1991	2	.90
Wilson	1988	2	.90
Writing			
Bos	1990	6	.55
DelaPaz	1995	6	1.06
Englert	1991	1	1.48
Englert	1991	1	.38
Fortner	1986	5	.36
Graham	1989	4	.67
Graham	1990	8	.45
Jaben	1983	4	1.50
Jaben	1987	3	.58
Kershner	1990	1	.03
King-Sears	1992	3	1.34
Lerner	1978	3	.14
MacArthur	1991	7	.78
Morgan	1991	1	.27
Reynolds	1986	8	.52
Sawyer	1992	2	1.77
Schulte	1991	1	.52
Welch	1992	1	2.11
Wong	1994	2	1.55
Vocabulary			
Bos	1985	1	1.62
Bos	1992	6	.99
Fiedorowicz	1987	2	.66
Gittelman	1983	1	.45
Leong	1990	3	.97
Lovett	1989	2	.39
Pihl	1990	1	1.04
Ratekin	1979	1	.75
Scruggs	1985	1	1.20
Wade	1987	1	.58
Wise	1997	1	.00

Author	Year	k^a	Mean
Attitude / Self-Concept			
Amerikaner	1982	5	.44
Darch	1986	2	1.62
Gittelman	1983	34	.19
Graham	1989	1	.00
Graybill	1984	2	.47
Guyer	1989	2	.00
Helper	1982	2	.05
Humphries	1992	1	2.57
Kendall	1982	3	.41
Kendall	1982	4	.94
Kershner	1990	1	.03
Lenkowsky	1987	1	1.70
Lerner	1978	1	.19
Lovett	1994	1	.15
MacArthur	1990	4	.42
Mathes	1993	5	.86
Moore	1987	2	.00
Naylor	1983	1	2.43
Omizo	1985	5	.67
Omizo	1986	5	.70
Pihl	1990	1	.58
Porinchak	1984	2	.23
Schunk	1985	1	.39
Scruggs	1992	1	1.12
Sheare	1978	1	.76
VanDaal	1990	3	1.08
Wanat	1983	2	.33
Whitman	1986	1	.17
Wong	1996	1	.41
Wong	1994	1	.15
Intelligence			
Argulewicz	1982	1	1.98
Ayres	1972	2	.96
Das	1995	8	.36
DeBoskey	1982	3	.06
Gittelman	1983	6	.23
Humphries	1992	5	.47
Mccollum	1974	1	.26
Nelson	1984	5	.74
Zieffle	1985	1	.19

Author	Year	k^a	Mean
General Reading (cont.)			
Brailsford	1984	1	.56
Carte	1984	1	.35
Commeyras	1992	3	1.34
Gittelman	1983	4	.64
Helper	1982	1	.10
Kennedy	1993	1	.28
Kim	1992	1	1.72
Lloyd	1980	2	.84
Losh	1991	3	.09
Maron	1993	3	.33
McCollum	1974	2	.31
O'Connor	1979	6	1.40
Schutle	1991	1	.24
Scruggs	1985	1	.42
Swanson	1992	1	.46
Word Skills			
Berninger	1991	2	1.19
Brown	1984	3	.72
Brown	1990	3	.57
Bryant	1979	4	.47
Chase	1984	6	.30
Das	1995	1	.43
DeBoskey	1982	1	.54
Fiedorowicz	1987	15	.46
Fletcher	1990	1	.82
Gittelman	1983	54	.92
Hurford	1990	1	.39
Hurford	1990	2	1.19
Kennedy	1993	4	.91
Kershner	1990	1	.93
Kerstholt	1994	18	.27
Lovett	1989	4	.47
Lovett[b]	1994	8	.78
Lovett[b]	1998	7	.92
Lovett-1	1998	8	1.50
Lovett-2	1998	7	.59
Lucangeli	1995	1	.08
Meyer	1982	1	.43
Olofsson	1992	5	1.53
Ratekin	1979	1	1.29
Scheerer	1981	1	1.22

Author	Year	k^a	Mean
Word Skills			
Smith	1989	3	.74
Torgesen	1997	1	.36
Wade	1979	8	.31
Wade	1987	2	.27
Wise	1998	2	.75
Global Achievement			
Ayres	1972	2	.19
Bay	1992	2	2.12
Brigham	1992	1	1.52
Bulgren	1988	1	.68
Carte	1984	2	.53
Gittelman	1983	8	.23
Kim	1992	2	.94
Losh	1991	1	.04
Pihl	1990	1	2.14
Simpson	1992	1	.71
Creativity			
Jaben	1985	3	.39
Jaben	1986	6	.75
Jaben	1982	2	1.38
Social Skills			
Balcerzak	1985	1	.29
Brigham	1992	1	.64
Chase	1984	5	.13
Graybill	1984	1	.33
Humphries	1992	2	.24
Kendall	1982	10	.40
MacArthur	1990	2	.56
Morgan	1991	5	.45
Pihl	1990	3	.79
Sheare	1978	1	.72
Simpson	1992	2	.37
Straub	1983	2	.82
Trapani	1989	1	.23
Perceptual Processes			
Chase	1984	3	.08
DeBoskey	1982	4	.98
Gittelman	1983	5	.25

Author	Year	k[a]	Mean
Perceptual Processes (cont.)			
Humphries	1992	18	.20
Lovett	1988	2	.34
Nelson	1984	1	.29
Somerville	1988	1	1.23
VanDaal	1992	1	2.18
Welch	1992	1	1.15
Zieffle	1985	1	.71
Language			
Das	1995	2	.41
Humphries	1992	5	.35
Losh	1991	3	.46
Lovett	1988	2	.27
Lovett	1989	1	.44
Naylor	1983	3	1.82
Olsen	1983	11	.39
Sowell	1979	23	.25
Stevens	1995	2	.45

SINGLE CASE STUDIES

Author	Year	k[c]	Mean
Cognitive Processing			
Blick	1987	4	.96
Ellis	1989	13	.82
Hallahan	1981	3	.71
Harris	1986	8	.87
Harris	1994	8	1.06
Hazel	1982	1	1.09
Lenz	1991	12	1.06
Maag	1993	18	.81
Prater	1991	5	1.01
Salend	1992	1	1.06
Seabaugh	1994	3	.81
Wood	1993	1	.88
Word Recognition			
Billings	1977	3	.48
Chiang	1980	4	1.11
Cochrane	1986	10	.85

Author	Year	k^c	Mean
Word Recognition (cont.)			
Daly	1994	8	.58
Darch	1985	4	1.03
Duvall	1992	5	.68
Fantasia	1982	12	.74
Idol-Maestas	1981	2	.37
Lahey	1977	2	.93
Lalli	1990	10	1.11
McCurdy	1990	4	.93
Roberts	1980	4	.64
Rose	1982	5	.92
Rose	1984	5	1.02
Rosenberg	1986	4	.29
Schiemek	1983	3	1.17
Swanson	1981	3	1.06
Swanson	1987	2	.38
Thorpe	1981	3	.84
Weidler	1986	12	.64
Weinstein	1992	3	1.09
Reading Comprehension			
Beals	1983	18	1.12
Danoff	1993	6	.99
Idol	1987	4	.98
Newby	1984	4	.42
Roberts	1980	2	.59
Swanson	1981	7	1.00
Swanson	1985	2	.79
Swanson	1985	1	1.14
Swanson	1987	4	.67
Vanden-Meiraker	1986	9	.65
Weidler	1986	12	.76
Spelling			
Cuvo	1995	5	1.37
Diveta	1990	2	.38
Kitterman	1984	30	.51
Rosenberg	1989	4	.62
Schiemek	1983	3	.90
Schumaker	1982	17	1.00
Swanson	1985	1	.72
Swanson	1985	2	1.20
Thorpe	1981	3	.70

Author	Year	k^c	Mean
Mathematics (cont.)			
Ayllon	1975	3	.99
Case	1992	16	.64
Chiang	1986	6	.81
Digangi	1991	2	.89
Dupaul	1993	1	.90
Fantasia	1982	36	.78
Hallahan	1979	1	1.14
Hutchinson	1993	84	.99
McIntyre	1991	1	1.14
Montague	1986	12	.89
Montague	1992	12	.88
Rivera	1988	8	1.13
Rosenberg	1989	5	.64
Vivion	1985	6	.92
Wood	1993	2	.63
Writing			
Ault	1990	8	1.15
Beals	1983	26	.76
Boyer	1990	9	1.08
Campbell	1991	8	1.12
Cole	1993	6	1.34
Dowis	1992	8	1.03
Duvall	1992	1	1.12
Graham	1992	8	1.03
Harris	1985	2	1.07
Kraetsch	1981	1	1.03
Martin	1995	3	.85
Montague	1994	26	.57
Wallace	1989	4	1.14
Zipprich	1995	12	.90
General Reading			
Ayllon	1975	3	.90
Word Skills			
Deno	1979	5	.74
Lahey	1977	1	.89
McNaughton	1997	2	1.14
Swanson	1981	2	.99

Author	Year	k^c	Mean
Global Achievement			
Ayllon	1975	6	.66
Barbetta	1993	6	.40
Bell	1991	6	.90
Bulgren	1995	47	1.11
Burkwist	1987	1	1.13
Darch	1985	4	.83
Hughes	1991	6	1.20
Social Skills			
Salend	1985	1	1.25
Whang	1984	12	.84
Perceptual Processes			
Blandford	1987	2	1.15
Hallahan	1979	1	1.08
Kosiewicz	1981	1	1.11
Kosiewicz	1982	2	1.22
Lahey	1977	2	.54
Tansey	1985	5	.50
Language			
Salend	1986	1	1.13

NOTES

[a]Number of dependent measures as a function of experimental conditions. *k* was reduced in some studies because of outliers.

[b]Study a priori divided into multiple independent samples.

[c]*k* (number of dependent measures) times the number of participants with learning disabilities. *k* is reduced when absolute ES for three baseline and treatment sessions were outliers. *k* is high if ES is based on group data or frequent number of dependent measures within a category.

Appendix E

Description of Studies

Author (year)	*N*	Selection criteria	Target domain(s)	Treatment(s)	Measures	Results
Ayres (1972)	84	All Ss were pretested with a battery of neuromuscular tests, portions of the Southern California Sensory Integration Tests, the Illinois Test of Psycholinguistic Abilities, the WRAT, and the SORT. The mean IQ scores for the two groups were 92.5 and 94.6. The Ss' range on the WRAT was Reading, 78.3–84.0; and Arithmetic, 87.6–87.9. On the SORT, the Ss' range of scores was 69.3–73.0. Characteristics included five syndromes of dysfunction: disorders in postural–ocular–bilateral integration, praxis, functions of the left side of the body, form and space perception, and auditory language function.	Reading Math	The experimental and control groups each had two groups: Generalized Dysfunction and Auditory Language Dysfunction. Experimental Ss received remedial activity to enhance specific types of sensory integration for 25–40 min/day, 5 days/wk, for 5–6 mo. The program was individualized, based on each subject's particular pattern of sensory integrative dysfunction (as determined from pretest scores). Control Ss received a comparable amount, in time, of classroom experience, without treatment.	WRAT, Spelling, Arithmetic, Reading (Jastak & Wilkinson, 1974) Slosson Oral Reading Test (SORT)	The experimental Ss, matched with control Ss for degree and type of sensory integrative dysfunction, showed greater gains than the control groups on academic tests after the intervention program, which was designed to enhance sensory integration. Ss with auditory–language problems but without other evident perceptual–motor involvement made significant gains, as did those with more generalized problems.

(*continued*)

Author (year)	*N*	Selection criteria	Target domain(s)	Treatment(s)	Measures	Results
Sullivan (1972)	82	All Ss had average to above-average IQ, with IQ scores ranging 90–131, and with means of 107.8 and 109.1. On the *Step Reading Program*, mean percentiles were 28–34. Oral Reading scores indicated Ss were from 1 to 15 yrs below grade level. Ss ranged in age from 8.3 to 18.0, with a mean age of 15.4, and they were in grades 4 to 12. Experimental and Control Ss were matched on the basis of age, grade, intelligence, and reading achievement.	Perceptual–motor skills Oral reading Reading comprehension	The experimental condition included perceptual–motor training and reading instruction; control Ss only received reading instruction. The intervention took place over 6 wk. The perceptual–motor exercises were conducted for 30 min/day within the 2-hr session. Three types of training exercises were used: (1) *Chalkboard exercises* (Kephart, 1962) consisted of four tracing exercises; (2) *Ocular pursuit exercises*, in which S followed a visual target while simultaneously performing walking, balancing, and creeping exercises, or walking on a balance beam; (3) *Sensory–motor exercises* consisted of exercises in balance, laterality, and directionality. The remaining 90 min were used for reading instruction.	Daily time in sec for each perceptual–motor exercise Comparison of reading comprehension and oral reading	Perceptual–motor training had no effect upon the reading comprehension of poor readers, although effects upon oral reading were close to significant.
Warner (1973) Dissertation	30	Ss were 4th through 6th graders ranging in age from 8.9 to 9.2. Their mean IQ score ranged 102.1–103, and reading achievement by grade level ranged 3.31–3.42	Math computation Oral reading Sight word vocabulary	The study investigated the effects of two types of remediation on LD children. The experimental condition included two groups of 10 Ss each. Group 1 utilized individualized teaching of intense remediation of deficits through tutoring. Group 2 involved consultant help within a classroom. Specific compensatory recommendations were given to the regular classroom teacher from a prescriptive educational diagnosis and plan under normal classroom conditions. Teachers were instructed to teach to the Ss' strengths. Ss met three times wkly over the course of the school. A no-treatment group (10 Ss) served as controls.	WRAT, Reading, Spelling, Arithmetic (Jastak & Wilkinson, 1974) DTLA Arithmetic, subtest 14 Gates–McKillop Diagnostic Reading Test, Spelling Gilmore Oral Reading Test, Reading (Gilmore & Gilmore, 1968) Slosson Oral Reading Test, Reading	There was at least a half-yr difference in language gain scores between Group 1 and the Control group. Significant differences in arithmetic achievement were also reported.

Belmont & Birch (1974)	58	Ss were 1st graders with an age range 5.8–6.8. Four groups of Ss were studied, and all had functioned most poorly in their grades on the New York City Pre-Reading Assessment Test and had been judged as having exhibited the poorest overall performance in their kindergarten grades. Each of the four groups included 15 Ss representing the lowest 20% of performers in the class as a whole on the New York City Pre-Reading Assessment Test and who had functioned most poorly in their kindergarten grades.	Word knowledge Reading comprehension	There were four groups, three experimental and one no-treatment control. The Ss met four times wkly over 7 mo. *Supplemental perceptual training* activities included discriminating, matching, tracing and copying geometric forms; figure–ground and perceptual constancy exercises; spatial organization and orientation exercises; walking board; and other balancing, coordinating, and rhythmical activities. The aim was to improve visual, auditory, and kinesthetic perceptual skills, memory, eye–hand coordination, spatial orientation, gross and fine motor coordination, and awareness of laterality, directionality, and sequencing of events. The goal of *remedial reading* was to use supplementary reading instruction to develop adequate visual and auditory recognition of letters and letter sounds, to develop automatic sound symbol associations, and to reinforce sight vocabulary taught in the regular classroom. With *placebo play*, Ss selected their own activities and the condition was non-teacher-directed. The teacher only interfered when children were disruptive or fighting.	WRAT, Reading (Jastak & Wilkinson, 1974) Metropolitan Achievement Test Gates–MacGinitie Reading Test (reading errors were divided into mispronounced and omitted words)	Supplementary perceptual training or remedial reading were no more effective than either placebo or no intervention in influencing the reading attainment of 1st grade children identified as being at risk for reading failure.

(continued)

Author (year)	*N*	Selection criteria	Target domain(s)	Treatment(s)	Measures	Results
McCollum & Anderson (1974)	48	Ss were chosen from three schools, two public schools and a parochial school, that offered classes for children with minimal brain dysfunction. An experimental and a control group were selected from each school. Each subject was diagnosed as having minimal brain dysfunction and/or a LD. Ss were 10–14 yr old. The range of IQ scores was 80–131, and the reading mean from the Slosson Oral Reading Test was 80.46.	Oral reading Reading comprehension Vocabulary	Ss in the experimental group received 10 group counseling sessions. The content centered on school problems, reactions to having a reading disability, teacher–pupil relationships, home problems, and reactions toward the special education classes. The therapeutic style was primarily Adlerian and the therapist concentrated on the goal mechanisms used by each S in order to master his environment and overcome feelings of inferiority. Control Ss did not receive treatment.	Gates Reading Vocabulary Slosson Oral Reading Test Gates Level of Sentence Comprehension	At the conclusion of the group counseling sessions, Ss in the treatment groups demonstrated significant increases in both oral and reading vocabulary skills. Mean scores on measures of sentence comprehension were not significantly different between treatment and control conditions
Waterman (1974) Dissertation	34	Ss, ages 8–14, with a mean IQ of 88 as measured by the WISC-R, SIT, and Stanford–Binet, and with mean achievement scores in reading of 3rd grade equivalent (WRAT).	Word recognition	There were 18 sessions total for all Ss. The treatment group received individualized tutoring using the Fernald Method (1943), a whole word approach that uses a multisensory technique for developing reading skills. This method is a four-stage process whereby the Ss move from word recognition to word comprehension to reading generalizations. Also included in the treatment was total body movement learning games (TBMLG). There were	WRAT, Reading (Jastak & Wilkinson, 1974)	No significant differences were observed between the experimental and control groups on the reading subtest of the WRAT.

				38 TBMLG available, from simple to complex. It is a physical education–type activity performed on two letter grids 10″ tall. Ss were told to locate a letter or sequence of letters by positioning self within the letters, thus using the total body. Control Ss received individualized tutoring using the Fernald Method only.		
Ayllon, Layman, & Kandel (1975)	3	LD Ss clinically diagnosed as chronically hyperactive; receiving drugs to control their hyperactivity. S 1 was 8 yr old, with WISC-R IQ of 118, enrolled in an LD class because of her hyperactivity, and had received Ritalin since she was 5 yr old. S2 was 9 yr old, with WISC-R IQ of 94, enrolled in an LD class, and received Ritalin for 1 yr. S3 was 10 yr old, with a WISC IQ of 103, enrolled in an LD class, and had taken Ritalin for 4 yr.	Hyperactivity	The study consisted of 35 sessions of treatment in the resource room during regular instruction. Each subject's daily level of hyperactivity and academic achievement, on and off medication, was directly observed and recorded before the behavioral program and following introduction of a contingency-management without the use of medication.	Hyperactivity: recorded on an observation sheet as present or not present Mathematics: 10 problems daily Reading comprehension: 10 questions daily	Each child performed behaviorally and academically in an optimal manner without medication.

(continued)

Author (year)	*N*	Selection criteria	Target domain(s)	Treatment(s)	Measures	Results
Glaman (1975) Dissertation	33	Ss were 6th through 8th graders with a mean IQ of 103.7 (WISC-R, Stanford–Binet) and significantly delayed achievement (Iowa Test of Basic Skills)	Math computation skills Analytical reasoning Visual–spatial reasoning	This study took place over three sessions and compared two groups. Both groups received the same treatment except that parts 1 and 2 were reversed. The first two sessions consisted of instruction and practice for 30–35 min and computational tests for 15 min. The third and final sessions occurred 3–10 days later with help and positive feedback given. Materials included a paper-folding test, a flow diagram of the possible manipulations of the triangle (Dienes, 1971), a listing of the notations of all six possible manipulations, a cardboard triangle with front and back axes marked, a chart showing single manipulations, and a copy of the 6 × 6 table with the results of an operation involving all possible pairs of the specific group to be studied. *Group A:* Comprehension of principles; Test 1 Rote Memory; Test 2 Transfer Task *Group B:* Test 1 Rote Memory; Comprehension of principles; Test 2 Transfer Task	Analytical reasoning ability Numerical (memory) ability Visual closure ability Visualization (paper-folding) ability Test 1; Test 2; Transfer Task	Of the 12 analyses performed, only 1 showed a significant difference. Ss with low visualization scores did significantly better on the transfer task when they received comprehension instruction first and memorized their "facts" later. No significant overall differences were noted between treatment group means.

Billingsley (1977)	8	WISC VIQ fell between ± 1 *SD* of the mean of 100.; DRS reading achievement was 1 ½ yr below grade placement	Oral reading	*Treatment 1—Self-imposed reinforcement:* Subject was told that for reading correctly he could receive chips to exchange for free time; the subject indicated the number of words to be read before receiving reinforcement. *Treatment 2—Externally imposed reinforcement:* Subject was treated the same as in Treatment 1, only reinforcement schedules were predetermined by the experimenter.	Words/min	Self-imposed scheduling consistently resulted in greater gains in median total response rates of oral reading for two Ss, while greater gains under external scheduling was found for two other Ss. Reliable differences in treatment effects were not observed in four of the eight cases. As a group, subjects chose the most lenient option on 111 of 136 self-imposed scheduling sessions.
Lahey, Busemeyer, O'Hara, & Beggs (1977)	2 2	LD Ss, aged 7–9, were chosen by asking school officials to refer Ss who had serious and pervasive perceptual problems, and by pretesting on tasks similar to those used in the BL phase. Ss were chosen on the basis of high frequency of errors in orientation and sequence in copying words, and "mirror writing" or "reversals." Psychometric data were not available.	Perceptual–motor skills	*Study 1*: Multiple BL design with an average of 8 BL and 11 treatment sessions with three probes. Ss met 4 days/wk, two sessions/day. The sessions took place in a separate room from the Ss' classroom. During BL, Ss were asked to practice handwriting. The task included making 15 copying responses/session. No feedback or reinforcement given. During treatment, Ss were asked to copy their first name five times, five different but similar four-letter words, and five geometric stimulus presentations per session. Ss were given corrective feedback and tokens. The three probe sessions were interspersed throughout the treatment and included no feedback or reinforcement.	Handwriting and shoe tying: number of correct responses Writing name: number of correct responses Reproducing geometric figures: number of correct responses	*Study 1:* When reinforcement and corrective feedback were introduced, substantial increases in the frequency of correct printings were found during both the treatment and probe sessions for both children.

(*continued*)

Author (year)	*N*	Selection criteria	Target domain(s)	Treatment(s)	Measures	Results
Lahey, Busemeyer, O'Hara, & Beggs (1977)				*Study 2:* A reversal design was used with one subject and included 12 BL sessions and 15 treatment sessions. A multiple BL across-responses design was used with the other subject and included an average of 22 BL and 15 treatment sessions. Study 2 was designed to replicate Study 1, using different strategies and Ss whose academic and behavior problems were more severe than Ss in Study 1. One subject was asked to copy his first and last name and 14 four- to six-letter words for a total of 15 responses per session. The second subject was asked to write 10 four- to ten-letter words and his first name twice for a total of 32 responses per session. Shoe tying was a second behavior. Modeling was included.		*Study 2:* Similar results were found using a reversal design in one case and a multiple BL across-responses design in the other. A substantial degree of generalization to handwriting in the classroom was found for one S, but weaker evidence for generalization was found for the other S.
Cartelli (1978)	48	Identified as LD based on Florida state guidelines; normal IQ, visual and auditory acuity, no primary physical handicap; below the 10th percentile in one or more academic areas; not severe emotional disturbance (SED); less than –2 *SD* on measures of basic psychological processes.	Language Reading	The *Key to Learning Series* , Kits I and II (Dinnan & Cowart, 1976), was used to train experimental subjects to acquire and apply paradigmatic language structures. The control group received only their usual LD program;. language training for the experimental group was provided for 19 consecutive school days, for about 2½ hr/day, approximately 45 to 50 hr total.	Metropolitan Reading Test; P/S Oral Inventory (Dinnan, 1971b); Stanford–Binet	Special training produced significant gains on all criterion measures as measured both at program completion and 10 wks later. The effects of training were also residual over time, i.e., experimental Ss made significantly greater gains from posttest to follow-up test compared to controls.

Lerner (1978) Dissertation	60	High school Ss with a mean age of 16.4, ranging 15.0–19.5; mean IQ was 84.53. Mean vocabulary score was 20.37 and mean comprehension score was 22.10 (California Achievement Test). Ss were in four remedial reading classes because they scored below the 4th percentile on the national norms of the Reading subtest of the CAT.	Oral reading Reading comprehension Phonics Written language	The purpose of the study was to compare the effects of a language experience approach and a basal-type approach to remedial reading instruction for severely disabled readers in a senior high school. Ss met daily for 45 min, although the total length of the intervention was not given. Procedures common to both experimental groups included individual classes divided into two groups. On a daily basis, each group alternated between working with an aide and worksheets, and working with the investigator and instructional activities.	Attitude toward reading Reading achievement in vocabulary and comprehension Writing mechanics (capitalization, punctuation, English usage, and spelling)	A language experience approach and a basal-type approach that essentially differed only in the sources of the reading material were equally effective in improving the reading achievement, attitude toward reading, and writing achievement scores of the experimental population.
Bryant (1979) Dissertation	42	Elementary LD readers with normal IQ and reading scores below grade level. Their mean PPVT score was 103. On the Spache Test, Ss were 1 or more yr below grade level. Mean age was 7.1, ranging 6.1–8.6.	Word recognition Phonics	Each of the 42 Ss served as his or her own control. For both treatment and control, sight words and letter sounds were taught, tested, and reviewed on each of the 6 days. Incidental learning in spelling and visual discrimination was also tested, and the same format was used for sight words. Ss were pretested twice on sight words and letter–sound associations to be sure these were unknown. On the first teaching and testing day, orientation and sight word practice took place. On each of the following 5 days, each child was taught 6 sight words/day, for a total of 30 scored words. Half of the words/day (3) were taught via the Visual, Auditory, Kinesthetic, Tactile Method	Sight word and letter–sound learning:: same day retention, 5–7 day retention, learning errors, learning time. Sight word learning:: same day spelling, 5–7 day spelling, visual discrimination from taught words, sequence and reversal errors with 5–7 day reading and 5–7 day writing.	Despite adequate reliability of the learning and retention measures, no significant differences were found between the two procedures at the .01 level of confidence on 14 of the 15 *t*-tests. A significant difference was found between teaching time in sight word learning, with VAKT procedures requiring approximately one-third more teaching time.

(continued)

Author (year)	*N*	Selection criteria	Target domain(s)	Treatment(s)	Measures	Results
Bryant (1979) (*cont.*)				(VAKT; Fernald, 1943). The other half of the words were taught by an equated, visual–auditory procedure without tracing and writing practice. Order was counterbalanced; time and number of word repetitions were not equated and were greater in the multisensory conditions. Teaching was continued to a criterion of two consecutively correct responses. Also taught were two letter–sound associations/day for 6 days, for a total of 12 sounds. One sound was presented daily via VAKT. The other was taught by an equated, visual–auditory procedure that omitted tracing and writing practice. Order was counterbalanced; time was not equated.	Letter–sound learning: same day spelling, 5–7 day spelling.	
Deno & Chiang (1979)	5	Severely LD Ss from grades 3–5; enrolled full time in a Child Service Demonstration Center for children with severe LD; previously classified as LD by a multidisciplinary team, had received service, and then failed in LD resource programs in their home schools; tested IQ within the normal range, with reading	Letter reversals	Each subject participated in two successive, short-duration experiments differing only with respect to pacing of the stimulus materials. Each experiment took place in a small, quiet area normally used for psychological evaluations. Ss were taken individually to this room, then seated across from the experimenter at a small table; rapport was established prior to intervention. A multiple BL design across subjects was used to determine the extent to which	Data were collected throughout all four experimental phases; Ss were presented with the task of naming lower-case letters from the set b, d, p, and q in timed (30 sec) and untimed trials. Measures for both experiments consisted of the percent of correctly named letters.	Overall, the results showed that reversal errors decreased sharply when incentives were introduced and, for some Ss, did not increase when incentives were removed. These findings suggest that reversals may be behaviors, which respond to training.

performance less than one-half that of their NLD peers; program enrolls about 25 elementary Ss at any one time, with those Ss representing .02 % of the elementary-aged population of a midwestern metropolitan school district; Ss in this study consistently reversed.		changes in incentive conditions would affect the Ss' reversal errors. During BL, the subject was presented with a series of letters printed on a card, and given 30 sec to name as many letters as possible. Letters were printed in random order in four rows of 16 letters each on the card; one-half the letters in each row were b, d, p, and q, and these letters were interspersed among 8 other letters from the alphabet. A stopwatch was used to time the 30-sec interval; the subject did not receive feedback on the number of letters correctly named. During the first phase with incentives, the subject was again required to name the letters using the same stimulus materials, but was told the experimenter would count the number of correctly named b, d, p, and q letters and give the S colored beads to be exchanged for pennies at the rate of 1 penny/10 beads after this phase. During the second BL, the subject was told that the task was the same, but that beads and pennies would not be given. During the second phase involving incentives, there were four more 30-sec trials wherein the subject was simply told beads and pennies would be given contingent upon correct responses.

(continued)

Author (year)	N	Selection criteria	Target domain(s)	Treatment(s)	Measures	Results
Hallahan, Lloyd, Kosiewicz, Kauffman, & Graves (1979)	1	A LD male, aged 7yr 11 mo, with attentional problems; performing 1 yr below expected grade level in reading and one-half yr below expectancies in arithmetic; identified LD according to school district following referral for attention problems; placed in special class at a public school.	On-task behavior Academic productivity	Daily observations occurred during handwriting and math seatwork tasks for 49 days. A combination of multiple BL across-responses and reversal designs was used; there were six phases, A BABCD, with BL during A phases and the B, C, and D phases consisting of different treatments. The first B treatment for math lagged behind that for handwriting by 7 days. A follow-up for math seatwork was also obtained 1 mo after the study conclusion. The first BL consisted of 10 days for handwriting and 17 days for math. During BL, the subject was told to sit in his seat and work on his seatwork assignments. During self-monitoring with tape 1, which lasted 13 days for handwriting and 6 days for math, the teacher told the subject she wanted him to help himself by keeping track of when he was paying attention. He was given a self-monitoring sheet with a picture of a boy reading a book and the question, "WAS I PAYING ATTENTION?" in large capitals at the top and two columns labeled "Yes" and "No." The teacher explained use of the self-monitoring sheet and a tape recorder with randomly spaced, audiotaped tones, which	On-task behavior: Defined as being seated with eyes focused on work; data were recorded as the percent of 6-sec intervals when subject was on-task. Academic productivity: Daily measures were taken of the subjects' academic performance. His academic responses were recorded in terms of rate, rather than % correct, since his major problem was in academic output rather than in errors. For handwriting seatwork, he was required to copy a variety of short stories for handwriting practice; his handwriting productivity was defined as the number of words correct when all letters in a word were legible and in	Self-monitoring with tape 1 and 2 substantially increased on-task behavior in both subjects during the multiple BL plus reversal portion of the experiment (ABAB). In the final phases, self-monitoring without tape and self-praise, a high degree of on-task behavior continued. Further, the 1-mo follow-up for math revealed on-task behavior at a level well above BL levels and well within the range of on-task behavior observed during treatment.

				prompted him to monitor his attention to task. During the BL 2 (6 days) the tape recorder and self-monitoring sheet were withdrawn during seatwork activities; inst ructions to self-monitor were not given. The second self-monitoring phase, identical to the first, was followed by a self-monitoring phase without the tape-recorded prompts. The following 8 days, the subject was simply instructed to occasionally ask himself if he was paying attention, then check under "Yes" or "No" on the self-monitoring chart. Throughout the study, the teacher praised him and others occasionally for being on-task. The subject and his peers could also earn a point for finishing seatwork on time; these points were not redeemable for back-up reinforcers.	correct order. For math seatwork, he was given times tables identified by the teacher as commensurate with his math achievement; math productivity was defined as the number of answers correctly written per min.	
Lorenz & Vockell (1979)	54	Ss were 2nd through 5th graders from eight schools, ranging in reading ability from 2.6 yr below grade level to 5 mo above grade level (PIAT); IQ scores ranged 79–113. Ss' actual instructional reading level ranged from 3.0 yr to 6 mo below grade level. All Ss attended a regular classroom for the majority of the school day.	Reading comprehension Word recognition	Experimental Ss met three times/wk for 30 min. The Neurological Impress Method (NIM) was used with the Ss. During 10 min of the half hour, Ss and teacher read aloud in unison. The study was conducted under conditions similar to Gardner (1965) and Heckelman (1969). Control Ss received traditional remedial reading techniques.	PIAT, Reading Comprehension WRAT, Word Recognition	An analysis of variance showed no significant differences among the Reading Comprehension and Word Recognition pretest, posttest, and gain scores for the experimental and control groups.

(*continued*)

Author (year)	*N*	Selection criteria	Target domain(s)	Treatment(s)	Measures	Results
O'Connor, Stuck, & Wyne (1979)	108	Ss were 2nd, 3rd, and 6th grade LD Ss 1 or more yr behind in reading and/or math achievement who were observed spending low percentage of time on-task.	On-task behavior	Groups of about 10 children from two schools participated in each of three 8-wk intervention phases. Ss met 5 days/wk for 8 wk from 8:30 A.M. to noon. For each phase, Ss met in the resource room during the morning and returned to their regular classes during the afternoons. In the resource room, the following highly structured conditions were in effect: strict behavioral principles, scientific application of positive reinforcement, individual timers for specific assignments, highly individualized daily academic assignments, charting of academic progress, and procedures for time-out. Eighty percent of the time each morning was devoted to individual assignments. A token system was used whereby the Ss received points for both academic performance and task-oriented behavior. Control Ss received no treatment; they remained in their regular classrooms. BL and postintervention data were recorded for their task-oriented behavior.	Walker Observation Scale Metropolitan Achievement Test, Reading and Math	Following the intervention, resource room pupils spent significantly more time on-task and achieved at a significantly higher level in reading and math than did their comparison counterparts. These advantages were maintained over a period of 4 mo after their return to regular classrooms on a full-time basis.

Ratekin (1979a)	115	Elementary pupils with LDs identification following state guidelines, including a comprehensive evaluation by a child study team. Criteria common to all five districts involved in three states included psychological testing, achievement and learning assessment, teacher observations, a social history, and a medical history. Neurological and perceptual testing results were frequently included. Ss thus identified were given the Gates–McKillop Reading Diagnostic Test and the Gates–MacGinitie Reading Test, Level A. All Ss scoring above 2.0, all 2nd graders scoring above 1.7, and all 1st graders scoring above 1.3 were eliminated from the pool. The remaining Ss were randomly assigned to either experimental or control conditions; attrition reduced the sample size to 89 (45 experimental and 44 control Ss).	Reading	All Ss worked on programmed lessons in groups of two or three under the supervision of a teacher or aide. Lessons were provided daily for up to 60 min; no other direct instruction in reading was provided, either in classrooms or in special programs. Materials and procedures were varied, with the experimental group receiving the Oralographic Reading Program and the control group instructed with the remedial program regularly provided at each location. The Oralographic Reading Program includes printed lesson sheets (60) and disks or tapes used with a Talking Typewriter or with a Talking Page and a Voice Mirror, printed reading materials, and record-keeping materials. This program is designed for individual pacing, and both auditory and visual feedback is available. Lessons are sequentially organized in a bottom-up, skills-based format. Review is provided. Ss were allowed to complete all 60 lessons, producing a range in the intervention time span of 7–16 mo of school. Upon completion of the program, each experimental child and each control group child was retested on the Gates–McKillop and the Gates–MacGinitie.	The vocabulary and comprehension subtests of the Gates–MacGinitie Reading Test and four subtests of the Gates–McKillop Reading Diagnostic Tests (oral reading, words flashed, words untimed, and common word parts) were administered at posttest. Various levels of the Gates–MacGinitie were given as a result of the wide ability range, with posttest administration varied as a function of final treatment date for each subject.	Due to lack of equivalence between the groups, the final data were analyzed using ANCOVAs with the pretest score as the covariate. Using this proced ure for each of the six reading subtests, statistically higher scores were revealed favoring the experime ntal children, supporting the superiority of the Oralographic Reading Program over remedial methods typ ically used. Age comparisons, however, only revealed a slight but nonsignificant trend among disabled children at younger ages. Comparisons between reading performance relative to type of equipment used did not reveal significant differences between the Talking Typewriter and the Talking Page.

(*continued*)

Author (year)	N	Selection criteria	Target domain(s)	Treatment(s)	Measures	Results
Ratekin (1979b)	89	Elementary Ss identified as LD according to state guidelines, including comprehensive evaluation by child study team. Ss scoring below cutoff scores on Gates–McKillop Reading Diagnostic Tests and the Gates–MacGinitie Reading Test, Level A, randomly assigned to experimental or control condition.	Reading	Experimental Ss received instruction using the Oralographic Reading Program. Components included lesson sheets, sound disks or tapes, printed reading selections, record-keeping materials, and presentation by either a Talking Typewriter or a Talking Page and Voice Mirror. Program was individualized, with Ss determining pacing, including item repetition for auditory and/or visual feedback and rehearsal of item elements. Multimodal, mastery-oriented learning activities targeted instructional goals including phoneme recognition, letter form discrimination, letter–sound relations, letter–sound blends recognition, sight vocabulary development, identification of complex letter–sound sequences, recognition of letter sequences in context, identification of letters and letter sequences response alternatives, and extended passage reading. Lessons included frequent review and teaching for transfer across lessons. Materials designed to develop reading skills from beginning to 3rd grade levels. Ss worked individually under guidance of a teacher or aide who simultaneously monitored two or three Ss for up to 60 min/day. Ss	Reading achievement assessed by the Gates–MacGinitie Reading Test, vocabulary and comprehension subtests, and the Gates–McKillop Reading Diagnostic Tests (oral reading, words flashed, words untimed, and common word parts subtests). Considering the wide range of reading performance, the level of the Gates–MacGinitie Reading Test administered varied. Each experimental subject, along with a randomly selected control subject, completed the posttest upon after the experimental subjected finished all program lessons.	An ANCOVA, using pretest scores as the covariate, supported the superiority of the Oralographic Reading Program over regular instructional methods for LD Ss. Comparisons indicated no significant differences existed between Ss receiving oralographic reading instruction via Talking Typewriter versus the Talking Page. Age comparisons revealed a slight, but insignificant, trend indicating that oralographic instruction is more effective with younger LD Ss.

				continued working until all 60 program lessons were completed; time to completion spanned 7–16 mo of schooling. Control Ss received the specialized reading intervention already being provided for disabled learners at each of the five locations included in this study.		
Sowell, Parker, Poplin, & Larsen (1979)	63	Ss were 1st graders in regular classrooms with normal intelligence and physical development; designated as being of low readiness for academic success based on scores obtained from standardized readiness tests and teacher perception of readiness for school-related tasks. Ss scored in the lowest 20% of their class on the readiness instruments and had been placed in the low reading group.	Psycho-linguistic abilities	The intervention was based on the Minskoff, Wiseman, and Minskoff (MWM; 1972) program that included psycholinguistic remedial activities centered around 12 psycholinguistic activities in Ss' deficit areas. Ss in the treatment groups met for 2.5 hr/wk over 12 wk. Control Ss received no treatment, but continued with their regular 1st grade curriculum.	Illinois Test of Psycholinguistic Abilities (ITPA; Kirsk, McCarthy, & Kirk, 1968) MWM Inventory of Language Abilities (Minskoff, Wiseman, & Minskoff, 1972)	Although Minskoff's stringent criteria were followed, attempts to train psycholinguistic abilities proved unsuccessful.
Wade (1979) Dissertation	76	LD Ss, ages 8–11; IQ scores (WISC-R or SIT) ranging 81–124.	Oral reading Reading comprehension Decoding Reading fluency	This study took place in the resource room during regular instruction. Treated Ss were divided into two groups and provided with Component Deficit Remediation and Academic Deficit Remediation. During treatment, both groups received 3 wk of Component Deficit Remediation and 6 wk of	Stanford Diagnostic Reading Test (SDRT; Karlsen et al., 1976)	The magnitude of effect sizes on measures of reading were greater for the Component Deficit Remediation Condition than for the Academic Deficit Remediation Condition.

(continued)

Author (year)	*N*	Selection criteria	Target domain(s)	Treatment(s)	Measures	Results
Wade (1979) (*cont.*)				Academic Deficit Remediation. Group A received the pretest before any remediation, and Group B received the pretest after the component remediation. During Component Deficit Remedial sessions, three 15-min tasks, which included a one-paragraph story, and a fourth task, homework, were instituted. Task 1 focused on remediation of a *Haptic Discrimination Deficit* using a modified Fernald Method to focus attention on tactile and muscle sensation. Task 2 was oriented toward developing *Visualization* skills through choral reading of a paragraph, flashcards of words with definitions, and an emphasis on word endings, syllabication, and inflections. Task 3 was directed toward developing *Figure–Ground* skills. The child read a story followed by the teacher reading to the child. The child then drew a picture about the story and titled it. Task 4 consisted of *Homework*. The Academic Deficit Remediation involved development of an IEP for each child based on their Stanford Diagnostic Reading Test (SDRT). Control Ss were also provided intervention using this method.		

Chiang, Thorpe, & Darch (1980)	8	Previously identified LD by school personnel according to state guidelines, including normal intelligence and a significant discrepancy between expected and actual achievement levels. The four tutors ranged in age from 10.4 to 11.3 and the tutees ranged in age from 7.9 to 10.0. On the Slosson Oral Reading Test, the tutors scored 1.8 yr below grade level, and the tutees scored 1.2 yr below grade level.	Word recognition	The study incorporated a multiple BL design and direct, daily measures as the dependent variable. Ss met for 15–20 min/day. BL sessions ranged 7–18 days, and the treatment was in effect for 6–17 days. The tutor was the older LD S in this study; the tutee was the younger LD S. During BL no treatment occurred. The teacher tested the Ss' word recognition performance daily on the respective word lists. During tutoring sessions, the tutor modeled the correct pronunciation of each word, and the tutee repeated it. The tutor then asked the tutee to say each word alone, without help, and the tutor corrected error responses. Flashcards were separated for misread words and the tutor modeled those words only. The tutor reinforced the tutee's correct responses with praise. Upon completion of the tutoring sessions, the teacher first tested the tutee, and then tested the tutor on reading their own word lists.	Daily measures of word recognition accuracy on two word lists, recorded in percentage correct	The cross-age tutoring procedure was mutually beneficial for the tutors and the tutees. During the intervention phase, all tutees improved their performance on reading 60 morphemes, while all tutors showed gains in reading multisyllable words containing one or more of the morphemes they had taught.
Kane & Alley (1980)	38	Incarcerated youths 12–17 yr old with identified LDs were selected in two steps. First, the Arithmetic, Comprehension, and Similarities subtests of the WISC-R (Weschler, 1974) or the WAIS (Weschler, 1955)	Computational mathematics	Tutors received 100 min of preservice training during the wk prior to the study. Training topics included classroom procedures, learning principles, direction giving, effective communication, computation instruction techniques, and strategies for dealing with problem	The WISC-R (Weschler, 1974) or the WAIS (Weschler, 1955) Compre-hension, Arithmetic, and Similarities sub-tests; the (SRA)	Posttest mean scores were not significantly different depending on tutorial provided, i.e., peer or teacher. Results indicated no significant differences between the two LD

(continued)

Author (year)	*N*	Selection criteria	Target domain(s)	Treatment(s)	Measures	Results
Kane & Alley (1980) (*cont.*)		were administered, followed by the SRA Assessment Survey's Multilevel Edition of the Achievement Series, Form E. Then the learning quotient formula developed by Johnson and Myklebust (1969) was computed for subjects with an IQ larger than 81. For sample inclusion, a learning quotient lower than 89 was required.		behaviors and attitudes. Teachers were provided with preservice and inservice training. Tutors were assigned to classrooms in pairs for two periods/day, one in each room. Computational math tutoring was provided by either a peer or a teacher for 8 wk, 45 min/day. Implementation of curriculum followed procedures outlined in the SRA teacher's guide.	Assessment Survey's Multilevel Edition of the Achievement Series, Form E	groups who were peer-tutored. Computational mathematics achievement test scores were not significantly different as a function of which of the two teachers provided instruction. No class differences were found as a function of teacher or composition differences.
Lloyd, Cullinan, Heins, & Epstein (1980)	23	LD Ss in self-contained classrooms; LD defined as severe educational underachievement based on individual and group standardized tests, with normal intellectual performance on individual ability test. Process deficits were not necessary for identification, although developmental deficits were frequently noted in perceptual, motor, and language abilities as indicated by various diagnostic tests. LD Ss from a single elementary school were randomly	Oral and written language skills	Applied behavior analysis for monitoring S progress was combined with direct instruction in academic skills for experimental subjects. Control classroom teaching methods typified those generally used in special education classrooms. *Experimental Group:* Direct instruction in reading and language skills was implemented through the *Corrective Reading Program* (Engelman, Becker, Hanner, & Johnson, 1978). Activities in this program emphasize vocabulary, sentence memory, logical reasoning, following directions, and common information. Small groups of experimental Ss from both experimental	The Slosson Intelligence Test (Slosson, 1971); the Gilmore Oral Reading Test (Gilmore & Gilmore, 1968), Comprehension subtest	Language comprehension was significantly higher among experimental Ss than controls following intervention. Experimental classrooms did not differ significantly. Means for the experimental group were .75 *SD* higher than control group means.

		assigned to one of three self-contained classrooms; experimental procedures were used in two classrooms, while Ss in the third class served as controls.		classes were clustered for instruction based on skill level similarity. *Control Group:* Instruction involved individual and small group lessons in language arts and arithmetic combined with some training in perceptual, perceptual–motor, and other basic psychological processes. The principle means of instructing language comprehension included teacher-devised lessons presented through chalkboard demonstration and worksheets. Materials were derived from a locally designed language program, *Teaching Activities* (Rockford Public Schools, 1977).		
Pihl, Parkes, Drake, & Vrana (1980)	90	Ss were 3rd and 4th graders selected as follows. The Pupil Rating Scale (Myklebust, 1971), the PPVT (Dunn, 1959), and the Metropolitan Achievement Test, Reading, Spelling, Math Computation, and Math Problem Solving subtests (Durost et al., 1955) were administered to 1,030 Ss. Of these, 176 scored above the criterion scores of 90 on the PPVT and below 90 on any one of the achievement tests. Of these 176 Ss, 35 were eliminated because English	Personal social behavior School grades (reading and gym)	Two groups received the services of a modulator (child advocate). Modulation services lasted 6 mo, after which all of the Ss in the three groups were posttested, and all principals and parents were informed of all test scores for all Ss. A third group was a no-treatment control group. *Group 1:* Ss were assigned to one of two modulators who were trained as teachers and provided the following coordinating services: (1) liaison on behalf of the subject with home, school, physician, and any other professional in contact with the subject or family; (2) psychoeducational, diagnostic, and achievement testing	Pupil rating scale: personal social behavior School grades in reading and gym	In the long run, the differential between groups seems to reflect a more positive self-attitude in those individuals who received modulation as well as deterioration in their responsiveness within the classroom. Treatment Ss did as well as the control Ss in grades.

(continued)

Author (year)	*N*	Selection criteria	Target domain(s)	Treatment(s)	Measures	Results
Pihl, Parkes, Drake, & Vrana (1980) (*cont.*)		was not their home language. Then 90 Ss were randomly selected from the remaining pool.		when required and not available through any other agency; (3) initiation of prescriptive remedial and home programs by means of convening case conferences with teachers, principals, psychologists, and parents; (4) coordinator of the suggested programs and feedback of progress to all relevant parties; and (5) periodic reassessment of the program with those involved in day-to-day contact with the subject. The role of the modulator was not treatment, but rather as serving as a catalyst in organizing treatment programs and maintaining contact to ensure treatment fidelity. *Group 2:* This was the school-informed group. Principals were informed of the Ss' ratings, achievement scores, and progress. *Control:* No treatment; school and parents were not informed of the Ss' test scores.		
Roberts & Smith (1980)	8	Ss ranged in age from 10.8 to 12.0 and attended the same self-contained LD classroom. All Ss had normal IQ, but scored 3 to 4 yr below grade level on the Gilmore Oral Reading Test (Gilmore & Gilmore, 1978), with a mean GE of 1.7.	Oral reading Reading comprehension	A multiple BL crossover design was used with four pairs of Ss. BL included three phases and 21–24 sessions. During BL, Ss read but received no praise for correct reading or question answering. The treatment condition spanned 34 sessions and included a combination of three tactics to increase reading rates: (1) *Instruction* The Ss were instructed to read	Oral reading: error rate (WPM) and correct rate (WPM) Comprehension: percentage correct	Improvement in either correct rate or error rate scores produced only mild increases in comprehension. When comprehension was targeted, correct and error rate scores were at desirable levels.

					as fast as possible, and to skip unknown words; (2) *Token Reinforcement* Tangible reinforcers, backed up by money, were provided based on improvement over BL; and (3) *Modeling with Drill* 10 words were taught before the Ss read. During the procedure, Ss read orally for 5 min and then responded to comprehension questions.		
Bryant, Drabin, & Gettinger (1981)	64	School-identified LD enrolled in classes for the neurologically impaired or in resource rooms. Ss randomly assigned to one of three groups.	Spelling		This intervention varied the number of phonemically irregular spelling words taught daily (i.e., three, four, or five words). Five teachers participated using a standardized method. Children were taught during 30–40 min lessons for 3 consecutive days; three of the nine words common to all three spelling lists were taught first each day, with additional words then presented to the four- and five-word groups.	WISC-R (Weschler, 1974); WRAT (Jastak & Jastak, 1965), Reading subtest; Slingerland (visual memory items); daily verbal recall tests following each unit of instruction	Mean total words learned was not significantly different. The group that received three words/ day correctly spelled a significantly greater number of the nine words that were common to all three groups. Ss from the four- and five-word groups spelled relatively more of the additional words correctly. Transposition errors increased with list size. Greater performance variance was observed in the four- and five-word groups.

(*continued*)

Author (year)	N	Selection criteria	Target domain(s)	Treatment(s)	Measures	Results
Hallahan, Marshall, & Lloyd (1981)	3	Ss enrolled in a self-contained LD classroom. Classified as LD and identified with attentional problems. Ss ranged in age from 10 to 11 yrs. The WISC-R scores ranged from 87 to 106, and Woodcock–Johnson Achievement Test scores ranged as follows: Reading, 65–81; Math, 81–82; Written Language, 69–78; and Knowledge, 81–90.	Reading	The effects of self-monitoring on attention to task during small group instruction were investigated. Three LD Ss with severe attention problems were taught to self-monitor their on-task behavior while participating in oral reading tasks. A reversal design was used that included 5 BL sessions, 16 treatment sessions, 5 reversal sessions, and 11 fade sessions. Ss met for 45-min sessions. *BL:* The oral reading comprehension lesson was presented in the standard manner. The observer collected data for the first 20 min of the 45-min session. *Self-Recording:* The self-contained class had two oral reading groups; Ss in this experiment were in one group. Instruction incorporated sequential progression through the SRA Corrective Reading Program. Skills included vocabulary development, use of analogies, deductive reasoning, and practice in subject–verb agreement. Most of the activities required that Ss respond chorally on cue. A token economy system was used and points were awarded for academic and behavioral accomplishments. Self-recording required that Ss to record their own attention to task in response to audiotaped cues. They were given wrist	Percentage of time on task	The results suggest self-monitoring procedures can be effectively employed during oral, small group instruction, and that positive behavioral changes can be maintained over a period of time following the gradual fading of external, procedural components.

				counters and a tape recorder. The teacher played a tape that emitted tones at random intervals. The tones were approximately 2 sec long with about 45-sec intervals between tones. Ss were instructed to ask themselves, "Was I paying attention?" at the sound of each tone. If on task, the S was to press a wrist counter button and continue with the lesson. If not on task, tthe S was to do nothing.		
Idol-Maestas (1981)	1	S was 21 yr old and required assistance with reading. Normal IQ, although the WISC-R Coding subtest was more than 2 *SD* below the norm. The S had never attended special education classes. The Sucher–Allred Reading Placement Inventory indicated independent reading level at 2nd grade, and instructional reading level at 3rd grade. No comprehension errors were made. The Basic Educational Skills Inventory and the Roswell–Chall Diagnostic Reading Test were given to determine word recognition problems. The S made word recognition errors because he did not attend to all the phonetic components within a given word.	Reading	A multiple BL design was used in order to monitor subject gains in any category, with and without instruction. A direct instruction approach was used to teach deficit phonic skills. Instructional targets were broken into four classes of vowel pattern characteristics: R-controlled vowels, short vowels, long vowels, diphthongs. Lists of words containing these patterns were used to measure skill acquisition after each vowel pattern was taught. In addition, four other sounds were taught: hard and soft C sound, consonant digraph CH, CH as K phoneme, and CH grapheme as SH phoneme. BL measurement was made with the first word list and lasted for four sessions. Treatment consisted of 16 sessions.	Acquisition of vowel concepts: R-controlled, short, long, diphthongs Acquisition of selected consonant sounds: C (K), C (S), CH, CH (K), CH (S)	The subject showed a 3-yr gain in oral reading in a 3-mo period.

(continued)

Author (year)	*N*	Selection criteria	Target domain(s)	Treatment(s)	Measures	Results
Kosiewicz, Hallahan, & Lloyd (1981)	1	An 11-yr-old boy with LD; attended a self-contained LD class in a public school; Ss in the classroom identified by resource teachers as having attention problems; identificationperselection procedures for special education and classroom characteristics met state requirements for LD programs.	Handwriting	A reversal design with multielement features was employed to compare the effects of S versus teacher choice; the study consisted of five phases spanning 81 school days. During 18 days of BL, the subject was told to neatly copy a paragraph, but was not given additional direction or instruction. After BL, one of two teacher-selected treatments followed on alternate days. The S was told to use one of the two methods as a means to improving his handwriting. One required self-instruction using a list of rules; the other involved self-evaluation through the use of a red marker to circle correctly produced words or letters in the paragraph. The teacher sat next to the S while he completed these activities. A phase of S-selected treatment choice followed with subsequent reversal back to teacher-selected treatment. The study ended with a repeated phase of the S's treatment selection.	Daily assignments were scored according to the following criteria: (1) correct letter formation, 1 point; (2) 1/8″ spacing between words, 1 point; (3) correct punctuation, 1 point; (4) incorrect spacing, letter omission, or added letters, −1 point; (5) no penalty for losing his place in the paragraph. The percent of points awarded divided by the total points possible was the dependent variable.	Results from the first 72 days of the study suggest that allowing the S to choose a handwriting improvement strategy was associated with better performance than was observed when the teacher determined which strategy would be used.
Kraetsch (1981)	1	A 12-yr-old boy attending a tutorial clinic at a university four times wkly for 1 hr; enrolled in a LD resource program at a public school for the remainder of the school day; average intelligence, and skills in reading in math at 5th	Written language	The study took place in a room with five study carrels, each large enough for the subject and a tutor, who conducted all experimental sessions; the experimenter trained, observed, and supervised the tutor during each phase to ensure that procedures were followed correctly. The resource teacher at the S's school gave	Written compositions were scored quantitatively using the following: (1) *P roductivity*, determined by the total words and sentences in each written passage; (2)	Adding the oral instructions increased this S's productivity; i.e., the number of words and sentences he produced. Overall, this S's written output increased by telling him to write as

grade level, but spelling skills were at 3rd grade level and he lacked skills in capitalization, punctuation, grammatic structure, and composition.	the oral directions during BL probing on a wkly basis in order to assess generalization. The effects of oral instructions and training on written language were examined using a reversal design. The S wrote four times/wk for 12 wk about randomly selected and ordered stimulus pictures; the second half of each tutoring period was devoted to the experiment. The tutor presented two pictures/section to the S who selected one as the writing topic for that session; pictures were not repeated. During BL, the tutor orally directed the S to pick one of the two pictures to write about; directions followed a format described by Myklebust (1965). Otherwise the S was left alone to write. During the next phase, the oral directions were altered by adding instructions to write as many words and ideas as possible about the picture. After a second BL condition, the treatment phase was repeated followed by a fifth phase, which combined a preliminary training session with the expanded directions. Training in this phase consisted of the tutor showing the S two sentences from his previous composition and demonstrating where adjectives and adverbs could be added. Throughout the study, the resource teacher at the subject's school asked him to write a story every Wednesday using the same BL conditions as the tutor.	*Words* , defined as any group of letters representing a spoken word; (3) *Sentence*, defined as a unit of thought whether incomplete, simple, or compound/complex; (4) *Sentence variety*, defined in terms of the kinds of sentences used; (5) *Adjectives*, defined as noun modifiers, excluding numbers, ordinals, possessives, articles, and quantitative words; and (6) *Adverbs*, defined as verb modifiers. Percentages were calculated and graphed for the first four variables, and the remainder were counted and graphed. Productivity was calculated according to the number of words and sentences used in each composition; a type–token ratio for vocabulary diversity was charted as well.	many words as possible in spite of his lack of skills in written mechanics. Although his stories were longer, he tended to express himself using simple sentences rather than complex or compound ones. Also, his writing tended to describe the pictures; he did not write stories with plots based on the pictures.

(continued)

Author (year)	*N*	Selection criteria	Target domain(s)	Treatment(s)	Measures	Results
Scheerer-Neumann (1981)	30	Ss were 3rd grade poor readers ranging in age from 8.10 to 10.3 (mean of 9.4); mean nonverbal IQ was 103 as measured by the Frankfurter Denkaufgaben; scores on the Zurcher Lesetest (reading test) were at or below the 25th percentile.	Oral reading fluency	This study was concerned with the utilization of linguistic structure in RD children. Only Experiment 2 is reported here, which examined how poor readers' performance with redundant stimuli can be increased when stimuli are grouped into syllables. Ss met for 30–45 min twice wkly for 12 sessions. Control Ss did not receive treatment. *Treatment sessions—Sessions 1 and 2:* Training in segmentation of spoken words and difficult grapheme–phoneme correspondences. *Sessions 3 and 4:* Spoken word segmentation, introduction to the differences between vowels and consonants, categorization of all graphemes, and writing vowels into syllable bows. *Sessions 5 and 6:* Segmentation first of a spoken word and then of the corresponding written word, finding vowels and marking syllable boundaries in written words, and training in complex graphemes (sch, ch, and qu). *Sessions 7 and 8:* Written word syllable segmentation, reading of short sentences, and training in common prefixes and suffixes. *Sessions 9 and 10:* Introduction to two-syllable segmentation rules, training in the rules of single words and short sentences, and	Oral reading fluency: error rates	On the posttest the experimental group committed significantly fewer errors than the control group ($p < .01$). An effect was reported of almost 40% error reduction after 12 training sessions.

				training in common prefixes and suffixes. *Sessions 11 and 12:* Introduction to the function of punctuation, training in syllable segmentation rules, and training to discriminate between the graphemes ei and ie.		
Swanson (1981)	3	*Experiment 1:* LD Ss attending a Colorado rural public school system; selection based upon teacher, referral, oral reading, and the PIAT (Dunn & Markwardt, 1975) Reading subtest; basic word-attack skills commensurate with reading recognition scores not used when reading words in paragraphs; reading below grade level, with a large discrepancy between oral reading and reading comprehension scores.	Reading rate Reading comprehension	*Experiment 1:* The study occurred in a clinical study at a university-based center; Ss were instructed by graduate students during 30-min sessions held five times wkly during the normal school day. A combination of multiple BL across-Ss and changing criterion designs was used to examine the impact of various contingencies on the oral reading errors in paragraphs and reading comprehension. Data were collected during the first 15 min of each session; each subject orally read typed excerpts from a 1st grade Laidlaw basal reader which were adapted to his/her instructional level. An audiotape was made of each session; the teacher also recorded the number of oral reading errors. After reading, 5–10 factual questions were asked. During BL, each S was directed to orally read, and was asked predetermined questions; for each error the S was directed to cover all but the initial letter, then to verbalize the sound of this letter. Correct sounds were	*Experiment 1:* Data for percent of oral reading errors and percent of comprehension questions correctly answered were collected and graphed.	*Experiment 1:* The introduction of self-recording and token reinforcement decreased the percentage of oral reading errors at the subject's instructional level, with no concomitant effect on comprehension.

(continued)

Author (year)	N	Selection criteria	Target domain(s)	Treatment(s)	Measures	Results
Swanson (1981) *(cont.)*				provided if needed. During the next phase, Ss were given individual charts on which to record their own errors; they were told that tokens would be provided for correcting oral reading errors, correcting their own reading errors before the teacher initiated sound-blending procedures, and performance at or below the error criterion established by the teacher; contingencies for comprehension performance were not in effect.		
Swanson (1981)	2	*Experiment 2:* Ss were drawn from an LD classroom; teachers noted Ss experienced considerable difficulty in reading assignment completion; teacher observation indicated excessive word analysis and word-by-word lip movement.		*Experiment 2:* The experimental design was the same as the first study. Passages from the Gates Peardon Reading Exercises (Gates & Peardon, 1965) were individualized according to each S's instructional level; each S worked on one passage/session and answered comprehension questions. Each S was told to read the selection completely. Prior training was given emphasizing: (1) content details mastery; (2) material evaluation; (3) sequence of details; and (4) reading material summarization. During BL (8 sessions), Ss read silently and answered 10–28 questions; a stopwatch was used to time silent reading. Teacher comments and actions were not contingent upon the	*Experiment 2:* Measures of reading comprehension were calculated as a ratio between number of correct and possible responses. The Ss' silent words/min were calculated as the number of words in the passage divided by the number of mins to read the passage. Reading performance accuracy data were collected by the teacher, who observed the Ss' silent reading	*Experiment 2:* Silent independent reading rate improved as a result of contingent free time and self-recording, but comprehension scores were only mildly effected.

				time required to read the passage. During the next phase, Ss were presented with individual record books and instructed to record the amount of time required to finish their daily reading assignment and their comprehension scores. Free time activities were available contingent on meeting study criterion.	and noted the amount of time spent. Words/min were determined by dividing the number of words read by the time lapsed. Ss used individual record books to record their own reading data.	
Swanson (1981)	8	*Experiment 3:* LD children within the normal range of intelligence (95–108) with reading comprehension percentile scores from 22% to 4% and reading recognition scores ranging from 53% to 1% on the PIAT; receiving special education services during the regular school.		*Experiment 3:* A multiple BL across-Ss design was used; order of treatment presentation was randomized for Ss grouped in two groups of four. Each S was given an assignment from the New Reading and Skill Builder Series (Reader's Digest, 1973) individualized to his/her instructional level; Ss read passages and answered questions during 50-min sessions. During BL, Ss were told to read an assignment and answer questions about the material read; responses were written by the Ss. No special contingencies were in effect for these sessions. During the next phase, self-recording and free time contingent on performance were introduced; Ss were given charts for graphing their own comprehension scores. A list of preferred activities was developed for each S; the same basic procedure was in effect for all children.	*Experiment 3:* Recording procedures were similar to those used in the second study. Reading comprehension was calculated as a ration between correct and possible responses; the teacher collected reading accuracy data. Response keys were used from the published materials	*Experiment 3:* Substantial comprehension improvements were associated with contingent free time and self-recording. Overall, the results from these experiments support the assertion that comprehension performance is only minimally impacted when not targeted as a dependent behavior

(*continued*)

Author (year)	*N*	Selection criteria	Target domain(s)	Treatment(s)	Measures	Results
Thorpe, Lampe, Nash, & Chiang (1981)	3	High school LD Ss; two freshmen and one sophomore. Ages ranged from 15.7 to 17.5; WISC-R IQ scores were 86, 93, and 91; WJPB reading levels were 2.6, 3.5, and 3.0.	Reading fluency	This study compared the effects of Visual–Auditory (VA) to Visual–Auditory–Kinesthetic–Tactile (VAKT) instruction. VAKT is a reading instructional technique that employs multisensory input simultaneous. A multiple BL design was used in this study where Ss met for 4–12 BL and five to sixteen 1-hr treatment sessions. BL: VA procedures were implemented exactly the same as the VAKT except the kinesthetic and tactile components were eliminated. Steps included: (1) Say the isolated vowels or vowel combination; (2) Say all of the assigned phonemes left to right; (3) Look and say phonemes rapidly; (4) Look and say the word fast; (5) Say the sounds in the words five times; and (6) Say the sound again fast. Treatment: VAKT steps were followed, including: (1) Mark and say isolated vowel or vowel combinations; (2) Underline and simultaneously say all assigned phonemes, left to right; (3) Look and say assigned phonemes; (4) Underline and say the word fast; (5) With the index finger, write the word on the desk five times and say the letters' assigned sounds simultaneously; and (6) Underline and say the word fast again.	Words read correctly Words spelled correctly	The three secondary LD Ss read more VAKT-instructed words at 1-wk, 3-wk, and 6-mo retention probes. The instruction did not differentially affect the spelling of words.

				The instructional procedure had four distinct, 4-day segments: (1) a BL (VA) across all Ss, (2) the VAKT implemented for all three Ss; (3) once VAKT was implemented for the S, it was continued through the rest of the 16-day experiment using 16 equivalent word lists, each containing 10 unknown phonetically regular words (1 list/day given to each S), (4) retention probes at wk 1 and 3 and 6 mo after the end of each instructional segment .		
White, Pascarella, & Pflaum (1981)	30	School-identified LD Ss from an inner-city school. Ss were randomly assigned to one of three conditions.	Comprehension	All Ss received instruction in groups of three or four from the same resource teacher. Lessons in both treatments occurred about three times wkly for 8wk total for a grand total of 21 lessons. Sessions lasted about 25–30 min each. Ss received either the Anagram/Word Grouping or the Sentence Study Treatment. Anagram/Word Grouping: Ss worked with packets of words that could be combined to make sensible sentences; Ss worked through progressively longer sentences as they experienced success with five- or six-word sentences. All vocabulary was at the 2nd grade level. The teacher provided modeling with explicit directions for focusing on key task aspects. Sentence Study: This treatment involved less individual interaction	Pretesting and posttesting was completed using two measures. The sentence construction measure involved the use of anagrams and word grouping, and required the construction of sentences from words out of packets. Set size ranged from 5 to 15 words. Testing continued until the S made three consecutive errors. Two different cloze tests were made from Getting the Facts	With sex, intelligence, and pretreatment test scores held constant, the anagram intervention accounted for a significant increase in the variance explained in sentence construction behavior. With the same variables held constant, the anagram condition also accounted for a significant proportion of the variance in the posttest cloze scores. However, a significant interaction between the cloze pretest results and experimental condition suggests that the impact of treatment depended on prior reading achievement.

(*continued*)

Author (year)	*N*	Selection criteria	Target domain(s)	Treatment(s)	Measures	Results
White, Pascarella, & Pflaum (1981) (*cont.*)				between the Ss and the teacher. Lessons covered material from the Holt Basic Reading System, levels 8 and 9. Instruction covered a variety of sentence patterning tasks. Each lesson began with teacher explanation and modeling, and continued with S worksheet completion.	(Boning, 1963) passages, 3rd grade level. Each test required the S to fill in 56 deletions (every fifth word).	In general, LD children with severe reading problems gained more from the anagram treatment and word group strategies than from the sentence study intervention.
Amerikaner & Summerlin (1982)	46	Ss were 1st and 2nd graders; LD based on discrepancy between aptitude and achievement.	Self-concept Behavior	Children in the Social Skills group attended 30-min sessions twice wkly. Relaxation Training Ss listened to prerecorded tapes for 30 min twice wkly. Control group members followed their regular routine. The intervention covered 6 wk total.	Primary Self-Concept Inventory (PSCI; Muller & Leonetti, 1974); Walker Problem Behavior Identification Checklist (WPBIC; Walker, 1976), WISC-R, WRAT	Relaxation training was associated with reduced acting-out behaviors. Improvements in social skills, and in self-esteem scores, were associated with social skills group participation. Effects were specific to treatment, and predictable.
Argulewicz (1982)	72	Ss were 3rd graders from eight elementary schools identified LD and currently enrolled in resource programs. Ss ranged in age from 8.7 to 9.11, with a mean age of 9.0 yr. The mean IQ score for the two treatment groups was 97. Ss were randomly assigned to one of two treatment groups or a control group.	Attending behaviors	One treatment group received training in attending behaviors by a direct instruction method. Ss in one treatment group were trained in physical attending or posturing behaviors: sitting squarely, leaning forward, focusing eyes on the person or object to which one must attend. Training included three steps: (1) Didactic—Ss were told which behaviors constituted attending, and were asked to state the three behaviors; (2) Modeling—	Attention: digit span (forward and backward) and memory for sentences Attending behaviors: percentages of visual contact, squaring, and leaning	Ss in Group 1 engaged in the behaviors with higher frequency than the groups that had not received the training. The group also scored significantly higher than the other groups on two of three tasks that are sensitive to attentional variation.

				Ss were shown illustrations of people in various attending positions and asked to identify which attending positions they recognized followed by the trainer modeling the behavior; and (3) Experiential—Ss practiced the attending behaviors, and the trainer asked the Ss after 10–15 min to describe the attending behaviors that were present or omitted and each subject practiced the behavior. The second experimental group received trainer modeling of the same physical attending behaviors for which Group 1 received training, but without direct instruction. Control Ss received the criteria measures of attention, but no treatment.		
Bryant, Fayne, & Gettinger (1982)	48	Enrolled in diagnostic-remedial classes in public schools. Ss' mean age was 10.1 yr, with a range of 7 to 11.75 yr. All treatment Ss demonstrated 10% or lower accuracy on a pretest of sight words to be taught and average intellectual functioning. Mean WISC-R score was 97, and mean WRAT Reading score was 2.2 grade equivalent.	Word recognition	This study evaluated the effect of applying a mastery learning model to sight word instruction for elementary children with LD. Experimental Ss met three times wkly for 30 min over 3 wks and received the following intervention. Lesson 1: Introduction of activities on 5 of the 10 words to be taught; mastery practice included Ss reading from cards, teacher recording for criterion purposes, and teacher modeling when errors were made. When a word was correctly read, it was temporarily dropped from the list. Misread words were recycled. Lesson 2: Ss reviewed the 10 words and practiced	Number of words read correctly	Ss could read less than 10% of the words on the pretest. The experimental group achieved over 90% accuracy on the posttest. This was higher than the average posttest performance of the comparison group (72% accuracy). Results suggest that a majority of LD children can reach mastery on sight words within a reasonable time framework if remedial principles are applied consistently.

(continued)

Author (year)	N	Selection criteria	Target domain(s)	Treatment(s)	Measures	Results
Bryant, Fayne, & Gettinger (1982) (*cont.*)				reading phrases and sentences with 10 training words until correctly read. Lesson 3: Silent and oral reading practice plus comprehension exercises on a short story with all 10 words. Control Ss did not receive treatment.		
Cornelius & Semmel (1982)	60	Ss were 3rd–8th graders with a mean age of 10.83. Mean WISC-R score was 101.50, and mean score on the Slosson Oral Reading Test was 3.5. All Ss were at least average in intelligence and 2 or more yr below grade level in reading.	Reading	The study included three groups of Ss. Two treatment groups met daily for twenty-four 1-hr sessions. Ss received individualized instruction while attending 5 wk of summer school. Methods and materials were selected on the basis of individual abilities and needs as determined from diagnostic testing. Group 1 attended the first 5 wk and Group 2 attended the second 5 wk of summer school. The control group received no treatment.	Slosson Oral Reading Test	Results support the position that LD Ss regress in their reading skills when they experience extended breaks in their educational programs. A 5-wk summer reading program during either the first or last half of the summer minimized this regression. The data also suggest that the largest proportion of the achievement regression occurs during the first part of the summer break in instructional programming.
DeBoskey (1982) Dissertation	23	Thirteen LD and 10 NLD Ss ranging in age from 9 to 12, with a mean age of 10.5. Ss' mean IQ score was 96.25.	Reading Math Spelling Visual–motor skills	Individualized remediation was provided based on deficits identified in the neuropsychological testing. Ss received treatment in addition to continued and regular assistance in the resource room. A number of techniques were utilized in the treatment, including:	WISC-R EEG recording WRAT Bender–Gestalt Spache Diagnostic Reading Scale	Neuropsychological posttesting indicated scores for the treated LD group showed a general trend of improvement greater than for the two control groups, but the differences were

				Showmanship—The teacher used an animated, more lively presence; Establishment of ground rules and penalties—5 min of sharing time was allowed, then a timer was set for the 40-min session to reduce impulsive behavior and verbalizations; Structure Sessions were organized beforehand; Frequent Change of Activities—Each S's lesson plans consisted of 12–20 different activities based on their deficits; Success-Oriented Activities—Activities were carefully planned so that success was expected 75–80% of the time; Frequent Review with Appropriate Instructional Materials—Individualized and concrete, based on the Ss' scores from the Halstead–Reitan Neurological Test Battery. Control Ss continued to receive assistance in the school resource room with no additional treatment.	Halstead–Reitan Neuropsychological Battery	not statistically significant. The overall Seiz and Reitan score (a general measure of neuropsychological functioning) was found to be significantly different for the treated LD group and the normal controls but not for the treated LD versus LD controls. The psychoeducational testing (WRAT, Spache, Bender) suggested the remediation technique had the effect of increasing the academic performance of the treatment group. The treatment group showed significant gains in reading, spelling, arithmetic, and copying geometric designs in comparison to the LD and normal controls.
Fantasia (1982) Dissertation	6	Ss were 4th to 6th graders; mean age was 10.11, with a range of 9.10 to 12.4. Mean IQ score was 86; mean scores on the Diagnostic Reading Scales were 1.8 (fall) and 3.0 (summer). Mean scores on Key Math were 2.5 (fall) and 3.1 (summer).	Math problem solving Computation skills	During 10 BL sessions, no instruction was provided. However, four skills were measured: target word problem computation, generalization word problem computation, oral reading of word problems, and basic fact computation. Treatment consisted of 20 sessions. Instruction focused on strategies for solving word problems and included	Word problems: answers/min correct; answers/min errors Reading: words/min correct; words/min errors Math facts: answers/min correct; answers/min errors	Direct instruction of formal analysis was effective in teaching LD pupils to accurately compute single-step addition and subtraction word problems containing extraneous information. In addition, pupils who had been taught formal analysis

(continued)

Author (year)	*N*	Selection criteria	Target domain(s)	Treatment(s)	Measures	Results
Fantasia (1982) (*cont.*)				five steps: (1) underline what the problem is asking; (2) circle the information needed to solve a problem; (3) state whether the problem gives the parts or the total and one part; (4) state whether to add or subtract; and (5) write the answer to the problem. Maintenance was the same as BL.	Word problems—generalization: answers/min correct; answers/generalized	to new problems. Finally, reading and math fact fluency alone did not affect accurate problem solving.min errors
Gettinger, Bryant, & Fayne (1982)	39	LD Ss enrolled in special education classes; 10% or lower accuracy on a spelling pretest; average intellectual functioning as documented by standardized testing during previous yr. Ss were randomly assigned to either experimental or control conditions following initial screening.	Spelling	The intervention consisted of eight sessions over a 3-wk period. The experimental group (*N* = 24) received lessons characterized by reduced unit size, distributed practice, and training for transfer. The comparison group (*N* = 15) received typical spelling instruction. Lessons focused on nine phonemically irregular words and eight phonemically regular words, with the lesson format varied. Controls received the same amount of instruction in the usual format. Experimental lessons began with instruction about regular words; the second lesson taught irregular words; the third lesson focused on list and sentence practice using the combined lists. Several teaching/practice activities were emphasized: oral spelling, single word presentation and practice, small instructional units each day (three–four	Spelling was measured 1 day before intervention and again on the last day of instruction. Two tests measured: (1) the number of correctly spelled words out of 17 words total, and (2) the amount correct of 12 transfer words. Daily criterion-referenced tests were given after each instructional unit; retention measures were given prior to each day's lesson.	At pretest, less than 10% of the words were spelled correctly by all the children. Following instruction, children in the experimental group achieved 80% accuracy on spelling words, and 75% accuracy on a delayed posttest of transfer words. The average posttest scores of the comparison group showed 60% accuracy on training words, and 50% accuracy on transfer words.

				words), practice to criterion, immediate corrective feedback after each dictation, distributed and cumulative practice, focus on difficult or misspelled word parts, and sentence writing practice. Besides these general strategies, training also differed by word regularity. Patterns of phonemically regular words were emphasized using visual cues and sound–symbol association, and training for transfer used nontrained words with similar patterns. Attention was not focused on grapheme–phoneme relations during instruction for regular words, but children were encouraged instead to develop exact representations of irregular words.		
Hazel, Schumaker, Sherman, & Sheldon (1982)	21	Three groups of adolescents participated in this study: LD adolescents enrolled in an alternative high school, NLD Ss attending the same school, and court-adjudicated youths on probation with a juvenile court. One group consisted of seven Ss classified as LD based on a three-step process: (1) assessment using selected subtests from the Woodcock–Johnson Psycho-Educational Battery and the WISC-R or WAIS; (2)	Social skills Social problem solving	A group skill-training program was implemented to evaluate the efficacy of training LD adolescents in social and problem solving skills. Ss were taught six skills, including giving positive feedback, giving negative feedback, accepting negative feedback, resisting peer pressure, negotiation, and social problem solving; training occurred in a multiple BL design across skills. The verbal and nonverbal components of each skill were detailed to the Ss. The problem-solving skill consisted of a noninteractive cognitive skill that required the subject to verbally describe a social problem,	Skill acquisition was evaluated through behavioral role-playing situations using novel, previously unpracticed situations. Behavioral checklist were used to assess performance of each skill during the role-playing situations; these checklists consisted of all steps needed for the skill listed sequentially. An observer recorded	All three groups demonstrated increased levels of the targeted skills following training. On the cognitive problem-solving skill, LD Ss experienced only a slight gain in comparison to Ss in the other two groups.

(*continued*)

Author (year)	*N*	Selection criteria	Target domain(s)	Treatment(s)	Measures	Results
Hazel, Schumaker, Sherman, & Sheldon (1982) (*cont.*)		demographic and other background information collected from school records; and (3) testing and other relevant information were presented to a validation team who reviewed the data and voted on whether each S should be included in or excluded from the LD group based on their judgment that the S did not exhibit any cultural, physical, or emotional handicaps but did evidence LD. The second group of Ss consisted of Ss in the same school excluded from the LD group by the validation team based on the procedures already described. The third group of Ss was composed of adolescents on probation with a juvenile court who wre referred by their probation officers for the social skills training.		generate three solutions, evaluate the consequences of each solution, then select and decide how to implement the best solution. The LD and NLD Ss were randomly divided into two groups which met for 2 hrs once a wk during school for 10 wks; the Ss on probation met in the juvenile court offices one night/wk. Except for the first one, all meetings started with a review of previously taught skills that consisted of the Ss performing verbal and behavioral rehearsals. Then a new skill was trained in the following steps: (1) introduction and description of the skill; (2) discussion of rationales which emphasized benefits of using the skill; (3) discussion of example situations; (4) Ss received a list of the skill components and the group discussed and gave rationales for each component; (5) modeling by the group leader in a role-play situation; (6) verbal rehearsal of the steps until Ss could name the steps in order; and (7) skill rehearsal using subject-selected situations. After each role-playing activity, the group leader elicited feedback from the Ss on their performance; role-playing continued until each subject had practiced the skill at least twice and met the criterion of 100% accuracy performing the skill without prompts.	each skill component performed using a 3-point rating scale; correctly performed steps were rated "2," approximations received a rating of "1," and failure to perform the step received a score of "0." These ratings were summed and divided by the total number of points possible, yielding a percentage of correctly performed steps. Prior to treatment, Ss were individually pretested and rated on each skill using the role-play situations; the tester read situations to the subject, telling himperher to behave as sperhe typically would in such a situation, and acted the other role(s) as needed. The same testing procedures were used wkly during treatment and at the end of the program.	

Helper, Farber, & Feldgaier (1982)	87	Ss were 2nd and 3rd graders participating in a therapeutic tutoring program; teacher nomination based on significant under achievement in reading; 5 mo below grade level on the WRMT; Full Scale IQs above 70 on the WISC-R.	Conflict resolution Behavior	Half the Ss were randomly assigned to an intervention designed to elicit production of alternate solutions to social problem situations. Tutors taught 14 lessons, although inconsistent implementation was noted. The rest of the Ss continued to receive only therapeutic sessions designed to reduce affective obstacles to learning.	Woodcock Reading Mastery Test; WISC-R; the Devereaux Elementary School Behavior Rating Scale; Bender Visual Motor Gestalt Test; Wepman Auditory Discrimination Test; Doehring Underlining Test; classroom sociometric ranking.	Measurable effects on amount of alternative problem solutions and negative classroom behaviors were not obtained. Reduced reading gains were observed for Ss in the experimental group. Pretest to posttest increases in the number of alternative problem solutions were associated with increased acting-out behaviors for both boys and girls.
Jaben, Trefflinger, Whelan, Hudson, Stainback, & Stainback (1982)	49	Ss between the ages of 11 and 12 identified as LD by a multidisciplinary team; achievement at least 2 yrs below age expectancies based on standardized tests; reading achievement of at least 3rd grade level; intelligence with the normal range. Ss were randomly assigned to either the LD experimental group or to an LD control condition.	Written expression Creativity	The intervention consisted of two 45-min lessons/wk for 14 wk total using the Purdue Creative Thinking Program which is designed to stimulate divergent thinking abilities related to verbal and figural fluency, flexibility, and originality. Instruction consisted of (1) 3–4 min instruction of a principle related to creative thinking, (2) a 10–12 min story about a famous American pioneer, and (3) three or four exercises related to the story content. Time of day and days chosen for the lessons were held constant for 14 wk. The least distractible area in the classroom was the area designated for Ss' independent completion of lessons. Assistance was provided for word recognition; responses were not corrected or graded. The lessons were stored in individual folders. Children in the control condition continued to receive their regular program.	Torrance Test of Creative Thinking (TTCT), Verbal and Figural subtests, Form A (Torrance, 1974) was given to all Ss as a pretest; figural subtests used included Parallel Lines and Picture Completion, and verbal subtests used included Just Suppose, Product Improvement, and Unusual Uses.	ANCOVA procedures were applied with posttest scores as the dependent variables and pretest scores as covariates. Analyses were computed for each of six subscores derived from the TTCT. LD subjects who received training obtained significantly higher scores on the verbal subtest than those who did not participate in the intervention. However, the figural aspects of creative behavior were not differentially affected.

(continued)

Author (year)	N	Selection criteria	Target domain(s)	Treatment(s)	Measures	Results
Kendall & Braswell (1982)	54	Ss were 3rd to 6th graders with IQ ranging 80–138 (PPVT). Treatment Ss were teacher-referred for exhibiting non-self-controlled behavior that interfered with academic and social performance. Ss were homogeneous in terms of having problematic impulsive classroom behavior, but the presence and extent of LD, aggressive behavior, and clinically hyperactive behavior was varied. To control for variations in rates of observed behavior across classrooms, nonreferred classmates were chosen and observed.	Cognitive–behavioral self-control	All Ss received twelve 45- to 50-min sessions twice wkly. Treatment Ss (27) were matched and paired with the control Ss (27). All Ss were exposed to the same training materials and received comparable rewards for participation. Sessions 1, 2, and 3: Each S was asked to select what would come next in a sequence and books from the Specific Skills Series (Barnell-Loft) Sessions 4, 5, and 6: A calculator-type math toy presented problems of increasing levels of difficulty and tangrams were used. Sessions 7 and 8: Playing checkers and interpersonal play situations. Sessions 9 and 10: Ss identified emotions of children displayed in pictures and gave possible reasons for the feelings. Sessions 11 and 12: Role-playing of problem solving in social situations, especially in non-self-controlled behavior specific to each subject. Cognitive–Behavioral Treatment Training in self-instruction (five problem-solving steps) via modeling, rewards for correct responses, response-cost for errors, and positive reinforcement. Behavioral Treatment: The same as Group 1 except no self-instruction. Attention Control Condition: The same materials as Groups 1 and 2, but no self-instruction, modeling, or contingencies.	Self-Control Rating Scale (SCRS; Kendall & Wilcox, 1979) Hyperactivity Scale (Conners, 1969) Therapists' ratings of improvement Matching Familiar Figures Test (MFF; Kagan, 1966) Wide Range Achievement Test (WRAT; Jastak, Bijou, & Jastak, 1965) Peabody Picture Vocabulary Test (PPVT; Dunn, 1965) Piers–Harris Children's Self-Concept Scale (Piers & Harris, 1969) Behavioral observations In-therapy measure (session summary sheet)	The cognitive–behavioral (C-B) intervention improved teachers' blind ratings of self-control, and both the C-B and behavioral treatments improved teachers' blind ratings of hyperactivity. Parent ratings did not show that treatment produced improvement. Several performance measures (cognitive style, academic achievement) showed improvements for the C-B and behavioral conditions, whereas only the C-B treatment improved children's self-reported self-concept. Normative comparisons and 10-wk follow-up provided additional support for the efficacy of the C-B treatment, whereas 1-yr follow-up data did not show significant differences across conditions. The data provide support for the inclusion of the cognitive component in the cognitive–behavioral intervention.

Kosiewicz, Hallahan, Lloyd, & Graves (1982)	1	S was 9.11yr old with attention problems and was attending a public school, self-contained, LD classroom. IQ scores (Woodcock–Johnson Cognitive Abilities Test; Woodcock & Johnson, 1977) were Verbal Ability, 94, Reasoning Ability, 89, Perceptual Speed, 83, and Memory, 110. On the achievement section of the same test, subject performed at the following levels: Reading, 5.5, Math, 3.6, Knowledge, 2.7, and Written Language, 2.4. Subject was reported to have difficulty with illegible written work.	Handwriting	The reversal design with multiple BL features took place from October to June during regular instruction in the S's resource room. The S completed two handwriting assignments/day. During the first BL (10 days), the S copied a list of words; during the second BL (15 days), he copied a paragraph. Treatment 1 (22 days) involved self-instruction. The teacher first explained and then modeled the five self-instruction steps which were listed on a card kept on the S's desk. No systematic reinforcement was provided other than what was previously normal for the teacher and S. Treatment 2 (6 days) involved self-instruction (S-I) and self-correction (S-C). In addition to the five self-instruction steps in Treatment 1, the S was taught how to correct by circling the errors on the previous day's work prior to copying the present day's work.	Percent correct handwritten letters	A set of self-instructions designed to provide the S with a strategy for writing appropriately was highly effective, as was a self-correction condition and a condition combining the two treatments.
Lloyd, Hallahan, Kosiewicz, & Kneedler (1982)	1	*Experiment 1:* A 9-yr-old boy identified as LD according to school district criteria, including average or above average ability and retarded academic achievement; observations prior to study indicated he was attending to seatwork tasks about 40% of the time.	Attention to task Academic productivity	*Experiment 1:* During BL, the S was instructed to independently complete math computation worksheets while seated at his desk. One point was available each day for completing all assigned math tasks; points were recorded on a chart at the back of the room, and were not redeemable for activities or tangible rewards. BL data were recorded for 7 days. During	*Experiment 1:* On-task behavior was measured by a 6-sec, whole interval recording procedure. Intervals were coded as "on" if the S was on-task throughout the interval; when off-task behavior was	*Experiment 1:* Self-assessment and self-recording were associated with higher levels of attention to task. In general, the two treatments were effective in increasing productivity.

(continued)

Author (year)	*N*	Selection criteria	Target domain(s)	Treatment(s)	Measures	Results
Lloyd, Hallahan, Kosiewicz, & Kneedler (1982) (*cont.*)				treatment, three different treatments were used daily. For about 1/3 of each treatment session, the S assessed his own attention to task. For another 1/3, the S assessed and recorded his attention to task. For the remaining 1/3 of each session, the S was not asked to either assess or record his own attention to task. The first two conditions were counterbalanced across the days of treatment. During a reversal phase, directions to assess and record task attention were withdrawn.	observed during any portion of a recording interval, the interval was coded as "off." Teacher praise comments were also recorded on the observation protocol as a plus for the interval in which they occurred. Academic productivity was noted as the rate of movements/min made while completing the assigned math tasks.	
	3	*Experiment 2:* Ss with LD enrolled in a semirural elementary school identified according to the same criteria used in Experiment 1		*Experiment 2:* To control for the possibility of multiple-treatment interference inherent in Experiment 1, the Ss in Experiment 2 were first required to assess their own attention to task, then a multiple BL across-subjects design was used to introduce the self-recording condition.	*Experiment 2:* A time-sampling recording procedure was used by an observer seated near the front of the classroom facing the Ss. The observer was cued to observe and record about every 2 sec, with observations made of the three Ss	*Experiment 2:* The results of this experiment were not consistent with those obtained from Experiment 1. While the effects of self-assessment on attention to task were minimal, self-recording was consistently effective for increasing attention to task. In terms of academic productivity, self-

					in sequential rotation. On-task behavior and academic productivity were coded according to the same criteria employed in Experiment 1.	assessment and self-recording did not have the beneficial effects observed in Experiment 1. Considering the results of both experiments together, the authors conclude that although self-assessment may improve attention to task, it appears that self-recording is a more effective technique. Because of the observed inconsistent effects on academic productivity observed in these experiments, it is not clear if academic productivity is more influenced by self-assessment or self-recording.
Meyer (1982)	58	Ss were 2nd–7th graders enrolled in special education classes. Mean age was 11.2, with a range of 7.1–14.1. Mean IQ score was 89.6, range 68–117. Mean reading score (WRAT) was 3.5. The Gray Oral Reading Test mean was 2.21, and the mean score on the Corrective Reading Placement Test was 17.40.	Phonics	Two procedures were examined for correcting oral reading errors during training in word-attack strategies in a naturalistic setting. Treatment lasted for 4 mo, where the Ss received daily, 45-min sessions. There were two treatments. Word Analysis: The teacher first determined if the misidentified word was regular, irregular, or a word with or without an ending, and then taught the correction approach for the word type. The Ss then repeated the list of words in	WRAT Gray Oral Placement Test	No significant differences were observed in oral reading accuracy between Ss taught using the word-analysis correction procedure and the word-supply correction procedure. Ss gained more than the norm samples on both the WRAT and the Gray.

(continued)

Author (year)	*N*	Selection criteria	Target domain(s)	Treatment(s)	Measures	Results
Meyer (1982) (*cont.*)				which the misidentified word occurred. Word Supply : The teacher corrected errors by telling the Ss the correct word after an error was made. Ss then repeated the word and practiced the list in which the word occurred until all words were correct. The procedure was the same for both groups with the exception of the above-stated differences. The first portion of the procedure was 10 min of word attack where new words and patterns were presented to Ss on the board. Then Ss read from the program text for 20 min. Teachers used a word-supply correction with all groups for errors made in this part of the lesson. The final portion was 10–15 min and consisted of individual checkouts. Individual Ss read 100-word passages aloud to a teacher or aide who tallied the number of errors made by each S.		
Omizo & Williams (1982)	32	LD children between the ages of 8 and 11yr classified LD according to the guidelines of the Texas Education Agency, 1976. Ss were from two school districts and attended special classes during a portion of the day. Excluded from the study were children whose IQ was below 90.	Attention to task Impulsivity Locus of control	Experimental Ss were matched with the control Ss. One experimental S and one control S went in pairs to the treatment that consisted of three sessions/wk for 8 wk. Treatment Ss listened to the relaxation tapes Peace, Harmony, Awareness (Lupin, 1977) and received visual biofeedback. These Ss received an overview of the tape, including novel terms, and were encouraged to relax to	Attention to task and impulsivity: Matching Familiar Figures Test (MFFT; Kagan et al., 1964) Locus of control: Nowicki–Strickland scale (1973)	Experimental Ss made significantly fewer errors on the attention-to-task measure and obtained significantly lower impulsivity scores.

				try to keep the numbers on the visual digital display of the biofeedback unit as low as possible. The Toomin 502A Electromyometer (EMG) was used to provide the biofeedback. Control Ss concurrently listened to tapes of a neutral story, about equal in length to the experimental subject's tape. Ss were hooked up to an inoperative biofeedback unit (i.e. no feedback was given, only the appearance of such.)		
Pany, Jenkins, & Schreck (1982)	12	*Experiment 1:* 4th graders, ages 9 to 10, participated in the study. Ss were from two classrooms and were selected according to their performance on a vocabulary screening test. Ss had to be able to read orally at least 75% of the experimental pretest items without error, but correctly identify no more than 10% of the word meanings on the initial screening test. Metropolitan Achievement Test Word Knowledge scores ranged 2.9–6.9, and Reading subtest scores ranged 2.9–8.0.	Word knowledge Reading comprehension	*Experiment 1:* An incomplete randomized block design wherein all Ss received each of four treatments. In each, two typed words and/or sentences were presented on small index cards. Ss read each card silently, then orally, then silently for three sessions. Treatment 1. Meanings from Context: No direct instruction on word meanings; Ss read two sentences. The first sentence contained a target word, the sentence contained a synonym of the target word. Treatment 2. Meanings Given: Ss read a sentence containing a target word; the experimenter provided both the meaning of the target word and a sample sentence using the word as it might be heard during daily experience. Treatment 3. Meanings Practiced: Ss read a single target word, the	*Experiment 1:* isolated-word vocabulary test, multiple choice vocabulary test, sentences paraphrase test, and a sentence anomaly test	Results from Experiments 1 and 2 indicated that the treatments were differentially effective in teaching synonyms for unfamiliar words. More meanings were acquired as a result of increased direct instruction. Average Ss learned some word synonyms under all conditions except a noninstructional control condition. However, LD Ss acquired fewer meanings across all conditions and seemed to require more direct instruction in order to produce learning. In both experiments,

(*continued*)

Author (year)	*N*	Selection criteria	Target domain(s)	Treatment(s)	Measures	Results
Pany, Jenkins, & Schreck (1982) (*cont.*)				experimenter stated a synonym and a sample sentence using a target word, and the Ss reported the target word and synonym. Two added words were presented to increase the task difficulty and to ensure that Ss attended to each word. Treatment 4. No Meanings Control: Ss read target words from an index card.		procedures that were differentially effective in teaching synonyms also produced differential transfer to sentence comprehension.
	6	*Experiment 2:* 4th and 5th graders aged 10–13 with LD; receiving reading instruction form the special education resource teacher. Scores on the Stanford Achievement Test Paragraph Meaning Subtest (1970) indicated that comprehension ranged 1.1–2.6 yr below grade level.		*Experiment 2:* Ss received 20 min of one-to-one oral reading practice with the teacher in the resource room. Oral or written responses to factual comprehension questions were given from the reading passages. All other procedures were identical to Experiment 1.	*Experiment 2:* same four measurements as in Experiment 1 plus isolated word-delayed test and a multiple choice-delayed test	
	10	*Experiment 3:* 4th graders with LD who were attending summer school. Metropolitan Achievement Test Vocabulary scores were below grade level; Word Meaning ranged from 1.7 to 5.8; Reading subtest scores ranged from 1.6 to 4.5.		*Experiment 3:* A within-subject design with two conditions. In each Ss practiced with the index cards until everyone could read with 100% accuracy. Then, Ss trained for four sessions on one of the sets of target words. Synonym Instruction: The experimenter showed a target word, said it and a one-word synonym, then stated a sample sentence containing the word. Ss individually	*Experiment 3:* isolated-word vocabulary test, multiple choice vocabulary test, sentence comprehension, sentence paraphrase, sentence anomaly, cloze test for stories that were read, and a story retell test	*Experiment 3* examined the effect of vocabulary instruction on comprehension of connected discourse. Vocabulary training transferred to comprehension of single sentences. However, on two of three measures of

				stated the word/synonym; the group repeated in unison. Words were trained to 100% mastery, then subsets were combined and individual test trials were given. No Instruction (control): Ss read only the target word; no synonym instruction was provided.		passage comprehension no effects were observed that were attributable to vocabulary instruction.
Rose, McEntire, & Dowdy (1982)	5	LD Ss ranging in age from 8.7 to 11.6 and receiving LD resource room instruction. All Ss had normal IQ, but were 2–4 yr behind in academic achievement. Mean scores on the Gilmore Oral Reading Test were 1.4, with a range of 1.2 to 2.0.	Reading	The relative effectiveness of two error-correction procedures, word supply and phonic analysis, on oral reading performance was investigated using an alternating treatment design. During BL, Ss' oral reading errors were not corrected. The 25 treatment sessions included two parts. Word Supply: While the S read, the teacher supplied the correct word after the learner erred. The S looked at the word and verbally repeated it. Phonetic Analysis: The S read aloud and was asked to look at various phonetic elements of the error word and told to "sound out" each element. After successfully doing so, the S read the word at the normal speed. Each BL and correction procedure was used daily on a random basis. Daily 2-min probes from the previous day's reading sample were measured.	Words read correctly/min	Increased oral reading rates were related to systematic correction procedures and the word-supply procedure was relatively superior to the phonic analysis method.

(continued)

Author (year)	*N*	Selection criteria	Target domain(s)	Treatment(s)	Measures	Results
Schumaker, Deshler, Alley, Warner, Clark, & Nolan (1982)	9	LD Ss in grades 8–12, and aged 12–18. IQ scores in the normal range, with deficits in one or more achievement areas, and did not displaying evidence of physical or sensory handicaps, emotional disturbance, or economic, environmental, or cultural disadvantage.	Error monitoring	A multiple BL design across three Ss was employed and was replicated twice with two more sets of three Ss each. The first S in each group received only one set of pretests before instruction began, the second S received two sets of pretests, and the third S received three sets of pretests. The teacher copied passages and inserted five capitalization errors, five appearance errors, five punctuation errors, and five spelling errors. Instruction consisted of the following steps (Alley & Deschler, 1979; Deschler, Alley, Warner, & Schumaker, 1980): (1) Test to determine S's current monitoring skills and discuss results with S; (2) Describe error monitoring strategy and rationale; Model strategy (verbal rehearsal of steps); (3) Verbally rehearse strategy without prompts; (4) Practice using teacher-generated, ability-leveled materials; (5) Provide feedback; (6) Test on teacher-generated passages; (7) Individual analysis of common errors; (8) Practice in S-generated paragraphs; and (9) Feedback and test on S-generated paragraphs. Procedures for detecting and correcting errors: read each sentence separately; ask COPS questions (Capitalization, Overall Appearance, Punctuation, and Spelling); when an error is found, circle it and put the correct form above the error.	Percentage of errors, ability level (detected and corrected) Percentage of errors, grade level (detected and corrected) Number of errors, before and after monitoring	Three replications of a multiple BL design across Ss demonstrated that improved performance did not occur until after each subject received instruction in the strategy. All of the Ss showed marked improvement in their first practice lessons immediately following instruction.

Sindelar (1982)	53	Ss receiving reading instruction in special resource programs; not all Ss were labeled RD; nominated by 17 resource teachers based on reading levels consistent with the materials used in the study. Ss were randomly assigned to one of four treatment conditions. The resource teachers whose Ss were assigned to the three tutorial conditions recruited, trained, and supervised the tutors for their own Ss. They were encouraged to secure competent readers of intermediate grade levels and to train more tutors than the number of Ss would require. The researcher supervised the teachers assigned to the small group condition. Twenty 15-min lessons were prepared for each of the four treatments.	Comprehension	*Oral Reading* (OR) practice was administered to individual Ss by tutors; it included positive reinforcement for correct reading, error correction, and S rereading of miscued words. Ss completing the passages before the end of 15 min reread it until the end of the time allocated. *Word Reading* (WT) training required the Ss' oral responses to words (200) presented on flashcards, with periodic reinforcement for accuracy, and tutor annotation of accuracy (+ or –). Words read correctly for three consecutive trials were dropped from the instructional set and replaced with new words, maintaining the set size at 10 over all 20 lessons. *HypothesisperTest* (HperT) training was based on procedures described by Dahl, Samuels, and Archwatemy (1973). For this group, 50 phrases were adapted from the OR passages by deleting the final words. Ss were individually taught four subskills requiring them to provide words consistent with (1) a preceding spoken context, (2) a preceding spoken context and the initial sound of the missing word, (3) a preceding written context, and (4) a preceding written context and the initial letters of consonant digraphs. Tutors periodically praised correct responses, corrected errors, and prompted slow responding.	Each child was pretested and posttested on four measures of reading performance; three nonstandardized tests (word reading, oral reading fluency, and cloze comprehension), and one standardized measure of comprehension, i.e., the Paragraph Meaning subtest of the Stanford Achievement Test (Kelly, Madden, Gardner, & Rudman, 1964).	The cloze comprehension data did not support the hypothesis that HperT instruction in a tutorial format would affect significant improvements in reading comprehension by disabled and poor readers. Support was obtained, however, for the comparability of this procedure to small group HperT instruction for teaching specific reading skills and for the efficacy of cross-age tutoring as a means of supplementing instruction.

(*continued*)

Author (year)	*N*	Selection criteria	Target domain(s)	Treatment(s)	Measures	Results
Sindelar (1982 (*cont.*)				*HperT Small Group Control:* The materials and procedures for these Ss were identical to those used in the HperT group, except where adaptations to small group use were needed.		
Sindelar, Honsaker, & Jenkins (1982)	1	*Experiment 1:* S was a 7-yr-old, 2nd grade girl referred to a special education resource program for remediation in math and reading; her achievement in both areas was mid-1st grade level; identified as LD according to state definition, including normal intelligence along with a central processing dysfunction.	Attending behavior	*Experiment 1:* The S read aloud 12 half-page segments from Book 5 of the Sullivan Programmed Reading Series during each session. She was praised after every one ot two lines read correctly, and she was required to verbally complete incomplete words or sentences; systematic error correction procedures were used. No systematic attempts were made during BL improve attending behavior; praise was contingent upon performance during all study sessions. The definitions and contingencies for reinforcement were made clear. During DRO1, a token economy was introduced with one token provided for each ½ page read without looking away. During RC1, the S received 12 tokens at the beginning of each session, with one token removed the first time she looked away on any ½ page. During DRO2, DRO1 conditions were reinstated. A return to response cost occurred in RC2.	*Experiment 1:* "Looking away" was the behavior targeted for intervention; this was defined as any head or eye movement away from the tutor's face or the page. The tutor tallied the frequency of "lookaways" using a recording form divided into intervals which corresponded to ½ page segments from the subject's basal reader. The tutor also timed each session to enable computation of a response rate, defined as the number of words read orally per min, which was not targeted directly for intervention.	*Experiment 1:* Differential reinforcement of other behavior and response cost were successful in reducing the frequency of looking away to well below BL levels, although performance was more stable under the response cost conditions. In addition, a decrease in looking away during oral reading was associated with increases in oral reading rate.

	1	*Experiment 2:* S was a 10-yr-old, behaviorally disordered girl attending a self-contained special classroom; placed in Distar Arithmetic 1 at about a 1st grade level. This girl was observed to look away frequently from the teacher's face or stimulus material.	*Experiment 2:* Distar arithmetic lessons were provided; token reinforcers and praise were given intermittently for task performance; tokens could be exchanged for recess time. Attempts were not made during BL to increase attending behavior. Praise and tokens were contingent upon task completion during this and all study phases. During DRO, the tutor played a cassette tape of tones randomly recorded at 15–165 sec intervals; a token and praise were given for looking at the appropriate place when the tone sounded, otherwise no token was given. Contingencies, exchange rate, and definitions of appropriate attending behavior were provided. During RC, 15 tokens were noncontingently provided prior to each session; one token was removed for each lookaway; smiles and praise were given for appropriate attending behavior.	*Experiment 2:* Looking away was again the behavior targeted for reduction. "Lookaways" were defined as any head or eye movement away from the tutor's fact or stimulus material, including looking at the tutor when the printed stimuli were presented. Excluded were lookaways during rote counting and periods when the tutor read presentation materials to herself. The frequency of lookaways were tallied on a wrist counter and session length was recorded. During DRO, the subject was observed to look frequently at the abacus on which her tokens were being recorded, which increased her rate of looking away; consequently, looking at the tokens was counted separately from lookaways as originally defined.	*Experiment 2:* DRO was associated with increased looking away, which was attributed to an increase in the subject's glances at the abacus used to record tokens earned. When lookaways directed to the abacus were excluded, inattentive behavior was slightly less than during BL. Under response cost conditions, the subject's inattentiveness decreased. Considering both experiments, the authors conclude that a simple respons–cost procedure proved an effective and easily managed method for improving attention. Differential reinforcement, in contrast, proved effective when nearly all lookaways were associated with nonreinforcement, but it failed to exert control over unconsequated lookaways. In addition, they recommend that reinforcement delivery be discrete to avoid increasing rather than reducing problem behaviors.

(*continued*)

Author (year)	N	Selection criteria	Target domain(s)	Treatment(s)	Measures	Results
Wong & Jones (1982)	120	Half of the Ss were LD from grades 8 and 9, with a mean age of 14.1 yr. They were receiving remedial reading services daily for about 30–60 min at learning assistance centers. Their WISC-R scores were in the normal range, and the results from the Nelson Reading Scales showed they were 3–4 yr below grade level. The other half of the Ss were normally achieving 6th graders.	Reading comprehension	This study investigated the hypothesis that insufficient metacomprehension is one possible cause underlying LD adolescents' comprehension problems, and that training them to monitor their understanding of important textual elements fosters metacomprehension and improves their comprehension performance. The study included one treatment group and a control condition; both consisted of LD Ss and normally achieving Ss. Self-Questioning Strategy: This treatment was designed to foster metacomprehension. Each S received an eight-page booklet with short, single paragraphs and was shown how to turn the main idea into a question. Ss then completed exercises, including underlining main ideas and formulating questions about them. Corrective feedback and direct instruction were used to develop the self-questioning technique. Control: Ss were provided with the same materials but received no training.	Number of ideas predicted Good questions generated Comprehension Recall Study time	Training substantially increased the LD Ss' awareness of important textual units, as well as their ability to formulate good questions involving those units. Training also facilitated their comprehension performance, but did not substantially increase normally achieving 6th graders' metacomprehension or comprehension performance. The differential effects of training on the two groups of Ss underscore the inactive nature of the LD Ss' reading as opposed to the active nature of reading in normally achieving 6th graders.
Branwhite (1983)	14	School-identified RD based on 20–40 mo retardation in reading achievement. Sample included Ss between 8.1 and 9 yr of age.	Reading	Phase 1: Ss divided into two groups received either direct instruction or diagnostic–prescriptive remedial reading instruction from the same reading specialist.	Schonell's Graded Word Reading Test (1972 revision); the DISTAR Reading II placement test	Direct instruction produced rapid and substantial gains. Effects were consistent within and between Ss. While both

				Phase 2: Both groups received direct instruction; Ss were given 35 min of instruction/day across both phases covering 110 days total.		treatments produced gains exceeding conventional growth rate prediction of 12 mo for a complete 200-day school , results from direct instruction were superior.
Fleischer & Jenkins (1983)	21	Ss were 4th and 5th graders; teacher nominated as LD based on performance 1 or more yrs below grade level in both reading comprehension and word recognition accuracy. Potential Ss read orally from basal series. Ss with word recognition from 88% to 90% and comprehension from 40% to 70% were randomly assigned to one of three groups.	Comprehension Word recognition	The same basal text was used for all Ss, with teaching method varied. Daily lessons were provided for 30 min each across a 4-wk intervention. *Word emphasis* involved oral reading and word drill correction. *Comprehension emphasis* consisted of verbal questions for each page and corrections for comprehension errors only. *Comprehension emphasis plus word emphasis* were combined for Ss in the third group.	Reading performance was assessed by three measures: oral reading accuracy was defined as the proportion correct of the final 100 words read; comprehension was measured by S's response to literal and interpretative questions following each story. A score was also obtained for oral reading accuracy of new words introduced in each story.	Reading comprehension was not differentially affected by these treatments. Word emphasis improved recognition of new words in isolation, but did not affect either word accuracy in context or comprehension. Less-skilled readers benefited the most from word emphasis.
Foster (1983) Dissertation	12	*Experiment 1:* Ss were 3rd–5th graders ranging in age from 9 to 12 with a mean age of 11.3 yr; all Ss had an average IQ.	Math	The effectiveness of two drill and practice methods, CAI and workbook, was compared using six LD and six NLD Ss. Both instructional methods provided highly structured drill and practice of multiplication facts, but differed on several important dimensions: immediacy of feedback, individually	Mean proportion of problems answered correctly Mean time per problem (in sec)	It was concluded that the highly structured nature of both modes of drill and practice eliminated differences in performance between the two groups. While computer and workbook instruction

(*continued*)

Author (year)	*N*	Selection criteria	Target domain(s)	Treatment(s)	Measures	Results
Foster (1983) (*cont.*)				tailored practice of problems, and mode of presentation. A combination group/single-subject methodological approach was employed to determine any idiosyncratic or group performance differences between drill and practice methods or any group differences between LD and NLD Ss. *Experiment 1:* Three conditions (A, B, C) which differed in the mode of instruction (CAI vs. workbook) and the subset of multiplication problems to be learned. Multiplication facts (3's to 9's) were divided into three subsets. At the beginning and end of each session quizzes were given and scores averaged. In both the CAI and workbook modes, Ss were allowed 8 min to complete the task. On the computer, visual feedback was given immediately on the screen. Auditory feedback was also given by a beeping sound when a point was earned. Ss had a 10-sec time limit. Extra points were given for accurate answers completed in less than 4 sec. For the workbooks, feedback was delayed until the next session. Condition A consisted of computer drill and practice given on Subset A. Condition B involved workbook practice on Subset B. Condition C consisted of computer drill and practice on Subset C.		differed on some basic structural features, these characteristics did not have a significant impact on S achievement.

	6	*Experiment 2:* Ss were drawn from Experiment 1.		*Experiment 2:* This experiment included two conditions on alternating schedules. Ss had one workbook and one computer session per day of instruction. Session format and modes of instruction were identical to Experiment 1. Session quizzes were administered providing a continuous measure of accuracy and time to complete the problems. Control Ss completed workbook exercises.		
Gittelman & Feingold (1983)	66	Teacher referral for poor academic performance; 7 to 13 yr old; no behavior problems in school; not hyperactive as defined by mean scores less than 1 on Conners Teacher Rating Scale, Hyperactivity Factor; English as a first language; WISC-R Full Scale IQ more than 80, Verbal IQ of at least 85, and Performance IQ more than 70; reading lag as measured by performance on the WRAT and the Gray Oral Reading Inventory below cutoff scores established for this study, i.e., VIQ 85–90 required a 2-yr reading lag, VIQ 91–95 required a 1.5-yr reading lag, and VIQ over 96	Reading	*Motivated Reading Remediation:* The Intersensory Reading Method, a phonics method devised by Pollack, was individualized depending on the child's reading level. The reading process was emphasized, supplemented by whole word recognition activities to avoid overreliance on phonetic word analysis. *Motivated Nonspecific Academic Tutoring:* This condition served as a control for effects related to increased attention, social contact, individual tutoring, and the like associated with remediation. This group received assistance with schoolwork based upon the child's academic difficulties. Materials were read to Ss unable to independently read, but no reading instruction was provided. Three professional reading teachers implemented the program. Remedial instruction was combined with positive	Basic reading: Pollack test of auditory discrimination and phoneme blending, and the Pollack test of basic reading skills (Pollack, 1969); the Monroe Auditory Discrimination Test (Monroe, 1932); the Roswell–Chall Auditory Blending Test (Roswell & Chall, 1959); the Roswell–Chall Diagnostic Reading Test (Roswell & Chall, 1959); and the Rosner Auditory Word analysis (Rosner & Simon, 1970)	Significant improvements in the reading achievement of Ss with RD were affected through the use of an intensive phonetic teaching method. Treatments were durable, with differences still noted up to 8 mo after treatment. Superiority of control group compared to treatment group on the Stanford Achievement Mathematics Computation subtest was attributed to special math tutoring provided to controls. This effect was not maintained at posttest, and special help with science and social studies did not produce

(*continued*)

Author (year)	*N*	Selection criteria	Target domain(s)	Treatment(s)	Measures	Results
Gittelman & Feingold (1983) (*cont.*)		required a delay of at least 1 yr. Exclusion criteria were also stipulated, including no significant psychopathology, no diagnosed neurological disorder, no gross family pathology, no uncorrected visual acuity defects.		reinforcement to facilitate acquisition of reading. Tutoring was initiated during the school , overlapping with academic instruction for at least 14 out of 18 wk of interventions. Ss received individual tutoring three times/wk across 18 wk. All treatments were free. Because a third group of Ss received reading instruction as well as methylphenidate at the same clinic, the two experimental groups in this study were given a placebo.	Reading and other academic tests: WRAT (Jastak & Jastak, 1965); the Gray Oral Reading Inventory (Gray, 1963); tests with phonetic content by Daniels and Diack (1973); Stanford Achievement Test Psychological tests: Matching Familiar Figures Test (Kagan et al., 1969); Visual Sequential Memory Test of the Illinois Test of Psycholinguistic Abilities (Kirk et al., 1968); Raven's Coloured Progressive Matrices (Raven, 1965); Purdue Pegboard (Purdue Research Foundation, 1948); Porteus Mazes (Porteus, 1950); Visual Motor Integration Test (Beery & Buktenica, 1967)	similar effects. Although the reading of LD Ss was improved, normal skill was not obtained, and teachers rated experimental Ss as more improved academically than controls.

					Behavioral assessment: Conners Teacher Rating Scale (Conners, 1969); a 13-item rating scale adapted from Rubin et al. (1966); Conners Parent Questionnaire (Conners, 1970); and the Home Hyper-activity Scale (Werry & Sprague, 1970).	
Gittelman & Feingold (1983)	61	Children between 7 and 13 referred by teachers due to poor academic performance; no behavior problems at school, not rated hyperactive as defined by Conners Teacher Rating Scale (Conners, 1969); English as primary language; WISC-R (Weschler, 1974) Verbal IQ of at least 85, Full Scale IQ of 80 or more, and Performance IQ above 70. Reading lag, as measured by the Wide Range Achievement Test (WRAT; Jastak & Jastak, 1965), and the Gray Oral Reading Test (GORT ; Gray, 1963), relative to IQ. The Stanford	Reading	All Ss received remediation coupled with the reinforcement methods described by Staats et al. (1967). There were three groups involved in this study, although results were only reported for two. *Motivated reading remediation:* While all Ss received phonics remediation via the Intersensory Reading Method (e.g., Pollack, 1967a, 1967b) treatment was tailored to each S's reading level. Whole word recognition was used to improve fluency; treatment did not involve perceptual or perceptual–motor training. *Motivated nonspecific academic tutoring:* This condition was provided to control for social–emotional and physical aspects of remediation. This group received tutoring in a variety of academic subjects	Basic reading: The Pollack test of auditory discrimination and phoneme blending, the Pollack test of basic reading skills (Pollack, 1969), the Roswell–Chall Auditory Blending Test (Roswell & Chall, 1963), the Roswell–Chall Diagnostic Reading Test (Roswell & Chall, 1959), the Rosner Auditory Word Analysis (Rosner & Simon, 1970), and the	Significant changes were obtained in the reading performance of children with RD following the intensive phonetic teaching program. Treatment effects were maintained up to 8 mo following the intervention, although the observed differences between groups diminished over the long term. The scores of control group Ss on the SAT math computation subtest, however, were superior to those of experimental Ss, a fact attributed by the authors to the special math

(*continued*)

Author (year)	N	Selection criteria	Target domain(s)	Treatment(s)	Measures	Results
Gittelman & Feingold (1983) (*cont.*)		Achievement Test (SAT; Madden et al., 1972) was used when a subject met study criterion on the GORT but not the WRAT. No significant psychopathology, no diagnosable neurological disorder, no gross family pathology, no uncorrected visual acuity defects.		depending upon each S's current academic problems. Tutors used each S's school texts along with various commercial academic materials. Materials were read to the Ss when needed but did not provide remedial reading instruction. *Reading instruction combined with methylphenidate:* Since this group was receiving medication to improve attention, all Ss in the above groups received a placebo. However, results were not reported for this group.	Monroe Auditory Discrimination Test (Monroe, 1932). Reading and other academics: The WRAT, GORT, SAT, and unspecified British tests with phonetic content by Daniels and Diack (1973). Psychological abilities: A continuous performance test; the MFFT (Kagan et al., 1969); a paired associate test; the ITPA, Visual Sequential Memory subtest (Kirk et al., 1968); Raven's CPM (Raven, 1965); the Children's EFT (Witkin et al., 1971); the Purdue Pegboard (Purdue Research Foundation, 1948); Porteus Mazes (Porteus, 1950); the VMI Test (Beery & Buktenica, 1967); the Draw-A-Person Test (Harris, 1963).	tutoring only received by the control group. Similar outcomes were not observed between the two groups for social science and science.

					Behavior: Teachers completed the Teacher Rating Scale (Connors, 1969), and a 13-item Behavioral Rating Scale (Rubin et al., 1966); after treatment, they rated Ss on global improvement in academic performance and behavior. Parents completed the Parent Questionnaire (Conners, 1970) and the Home Hyperactivity Scale (Werry & Sprague, 1970), which was also completed by the social worker.	
Jaben (1983)	49	LD Ss with reading skills of at least 3rd grade level; enrolled in self-contained, intermediate-level LD classrooms. Formal diagnosis by LDs specialists as LD. Ss were randomly assigned to either a treatment or a control condition.	Written expression Creativity	The Purdue Creative Thinking Program was administered for two 45-min lessons/wk for 14 wk to the experimental Ss. Control Ss continued to receive writing instruction typical to LD classrooms. The Purdue Creative Thinking Program is designed to encourage divergent thought processes in the area of verbal and figural fluency, flexibility, and originality.	Pretest and posttest data were collected of fluency, flexibility, and originality in written expression using the Torrance Tests of Creative Thinking (Torrance, 1974). Reading ability was determined by performance on the Passage Comprehension and Word identification subtests of the WRMT (Woodcock, 1973).	Scores for verbal fluency, flexibility, and originality were significantly higher for the experimental Ss than for the control Ss as measured by an ANCOVA. The adjusted means for total creativity also revealed significantly higher performance for trained LD Ss.

(*continued*)

Author (year)	*N*	Selection criteria	Target domain(s)	Treatment(s)	Measures	Results
Leon & Pepe (1983)	37	Preliminary stage: Eligibility initially determined by teacher; eligibility for inclusion based on state special education certification in either LD or EMH, teaching assignment in resource room for mildly handicapped Ss at elementary school. Twenty-two special education teachers from a single district met the eligibility criteria at this stage. Ten were selected randomly for the study, then randomly assigned to either intervention or contrast conditions. Ss inclusion criteria: LD or EMH Ss 9 to 12 yr old; diagnosed LD or EMH according to New Mexico State Standards for Special Education (1975); a minimum of 2 yr below age expectancies in math documented by prior testing. All Ss were included who were enrolled in participating teachers' classes and who met these criterions.	Metacognition Mathematics	Both groups of teachers were trained in subject selection, arithmetic skills development, usage of the KeyMath Diagnostic Arithmetic Test (KMDAT), the curriculum, and criterion-referenced measurement. Teachers assigned to implement the self-instruction intervention received additional training on the KeyMath Diagnostic methods to encourage the usage of self-instructional procedures. The same curriculum was used for both groups of Ss. Lessons were clustered into modules according to arithmetic functions being taught. Each module included a criterion-referenced test, a rationale, training alternatives, and a vocabulary/concept test of prerequisite skills. All Ss met the 80% mastery criterion for the vocabulary/concept test prior to intervention. Training duration was held constant for both groups at 15 min/day throughout the 7-wk intervention. Testing, curriculum placement, and instruction occurred during this time frame. Curriculum was individualized for all Ss based on KMDAT pretesting. Experimental Ss received training in self-instruction based on the model of Meichenbaum and Goodman (1969, 1971). Contrast Ss received individualized instruction only.	The KMDAT (Connolly, Natchman, & Pritchett, 1971); a criterion-referenced vocabulary concept test; criterion-referenced, curriculum-based measures for each training module instructed during intervention.	Significant posttest differences favoring the self-instructional group on the KMDAT operations subtest. Superior performance on the generalization measure by the self-instructional group. LD Ss scored higher than EMH Ss regardless of method. Significant improvement was noted for both groups over the intervention period.

Naylor & Pumfrey (1983)	60	Junior high Ss labeled at educational risk based on low reading attainment, operationally defined as a reading quotient on the Young Group Reading Test (Young, 1968) of 80 or less. All the Ss in grades 7 and above were screened, yielding 169 potential Ss with scores below the cutoff point. The study sample was then drawn randomly from the four junior highs with the highest referral rates in the participating district. Intelligence within normal limits was identified by Raven's Coloured Progressive Matrices (Raven, 1952). Exclusionary criteria included immigrant status, identified physical or sensory handicap, and/or emotional problems. Ss were randomly assigned to one of three groups; treatments were supervised by a teacher at each of four schools; there were five Ss in each group at each school.	Psycholinguistic processes	The study was divided into three stages. During Stage 1, the Ss were assessed individually on the ITPA-R (using the Mittler, Ward, & Rosen, 1970, wording suggestions), on the Raven's Coloured Progressive Matrices (Raven, 1952), and on the Burt (Rearranged) Word Reading Test (Vernon, 1938), followed by group testing with the Young Group Reading Test. Stage 2 involved Ss in 24 sessions of intervention in one of three treatment programs. In one group, remediation of basic processes according to the general guidelines and specific suggestions of Kirk and Kirk (1971) was provided. A second group completed activities drawn from a representative sample of those described in Manual II of the Peabody Language Development Kit (Dunn & Smith, 1976). The third group consisted of control Ss who participated in a simple number program. Ss received two 45-min sessions of remedial teaching/wk for 12 wk. Following treatment, the Ss were retested on all the criterion tests.	Pretests and posttests included individually and group administered instruments. These measures included the Young Group Reading Test (Young, 1968), Raven's Coloured Progressive Matrices (Raven, 1952), the Burt (Rearranged) Word Reading Test (Vernon, 1938), and the revised ITPA (Kirk, McCarthy, & Kirk, 1968).	Prior to the experiment, all three groups showed almost identical patterns of psycholinguistic ability. Following treatment, a significant increase in psycholinguistic function was apparent among the groups of children receiving the Kirk- and the Peabody-based training, with the Kirk-trained Ss demonstrating the highest levels of language usage at the automatic level. In addition, evidence supporting the diagnostic validity of the ITPA-R was obtained.

(continued)

Author (year)	*N*	Selection criteria	Target domain(s)	Treatment(s)	Measures	Results
Olsen, Wong, & Marx (1983)	45	Middle-class Ss enrolled in 5th grade at eight suburban schools; two to four normal achievers and four to seven LD Ss were randomly chosen from each school. All Ss were 10.0 to 11.8 yr old. A pool of partner Ss was formed by randomly selecting Ss from the schools' class registers. These Ss shared the same ethnic and SES characteristics as the experimental Ss, but were chosen from 1st graders to ensure nonpeer status. These children served as an audience for Ss from the other groups. *Normally achieving:* 15 Ss reading at grade level as identified by teacher observation and recent scores on the Canadian Test of Basic Skills (CTBS; King, 1976) given within the 3 mo prior to the experiment with normal IQ as determined by scores from the Peabody Picture vocabulary Test (Dunn & Markwardt, 1965).	Language Metacognition	*Experiment 1:* Each S was tested individually. After administration of the PPVT, the examiner taught the Mancala game to the child, after which the child practiced teaching the game to the examiner. The child's peer partner was brought into the room after the subject learned the game procedures enough to teach them to someone else. The child then taught the game to the peer. Their interactions were audiotaped, and the examiner remained in the room. After the game was played, the peer left the room and the Ss answered five questions about teaching the game. The Ss were then required to teach the game to a 1st grader using the same procedures. All pretest sessions followed this routine, taking between 30 and 40 min/experimental S. *Experiment 2:* The effects of training LD Ss to be more aware of pragmatic restraints on sociolinguistic interactions were examined this phase. The same LD Ss who were involved in the first experiment were randomly assigned to either a training or a control group. Control Ss received equal exposure to the examiner the Mancala game by engaging in an irrelevant activity.	*Ability and achievement:* Recent CTBS scores were used to identify Ss reading achievement for group assignment. The PPVT was individually administered during the first study session to document normal ability. *Language:* Linguistic complexity was measured by counting the total number of words used, the number of words excluded for being repetitious or nonmeaningful, the number of t-units (transformations in one utterance of complete meaning), the number of words in t-units, and the total number of complexities in 11 linguistic categories. A linguistic complexity ratio was calculated by dividing	*Experiment 1:* Reliable differences occurred on 3 of the original 11 linguistic variables. Normally achieving Ss used more adjectives, more prepositional phrases, and more tag questions. It was concluded that these findings are indicative of specific rather than general communication deficits. No reliable Groups x Partners interactions were observed, suggesting that both LD and NLD children were able to modify their language equally well for younger children. LD children articulated less pragmatic awareness than was observed with NLD children, as suggested by the lack of main effects for partners. Data analyses indicated that the LD Ss used fewer pragmatic strategies than were displayed by the NLD Ss. These findings indicate that

	LD: 30 Ss reading one or more levels below grade 5 as determined by teacher identification and recent scores on the CTBS with normal IQ as measured by the PPVT.		Experimental Ss were trained to use planful strategic behavior during the instructional portions of the game. Training occurred over 3 successive days, with 30-min sessions provided daily. Three main strategies were instructed: main ideation, subordinate ideation, and sequencing. Each session involved discussion of the general value of planfulness and ended with review of the strategic behaviors used during the session. Pretesting and posttesting followed the same format described for Experiment 1.	the total number of linguistic complexities by the total number of t-units. Three minutes of communication were analyzed for each category. Awareness was evaluated along three dimensions, two behavioral and one covert, measured in the contexts of speaker-to-peer and speaker-to-younger-child dyads. The overt dimensions of language modification according to audience age and strategic planfulness were measured by analyses of dyad transcripts. The covert dimension of pragmatic awareness was measured by scoring questionnaire responses.	LD Ss are less organized when presenting information and include fewer subordinate details in their explanations. *Experiment 2:* Pragmatic strategy training increased LD Ss pragmatic awareness and use of pragmatic strategies, although maintenance was limited and transfer was not obtained.

(*continued*)

Author (year)	N	Selection criteria	Target domain(s)	Treatment(s)	Measures	Results
Omizo & Cubberley (1983)	60	Ss enrolled in four classrooms for children certified as LD according to the guidelines established by the Texas Educational Agency (TEA, 1976). Ss were randomly assigned to experimental and control conditions using a random numbers table. The experimental group was divided into two groups with 15 Ss/group.	Self-concept Locus of control	Two teachers were trained by a certified reality therapist during an 8-hr workshop, including demonstration and practice in the conduct of class meetings. Class meetings were also demonstrated within classrooms. The therapist visited classrooms to ensure that meetings were adequately conducted as well. The importance of developing a personal identity and active involvement in the psychological and social environment were emphasized. The provision of positive, authentic, and open conditions conducive to development of positive self-concept was highlighted. Teachers were taught to avoid focus on past failures, and to accent the positive and future success potential instead. Teachers were instructed to focus on behaviors instead of attitudes, especially in terms of modifying behaviors to enhance opportunities for future success. The provision of meaningful learning opportunities and the avoidance of punishment and reinforcement for failures were final concepts. Teachers applied these principles during classroom meetings held twice wkly for 11 consecutive wk.	All Ss were administered the Dimensions of Self-Concept (Michael & Smith, 1978) and the Nowicki–Strickland Locus of Control Scale (Nowicki & Strickland, 1973) 1 wk prior to the first treatment session and again 1 wk following intervention.	Data from the Academic Interest and Satisfaction subscales of the DOSC indicated that the experimental Ss were more interested and satisfied with their school experiences than the control group Ss. Results also supported enhanced academic aspirations for LD Ss receiving the treatment, as well as lower anxiety scores. Experimental Ss did not differ significantly from control Ss on the Leadership and Initiative, Identification vs. Alienation, and Locus of Control measures, although the direction of as was consistent with expectations. This study provided support for the use of Reality Therapy classroom meetings to improve several aspects of self-concept in LD Ss.

Schimek (1983)	1	An 8-yr-old female retained in 1st grade was selected for this intervention; normal intelligence with a visual–motor integration age was identified by a social history, a Bender–Gestalt, a WISC-R, figure drawings, and a House–Tree–Person. Testing by the LD teacher subsequently confirmed an impulsive response style and problems in visual–motor and auditory–oral analysis, and in synthesis and sequencing of material.	Oral reading	Errorless discrimination training (EDT) was incorporated into a single-subject ABCD design to: (1) improve auditory discrimination of ch, th , and sh; (2) increase oral reading of words containing these digraphs; and (3) correct writing of words containing these digraphs. Training and evaluation took place within a 3-wk period; posttesting occurred 6 wks after the original training and evaluation. Intervention occurred for 15–20 min daily, with the child seated at the trainer's desk in the LD class. A token system was used, with a backup reinforcer of allowing the S to read to younger children. During BL, the digraphs were presented in a list of 30 words on a blackboard for 3 consecutive days. To establish the auditory–visual discrimination level, the child was directed to find and circle each word as dictated by the trainer; then she read the list, the list was erased, and she was asked to write the words from dictation. Intervention consisted of EDT of the three digraphs in sequential order determined according to the child's prior success with each. Each digraph was presented as a visual cue, the child was asked to repeat its sound, then the visual cue was gradually faded. EDT for of each occurred for 3 consecutive days,	The percent of correct responses to the auditory and written tasks were recorded.	Correct responses to the auditory tasks increased from an average of 23% during BL to an average of 90% during the final 3 days of intervention. Oral reading accuracy of all three digraphs ranged from an average of 17% correct before intervention for to 100% following treatment.

(continued)

Author (year)	*N*	Selection criteria	Target domain(s)	Treatment(s)	Measures	Results
Schimek (1983) (*cont.*)				with continuation of the one already new and presentation of each new one. The child earned plastic chips for each correct response; she was allowed to read to younger children after accumulating eight chips; earned chips were returned when accuracy was below 80% correct.		
Straub & Roberts (1983)	35	Children in grades 2–6 labeled by their school district as LD based on a substantial discrepancy between predicted and actual grade placement in academic subjects with IQ scores within normal limits; disability not primarily the result of sensory and/or emotional problems. All Ss completed the PONS test, then were randomly assigned to the experimental or the control group, with stratification applied on the basis of sex.	Social interaction ability	Experimental Ss received 4 wk of social awareness training that emphasized nonverbal communication. Twenty-min lessons were provided daily with the goal of sensitizing the Ss to appropriate use of nonverbal behaviors. Recognition of basic emotions was stressed first; attributions comprised the second focus. After the 4-wk intervention, Ss were placed on a 4-wk maintenance schedule during which a 20-min review was conducted each wk. Control Ss received a daily 20-min instructional enrichment activity related to their current studies.	The Profile of Nonverbal Sensitivity (PONS)—short form (Hall, Rosenthal, Archer, DeMatteo, & Rogers, 1977) is a 220-item test of decoding nonverbal behaviors presented through various modes. The present study used the 44-item short form. Silent videotape of forty 2-sec scenes is presented which display a woman expressing either positive or negative affect with dominant or submissive expression. Ss decide which of two choices best describes the scene. Slight revisions were necessary for this	Peers rated the trained Ss higher than the control Ss on the PAS. According to results from the SAR, peers gave more positive ratings to trained Ss. In addition, no main effects for trainer were observed, nor was there an interaction between treatment and trainees. The results suggest that training to improve affect awareness has positive effects on the social interactions of LD children.

study as some content was believed inappropriate for young children.

Social affect rating (SAR): This consisted of three questions, each illustrated by a simple line drawing, concerning interpersonal affect expressions. There were four possible answers for each question where a peer is rated along a 4-point continuum from "always nice" to "always mean."

Modified Peer Acceptance Scale (PAS): Peer acceptance of LD Ss was measured using a modification of this instrument by Bruinicks (1978). Class members rate every other member in terms of the extent to which others wish to have this person as a friend; the format is forced choice. An alphabetical class is used for the answer sheet, with simple line drawings added to illustrate the choices, along with a verbal choice description.

(continued)

Author (year)	N	Selection criteria	Target domain(s)	Treatment(s)	Measures	Results
Wanat (1983)	30	Ss were 10th–12th graders enrolled in an LD resource program. Identification began with a test battery including the Bender–Gestalt, the Detroit Tests of Learning aptitude, the Draw-A-Person Test, the WISC or the WAIS, the WRAT, and the Peabody Individual Achievement Test. Placement was then determined by consensus of a team consisting of teachers, parents, and school support staff. Ss who met these criteria were randomly assigned to either experimental or control groups.	Social skills	Each S received 1–3 hr of assistance/day in the resource room. Only the experimental Ss received the social skills treatment, People Success. Control group Ss participated in other classes at that time. Treatment sessions lasted 55 min/day for 80 consecutive school days. The teacher, who was already familiar with the materials, delivered the treatment. Sixteen units of the Interchange Human Development Program were presented, with one unit presented each wk of instruction. Supplemental filmstrips were presented periodically to 15 Ss seated in a circle with the instructor attended each daily session. Following vocabulary introduction, discussions were conducted which centered on specific issues. The remainder of each wk was spent reviewing vocabulary, viewing filmstrips (when applicable), and completing experience sheets.	Ss in both groups were pretested and posttested on the Fundamental Interpersonal Relations Orientation-Behavior (Schutz, 1978) and the Piers–Harris Self-Concept Scale (Piers & Harris, 1969).	Significant differences between the experimental and control Ss were obtained in comparisons of the Piers–Harris Self-Concept Scale. No significant differences between the two groups were observed for GPA.
Brailsford, Snart, & Das (1984)	24	LD Ss, ages 9 to 12, in resource room programs, with IQs above 85 (as measured by the Canadian Cognitive Abilities Test) and reading comprehension scores below	Information-processing strategies Reading comprehension	Regular reading instruction continued in the classroom. All Ss received 15 hr of additional remedial assistance. The experimental group was seen 30 min/day in pairs, with intervention focused on enhancing simultaneous and	Information-integration theory battery of tests (Ashman & Das, 1980; Das et al., 1979); the Gates–MacGinitie	Significant improvements for both groups in reading, but the experimental group had significantly higher scores on the cognitive measures and the Standard

		the 35th percentile (Gates–MacGinitie Reading Test, Level D). Children were assigned to either an experimental or a control group.		successive synthesis and verbalization during task performance. Controls received 30 min of reading instruction/day in small groups.	Reading Test (Comprehension subtest); the Standard Reading Inventory (McCracken, 1966); pre- and postintervention administration using alternate forms.	Reading Inventory measure of reading instructional level following intervention.
Brown & Alford (1984)	20	LD children receiving instruction in self-contained LD classrooms in a large metropolitan school district; placed after a rigorous diagnostic exam by qualified school psychologist based on history of learning problems; pediatric exam negative for other major diseases and obvious physical defects. All Ss identified by their teachers and qualified psychologists as having severe overt attentional problems; demonstrated deficits on the attention–concentration factor of the WISC-R (Wechsler, 1974). Ss also scored more than two grade levels below expectancies on the WRAT (Jastak & Jastak, 1975).	Attentional deficits	Ss were randomly assigned to either a training or control group. Trained Ss (9) received a package of cognitive self-control procedures. The program spanned a 2-mo period during which Ss were seen individually for two 1-hr sessions each wk, for a total of 16 sessions. Ss were trained to process information and selectively attend to visual discrimination problems more effectively using a variety of materials and exercises. Task and material selection followed the criteria defined by Douglas (1976): (1) training materials overlap as little as possible with tests used to assess training effects; (2) training materials/tasks should be varied and interesting, facilitating strategy generalization; (3) there should be several examples of each task type, and these should be arranged in ascending order of difficulty. The materials were	A battery of measures was administered to the training group prior to intervention, at the end of training, and 3 mo after training ceased. Measures were selected to meet one or more of the following criteria: (1) successfully discriminated between normal and LD children in prior research; (2) widely used in clinical practice to diagnose LD and related disorders; (3) closely related to academic achievement.	Cognitive self-instructional training was associated with improved performance on measures of reading, attention, and inhibitory control. In addition, maintenance was demonstrated for up to 3 mo following training.

(*continued*)

Author (year)	*N*	Selection criteria	Target domain(s)	Treatment(s)	Measures	Results
Brown & Alford (1984) (*cont.*)				similar to those used by Egeland (1974), including match-to-sample tasks using arithmetic and reading problems; match-to-sample tasks using drawings; component analysis training; detail analysis training; memory training; visual sequence training; and self-verbalization procedures. Control Ss (7) were not trained using these exercises and materials.	Measures in the assessment battery included attention tests from the DTLA (Baker & Leland, 1967), WRAT (Jastak & Jastak, 1974), and MFFT (Kagan, 1966).	
Carte, Morrison, Sublett, Uemura, & Setrakian (1984)	87	LD children receiving special education, ages 6–11, with normal/average IQ scores as measured by the WISC-R (short form), yet not achieving academically at a level commensurate with their intellectual ability. Ss were, on average, performing more than 1 *SD* below intelligence level on reading comprehension as measured by the Gates–MacGinitie.	Reading comprehension General academic achievement	Experimental Ss (46) participated in an individual program with a registered occupational therapist. Emphasis was directed toward equalization and integration of tactile proprioceptive and vestibular systems with bilateral coordination and motor planning. Therapy was provided twice wkly for 45 min for a total of 66 sessions. Control Ss (41) received no treatment. A matched pair design was used.	Gates–MacGinitie, Reading Comprehension WRAT, Reading, Spelling, Arithmetic Target test Underling Tests Southern California Postrotary Nystagmus Test (duration in sec)	After 9 mo of individual sensory integration (SI) therapy, no systematic effects on any of the dependent variables were discernible. However, modest improvement was observed in academic and perceptual function in both therapy and control groups.
Chase, Schmidt, Russell, & Tallal (1984)	54	Ages ranged from 8.0 to 13.11, with a mean age of 11.1. Mean WISC-R score was 102.4, and mean reading quotient was .73 (Reading Age × 100 per Chronological Age × Full Scale WISC-R IQ).	Reading Writing Spelling	Ss in the Piracetum treatment group received 3.3 grams of Piracetum daily, 5 ml (1.65 grams) before breakfast and 5 ml (1.65 grams) before the evening meal over 12 wk. Ss in the placebo group received a matching dose of placebo syrup.	Gilmore Oral Reading Test, Accuracy, Reading Comprehension, and Reading Rate; Gilmore Composite Reading, Accuracy	Compared to the placebo control group, individuals treated with Piracetam showed statistically significant improvements above their BL scores on measures of effective

					and Comprehension; WISC-R Digit Span; Gates–McKillop Syllabication Test; WRAT Spelling; Words Written; percent of Spelling Errors; Rapid Automatized Naming Test (RAN; Denckla & Rudel, 1976) Color, Letter, Number, Object; Visual Repetition, Long, Short and Criterion (Tallal); 75 msec Tone Repetition: Long, Short, Criterion; BA/DA Sound Repetition, Long, Short, and Criterion; Token Test (DeRenzi & Vignolo, 1962); Paired Associates Memory	reading accuracy and comprehension, reading speed, and writing accuracy. The medication was well tolerated, and all medical examinations showed no untoward effects.
Dixon (1984) Dissertation	60	Ages from 7 to 13 yr with a mean age of 10.04. Mean IQ score (WISC-R) was 96.03 with a range of 80 to 112. Reading at least one deficient. WRAT reading mean was 91.63; GORT grade	Reading comprehension	This study investigated the effects of using a questioning strategy with LD Ss to increase discussion participation and to increase reading comprehension. Ss in the treatment condition met for fifteen 30-min sessions. During half of the sessions, Ss read stories either silently or	Critical responses to reading S–teacher interaction	There were significant differences between the two groups, the teachers in the workshops asked significantly higher cognitive level questions that led to S response with

(continued)

Author (year)	N	Selection criteria	Target domain(s)	Treatment(s)	Measures	Results
Dixon (1984) (*cont.*)		equivalent mean was 1.97. On the SAT, Ss' mean grade equivalent scores were: Vocabulary, 3.54; Reading Comprehension, 2.94; Spelling, 3.15; Word Study Skills, 2.77; and Language, 2.89.		orally. The rest of the session involved teacher–S interaction discussion groups, which were recorded with TICOR.		higher level answers. There was no difference between the two groups in their performance on the written comprehension tests.
Gelzheiser (1984)	80	Sixty LD Ss classified by school evaluation teams, including teachers and psychologists. LD Ss received instruction either in the resource room or a self-contained classroom. Twenty NDL private school Ss provided normative comparisons. Ss ages were between 12 and 14.5 at pretest; WISC-R between 90 and 125; there was no history of emotional disturbance. LD Ss were randomly assigned to one of three treatments.	Memory strategies	LD controls received no treatment. One experimental group learned Rules Only, and another received Rules Instruction augmented by prose examples. All NLD Ss were assigned to a no-treatment control condition. There were four study phases over a 3-wk period: pretest, informational phase (two lessons), individualized training (three lessons), and posttest. The pretest, posttest, and each lesson occurred on different days; controls only took the pretest and posttest. Only the first lesson of the instructional phase was varied for experimental Ss; correct recall was rewarded. The pretest phase lasted 35 min and consisted of two tasks, recall of information from a passage and recall of pictures. In phase 2, Ss were taught to recognize the problem isomorph (Brown et al., 1983) and to derive categories	Recall was pretested with a deck of pictures that could be categorized into four groups of six cards each; a second deck of comparable difficulty was used for posttesting. Two passages were also used at pretest, then again at posttest, as a measure of transfer. Each passage was categorical and factual, containing four paragraphs labeled by subtitles. Paragraphs began with topic sentences that were then followed by five additional sentences. Prose	Picture recall: Gains in the use of sorting and clustering by LDs followed intervention. More strategic behavior was coincident with improved recall. The strategies used by instructed LD Ss were no longer observably different from those used by NLD Ss, nor was their recall different. LD controls continued to show poor performance on measures of strategy use and recall. Passage recall: Training affected skill transfer from pictures, words, and phrases to recall of facts from passages; instructed groups were more likely to

				during the first 20-min informational lesson. Rules Only Ss used examples of pictures, words, and two word phrases to identify categories. Rules-plus-prose Ss received the same lesson, but one of the word lists and a prose list and two more prose examples were used during instruction and for a quiz after instruction. The second informational lesson, also 20 min long, taught Ss four rules for studying information taxonomically arranged, i.e., sort to study, study, name the groups, and cluster for recall; this lesson was also followed by a quiz. Phase 3 consisted of three individualized lessons. Ss used the four rules to study categorical decks of pictures, words, and two-word phrases. Feedback regarding percentage correct, degree of clustering, and incentives earned was given after each recall trial. Direct instruct to use strategies was systematically faded across trials. The individualized lessons lasted 35, 60, and 40 min, respectively. Posttesting followed several days later.	recall was assessed again at posttest by these measures. The Organization score was used to assess strategy usage. A rating was obtained for the amount of notes saved to cue recall. An adjusted ration score was calculated reflecting degree to which clustering was used during recall. The total number of correctly recalled items yielded the recall score.	sort, save paragraph subtitles as notes, and cluster for recall. In contrast to pictures recall, instructed LDs did not recall as many facts as NLD controls even though their strategy use was increased. Only LDs who received the most explicit instruction recalled more then the NLD controls.
Graybill, Jamison, & Swerdlik (1984)	16	LD resource room Ss identified as impulsive based on the Matching Familiar Figures Test (Kagan et al., 1964) and the Devereaux	Behavior Cognitive behavior modification	Experimental Ss received 4 wk of individual Verbal Self-Instruction (Meichenbaum) to learn how to use language mediation to control their own behavior. Resource teachers delivered	The Matching Familiar Figures Test (Kagan et al., 1964); the Devereaux Elementary School	Significant differences were observed on the posttest Matching Familiar Figures Test, indicating that measurable changes in

(continued)

Author (year)	N	Selection criteria	Target domain(s)	Treatment(s)	Measures	Results
Graybill, Jamison, & Swerdlik (1984) (*cont.*)		Elementary School Behavior Rating Scale (Spivak & Swift, 1966). Ss rated impulsive were randomly selected for either the experimental or the control condition.		instruction in the resource room. The teacher first demonstrated problem solving covertly, then transferred problem resolution to the S. Verbalization was gradually faded until the child could work through the problem independently using covert than overt speech. The program for control Ss was unchanged.	Behavior Rating Scale (Spivak & Swift, 1966); the Piers–Harris Self-Concept Scale (Piers & Harris, 1969); and Burk's Behavior Rating Scale (Burks, 1968)	impulsivity can be induced by teachers in classroom settings. However, the meaningfulness of these results was questioned because there were no significant differences between the posttest ratings by teachers of S impulsivity.
Kerchner & Kistinger (1984)	37 (2)	Ss were LD 4th, 5th, and 6th graders in the resource specialist program (RSP). This study was conducted in three RSP classrooms using existing groups; composition was similar for SES levels, though varied by grade level distribution.	Writing	The Ss in one class served as experimental Ss. They received about 7 mo of instruction that combined the process approach to writing with word processing on computers using the Bank Street Writer program. The intervention for one control group emphasized the language experience approach, but computers were not used for word processing. The second control condition employed reading groups using a variety of texts, concentrating on the development of spelling skills through a teacher-directed sentence dictation program.	The Test of Written Language (TOWL; Hammill & Larsen, 1978) and the WRAT-R were administered to experimental and control Ss at pretest and posttest.	Superiority of the process approach to writing instruction was supported by significant main effects for Thematic Maturity, Word Usage, Style, and the Written Language Quotient when TOWL scores were analyzed by an ANCOVA with posttest scores as the dependent variables.

Kitterman (1984) Dissertation	5	Ages ranged from 10 to 11; mean WISC-R score was 91.8, with a range of 80 to 102. The WRAT reading mean score was 76.6, with a range of 73 to 82.	Spelling	The study included four conditions: BL, traditional paper and pencil tasks; Unmasked and Errors Verified (UEV); Masked and Errors Verified (MEU); and No Written Responses (NWR) Each S was given his or her own list of spelling words, 10/session (four word lists, 40 words). The treatment involved CAI. Each word was pronounced, used in a sentence, and pronounced again using an audio cassette. The S had three attempts to spell the word correctly. When incorrect, the computer showed both the correct and incorrect letters in different colors on the screen. An auditory and visual response confirmation was presented at the conclusion of the exercises for each word. The S received a printout of the correct and incorrect words. Each condition lasted for five sessions.	Percentage of correct words on first attempt and on computer Length of session, mean response time Number of sequences	Microcomputer presentation of the spelling words did not effectively enhance achievement over that of paper and pencil. The use of error verification procedures with the microcomputer format did not result in more efficient learning. Rather, these subjects learned more quickly without the verification procedures. Informal observations further indicated that the Ss ignored the cues provided for verification. Informal observations also indicated that attention-to-task behavior was enhanced by the microcomputer.
Kunka (1984) Dissertation	110	Ss were 4th through 6th graders with average IQ; achievement information was not available.	Math computation	Treatment consisted of the Speak and Math program. Ss used Level 1 for all four basic math operations, and used Level 2 for addition/subtraction only. Ss in the Versator (control) condition used only two number positions in both the addition/subtraction mode and the multiplication/division mode. Ss met for 11 wk, three times wkly for 20 min.	Written Math Achievement Test: Visual, Auditory, and Mixed Timed Orally Administered Math Achievement Test: Visual, Auditory, and Mixed	Analysis of variance indicated there was a mean gain in math achievement across all groups, regardless of treatment or modality. There was no significant interaction between modality groups and achievement, no significant

(continued)

Author (year)	*N*	Selection criteria	Target domain(s)	Treatment(s)	Measures	Results
Kunka (1984) (*cont.*)						main effect of dominant learning modality, and no significant main effect for treatment using the written math test as a measure of math achievement. There was, however, a significant main effect for treatment using the orally administered, timed test as a measure of math achievement, with the Versator group achieving significantly greater gains than the Speak and Math group.
Manning (1984)	100	Ss were 3rd graders identified as reading 1.5 yr below grade level expectancies, with intelligence within the average range. None of the children were receiving special education from a specialist with LD certification. Ss were randomly assigned to one of four conditions.	Oral comprehension Cognitive strategies	All four conditions were under the researcher's supervision. Three schools were involved in the study; classroom space was used at two of them, and the library was available at the third. Teacher orientation was provided during the first wk. Treatment was implemented during the second and third wks. Thirty-min sessions daily for 10 consecutive school days, totaling 5 hr intervention/S, was provided. In the experimental conditions, Ss were trained to use cognitive strategies, practiced applying the strategies, then compiled a booklet which represented their	The Gates–MacGinitie Reading Test (Gates & MacGinitie, 1972) and the Short Form Test of Academic Aptitude (Sullivan, Clark, & Tiegs, 1970) were administered to establish study samples. The Boehm Test of Basic Concepts (Boehm, 1971) was administered to assess training effects.	Cognitive strategy training resulted in significant improvements in the oral comprehension of Ss in all three experimental conditions. In addition, training appeared to differentially affect the development of literacy foundation skills since all three experimental groups obtained significantly higher mean scores than the control group at posttest. Since the

cumulative written experiences during the study. Cognitive Monitoring (CM): Ss were taught to ask themselves questions while listening to stories, instruction, directions, and the like. Training involved verbal repetition of questions gradually faded until Ss were trained to covertly monitor their own comprehension. Markman's essays (1978) were used for training following her protocol. Creative Problem Solving (CPS): Ss learned and applied the five steps of creative problem solving (Osborn, 1963; Parnes, 1967). Combination CM and CPS: Streamlined versions of CM and CPS were used during the first eight sessions, with four CM sessions followed by four CPS sessions. The two methods were synthesized for the last two sessions in the form of a soliloquy technique (Torrance & Myers, 1970). Control Ss received typical directions from the researcher, then completed age-appropriate art activities in sessions of the same duration and covering the same span of days as the experimental treatments.

strategies trained appear to affect processes necessary for skills assessed by the Boehm, these results may be attributed to second-order effects. combining the self-regulation strategy with training problem solving produced the strongest results, and using CPS alone had the weakest effects, although CPS Ss outperformed controls.

(*continued*)

Author (year)	N	Selection criteria	Target domain(s)	Treatment(s)	Measures	Results
Mathews & Fawcett (1984)	3	Ss were high school seniors who had been formally identified by high school personnel; enrolled in at least 1 credit in the high school's learning center classroom. IQ range on the WAIS was 91–96. The range on the Woodcock–Johnson Pscyhoeducational Battery, Writing subtest was 2.5–5.1.	Job applications Resume writing	Behavioral instruction procedure designed to teach the skills involved in completing employment application materials were evaluated using a multiple BL design. During BL, Ss were given three different applications and were asked to fill them out. In the first session, the Ss were also asked to write a resume after having read a one-paragraph description of the purpose of a resume. After BL, Ss were given nine sessions of training in application completion and resume writing. Ss were then asked to write a resume and complete nine additional employment applications.	Number of correctly completed items on job applications	Training was effective in teaching employment application completion and resume writing skills to three LD Ss. Rating data obtained from potential employers suggested that training improved the appearance and content of the application materials. In addition, the employers viewed applicants as better qualified for employment after training and indicated that they were more likely to invite the applicants to participate in a job interview.
Porinchak (1984) Dissertation	51	Ss were selected on the basis of their scores on the CISC-R and reading test scores extracted from their educational records. They were placed into either an average or below-average group. All subjects had a diagnosed reading disability.	Reading achievement	The experimental group received 20 min of diagnostic/prescriptive individualized instruction in the reading lab in addition to 20 min of computer interaction in reading. No specific computer software was listed. Control Ss also received 20 min of diagnostic/prescriptive individualized interaction in the reading lab in addition to 20 min of traditional instruction in reading. Control S materials paralleled, although not identically, those used by the	Metropolitan Reading Survey, Form K (Intermediate level) S views on reading Piers–Harris Self-Concept (Children's)	The main effect was significant (.05) with regard to reading achievement of the average group. The main effect was not significant with regard to CAI treatment and reading achievement. The interaction between reading achievement, CAI treatment, and intelligence was insignificant. Significant main

				experimental group. Computers were not used by controls. Both groups received two sessions/wk, although total length of study was not given.		effects and interactions were not obtained in comparisons of attitude toward reading, CAI treatment, and intelligence. There was no main effect for self-concept, and interactions involving this variable were not observed. There was a significant (.10) difference with regard to learner preference toward mode of instruction, with the computer most often reported as preferred. CAI and traditional methods appeared to be equally effective for the average S. For the Below-average S, CIA appeared to be more effective, but not significantly so.
Rose & Sherry (1984)	5	Ss were 8th and 9th graders with LD receiving resource room instruction in junior high school. Near-normal intelligence scores on the WISC-R, but at least 4 yr behind in academic achievement, having been retained at least once.	Oral reading	An alternating treatment, single-subject design was used to investigate the relative effects of two oral reading previewing procedures. In one, the S read passage silently first, then aloud. In the other condition, the S listened and followed along as teacher read aloud prior to the S reading the passage. During BL, each S read the passage without preview or practice.	Rate of mispronunciations, omissions, substitutions, and unknown words while oral reading	In four of five cases, results showed that systematic prepractice procedures were related to higher performance levels than was BL with no prepractice. Differential effects were noted. The listening procedure was related to higher rates of words read correctly than was the silent procedure.

(continued)

Author (year)	*N*	Selection criteria	Target domain(s)	Treatment(s)	Measures	Results
Rudel & Helfgott (1984)	59	Dyslexic Ss between the ages of 8 and 13 were included if they met the following criteria: WISC-R IQ scores 80+, with either Verbal or Performance scores greater than 90; and reading quotient (RQ) at least 1 *SD* below the expected level.	Memory	A double-blind 12-wk trial of Piracetum versus placebo was undertaken to detemine whether the drug treatment would selectively improve the verbal learning of dyslexic boys	Meimark Memory Strategies Test, Organizational Strategies Items recalled	Ss in the drug treatment group learned more of the items posttreatment than pretreatment, and retained more of them after a 25-min delay, than did the placebo group. The drug did not influence the strategy employed during study periods or the order in which the tiems were recalled.
Sinatra, Stahl-Gemake, & Berg (1984)	40	Ss were 2nd to 8th graders enrolled in a university reading clinic; 11 Ss had been retained in one or more grades, primarily due to reading deficits. Mean Slosson IQ score was 91, mean WRAT (1878) Word Recognition score was a GE of 4.0, and the mean score on the Nelson Reading Test (1977) was a GE of 2.5.	Reading comprehension	This study compared the effects of two treatments on reading comprehension. *Semantic Mapping Readiness Approach* (Experimental Group, 27 Ss): Instruction was sequenced. (1) Five map readiness presentations were given wherein teachers and Ss developed the vocabulary and key concepts for the mapping categories; (2) Each S was given the purpose question for reading and read the selection silently; and (3) Each S answered 10 comprehension questions. One of three map types was used, depending on the organization of the reading selection: (1) the *Episodic Web* was used for a story with narrative content; arrows were used in a flow chart	Comprehension questions at the end of each reading passage	For all of the Ss, comprehension scores were significantly higher (.05) using the semantic mapping approach. However, no significant differences were found between the semantic mapping technique and the verbal readiness approach in relation to the main idea, inferential question, and detail questions

				manner to link episodic information; (2) the *Thematic Map* relates elements and details about persons, places, or things arrayed around the central theme; and (3) the *Classifaction Map* (Pearson & Johnson, 1978) was used for expository discourse involving concepts and examples. *Verbal Readiness Approach* (Control, 13 Ss): Ss received a traditional directed reading program. Sequence included: discuss new content, introduce new vocabulary orally and visually, form a purpose question, read silently and answer 10 multiple choice questions.		
Tollefson, Tracy, Johnson, Farmer, & Buenning (1984)	61	Junior high Ss receiving resource room services for at least one 50-min period/day. Identified by a three-step sequential decision-making process: (1) teacher referral and screening by a teacher with LD certification; (2) individual testing by the school psychologist; and (3) if test results indicated a discrepancy of at least 2 yr between ability and performance, the S was placed in the resource program through a formal staff meeting. Ss in this study	Goal setting Personal responsibility	The five teachers involved in this study attended a 1-day workshop that covered the concepts of realistic goal setting, use of feedback, and accepting personal responsibility. Teachers participated in all activities that were used later with the Ss, yielding ideas for modification as needed. Two achievement games (a basketball game and a baseball game) were used to measure Ss goal-setting strategies and to familiarize them with the data collection methods for this study. In each game, the Ss selected performance standards, predicted their own performance, then charted their actual scores. During the next phase of the study, each S was given a booklet of	The Intellectual Achievement Responsibility Scale (IAR; Crandall, Katovsky, & Crandall, 1965) was administered to both groups as a pretest and posttest. The respondent is presented with either a positive or a negative achievement situation and is required to choose between two attributions, one internal and one external. The score gives the	LD Ss as a group did not set realistic goals at the beginning of the study. Significant increases were observed in several S's usage of realistic goal setting as a result of treatment. Ss' overall ratings of the project were positive. However, transfer was limited because a small group of Ss were unable to see the connection between using the strategy successfully in the project and using the strategy to improve school performance.

(*continued*)

Author (year)	*N*	Selection criteria	Target domain(s)	Treatment(s)	Measures	Results
Tollefson, Tracy, Johnson, Farmer, & Buenning (1984) (*cont.*)		had WISC-R Full Scale IQs ranging between 1 and 2 *SD* below their grade placement on the mathematics and language subtests of the ITBS. LD Ss were randomly assigned within each of four junior high school resource rooms to either an experimental or a control group.		contracts and $100 in play money to invest. Each S was assigned to work in wither reading or math depending on the area most needing improvement. Ss selected 10 words or math problems each wk from a list of 20 judged moderately difficult for this study by the teacher. Ss predicted how many they would answer correctly on a test the following wk and charted their own prediction. This goal was written in a contract, along with a plan for goal attainment. Next, each S deposited an investment in a bank book, with the greatest returns possible when goals were achieved. After a test the following wk, Ss charted their actual scores and completed an evaluation section in their contracts, giving a causal explanation for each outcome, then modified their study plans as necessary. Play money payoffs were also made, and the beginning procedures were repeated for four phases total. Following the final treatment phase, posttesting began.	number of achievement situations where the persona takes responsibility. The Task Attribution Questionnaire (Tollefson et al., 1979) was administered as a posttest to the experimental group only to measure success expectancy and attribution for actual school performance. The subject predicts his/her performance on a verbal or quantitative task, is given feedback, and then explains the factors responsible for the actual performance. The Evaluation of Treatment Inventory (Tollefson et al., 1979) includes three multiple choice items that require participants to report their feelings about and evaluation of the project.	There were significantly more effort attributions made for success and for failure than for ability, task difficulty, or luck attributions during the contract phase of the study. The end-of-project attributions were similar. Overall, the experiment was successful in teaching LD adolescents to set realistic achievement goals, to expend effort pursuing those goals, and to accept personal responsibility for achievement outcomes.

Trifiletti, Frith, & Armstron (1984)	28	LD Ss attending a private school; selection criteria included current diagnosis of specific LD according to state guidelines, and math difficulties documented by a least a half grade deficit on the KeyMath Diagnostic Arithmetic Test. Ss were randomly assigned to an experimental or a control group.	Math skills	Two resource room teachers were involved in the study. Both received the pretest results and it was assumed that both taught skills that were deficient prior to the intervention. They were also given the pretest results of the criterion-referenced assessment included in the computer program used by the Ss in the experimental group. Both groups received 40 min of instruction daily for 1 academic yr. Experimental Ss received CAI while controls received daily math instruction from their resource teacher for the same amount of time. *Computerized Instruction:* Experimental Ss received computerized tutorial instruction, drill, games, assessment, or work problems on deficient skills identified during preassessment. Computerized drill and computerized assessments generated reports listing the S's speed and accuracy on each skill. Ss worked on three to five deficient skills simultaneously, In addition, paper and pencil homework sheets were assigned based on each S's target skills.	The KeyMath Diagnostic Arithmetic Test (Connolly, Natchman, & Pritchett, 1971) was administered as a pretest and as a posttest; the Spark 80 Criterion Referenced Mathematics Assessment was administered prior to treatment.	Ss in the CAI group learned almost twice the amount of new math skills as the resource instruction group, both at the end of the first semester and for the whole yr.
Whang, Fawcett, & Mathew (1984)	2	High school identified as LD and enrolled in at least 1 credit hour in the school's learning center. Both Ss were 17 yr of age. Their WAIS scores were 85 and 89. Both Ss received a $30 incentive payment for participation.	Social skills	A multiple BL design across skill categories was used in this study. During BL, the performance of each trainee was observed for each of six social skills. No specific instructions or feedback were provided in how to respond in the job-related situations. During treatment, Ss used a *Role-Playing Evaluation Script*	Observations were mad to document the percentage of occurrence for each of the trained skills: accepting a compliment, providing a compliment, accepting an	The procedures were effective in increasing the level of job-related social skills performed by the participants in analogue situations. Direct observations of performance taken at the

(*continued*)

Author (year)	*N*	Selection criteria	Target domain(s)	Treatment(s)	Measures	Results
Whang, Fawcett, & Mathews (1984) (*cont.*)				(Mathews et al., 1980) with six social interaction situations: providing a compliment, accepting an instruction from a supervisor, accepting a compliment, accepting criticism from a supervisor, providing constructive criticism, and explaining a problem to a supervisor. After three observation sessions, training to mastery was administered for the first and fourth skills. After the sixth observation session, training was conducted for the second and fifth skills. Training for the third and sixth skills occurred after the ninth observation session. Sessions were videotaped and rated. Follow-up, 4 wk after training, included one observation session for the six skills.	instruction, accepting criticism, providing constructive criticism, providing constructive criticism, and explaining a problem.	adolescents' place of employment suggest some generalization of training effects to actual work environments.
Beals (1985) Dissertation	9	LD students ages 14.7–16.8, with a mean IQ of 90.1 (WISC-R). Mean achievement scores in Reading = 17.78, Math = 11.63, and Writing = 14.29 (expressed in percentiles; no instruments were named).	Cooperative skills Reading Writing	Three groups, A, B, and C, and a no-treatment control group were included: *Group A, Writing Intervention*—instruction in two writing strategies, sentences and error monitoring. *Group B, Reading Intervention*—instruction in two reading strategies, self-questioning and paraphrasing. *Groups A and B, Cooperative Skills*—training took place in both groups over 5 days and included four parts: (1) *Orientation*, three types of goal structures	Percentage of sentences completed Error monitoring Percentage correct on comprehension tests Paraphrasing	LD Ss mastered specific learning strategies in a large group setting. However, the LD Ss had difficulty maintaining the skills.

				(competitive, individualistic, and cooperative); (2) *Activation,* Winter Survival Exercise (Johnson & Johnson, 1975); (3) *Skill Training* (Social Skills Associates, 1983), Ss learned to give help and feedback to each other; and (4) *Prestrategy Training* (Johnson & Johnson, 1975), developed Ss commitment to working in a group and perception questions. *Group C, Regular classroom*—with LD, low achieving, and high achieving students. Scoring focus was on the LD Ss. The three categories of Ss were combined together in groups for cooperative learning in either reading or writing skills. *No Treatment Control Group* was pretested in reading and writing with the same pretests as the intervention groups, but received no strategy training.		
Bos, Anders, Filip, & Jaffe (1985)	50	High school students with LD. IQ range, 85–115; reading range, from 3 to 7 yr below grade level according to district records. To further ensure that the two groups were similar in reading comprehension and intelligence, all Ss were given the passage comprehension subtest of the WRMT (1973) and the Standard Progressive Matrices (Ravens, 1960).	Reading comprehension	This study included one treatment and one control group. Experimental Ss were taught Semantic Feature Analysis (SFA), a content-area vocabulary and reading comprehension strategy. The procedure was based on another of these authors' empirical studies (1984), to which the reader was referred. No further information was provided regarding the treatment. Control Ss were instructed to use the Vocabulary Look Up (VLU) approach to find dictionary definitions for difficult words from reading passages.	Content area vocabulary Content area concepts	SFA was an effective strategy for teaching LD adolescents content area concepts, related vocabulary, and passage comprehension. Results of the follow-up study suggest that learning effects are long term.

(continued)

Author (year)	N	Selection criteria	Target domain(s)	Treatment(s)	Measures	Results
Carter (1985) Dissertation	40	Students aged 8.7–12.0 with a mean IQ (WISC-R) of 104, and scoring 1 SD or more below grade level in Reading (Woodcock–Johnson).	Reading	In both the experimental and control conditions, Ss sat around a table and read orally with immediate corrections on miscues. No phonic analysis or word attack was used. The study took place over 15 wk. Experimental Ss (20) were taught semantic mapping by receiving the text after they had developed the map on the chalkboard with teacher-supplied words inserted while Ss supplied the others. Then the text was given to the Ss, who read orally. The semantic map remained on the board until session's end. Control Ss (20) were taught using the SQ3R method. These Ss surveyed the material with instructor guidance to discuss the major topics. Overview of the story was done orally while surveying the pictures. All Ss were also tested for immediate recall of a reading passage in addition to recall of the same passage 2 and 7 days later.	Immediate recall 2-day recall 7-day recall	Significant differences occurred five times and neared significance six times. In each instance, the semantic mapping group had higher mean scores, leading researchers to the conclusion that semantic mapping was a more effective method than SQ3R for teaching reading comprehension (long- and short-term recall) to LD Ss.
Darch & Gersten (1985)	4	LD Ss aged 7.8–8.3 yr; met state guidelines for placement in an LD classroom. Each of the Ss had failed to learn basic reading skills associated with the 1st grade curriculum.	Oral reading	The reading class met 45 min/day. The first 20 min were used for the interventions for 25 school days. During BL, material was presented from Distar lessons. The teacher only indicated to Ss if answers were correct or incorrect. If incorrect, the teacher modeled the	Percent of correct responding to teacher questions Percent of on-task behavior	Increases in teacher presentation rate and increased use of praise lead to improvement in levels of on-task behavior and correct student responding. Each of the variables in

				correct response. Teacher pace was controlled as she/he paused 5 sec between the end of a S's response and the next part of the instruction. A modified reversal design was used with the four Ss in a reading class. The intervention incorporated the *Distar Reading I Program* (Engelmann & Bruner, 1975). The teacher systematically varied the rate of instructional presentation (rapid vs. slow pace) and frequency of praising (praise vs. no praise). The 5-sec pause used during BL was eliminated.		isolation had an effect. Praise appeared to be more powerful than presentation rate. The combination of thetwo variables had the most powerful effect.
Englert, Hiebert, & Stewart (1985)	22	Students enrolled in 11 resource room programs. Resource room teachers were asked to refer two students from their classrooms who performed at about the same 2nd grade reading level, lacked skills in reading and spelling basic sight vocabulary, and were proficient in their rhyming ability. Ten of the 11 Ss in the treatment group had 90+ IQ.	Spelling	Two groups were used in this intervention which took place in 10-min sessions, three times/wk, over 4 wk. Experimental Ss were taught a strategy for spelling new words by using spelling patterns from known words. They were taught a rhyming rule, i.e., when words rhyme, the last parts are often spelled the same. Experimental Ss were then taught an analogy strategy. First, two to three words were introduced from the Ss individual word list. Then, while looking at the word, the S spelled it. Next, the S spelled the word aloud from memory. Finally, the S wrote the word from memory two times. Ss were given practice transfer words as they found a	Spelling common words Spelling uncommon words Reading uncommon words Reading sight words	Performance of experimental Ss was significantly superior to that of control Ss in spelling both high-frequency sight words and an untrained set of transfer words. However, there was no significant difference between groups in their ability to read sight words or to read transfer words. The authors assert that these findings support the notion that direct instruction in an analogy strategy (comparing

(*continued*)

Author (year)	*N*	Selection criteria	Target domain(s)	Treatment(s)	Measures	Results
Englert, Hiebert, & Stewart (1985) (*cont.*)				given word that rhymed with the auditorially presented word. Control Ss learned to read and spell sight word vocabulary via direct instruction. The teacher said the word while presenting the printed stimulus. The teacher and S next said the word in unison. Then the S said the word independently. The Ss learned to spell the sight words in a two-step presentation. First, the S spelled the new word while looking at the printed word. Then, the S wrote the word from memory twice.		unfamiliar words with known words) can assist mildly handicapped students in spelling new words.
Harris & Graham (1985)	2	LD students receiving resource room services; identification as LD by the school district, IQ scores between 85 and 115 on both the Slosson Intelligence Test and the PPVT, achievement at least 2 yr below grade/age level in two or more academic areas, absence of any other handicapping condition, and interviews with the resource room teacher indicating composition problems. The TOWL was also administered to both Ss.	Composition skills	Training effects on three composition aspects (number of different *action words*, *action helpers*, and *describing words*) were investigated in a multiple BL across-behaviors design nested within a multiple BL across-Ss design. Two instructors received training and practice applying the experimental procedures; each was assigned to one S for the experiment duration. Detailed plans were provided; each step of the daily plan was checked as it was finished. Black-and-white pictures were mounted on a poster, then randomly ordered and preassigned for each day of instruction. Each instructor met with a S in a quiet	Before the experiment, both instructors completed training and guided practice in scoring the response measures: number of different *action words*, *action helpers*, *describing words*, and total number of words. Quality ratings were independently obtained at the end of the study. *Action words* were defined as words expressing either a	The Ss use of the parts of speech selected for intervention increased substantially above baseline, as did mean number of words per story. In addition, stories written after training obtained substantially higher quality ratings than BL compositions. Generalization and maintenance probes completed up to 14 wk following training continued to reflect improvements.

area for 45 min two to three times/wk. Learner and task analyses were used to construct task-specific and metacognitive strategies that were instructed using CBM procedures (Harris, 1982; Meichenbaum, 1983). Instructional steps and training components included: (1) introduce task-specific strategy, (2) review current performance level, (3) describe the learning strategy, (4) model the strategy and self-instructions, (5) master strategy steps, (6) perform controlled practice of strategy steps and self-instructions, (7) train data collection, (8) maintenance and generalization. After each S completed the instructional steps for action words, instruction for action helper began at the first step; describing words were taught last.

physical or mental movement, act, or occurrence. *Action helpers* were defined as words that modify a verb and express how something is done. *Describing words* were defined as adjectives that modify nouns and tell the quality or quantity of the thing named. *Total number of words* was defined as the number of words written that represented spoken words, without regard for misspellings. Quality ratings were completed for stories written on the last 2 BL days and the last 2 training days in each phase. The accuracy of students' self-assessments on the number of different action words, action helpers, and describing words was determined through correlations between the students' and instructor's original scores on a measure.

(*continued*)

Author (year)	N	Selection criteria	Target domain(s)	Treatment(s)	Measures	Results
Jaben (1985a)	52	Students from 5th and 6th grade classrooms for the LD; aged 11–12; able to read at the 3rd grade level at least; formally diagnosed LD by a multidisciplinary team; a minimum of 2 yr underachievement based on normative standards; IQ within normal limits; enrolled in intermediate level, self-contained classrooms. LD Ss were randomly assigned to either the treatment or the control condition.	Drawing Creativity	Control Ss continued to receive their regular program. The experimental treatment consisted of the Purdue Creative Thinking Program (PCTP) for two 45-min lessons/wk over a period of 14 wk; the PCTP has 28 audio tapes and printed materials designed to stimulate divergent thinking, figural and verbal fluency, flexibility, and originality. Components have three parts each: (1) a 3–4 min lesson that teaches a principle related to creative thinking, (2) a 10–12 min story about a famous American pioneer, and (3) three or four exercises related to content of the story.	Ss completed the Torrance Tests of Creative Thinking (figural booklet), Form A, before the onset of the instructional program. Subtests used for the pretest were Picture Completion and Parallel Lines since these subtests assess fluency, flexibility and originality as related to drawing. Within 1 wk after instruction was complete, the Torrance Tests of Creative Thinking (figural booklet), Form B, was given as a measure of divergent training effects on creativity.	The posttest scores were analyzed with ANCOVA procedures, with the pretest scores as covariates. Separate analyses were performed for figural fluency, figural flexibility, and figural originality. Support was obtained for use of the PCTP to raise LD students' scores on figural flexibility and figural originality, but significant improvement was not observed for figural fluency.
Jaben (1985b)	52	Ss were 5th and 6th grade students; formally diagnosed LD by a multidisciplinary team; at least 2 yr underachievement based on	Productive thinking	Training consisted of two 45-min lessons/wk for 14 wk using the Purdue Creative Thinking Program. Control Ss continued with their regular intervention program. All Ss were pretested with	The WISC-R (Weschler, 1974); the Peabody Individual Achievement Test, Reading	An ANCOVA procedure was applied with posttest Torrance scores as the dependent variables, with groups as factors and

		individual standardized testing; intelligence within normal limits; reading at least 3rd grade level; middle SES. Ss were randomly assigned to either a training or a control group.		Form A of the Torrance Tests. Posttesting occurred within 1 wk after completion of the training program.	Comprehension and Word Recognition subtests (Dunn & Markwardt, 1970); the Torrance Tests of Creative Thinking (figural subtests), Forms A and B, Picture Completion and Parallel Lines.	pretest scores as covariates. Significant effects for training were observed for figural flexibility and figural originality. Differential effects were not obtained for figural fluency.
Lovitt, Rudsit, Jenkins, Pious, & Benedetti (1985)	112	Students in each of seven classes were rank-ordered by test scores accumulated during the school yr in which the experiment was conducted, then divided into high, medium, and low achievement groups. Two Ss were selected from each ability group within each class to form the experimental group; at least one LD S was included in each low group. *Experimental Group:* 42 Ss were randomly selected by assigning numbers to each S, then asking the teacher to select two numbers from each within-class group. *Control/Contrast Groups:* high (25), medium	Science	Curriculum specialists designed adaptations for a 7th grade science test chapter in consultation with the participating teachers. Both teachers selected the Study Guide (SG) and Precision Teaching (PT) methods and rejected the Visual Spatial method as incompatible with their teaching styles. Control and contrast Ss received their regular textbook assignments, lab exercises, and readings from a supplemental science magazine. Experimental Ss were instructed in an adjoining room for 10 min/day for 10 consecutive school days. *Precision Teaching:* Paired Ss read isolated words from a vocabulary drill sheet to each other in a 1-min timed format, then wrote down the number of words read. The second day of PT consisted of timed samples of filling in	A 29-item multiple choice test was administered as a pretest and again on day 9. Two write-facts assessme nts were given on day 5 and day 10 where Ss were prompted to write as much as they could recall of previously instructed topics for 10 min.	Both adaptations were successful with Ss of all achievement levels when presented through the collaborative model. Surveys completed by control Ss indicated Ss thought that all Ss should have been in the study, they disliked the write-facts tests, and they felt that more hints during assessment would have been helpful. Survey responses of the experimental Ss suggested they believed that the two methods helped, the study should be extended, the write-facts tests should be eliminated (although some suggested making the tests

(*continued*)

Author (year)	*N*	Selection criteria	Target domain(s)	Treatment(s)	Measures	Results
Lovitt, Rudsit, Jenkins, Pious, & Benedetti (1985) (*cont.*)		(27), and low (18) achieving Ss in each classroom were selected as controls using the same procedures described above; the remaining Ss served as contrast Ss. The treatment conditions were randomly scheduled into participating teachers' classes, with first period determined by a coin toss with successive periods alternating. Ss were rank-ordered by classroom tests taken up to that point of the yr, then divided into high, medium, and low groups; two Ss were then randomly selected from each ability group to form experimental groups; at least one LD S was included in each low group; three subgroups were selected as controls; the remainder were contrast Ss.		blanks on a worksheet from which key words were omitted. The worksheet was placed under an acetate sheet and Ss used a special pen to write. The remaining days followed this procedure using different worksheets. PT tasks were implemented by the project coordinator. *Study Guides:* This task was implemented by the teachers while the project coordinator supervised the other Ss in another room. The first day consisted of orientation to the project. Ss were provided with folders containing two types of worksheets the next day, (1) a framed outline of the chapter's main ideas sequentially organized, and (2) vocabulary exercises. Key words were omitted, and Ss were asked to fill these in as the teacher lectured. Ss were required to supply words, to supply definitions, or to match words to definitions. The method used was mainly lecturing.		easier and more specific), and the timed practices should be increased (a few wanted more lab time).
Nelson (1985) Dissertation	24	LD boys aged 7–11; selected from three Alameda, CA, elementary schools; identified as impulsive from MFFT scores; normal intelligence,	Impulsivity	Ss were assigned to one of three groups using a randomized block design; all participated in six, half-hr sessions, distributed once/day, 3 days/wk for a 2-wk period.	The efficacy of treatment conditions was assessed by seven dependent measures, including the MFFT	Significant differences were obtained between the groups that demonstrated the superiority of the CSI treatment. Ss in the CSI

		but functioning 2 or more yrs below expectancies in one or more academic areas. All Ss enrolled in special classes for Ss with LD.		*Cognitive Self-Instruction (CSI):* Treatment combined elements of Meichenbaum's Cognitive Self-Instruction (1971) and Egeland's scanning strategies (1974); Ss received behavior control training proceeding from overt verbalization modeling through covert self-verbalization. *Materials Practice (MP):* Same number of sessions, with exposure to same materials without training, modeling, or guidance; Ss worked independently with the training materials. *No Treatment Control (NTC):* Ss did not receive training or materials practice; sessions were spent talking to training or working on activities of own choice.	(Kagan et al., 1964); the WISC-R (Weschler, 1974) Performance IQ and the Picture Arrangement, Object Assembly, Block Design, and Coding subtests; and the Porteus Mazes.	group obtained significantly higher scores on MFFT latency; MFFT errors; and WISC-R Performance IQ, Picture Arrangement, and Object Assembly. Overall, the results suggest that impulsivity is a modifiable characteristic of LD boys.
Omizo, Cubberley, & Omizo (1985)	60	Children certified LD by the Texas Education Agency (TEA, 1976); with IQ scores above 90; aged 8–11. Ss were randomly assigned to two groups which were then designated experimental or control by a coin toss. Experimental Ss were divided into three groups of 10 children each; similar format and content were used for all three groups.	Self-concept Locus of control	Experimental Ss met for about 1 hr, twice a wk, for 12 wks. Pretesting and posttesting brought the total wks to 14. The intervention consisted of group instruction in Rational–Emotive Education (REE) facilitated by a trained leader. Activities involved peer group instruction, tutoring, exercises, games, and lectures about REE principles. Objectives included acquisition of the REE format; acquisition of basic problem-solving skills; understanding the influence of thoughts on feelings;	Ss were administered the Dimensions of Self-Concept Scale (Michael & Smith, 1978) and the Nowicki–Strickland Locus of Control Scale (Nowicki & Strickland, 1973) 1 wk prior to the intervention and again 1 wk after the last study session.	A MANOVA of the posttest data revealed significant differences between the experimental and control groups. Post hoc univariate *F*-tests and discriminant function analyses indicated that Level of Aspiration, Leadership and Initiative, and Anxiety were significant discriminators, with experimental Ss

(*continued*)

Author (year)	N	Selection criteria	Target domain(s)	Treatment(s)	Measures	Results
Omizo, Cubberley, & Omizo (1985) (*cont.*)				understanding that feelings are not expressed identically; transfer of learning to various life situations; coping strategy development; expressing feelings concretely and accurately; learning to support, empathize with, and encourage others; and learning to identify and dispute irrational thoughts. Control group Ss met twice/wk in small groups and listened to short stories to control for the effects of this type of participation.		having higher scores for Level of Aspiration and Leadership and Initiative, and lower scores for Anxiety. Ss receiving the experimental treatment also evidenced significantly more internal locus of control orientation. REE therefore appears to be effective in encouraging LD Ss to increase three positive aspects of self-concept and to develop a more internal locus of control.
Portsmouth, Wilkins, & Airey (1985)	26	Ss attending a day school for children with moderate learning problems; drawn from classes with ages ranging from 8+ to 15+; selection based on reading level at least 2 yrs below age expectancies. After being grouped into pairs, 28 Ss were matched on the Stanford C Reading Test of Reading Accuracy, then each S in the 14 matched pairs was randomly assigned to either an experimental or a control group (attrition reduced the	Reading	Parents of all Ss were asked to participate with their children in this intervention. After Ss were assigned to the experimental group, their parents were interviewed one family at a time and the study was explained to them, including their role as home tutors. Each family received a booklet of guidelines for parents' reference at home. Parents and children worked together for 20 wks, recording the frequency of at-home reading sessions in the booklet. Ss were tested three separate times after 4, 12, and 20 wk of the project. Parents were also interviewed at these times.	The Neale Reading Test (Reading Accuracy, Reading Rate, and Reading Comprehension subtests) and the English Picture Vocabulary Test were administered as pretests, then as posttests during the study at the end of 4 and 12 wk of intervention, and finally at the conclusion of the study.	Reading accuracy improved significantly for the experimental group. Most of the experimental Ss made 4–7 mo reading gains. The majority of control Ss made gains between 0 and 3 mo. The experimental Ss maintained their reading gains throughout the intervention period. While statistically significant differences on final posttests of reading rate

		sample size to 26). Experimental and control Ss were then group-matched by scores on the Neale Reading Accuracy Test, the English Picture Vocabulary Test, and their IQ scores (obtained from school records).				were not obtained, the experimental group gains were better than those of the control Ss on all final posttests of reading rate, reading comprehension, and listening vocabulary. The mean experimental group gain in reading age, i.e., over 1 mo/mo of intervention, was greater than typical gains made by children in this type of school.
Scruggs & Tolfa (1985)	16	LD Ss in 2nd and 3rd grade in special education classes; classified according to national, state, and local standards; identification criteria included a 40% discrepancy (expressed in standard scores) between ability and achievement in at least two academic areas. Current IQ scores were not available in study, although all Ss were reported to function within normal limits. Ss were individually matched based on grade and prior yr achievement scores, then randomly assigned to either a training or a no-treatment control condition.	Test-taking skills	Experimental Ss received strategy training with materials similar in format to the Word Study Skills and Reading Comprehension subtests of the Stanford Achievement Test. Eight scripted lessons were provided through direct instruction methods; items were similar, but not identical to, those on the Stanford. Specific strategies were taught for each subtest. Instruction for the experimental Ss occurred in four 20-min sessions each wk for 2 wk total. The first seven lessons were content-specific, and the last session was a general review.	The Stanford Achievement Test (Kelly, Madden, Gardner, & Rudman, 1964). Prior yr scores were used to construct the study sample. Posttest scores were obtained from current yr testing.	LD Ss trained in test-taking skills obtained significantly higher scores than their untrained LD peers on the Word Study Skills subtest but the two groups were not differentiated by the Reading Comprehension subtest scores at posttest. The mean effect size for trained Ss for the Word Study Skills subtest (1.01 *SD* unist) as well as the total score effect size (.63 *SD* units) were substantially larger than those previously observed in the research. This study provided additional support for efforts to improve the test-wiseness

(*continued*)

Author (year)	N	Selection criteria	Target domain(s)	Treatment(s)	Measures	Results
Schunk (1985)	30	Ss were 6th grade children from two middle schools; previously identified as LD in mathematics by the school district according to state guidelines; receiving special education services daily. IQ scores within normal limits (85–115) on the WISC-R (Weschler, 1974), and mathematics scores on the Woodcock–Johnson, Revised (Woodcock & Johnson, 1977) from 1 to 1.5 SDs lower than their WISC-R scores. The final criterion was nomination by the resource room teacher. Following the pretest, Ss were randomly assigned by sex and school to one of three treatment groups.	Self-efficacy Math	All Ss received 45-min training sessions over 5 consecutive school days. They worked on a packet consisting of seven sets of materials ordered from least difficult to most difficult. The format for these sets was identical. Page 1 contained directions and examples; there were similar problems to solve on the next six pages. Ss were seated individually by an adult proctor in the resource room; distance between Ss was maintained to avoid contact. The proctor reviewed the directions, then instructed the Ss to complete the pages in order. Careful work was emphasized, then the proctor moved out of view. The Ss solved problems alone and did not receive feedback about accuracy. *Self-Set Goals:* At the beginning of each session, the proctor suggested a goal-setting strategy and encouraged the student to set a goal, then moved out of sight. *Assigned Goals:* The proctor established the minimum number of pages to complete. *No Goals:* These children received the math training, but no goal instructions.	Self-efficacy: An instrument developed by the author in previous research was employed; scores ranged from 10–100 in 10 unit intervals from high uncertainty (10) through intermediate values (50–60), to complete certitude (100). Practice was provided wherein children judged their certainty of successfully jumping progressively longer distances. Each child was then shown 25 sample pairs of subtraction problems for about 2 sec/pair, then he/she circled an efficacy value indicating his/her degree of certainty that the problem could be solved. Subtraction skills: 25 problems ranging from 2–6 columns which measured the Ss' independent math skills on problems of varying degrees of difficulty.	Participation in establishing goals enhanced self-efficacy and math skills of LD Ss, with the strongest effect on self-efficacy observed in the group that established their own goals.

Swanson (1985)	1	A severely hearing-impaired child identified as having behavioral and learning difficulties was the S in this study. The S was receiving special education services in a self-contained class. IQ was estimated between 80 and 90, and reading comprehension and spelling scores on the PIAT were below the 15th percentile. Conduct problems included defiance of authority, attention seeking, and hyperactivity.	General academic achievement	Two experiments were conducted, although only Study 1 is reported. A multiple BL across-tasks design was used. During BL, normal classroom procedures were in effect, including individualized classroom learning activities, tutoring on corrective reading and spelling, and tokens (points) for correct academic performance and appropriate conduct. During treatment, self-instructed global strategies were coupled with explicit instruction on task components in reading and spelling. Tokens were given for correct academic performance and for appropriate conduct. Self-instruction was taught through sign language due to S's hearing loss. Materials included: *Merrill Linguistic Readers*, *Scientific Research Associates* (SRA), *Barbe Word List*, *Dolch Word List*, and reading comprehension passages. Generalization included three phases: (1) *Setting*—environmental changes included different room color, desks, and seating arrangements; (2) *Person*—teacher was new to the academic tasks, but the subject area was familiar; and (3) *Task*—activities were similar in content, grade level, procedure, and materials used during BL, but reading comprehension materials were different.	Spelling: percentage of correct responses	The findings lend evidence to the clinical utility of cognitive–behavioral training with handicapped children on academic tasks.

(continued)

Author (year)	*N*	Selection criteria	Target domain(s)	Treatment(s)	Measures	Results
Swanson & Scarpati (1985)	2	*Experiment 1:* Ss were selected from a special education self-contained classroom in a university laboratory school. S1 was a 9th grader, aged 14.6. His IQ score was 99 (WISC-R) and his academic scores included (in GE): reading comprehension, 4.4 (WRMT), and spelling, 2.8 (Peabody Individual Achievement Test). S2 was an 8th grader, aged 13.8. His IQ score was 93 (WISC-R), and his academic scores were reading comprehension, 3.9, and spelling. 2.9 (both scores GE from the Peabody Individual Achievement Test).	*Experiment 1* Reading Spelling	*Experiment 1:* A multiple BL was used to train Ss in the use of self-instruction. During BL, Ss were engaged for 45 min in individualized classroom learning and tutoring. Tokens were given for correct academic performance and for appropriate conduct. During treatment, *Self-Instruction* (S-I) was taught individually. Treatment took place in the same time period and setting as BL and the token system was the same as in BL. S-I followed the verbal modeling procedure of five steps (Meichenbaum & Goodman, 1971). The teacher verbally modeled the general error-monitoring strategy. Ss were also given specific questions to ask themselves. For example, "How do I understand this passage before I read it? I need to ask myself the questions who, what, when, where, why, how." Similar questions were asked for spelling.	*Experiment 1* Comprehension and spelling: percent of correct responses.	For both experiments, self-instruction training impromved academic performance. Generalization occurred across setting, person, and task in Experiment 1 and across setting in Experiment 2. It was concluded that successful academic performance occurs when self-instructional statements integrate global strategies while simultaneously directing attention to task specific information.
	1	*Experiment 2 :* S was a 13-yr-old selected from a self-contained class for the severely educationally handicapped. His IQ score on the Peabody Picture Vocabulary Test was in the	*Experiment 2* Math	*Experiment 2:* Similar to Experiment 1, but focused on math with S-I. A reversal design was used. S was given 10 problems daily on a worksheet; the task required carrying 2- and 3-digit arithmetic problems. During BL 1, the S completed a math sheet each day; and	*Experiment 2* Math: percent of correct responses	

		range 85–100, with a math achievement score below the 8th percentile (WRAT).	received a	token for each correct response. During the S-I treatment, individual instruction and tokens were provided. The teacher gave one verbal prompt for each component of S-I, e.g., "What is it you have to do?" During BL 2, S-I training was eliminated. The S was told not to talk aloud. All other procedures were the same as BL 1. During the second treatment phase, S-I was reimplemented using the same procedures as the first S-I phase.		
Tansey (1985)	8	Six of the Ss were formally diagnosed as LD, and were in classes for the neurologically impaired. The other two Ss were diagnosed as being perceptually impaired and hyperactive, respectively. Ss ranged in age from 7.11 to 15.3 yr. Four of the Ss' WISC-R IQ scores were between 76 and 85, while the other four scored between 102 and 116.	Brainwave activity	A multisubject A-B-A experimental design was utilized to assess the impact of operantly conditioned increases of the 14 Hz neural discharge rhythm, as monitored over the sensorimotor (Rolandic) cortex of the brain, where the active electrode was situated so as to maximally facilitate bilateral hemispheric transactions and conditioning. In search of relations between monitored cerebro–cortico–neural events and ongoing behavior, the pretreament BLs, against which to evaluate the effects of hypothesized altered cerebral function, were selected ad follows: an assessment of each S's LD and the administration of the WISC-R. The SS were provided with long-term, symptom duration,	EEG readings	Observation of the changing brainwave signatures showed a tendency for decreased slow wave activity concomitant with increases in fast wave activity, for cases with a Full Scale IQ within the range 76–85. Ss with a Full Scale IQ within the range 102–116 exhibited increased amplitudes over most of the monitored bands, but with the increases being much less at the slower frequencies. It is noteworthy that four Ss with significant Verbal and

(continued)

Author (year)	*N*	Selection criteria	Target domain(s)	Treatment(s)	Measures	Results
Tansey (1985) (*cont.*)				sensorimotor rhythm biofeedback (SMR) training for the remediation of their LDs. Simultaneous recording of five frequency bands of brainwave activity (5 Hz, 7 Hz, 10 Hz, 12 Hz, 14 Hz) was completed, intended to provide a glimpse of the "brainwave signature" reflective of the dynamic and synergistic processes involved in cerebro–neural activation and the brain's global response to such an alteration in the sensorimotor subnetwork. Each weekly session began with a 10- to 15-min review of each S's status the previous wk. Biofeedback training lasted 30 min. Ss were reclined with eyes closed when the instructions were presented. They were instructed to let themselves become hollow and heavy, and let the beeps come out. Intermittent, positive reinforcement was provided every few min for beep production. Every 10 min, the initial-orientation instructions were reported. Ss received a tangible reward (Matchbox car) at the end of each session, contingent upon having had many beeps come out. The control condition was the precondition, or BL.		Performance score discrepancies exhibited no less tha a 40% greater increase in the lower of the two IQ scores; indicating that this SMR training procedure also resulted in an increased symmetry in the interhemispheric interactions reflective of the higher cortical functions for these no longer LD Ss.

Vivion (1985) Dissertation	6	LD Ss were aged 10–12 attending an elementary special education resource program and mainstreamed in grades 4 to 6. They had normal intelligence and good oral language, and manifested their disability in an inability to read with comprehension. On the Clinical Evaluation of Language Functioning (CELF), Ss' average percentile range in processing was 69–99, and on production was 48–80. The Stanford Diagnostic Reading Test indicated the following results: Auditory Vocabulary, average or above average; Reading Skills, stanines 4 to 6; and Reading Comprehension, stanines 1 to 3. The Durrell Analysis of Reading Difficulty (DARD) indicated (in GE): Oral Reading, 3L to 3H, and Listening Comprehension, 3L to 3H.	Reading comprehension	The experiment analyzed the effect on literal reading comprehension of providing instruction in the application of psycholinguistic strategies used intuitively in apprehending meaning in discourse. A multiple choice cloze procedure was used to implement the investigation in a multielement BL design. The design involved repeated measurement of a behavior under alternating conditions of the independent variable. During BL, two passages were presented, one of which was one level above the preinstructional level and one of which was two levels above the preinstructional level. The Ss were asked to read and complete a multiple choice cloze exercise. After each completion, prompts were given regarding the correctness of each response. Praise was givin for a correct response. If the response was incorrect, the researcher circled the correct response in red pencil. During treatment, the teacher taught a concept lesson and trained Ss to use the *Strategies for completing Cloze Passages* checklist, defined "strategy" and "cur," presented strategies to be learned in checklist form (to be read during instruction and again later for self-instruction), and provided examples of strategies. Trained strategies	Comprehension questions: mean percentage correct SDRT (Form X) DARD	All Ss made use of the strategies to varying degrees in determining cloze replacements. Although there was considerable intra- and inter-S variability in BL and instructional condition data, literal reading comprehension was generally higher for all Ss during the instruction condition. All Ss evidenced an increase in literal reading comprehension from pre- to posttest of 1–2 grade levels. Comparisons of BL and instruction data indicated that practice with the cloze procedure was not as effective in increasing literal reading comprehension as discussion of the psycholinguistic strategies. It was concluded that RD children with good oral language may increase in literal reading comprehension when given instruction in the application of psycholinguistic strategies.

(*continued*)

Author (year)	*N*	Selection criteria	Target domain(s)	Treatment(s)	Measures	Results
Vivion (1985) *(cont.)*				included meaning, restating, phonics/word analysis, scanning, and parts of speech. Next, Ss completed *First Reading* (R1). Each S was directed to look at the first of two cloze passages and read through the passage silently, without stopping to replace deleted words. Multiple choice answers were covered. Passage content was discussed with the researcher, and supporting phrases were underlined. The S was directed to read the passage again, and to guess words that could make sense in the blanks. During the *Second Reading* (R2), each S was directed to reread the passage again silently, with the multiple choice answers visible. The S looked for the answers while reading. Feedback was provided after each sentence and correct strategies were discussed. The S was then asked to retell the passage content without looking at the text. The materials included the *SSPED Test Development Notebook,* the *Cloze Training Manual,* and the *Multiple-Choice Cloze Exercises Handbook.*		

Wilsher, Atkins, & Manfield (1985)	46	Dyslexic boys aged 8–13 referred to the Language Development Unit of Aston University; 42 had both reading and spelling problems, 4 had only spelling problems; all were of above-average ability, and were diagnosed by the clinical procedures defined by Thomson (1979). Criterion for inclusion included (1) WISC-R Full Scale IQ > 90; (2) discrepancy between mental age and reading age of more than 2 yr; (3) English as the primary language; (4) no emotional disturbance; (5) no educational deprivation; (6) no significant hearing impairment; (7) no significant sight impairment; (8) no gross neurological defect. Piracetam blood levels were verified under blind conditions prior to treatment.	Reading	Ss were administered 10 ml of syrup daily of either Piracetum or a placebo in a double-blind, parallel experiment, for a period of 8 wk.	British Abilities Scales (B.A.S.) Word Reading Test (Elliot, Murray, & Pearson, 1978): a word identification-task yielding a percentile standardized score Neale Analysis of Reading Ability (Neale, 1966): a passage reading test that analyzes reading rate and accuracy, producing a standardized test age (i.e., reading age) Free writing: Ss were given 5 min to write an essay. Measures of improvement on this writing sample were number of words written and percentage of spelling mistakes.	Significant treatment effects were not obtained. However, within-S analyses revealed significant improvements in reading rate and accuracy in Ss who received Piracetum. In addition, stratifying the Ss by reading age revealed that children with higher reading ages initially who received Piracetum improved significantly compared to similar Ss who received the placebo.
Zieffle & Romney (1985)	30	LD children volunteered to participate; each was a minimum of 2 yr below grade level. Ss were randomly allocated to one of three groups; two groups received treatment and one group served as controls.	Impulsive and inattentive behavior	Both treatment groups received ten 30-min sessions spaced over 3 wk. One group was trained to use self-instruction to clarify task requirements and impose verbal control over task performance. The second experimental group was trained to systematically tense and relax	Four instruments were selected for their sensitivity to impulsivity and inattention. Each child was given these tests in the same order: Porteus Mazes	A significant interaction between group and treatment was obtained from a repeated-measures ANOVA, with the two treatment groups performing better than the

(*continued*)

Author (year)	*N*	Selection criteria	Target domain(s)	Treatment(s)	Measures	Results
Zieffle & Romney (1985) (*cont.*)				various muscle groups. The control group continued with their regular program.	(Porteus, 1965), the Matching Familiar Figures (Kagan, 1966), and the Coding and Digit Span subtests of the WISC-R (Weschler, 1974).	controls on posttesting. However, support was not obtained for the superiority of one treatment group over the other.
Balcerzak (1986) Dissertation	40	Ss ranged in age from 9.6 to 12.4, had IQs ranging from 85 to +115, and averaged 87.75 on the KABC, which was used to identify Ss' strengths in sequential and simultaneous processing abilities.	Reading Mathematics Self-concept	Experimental Ss received instruction for 15 wk. Instruction was based on Ss' preferred learning style, step-by-step sequential processing, holistic simultaneous processing, or a combination of the two. Sequential processing lessons emphasized the presentation of information through a step-by-step gradual approach to teach the overall concept or skill. Steps included: break tasks down into steps; S verbalizes the strategy; state the rules; present tasks in a concrete fashion with manipulatives, pictures, models, diagrams, graphs; and emphasize visualization and imagery. Control Ss continued regular classroom instruction.	WRMT Piers–Harris Self-Concept Scale Mathematics scores	There was a significant increase in posttest mathematics scores over pretest mathematics scores for the experimental group as opposed to the control group. Improvement in reading achievement for the experimental group reached significance when compared to the control condition. There was no significant difference between the two groups on the self-concept scale measurement.

Chan & Cole (1986)	72	Ss enrolled in remedial classes or clinics; LD defined as ability within normal limits, with reading skills 2 or more yr below average expectancies for chronological age; excluded children with severe emotional disturbance (SED), physical, and/or sensory handicaps. Regular class Ss were matched with LD Ss on reading level; selected from 3rd grade classes at the same schools.	Metacognitive skills Reading comprehension	Groups of four to five Ss, clustered by age, received training a half-hr/day for a total of 4 days; there was one teacher for all Ss. Training sessions followed the same procedure for all groups: (1) strategy introduced using a toy robot followed by practice with a story booklet, (2) review and practice with another story booklet, (3) and (4) the same as the second session, but two passages were covered. Ss in the Self-Questioning Only condition were taught to generate questions about test. Ss in the Underlining Only group underlined interesting words, then generated questions about the words. Ss in the Read–Reread condition read the story twice to control for the extra time required for strategy training in the other conditions. Ss answered comprehension questions after each story. For the first three sessions, reference to test was allowed. Correct answers were provided during Sessions 1 and 2 when needed.	St. Lucia Graded Word Reading Test (Andrews, 1973); comprehension tests (multiple choice format) derived from story booklets used to train strategies; verbal reports regarding strategy use A comprehension score was calculated after session 3. To assess recall, questions were answered after session 4 without referring to the test. The next day, transfer was measured by uncued responses to questions about two more stories.	LD Ss in all three experimental conditions performed significantly better than those in the control group, although this effect was not obtained from the normal Ss. Differential effectiveness for the three strategies was not observed. Spontaneous transfer of the strategies by the LD Ss was not observed, although limited use of underlining was reported.
Chiang (1986)	6	Ss were 4th graders enrolled in a summer tutoring program. Mean age was 10.3. Ss were previously identified as LD by a public school multidisciplinary team according to the criteria set	Multiplication skills	The experiment consisted of three phases: BL, computer-assisted instruction (CAI), and transfer. During BL, girls received 4 days of 1-hr BL sessions, while boys received 3 days. Flashcards and math games were used, along with 4-min timings of	Multiplication facts: accuracy rate	Results of the daily 4-min timings of each S's multiplication facts indicated that about 12 days' drill and practice on a computer yielded an average gain of 4.7 and 6.1

(*continued*)

Author (year)	*N*	Selection criteria	Target domain(s)	Treatment(s)	Measures	Results
Chiang (1986) (*cont.*)		forth in PL 94-142. All Ss had been referred to the tutoring program to learn multiplication facts.		multiplication facts using worksheets from a computer program, Fact Sheets (Smith, 1982). Treatment consisted of CAI, and instervention was provided for 1 hr daily for 11 days. Various computer math programs were used, including Multiplication Table (Society for Visual Education, 1983), Micro Multiplication (Hayden Software, 1983), A Treasure Hunt of Facts (Josten Learning System, 1984), and Meteor Multiplication (Chaffin & Maxwell, 1982). CAI also included the use of a voice synthesizer. Transfer sessions (12) incorporated CAI activities and timings from Phase 2. Four-min timings on worksheets were used to measure the degree of transfer.		facts/min for the girls and boys, respectively, as evidenced by their worksheet performance.
Cochrane & Ballard (1986)	5	Ss were identified by senior school staff as needing special assistance, primarily on the grounds of failure to show progress in reading after 2–4 yr of schooling. Ss ranged in age from 7.9 to 10.1. Three Ss showed limited progress in academic skills and were considered as probably eligible for placement in a special class for backward	Reading fluency	A psychologist and a teacher worked together to establish a remedial reading program for the Ss. Effects of this program were evaluated using a single-S design. During BL, no treatment was provided; initial data were collected over a 4-wk period. During the intervention phase, each S was individually taught for 5—6 min/day. *The Mangere Home and School Program* (Glynn, McNaughton, Robinson, & Quinn, 1979) was used with S1 and S5. The teacher delayed	Reading: accuracy and self-corrections	Repeated measures data showed marked increases in reading skills and book reading levels, and a substantial increase over zero BL levels in independent reading during class reading time. The teacher commented favorably on the consultation model used and agreed with parents'

		children. One S had been retained for 1 yr in the junior class because of slow progress, and continued to demonstrate limited academic skills. The final S suffered from cerebral palsy and received ongoing physical therapies with the school.		attention to errors, used specific prompts for unknown words, and praised self-correction and accurate reading. Three successive interventions were used for Ss 2, 3, and 4, who were being considered for the special class for backward children. *The Otara Five Minute Reading Programme* (Otara FMRP; Awatere, 1982) was used as a temporary deviation from reading meaningful text to learning letter names and sounds, sight words, and reading sentences. The teacher also wrote the S's dictated text which then became the reading text. A reading log system for all Ss. Reading aloud to an adult facilitated independent reading. Each day, Ss were required to select and read three books, and then record the date and titles in a folder entitled *Maintenance Phase.*		observation that significant reading gains had been made by their children.
Darch & Carnine (1986)	24	Ss were 4th, 5th, and 6th graders; school-identified by a multidisciplinary team; assignment by stratified random sampling; IQ within normal limits, depressed reading achievement.	Literal and factual comprehension of science and social studies material.	Instruction was delivered in an LD classroom by the same teacher. Sessions were about 50 min for each of 9 consecutive school days. All Ss were taught the same content; information organization was varied for each group. Content was presented by visual display with a scripted description by the teacher for Group 1. Content instruction via text was provided for Group 2. Initial instruction was followed by review and group study sessions. There were three units of instruction total, with three lessons each.	All measures were developed for this study, including five tests of material taught, i.e., pretest, probe tests (three), posttest, transfer test. There was also a S attitude measure.	There were significant positive effects for the group taught with visual displays. No significant differences were obtained on the transfer test. Results from the S attitude questionnaire did not support Ss' preference for either teaching method, nor did they suggest that S attitudes about the group study procedure varied by group.

(continued)

Author (year)	*N*	Selection criteria	Target domain(s)	Treatment(s)	Measures	Results
Darch & Eaves (1986)	22	Ss were LD 9th, 10th, and 11th graders identified and placed in special classrooms. They had difficulties in reading comprehension. Ss were randomly assigned to one of two groups.	Comprehension of science concepts	The same teacher delivered instruction in LD resource classroom. Each of three units was covered for about 50 min/day for 4 consecutive school days. The same content was provided to both groups. Procedures were varied according to mode of information presentation. Visual Display: Information was organized by visual spatial display of unit concepts. Ss received copies of the display during Session 1, following along while the teacher described the conceptual relationships using a detailed script. During Sessions 2–4, they reviewed the concepts using a blank and a labeled display. Sessions 2–4 ended with cooperative group study in a game format. Text: Material was presented in a typical format, i.e., text with teacher-initiated group instruction. The teacher introduced the topic in Session 1, followed by S text reading interspersed with comprehension questions. Each session ended with group study focused on generating text related questions and group discussion.	Six tests were developed for this study: Unit tests were 5-item probes following each subunit. The posttest was a 10-item measure of total intervention. The maintenance test was a 10-item measure.	The visual display technique was more effective than the text method for teaching LD Ss, as documented by the unit tests and the posttest. Visual display Ss remembered more key concepts than did Text Ss as measured by the posttest; both groups performed poorly on both the maintenance and the transfer test.

Darch & Gersten (1986)	24	LD Ss enrolled in high school resource classes; school-identified based on a significant discrepancy between expected and actual achievement. Ss were randomly assigned to one of two treatments.	Reading comprehension	Instruction was delivered in the resource room. Fifty-min daily sessions were provided for 9 days total. The same teacher instructed both groups. Ss in the Advance Organizer group were provided with an outline/overview of important facts and concepts from each unit prior to text reading; method followed a direct instruction format. About 15 min of preteaching stressed systematic rehearsal of facts and concepts, with Ss responding to explicit questions and teacher modeling correct responses when errors occurred. Text was read aloud by individual Ss, with the teacher providing words as needed. Each period ended with independent study time. The Basal (Control) treatment followed the style typically suggested in teacher guides, i.e., loosely structured motivational activities introduced in a lecture-and-discussion format, followed by S reading of text. Independent study completed sessions for this group as well.	WRMT; three measures developed for this study, i.e., a 6-item pretest, three 6-item unit tests, and a 9-item posttest.	Mean group performance on the pretest was not significantly different. Analysis of the unit tests revealed significantly higher scores for the Advance Organizer Ss. Performance increased slightly for both groups over time, but the effect was not significant. Ss in the Advance Organizer group approached mastery on the posttest, while Basal Ss performed more poorly, and this difference was significant as well.
Fiedorowicz (1986)	15	All of the Ss met rigorous criteria for a reading disability. Mean age was 11.2; mean IQ was 97.2; and mean reading score on the WRAT was 3.9. Ss displayed one of three reading disability subtypes as treated in this study.	Oral reading Decoding skills	Ss met for forty-three 30-min sessions and formed three subgroups: Oral Reading, Associative, and Sequential. On the rationale that CAI training procedures emphasizing accuracy and speed of response to letters, syllables, and words would improve reading skills, the Ss were involved daily in CAI training for 2.5	Oral reading: accuracy and speed Auditory visual matching to sample: accuracy Word Recognition Phonetic knowledge	CAI training procedures were not only effective in improving component reading skills, but there was also a transfer of training to achievement measures of reading word recognition. This study lends support

(continued)

Author (year)	*N*	Selection criteria	Target domain(s)	Treatment(s)	Measures	Results
Fiedorowicz (1986) (*cont.*)				mo. Two schedules of testing and training allowed for an untrained control group and a follow-up group. Type O Ss were trained in the oral reading procedure. Ss read aloud, as accurately and quickly as possible, while stimuli were presented on the screen. Type A Ss were trained in the auditory–visual matching-to-sample method. These Ss matched an auditory sample with the correct visual item presented as three choices. Type S Ss were trained either as Type O or Type A above. These Ss matched a visual sample with the correct visual items presented as three choices. The three conditions all included: 50 stimulus items or trials for one run, 10-sec latency limit per trial, 0 second intertrial interval, 300 msec presentation of correct response signal, 1500 msec presentation of incorrect response signals with correct item presented. Ss trained on one type of stimulus item before moving on the to the next item. Stimuli included CV and VC syllables, CVC syllables, CVC words, CVVC syllables, CVVC words CVCV syllables, and CVCV words. Two criteria were used: accuracy and latency.		to the hypothesis that training according to subgroup classification, using training procedures that incorporate an application of the automaticity theory and a combination of task-analytic and process-oriented models, is an effective training approach for RD children.

Fortner (1986)	49	Ss were 3rd through 6th graders enrolled in LD classrooms; aged 9.5–12.5 yr; identified LD by a multidisciplinary team using multiple measures to compare intellectual ability and academic achievement.	Writing	A nonequivalent control group design was used. The Torrance Test of Creative Thinking (TTCT; Torrance, 1974) and the Test of Written Language, Story Section (TOWL; Hammill & Larsen, 1978) were given to both groups as a pretest. Experimental Ss spent about 15 min/day, 3 days/wk, completing tasks from New Directions in Creativity (Renzulli, 1973), a curriculum designed to stimulate creative, productive thinking, with another 15 min spent sharing and brainstorming. Control Ss continued with traditional instruction.	Torrance Test of Creative Thinking (TTCT; Torrance, 1974) and the Test of Written Language, Story Section (TOWL; Hammill & Larsen, 1978); Test of Written Language, Story Section (TOWL; Hammill & Larsen, 1978)	Creative, productive thinking activities correlated significantly with written expression improvement. While mean differences scores between pretest and posttest revealed gains by experimental Ss for every dependent variable, significant effects were only observed for number of thought units, subordinate clauses, and thematic maturity.
Graves (1986)	24	Ss were nominated to participate in this study by their resource room teachers on the basis of identification as LD; having scored at least 2 yr below grade level on a standardized reading comprehension test administered by school personnel; no gross neurological or sensory deficits; within the normal range on the IQ test; and in 5th through 8th grades. Mean age was 12.4, and mean WISC-R IQ score was 98.87. Mean reading score on the Stanford Diagnostic Reading Test or on the WRMT was 3.45	Reading comprehension	Ss met for four training sessions. Group 1 Ss received Direct Instruction and Metacomprehension (self-monitoring) training. The S was to check on a sheet of paper when she/he was half-way through reading the story. This was to help prompt the S to ask her-/himself if she/he understood what the story was about. The teacher used the direct instruction approach in teaching and modeling how to discern the main idea of a story. Group 2 Ss received Direct Instruction only. Group 3 Ss served as controls. These Ss were only told that they were going to learn about finding main ideas.	Reading aloud and silently: a 10-item posttest Reading aloud and silently: a 10-item test 1 wk after the last silent reading test	Both metacomprehension (self-monitoring) plus direct instruction and direct instruction alone were significantly more effective than the control training condition. In addition, metacomprehension plus direct instruction was more effective than both direct instruction alone and the control condition in improving reading comprehension.

(continued)

Author (year)	N	Selection criteria	Target domain(s)	Treatment(s)	Measures	Results
Harper (1986) Dissertation	9	Ages from 11.5 to 13.5; enrolled in grades 7 and 8. IQ ranged 72–109. Reading scores ranged 2.0–5.9. Instruments were not named.	Attention to task	The study had an alternating treatment design. BL consisted of 1–4 days during which measurements were taken with reading comprehension and paper and pencil tasks. Ss alternated between CAI (Comprehension Power, 1981) and workbook (Readability Comprehension Series, 1980). During CAI and workbooks, the focus was on silent reading comprehension. Ss met for sixteen 60-min sessions. Maintenance was measured after 4 days.	Percentage of comprehension questions answered correctly. Attention to task	For eight of the nine Ss, the computer was the most effective treatment in terms of productivity. No differences were found in terms of the effectiveness between computer and workbook instruction as it relates to attention to task. Eight of the Ss preferred the microcomputer to traditional workbook instruction. Eight felt they learned more on the computer. Finally, six stated that if given a choice between computer and workbook instruction to practice reading comprehension skills, they would select the computer.
Harris (1986)	4	LD Ss between 9 yr 10 mo and 10 yr 6 mo receiving services in a self-contained class at a suburban elementary school. WISC-R IQ scores between 85 and 115, with achievement scores at least 2 yr below grade or	On-task behavior Academic response rate	Interventions were implemented using a counter-balanced multiple BL design, with intervention order reversed for the last two Ss. During BL, and subsequently, Ss were directed to begin work immediately, and were reminded to file their papers at the end of the period. During the *self-monitoring of*	During the *self-monitoring of attention* condition, the S recorded check-marks under the words "yes" or "no" on a paper labeled "Was I paying	*On-task behavior:* On-task scores during BL ranged from 32% to 57%. During self-monitoring of attention, scores ranged from 77% to 91%. During self-monitoring of productivity, mean scores ranged from 75% to 98%.

age level in two or more academic domains. Nominated by teacher as having significant difficulties in attention and productivity.	*attention* condition, procedures described by Hallahan, Lloyd, Kauffman, and Loper (1983) were used. First, the teacher conferenced with the S, defining and explaining the importance of paying attention, then the teacher explained the self-monitoring strategy, including directions for recording task attention following random presentation of a tape-recorded tone during task completion. The Ss then used the procedure independently 5 days/wk. During the self-monitoring of productivity condition, the S and teacher discussed the meaning and importance of spelling practice, then the teacher described a strategy for increasing the amount of spelling practice. This involved counting the number of times spelling words had been written during the practice period, then recording this number on a graph in the spelling file. This procedure was also used independently following training, and was in effect 5 days/wk thereafter. The researcher or the teacher checked accuracy without the Ss knowledge. The choice condition occurred after data collection was completed under both the above conditions. During this period, collection of on-task and productivity data continued.	attention?" New recording sheets were used daily, then were filed in each S's spelling file. During the *self-monitoring of productivity* condition, the S recorded the number of spelling words written during each practice period on a graph which was kept in his or her spelling file. During the choice condition, each S selected one form of data collection.	*Academic productivity:* During BL, mean academic productivity scores ranged from 14 to 32 practices. Self-monitoring of attention produced scores ranged from 27 to 44. Productivity monitoring resulting in mean scores ranging from 47 to 78. Clear differences between the two practices were only apparent for one S. All four Ss selected self-monitoring of productivity as the preferred strategy. Overall, both strategies produced meaningful increases in on-task behavior. The effects of these strategies on academic productivity were less clear due to conflicting results among these Ss. In sum, the results support self-monitoring as a powerful strategy for increasing both on-task behavior and academic productivity.

(continued)

Author (year)	N	Selection criteria	Target domain(s)	Treatment(s)	Measures	Results
Jaben (1986)	98	Ss with behavior disorders and LDs placed in self-contained, intermediate classrooms for Ss with LDs. Aged 11 to 12, reading skills at least 3rd grade level, IQ within normal limits, and diagnosed by school specialists as either behavior disordered (BD) or LD. Ss were selected from an urban, middle SES population, then randomly assigned to an experimental (LD or BD) or a control group.	Written expression Creativity	Treatment consisted of the Purdue Creative Thinking Program administered in two 45-min lessons/wk for 14 wk. The program is designed to encourage divergent thought processes in the area of verbal and figural fluency, flexibility, and originality. Time of day for instruction and days chosen were held constant across the groups. The least distractible area of each classroom was selected for independent lesson completion. Answers were not graded for accuracy; and mechanical and grammatical errors were ignored. Assistance was provided for word recognition difficulty. The usual class curriculum continued for control Ss.	Pretest, posttest of fluency, flexibility, and originality in written expression using the Torrance Test of Creative Thinking (Torrance, 1974), alternate forms. Measures included the figural subtests, Parallel Lines and Picture Completion, and the verbal subtests, Just Suppose, Product Improvement, and Unusual Uses.	Using the posttest Torrance Test scores as dependent variables, and pretest scores as covariates, ANCOVA procedures were applied. Trained LD and BD Ss obtained significantly higher scores on the verbal and figural subtests than untrained Ss, with the exception that adjusted means for LD S's figural fluency did not vary significantly.
Lovitt, Rudsit, Jenkins, Pious, & Benedetti (1986)	202	Ss were 7th graders with LD (13) and SLD (17) enrolled in seven mainstream physical science classes in a middle-class to upper-middle-class area in Washington. LD Ss were identified according to state criteria, i.e., functioning level of two-thirds or below expectancies based on comparison of ability and achievement scores. Ss were	Science	Eight chapters from a Laidlaw physical science text were assigned during this study, although data were only collected for the middle six chapters. Study material format was varied for experimental Ss, following either the Precision Teaching or Study Guide method. These techniques were implemented in both the resource room and the regular science classrooms. Ss were enrolled on a semester schedule in classes taught by three veteran science	Ss were tested before and after each chapter was instructed. One test was a 24–29-item exam provided by the text publisher. A write-facts assessment was developed for this study which required Ss to record three major and three related cues about	Typical and LD Ss scored better on curriculum-based measures for adapted chapters. Both adaptations were associated with significantly improved performance. Pairwise comparisons of mean chapter scores significantly favored the adapted chapters with only two exceptions, and in these

		labeled specific LD when their scores on group-administered reading tests were at least 3 yr below grade level expectancies.		teachers and one intern. Study skills instruction was provided in the resource room for 50 min/day, with 10 min spent completing exercises and framed outlines presented by the science teacher in the regular classroom. The project coordinator explained the adapted materials to the teachers prior to implementation, then incorporated the materials into instruction while the teachers observed on the first day of intervention. The roles were reversed on subsequent days.	chapter topics. This information was used to assist Ss in generating as many topic related facts as possible in 2 min.	cases the means for the adapted chapters were higher but not significantly so. This study supports the use of curriculum modifications that incorporate precision teaching and study guide methods for all Ss.
Montague & Bos (1986)	6	High school Ss aged 15–19. Their mean IQ score on the WISC-R or WAIS-R was 93.8, with a range of 85–102. The results from the Woodcock–Johnson Psycho-Educational Battery placed Ss at least at the 4th grade reading level.	Math problem solving	This study investigated the effect of teaching an eight-step cognitive strategy on verbal math problem-solving performance. The multiple BL design included BL, treatment, generalization, maintenance, and retraining sessions. During BL, test scores and time required for test completion was recorded. Treatment procedures included (1) strategy acquisition training, (2) strategy application practice, and (3) testing sessions during which data were collected for the dependent measures. An eight-step verbal math problem-solving strategy was taught that included the following components: read problem aloud, paraphrase problem aloud, visualize problem, state the problem,	Number of correct problems Minimum required for test completion	Overall, the Ss demonstrated improved performance on two-step verbal math problems. Maintenance and generalization of the strategy were evident. This study provides an alternative teaching methodology that focuses on cognitive strategy training to improve the verbal math problem solving of LD Ss.

(*continued*)

Author (year)	N	Selection criteria	Target domain(s)	Treatment(s)	Measures	Results
Montague & Bos (1986) *(cont.)*				hypothesize how many steps are in the problem, estimate, calculate, and self-check. Generalization and maintenance measures including 10 three-step verbal math problems were given on the day following the final treatment and another test given 2 wk later which included 10 two-step verbal math problems. A final test of two-step problems was given 3 mo later.		
Omizo, Lo, & Williams (1986)	60	Adolescents aged 14 –18 in grades 9–12 certified LD according to Texas Education Agency (TEA, 1976) criteria, i.e., ability average or above with achievement in one or more subjects 2 or more yr below grade level. Ss were assigned to two groups using a random numbers table. One group received the experimental treatment, and the other group watched films for the same length of time.	Self-concept Locus of control	Ss in the treatment group received two 1-hr sessions/wk of Rational–Emotive Education (REE) for 6 wk. REE group sessions were conducted by two counseling graduate Ss trained and supervised by a school psychologist. Ss met after school for sessions, which were held in high school classrooms. REE sessions include two activities focused on the development of feelings, expression of feelings, and discrimination between rational and irrational feelings.	The Dimensions of Self-Concept Scale, Form S (DOSC; Michael & Smith, 1978), and the Rotter Internal–External Scale (Rotter, 1966) were given 1 wk prior to the study and again 1 wk after the last treatment. The same forms were used as pretests and posttests. All tests were given by a high school guidance counselor.	Although a MANOVA on pretest data indicated initial equivalence for the two groups, posttest analyses revealed significant differences in terms of level of aspiration, anxiety levels, leadership, and initiative as measured by the DOSC. The locus of control measure reliably discriminated between the two groups, with experimental Ss evidencing a more internal orientation of control.

Reynolds (1986) Dissertation	54	Ss were chosen from grades 6–8 in a resource room. The mean IQ was 96.4. Achievement information was not specified.	Writing skills	There were two groups, each with 18 Ss. The two groups were the same except that the order of treatment was reversed. Ss were taught the three stages of writing (prewriting, drafting, and revision). Ss wrote about topics about which they could express an opinion. Two revision strategies were taught: *COPS* (Capitalization, Overall appearance, Punctuation, Spelling) and *Evaluative and Directive Phrases*. Control Ss (18) received no treatment.	Writing: content and mechanics	Although there were no significant differences in the three groups on the pretest, there were significant differences following treatment. In both treatment groups, the posttest mechanics subscore is appreciably higher than the content subscore. The treatment groups showed improvement in both contents and mechanics.
Rosenberg (1986)	4	Adolescents with diagnosed reading problems. Ss were identified as LD based upon the following: (1) IQ of 80 or more based on the WISC-R or the Stanford–Binet administered by a certified school psychologist; (2) learning problems not primarily the result of hearing or vision problems; (3) learning problems not a result of emotional problems; and (4) a severe discrepancy between ability and achievement.	Oral reading	This study evaluated the relative effectiveness of three error-corrections procedures (word supply, drill, and phonic drill rehearsal) on the oral reading of middle-school Ss with LD. A teacher was recruited and trained in the study methods. Experimental procedures were implemented in an LD resource room at a university-based laboratory school. Word supply involved teacher provision of correct words following errors, after which the S repeated the supplied word and continued reading. Drill consisted of teacher provision of correct words and S repetition, followed at the end of reading by drill of the error words until the S correctly read all missed words from	Data were collected using two measures: percent correct of error words from reading the previous day and reading fluency. To obtain the former, each S read a list of the words missed the previous day; the number of words read correctly from this list was then divided by the total words listed. Reading fluency was evaluated by rereading the	During phase 1, the drill method was more effective and efficient than either a word-supply method or a phonic-drill rehearsal strategy on a measure of isolated error-word identification. Drill was also superior on a measure of oral reading. In sum, drill was the most efficient method of the three according to both dependent measures. Results from the second phase indicated that drill was superior to phonic drill

(*continued*)

Author (year)	*N*	Selection criteria	Target domain(s)	Treatment(s)	Measures	Results
Rosenberg (1986) (*cont.*)				index cards on two trials. Phonic drill rehearsal was similar to the word supply and drill conditions with the addition of attention to the phonetic elements of errors by way of a systematic covertization procedure. First, the teacher sounded out each element of the error word printed on an index card while the S observed. Then, the teacher and S read the card in unison by sounding out the word together. Next, the S sounded out the word alone, both aloud and in a whisper. Finally, the S read the card, sounding out the error word independently, and then read the word aloud at normal speed. This condition continued until the S read the entire deck of daily error words correctly on two consecutive trials. An alternating-treatments design was used with two phases and 40 sessions total. During the first phase, word supply and drill conditions were alternated; in the second phase, drill and phonic drill rehearsal were alternated. Treatment occurred daily during regularly scheduled reading periods; Ss read a 150–200 word passage from the Barnell–Loft Specific Skills program. Errors were recorded as the S read.	previous day's passage and computing how many words per min were correctly read. The ordering of the two measures was alternated according to a randomly selected, prespecified schedule.	rehearsal as measured by the measure of oral reading rate. However, no differences were observed between the two methods as measured by drill of the isolated error words. Overall, it appears that the drill procedure was the most efficient and cost effective of thethree methods used in this study.

Salend & Lamb (1986)	6	Ss labeled LD by placement teams in accordance with New York State guidelines; attending resource room programs for remedial assistance in reading and math in addition to regular class placement.	Inappropriate verbalizations	An interdependent, group-managed response-cost system mediated by free tokens was used to decrease inappropriate verbalizations of two groups of Ss identified as LD. The study occurred in a resource room for both groups; 30-min treatment sessions took place during the groups' daily reading periods. Two activities were completed during reading periods: word recognition and reading comprehension. During word recognition activities, all Ss read in unison words printed on the blackboard. During reading comprehension activities, Group A completed oral reading and comprehension questions from the SRA Corrective Reading Series (Decoding C), while Group B completed oral reading and comprehension questions from Decoding B materials from the same series. A reversal design was employed. During BL, the number of inappropriate verbalizations were counted during both groups' daily reading period. The teacher made no responses or attempts to influence these behaviors. Then, the interdependent group-managed response–cost system was implemented following teacher explanations to Ss of the target behavior, intervention, and consequences for successful performance. Next, BL conditions were replicated followed by a return to the experimental conditions.	The number of inappropriate verbalizations engaged in by both groups were counted and graphed. At the beginning of each intervention session, the groups received tokens representing how many inappropriate verbalizations could be made by group members before reinforcers were taken away. If any tokens remained at the end of the session, the groups received 15 min of free time. The tokens remaining after each session were also counted and their number graphed.	Substantial decreases in the inappropriate verbalizations of both groups were observed when the intervention was delivered in a resource room.

(*continued*)

Author (year)	*N*	Selection criteria	Target domain(s)	Treatment(s)	Measures	Results
Schunk & Cox (1986)	90	Middle school Ss, 6th–8th grade, classified LD in math by school specialists according to Texas Educational Agency (TEA, 1983) criteria. Selection followed a two-stage evaluation process: initial assessment of S's physical condition, typical behavior, intelligence, and emotional stability as measured by the WISC-R (Weschler, 1974); and the Stanford Achievement Test. BD criteria included display of deficiencies in social or emotional function, as a primary indicator, which interfered with performance. All Ss were receiving services in adaptive academic environments. Ss were stratified by grade level and handicapping condition, then randomly assigned to either a training or a no-treatment control condition.	Math problem solving Self-efficacy	This study investigated how verbalization of subtraction with regrouping operations influenced LD Ss' self-efficacy and skillful performance, and also explored how effort–attributional feedback affected these achievement behaviors. Ss met for 45-min sessions on 6 consecutive days. The study included two treatment groups and one control condition. All three groups received the same math problems to solve. Group 1 Continuous Verbalization—Ss were told to verbalize each step of problem solving as they performed the math tasks. Group 2 Discontinued Verbalization—Ss were told to verbalize for the first three sessions and told not to verbalize for the last three sessions. Group 3 No Verbalization (control)—Ss performed the math tasks without instructions to verbalize. All Ss were periodically monitored and either received effort feedback ("You've been working hard") during the first or second half of training, or no effort feedback.	Self-efficacy Subtraction skill Attributions: ability, effort, task, and luck Training performance: number of problems completed	A 3 × 3 multivariate analysis of covariance was performed. Continuous verbalization led to higher self-efficacy and skillful performance than did discontinued verbalization or no verbalization. Providing effort feedback promoted these achievement behaviors more than was observed when verbalization was not elicited. Effort feedback during the first half of training enhanced effort attributions.

Scruggs, Mastropieri, & Tolfa-Veit (1986)	85	LD and BD Ss in 4th, 5th, and 6th grade at a metropolitan school classified according to national, state, and local standards. LD identification criteria included a 40% discrepancy (expressed in standard scores) between ability as measured by the WISC-R (Weschler, 1974) and achievement in two academic areas from the Stanford Achievement Test. BD criteria included display of deficiencies in social or emotional function, as a primary indicator, which interfered with academic performance. All Ss were receiving services in academic environments structured to meet their special needs. Ss were stratified by grade level and handicapping condition, then randomly assigned to either training or a no-treatment control condition.	Test-taking skills	This study replicated previous findings by Scruggs and Tolfa (1985) and Scruggs and Mastropieri (1986), extending their research into mathematics test-taking skills, and to the upper elementary grades. Experimental Ss received training in small groups (1–6) from one of three trained experimenters. There were five sessions for 20–30 min/session. Session 1 consisted of instruction and practice using a separate answer sheet to mark answers indicated by an arrow in a practice test booklet. The next two sessions focused on training strategies specific to taking reading subtests. The last two sessions covered specific math test-taking skills. On all subtests, Ss were trained to work quickly and carefully, to check answers when time permits, to answer every question, to eliminate answers known to be wrong, to use prior or partial knowledge, and to become familiar with all test format demands. The posttest was administered 1 wk following treatment. Control Ss did not receive treatment.	Stanford Achievement Test (Kelly, Madden, Gardner, & Rudman, 1964)	Trained Ss outperformed controls on word study skills and mathematics subtests with complicated formats. The effect sizes obtained for scores on these subtests were larger than those obtained by nonhandicapped children. Smaller effects were obtained on the reading comprehension and word problems subtests. There was an interaction by handicapping condition on the mathematics concepts subtest, which the authors suggest may be attributable to the BD Ss benefiting from training techniques that enhanced concentration and sustained attention. Overall, the results suggest that BD and LD Ss may have more knowledge than they typically demonstrate on standardized achievement tests.

(continued)

Author (year)	N	Selection criteria	Target domain(s)	Treatment(s)	Measures	Results
Smith & Friend (1986)	54	LD adolescents who met district criteria for placement in special education, i.e., a discrepancy of at least 21 points between aptitude (WISC-R; Weschler, 1974) and achievement (Woodcock–Johnson Psycho-educational Battery; Woodcock & Johnson, 1977) measures based on NCEs; scored at least 4.0 on the WRAT reading subtest (Jastak & Jastak, 1978). Comparisons were made to ensure initial equivalence of the experimental and comparison groups since random assignment was not possible.	Instructional prose recall	There were seven sessions in this intervention. First, Ss were pretested by the special education teachers. Then, experimental Ss completed five text structure lessons the following wk in four 50-min sessions. The comparison Ss spent the same amount of time studying problem solving. All instruction was provided in the Ss' special education classrooms by two experienced teachers not employed at the schools. These teachers followed written procedures to ensure standard delivery of content. They also administered the posttests following the final treatment session.	A pretest, posttest, and delayed posttest were constructed consisting of three short passages (91–134 words). Ss were asked to specify the text structure in an open response format. Each task required recall of four out of five structures used in each lesson. One longer passage (211–247 words) was included on each test which required text structure identification and completion of a free recall task. All test passages contained history/social studies content ranked at 9th and 10th grade reading levels by the Dale–Chall (1948) readability formula.	Training in the text structure usage strategy significantly improved S's recognition of these structures and their recall of instructed content, with this effect remaining stable over at least one week. Recall protocols revealed strategy use by experimental Ss during the reading and recall tasks.

Weidler (1986) Dissertation	4	Mean age was 10.6, ranging from 9.4 to 11.4. The mean score on the Otis–Lennon Test of School Ability was 100.75, with a range of 96 to 111. The reading mean on the CAT was 3.4, with a range of 1.3 to 4.3.	Reading comprehension	This multiple BL study investigated the effect of cognitive self-instruction on the comprehension monitoring failures of poor readers. Treatment involved Ss reading from SRA reading lab materials. The Reading Miscue Inventory (RMI; Goodman & Burke, 1972) was used for recording two areas of miscues, grammatical relationships and comprehension. Each reading selection was transcribed into a worksheet format for the coding of miscues. During BL, each S read one selection aloud from the SRA lab; selections were matched to the S's instructional level. Oral miscues were recorded. No prompts or interruptions occurred. During the first treatment phase, Overt Self-Instruction (S-I) training was provided. The experimenter read aloud one of the SRA selections that was previously read by the S during BL. The experimenter reiterated the same miscues made by the S and applied appropriate correction strategies using overt S-I. After modeling correction strategies, the experimenter helped the S progress through a new selection by pointing out miscues and encouraging S-I. The S then read a new SRA selection aloud and applied S-I with the experimenter's aid. The miscue analysis was conducted only on this final step.	Grammatical Relationships: Strength Miscues, Partial Strength Miscues, Weakness Miscues Reading Comprehension: No Loss Miscues, Partial Loss Miscues, Loss Miscues	In the area of Grammatical Relationships, at the point CSI was introduced, for three Ss there was an increase in Strength miscue level and a decrease in Weakness miscue level indicating a shift toward higher-quality miscues. After total intervention, all four Ss showed a higher mean number of miscues classified as higher-quality (increase in Strength miscues/decrease in Weakness miscues). In the area of Comprehension, when CSI was introduced, three Ss showed an increase in No Loss miscue level and a decrease in Loss miscue level, again indicating a shift toward higher-quality miscues. After total intervention, all four Ss showed a higher mean number of miscues classified as higher-quality (increase in No Loss miscues/decrease in Loss miscues).

(continued)

Author (year)	*N*	Selection criteria	Target domain(s)	Treatment(s)	Measures	Results
Weidler (1986) (*cont.*)				During the second treatment phase, Semi-Overt Self-Instruction was provided. The experimenter again modeled the S-I procedure by whispering. The S practiced the procedures and then applied the semi-overt S-I on a new SRA selection. The miscue analysis was conducted only on this step. During the third treatment phase, Covert Self-Instruction was trained. For each session, the experimenter modeled the procedures, which were identical to the previous procedures except that S-I was to be "thought" rather than spoken aloud.		
Whitman (1986) Dissertation	72	Middle school and high school Ss with a mean IQ score of 86 as measured on the WISC-R	Math	This study took place over 4 wk and included 12 sessions, 40 min each, and met three times/wk. The experimental group used CAI for math with educational math games software. The control group also used CAI for math practice, but with drill and practice software. Both groups went to the computer lab.	Computer-generated math exercise	The data collected demonstrated CAI drill and practice to be more effective in teaching computation skills to EMH Ss. No difference was observed in the mathematics achievement performance of LD and EH Ss using the two types of CAI.

Blandford & Lloyd (1987)	2	Two LD Ss participated in this study. Both were determined eligible for LD services on the basis on guidelines in PL 94-142. S1 was 11.4 yr old and S2 was 10.6 yr old. Ss were in grades 4 and 5. S1 had a WISC-R IQ score of 104 and his Woodcock–Johnson Achievement Test scores ranged from 2.5 to 5.2. S2 scored 112 on the WISC-R and had scores ranging from 2.2 to 3.5 on the Woodcock–Johnson Achievement Test. S1 exhibited poor cursive handwriting skills. S2 performed independent seatwork hastily and sloppily. He had poor cursive handwriting skills as well.	Handwriting	A multiple BL design was used to analyze the effect of self-instruction on handwriting. During BL, which lasted between 7 and 12 sessions, Ss were only instructed to write neatly. During treatment, which lasted between 11 and 16 sessions, Ss wrote in their journal for 5 min about a topic of their own choosing. A card showing seven self-instructional questions designed to prompt Ss to think about important aspects of handwriting was provided to the two boys. The Ss checked which questions did not apply, e.g., "Am I sitting correctly?"	Assessments were made daily of the boy's handwriting performance, including letter formation, letter proximity to the line, letter height, and word spacing.	The Ss' handwriting improved markedly when the card was introduced. These improvements persisted over time while the card was still available for review, and were even maintained after the card was no longer available. Data from the regular classroom for one of the boys showed that his handwriting also improved in that setting.
Blick & Test (1987)	12	High school Ss in grades 9–12, between the ages of 15.4 and 18.2. Ss included nine LD, two educable mentally handicapped, and one emotionally handicapped S. IQ scores range 55–101 (WISC-R, WAIS-R, or	On-task behavior	A multiple BL design across groups was utilized. The teacher/experimenter collected BL data in each class for 5 days before introducing Intervention 1 to Class A. BL lasted from 5 days (Class A) to 17 days (Class C). Treatment lasted for an average of 23 days across the three groups (Class A, B, C) and four	Percentage of on-task behavior Accuracy in recording	Results suggested a functional relationship between the intervention and increased on-task behavior. Changes were maintained after audible cues were faded. S accuracy data showed a

(continued)

Author (year)	*N*	Selection criteria	Target domain(s)	Treatment(s)	Measures	Results
Blick & Test (1987) (*cont.*)		PIAT). PIAT Reading Recognition scores range 2.3–6.6, and PIAT Reading Comprehension scores range 2.8–8.8. All Ss exhibited some off-task behavior and self-monitored their own behavior.		interventions. The experiment took place in the resource room in the regularly scheduled 55-min class periods. *Intervention 1: 5-min self-record.* Ss recorded on-task or off-task behavior at the sound of the cue "record." Every 2 days, Ss were reminded of the four target behaviors and the need for accuracy, but only at the beginning of the class period. The teacher also recorded. *Intervention 2: 10-min self-record.* Ss recorded their behavior only four times each class period, after the verbal cue "record." The teacher however, recorded behavior every 5 min at the chime and at the cue "record." Every 2 days, Ss were reminded of the target behaviors and need for accuracy. They were not told the length of the intervals. *Intervention 3: Partially faded cue, self-record.* The third cueing tape was used. Ss recorded at the verbal cue, "record," given at 20 and 40 min, and at the times designated on their recording sheets. The teacher recorded every 5 min. Ss received the same reminders as in earlier phases.		relationship between increased on-task behavior and accurate self-recording. Anecdotal data indicated that Ss' academic performance improved in both training and nontraining settings.

				Intervention 4: No audio cue, self-record. The recording sheets had 4 blocks, each with clock times at 10-min intervals added underneath. Ss were told they were now able to monitor their own behavior without the verbal cue, and that they were expected to record their behavior at appropriate times. Reminders of behavior and accuracy were given. The teacher recorded at 10-min intervals.		
Burkwist, Mabee, & McLaughlin (1987)	1	S was a 13-yr-old LD female enrolled in a junior high school resource room. The S's IQ score was 81 (WISC-R), and her grade equivalency academic scores as measured by the PIAT were: Math, 4.4; Reading Recognition, 3.8; Reading Comprehension, 4.5; and Spelling, 3.8.	Inappropriate verbalization	The study was a minireversal and changing criterion design with 14 days of BL 1 and 1 day of BL 2. The treatment lasted for 134 days. During the BLs, no daily report card was in effect. Treatment consisted of a report card, sent home daily, which was in effect for inappropriate verbalizations. Points earned and lost, daily grades, assignments completed, incomplete assignments, and social behavior were all reported. Seven treatment phases were used with a stepwise change in criterion for inappropriate verbalizations. A daily criterion rate for inappropriate verbalizations and consequences (rewards) for meeting criterion were established	Inappropriate verbalizations: frequency counts	While the daily report card was in effect, the frequency of inappropriate verbalizations decreased. The behavior increased when the criterion was raised. A replication of a lower criterion again reduced the frequency of inappropriate verbalization.

(continued)

Author (year)	*N*	Selection criteria	Target domain(s)	Treatment(s)	Measures	Results
Cosden & English (1987)	12	LD Ss participating in a summer school program. Each S attended a special day class for mildly handicapped Ss during the school yr. Ss ranged in age from 9.1 to 12.9, and were in grades 3 to 6. Mean IQ score was 90.11, mean math achievement score was at a 3.5 grade level, and mean reading score was at a 2.9 grade level. All Ss were administered the Piers–Harris Children's Self-Concept Scale and the Intellectual Achievement Responsibility Questionnaire (IAR). A median split on the test scores was used to stratify Ss with higher self-esteem and lower self-esteem, and those with an internal locus of control and an external locus of control.	Self-concept Locus of control	Two studies were conducted; only Study 2 is reported here. Ss were paired with each other to create six dyads of classmates. Ss in each dyad were in the same grade and within a yr of each other in age. The treatment condition involved Ss working in dyads at the computer. Ss spent 10–12 min on the computer with Teasers by Tobbs (O'Brien, 1984). Half of the sessions were in dyads (treatment), while the other half involved Ss working individually (control condition). Ss selected the level of difficulty on the computer. S responses were recorded online by a research assistant.	Productivity Help-seeking Problem-solving: difficulty level of selected problems and solution accuracy.	Patterns of problem selection, help seeking, and performance accuracy appeared more due to S competence in math than a function of grouping or other personality characteristics. While grouping did not have the anticipated positive consequences, neither did it have a negative impact on performance.
Darch & Kameenui (1987)	25	LD Ss enrolled in a university summer school program; disabilities identified by local schools; obtained scores below 6 on an 11-item screening test	Critical reading skills	Ss in both experimental groups studied from the same text. The same teacher provided instruction for 40 min/day for 12 days total. Three critical skills were taught; method was varied. *Direct*	Three measures were developed to assess acquisition of the critical reading skills taught. The *Argument*	Support was obtained for the superiority of direct instruction over the discussion/workbook approach for teaching

		of critical reading skills taught in the study. Ss were randomly assigned to one of two experimental groups.		*Instruction* involved involved rule presentation of skills, with explicit error correction procedures, followed by guided practice that was gradually faded. *Discussion/Workbook* sessions began with discussions (without formally stated rules), then Ss completed workbook assignments independently.	*Analysis Test* involved detection of false causality, faulty generalization, and invalid testimonial. The *Embedded Argument Analysis Test* required detection of the same types of faulty reasoning in longer passages. The *Skill Classification Test* required Ss to identify the rules used to locate invalid arguments or opinions in text.	critical reading skills to LD Ss, although literal comprehension was not differentially affected by the two methods. However, neither group achieved mastery levels or transfer.
Fiedorowicz & Trites (1987)	115	RD Ss, age range of 7.9–14.4. IQ scores (WISC-R) range 95.1–98, and reading recognition scores (WRAT, SORT) range 2.8–3.3 yr below grade level. Ss were chosen on the basis of three reading disability subtypes: Oral Reading, Intermodal-Associative, and Sequential, labeled in this intervention as Type O, Type A, and Type S.	Reading	This intervention included twenty-eight 30-min sessions over 4–6 mo, and took place during regular instruction in the resource room. Ss were divided into five groups: Type O, Type A, Type S (all three of which were autoskill-trained), a no-treatment control group, and an alternative computer control group. The autoskill-trained groups included increasing the accuracy of response and decreasing the latency of response for the most deficient component reading skills. The three treatment groups received 56 hrs of intervention, while the control groups received 30 hrs. *Type O* Ss were	WRAT-R Reading Subtest G-E Phonetic knowledge phonic syllables Phonic words SPIRE Paragraphs: Word Recognition Oral (Errors, Latency, Retention, Comprehension), and Silent (Latency, Retention, Comprehension)	The autoskill-trained Ss made significant gains in reading word recognition, phonetic skills and importantly, paragraph reading. In addition, teacher and S evaluations of the program were quite positive. The major conclusion was that systematic training of deficient component reading skills according to subtype classifications does improve reading skills in

(*continued*)

Author (year)	*N*	Selection criteria	Target domain(s)	Treatment(s)	Measures	Results
Fiedorowicz & Trites (1987) (*cont.*)				trained on the *Oral Reading* procedure, including words, phrases, sentences, and paragraphs. Type A Ss were trained on the *Auditory–Visual* matching-to-sample procedure. *Type S* Ss were taught the *Visual Matching-to-Sample* procedure. All Ss were trained using CV and VC syllables and words. Ss were trained to criterion on 1one subtest before moving on to the next subtest. *No-Treatment Control* Ss were untrained and received no specific intervention. The *Alternate Computer-Trained Control* Ss were provided with computer programs that drilled some aspect of language arts development.	Projected grade level: Oral (Errors, Latency, Retention, Comprehension), and Silent (Latency, Retention, Comprehension) QASOR CLOZE: Word Recognition (Meaning, Graphic Sense, Fluency), and Projected grade level (Meaning, Graphic Sense, Fluency)	general. All subtypes of Ss made gains in reading word recognition and comprehension of paragraphs at the projected grade level.
Howell, Sidorenko, & Jurica (1987)	1	A 16-yr-old male sophomore in an urban high school. S was placed in special classes in 1st grade based on assessment by school psychologist indicating severe discrepancies between achievement and ability due to a psychological processing disorder. Testing indicated normal hearing, vision, and motor skills, along with evidence of both auditory and	Multiplication facts	The effectiveness of computer use on acquisition of multiplication facts was investigated in two studies. During the first study, a reversal design was employed wherein two BL periods of three nonintervention sessions were followed by three and four sessions, respectively, of computer drill and practice. A commercial math program called *Galaxy Math* (Random House, Inc., 1984) was used, which involves the S racing against time to answer randomly generated multiplication	During Study 1, records were made of the number of errors/20 multiplication problems and the average amount of time to complete the problems were recorded during each session; BL data were gathered from a random sample of 20	During Study 1, an initial increase in correct responses and a corresponding decrease in the amount of time to response was observed for both drill-and-practice and tutorial software, but this effect was not durable, with both errors and response time increasing when the S was returned to BL conditions. During Study

		visual processing disorders. Testing at the time of study indicated a Full Scale IQ of 112 (WISC-R; Wechsler, 1974), and 5th grade level mathematics (Woodcock–Johnson Psycho-Educational Battery; Woodcock & Johnson, 1984) with specific difficulties in recall and reproduction of multiplication facts. Discussion with the resource teacher also revealed the S was using an inefficient strategy to solve multiplication problems.		problems. After probing indicated that the S had not maintained the gains from this program, a second study was designed. Treatment consisted of integrating a tutorial-based computer program, *MemorEase* (Mind Nautilus Software, 1985) and a specific teacher intervention strategy, involving instruction of "the rules of 9s," on timed and untimed tests of the same multiplication problems within a multiple BL withdrawal design.	multiplication problems presented to the S using pencil and paper. During Study 2, records were made during each BL and intervention session of the number of errors/20 multiplication problems under timed and untimed conditions. For BL data, a random sample of 24 multiplication problems from the 6–9 times tables was presented to the S with pencil and paper. Intervention data were gathered by observing and recording the S's performance while answering 20 randomly generated problems on the computer.	2, combining the software with direct teacher intervention enabled the S to unlearn the ineffective problem-solving strategy, learn a new solution strategy, and use the software to practice and incorporate new knowledge and skills.
Idol & Croll (1987)	5	Intermediate-aged elementary Ss with mild learning handicaps and poor comprehension participated. Ss were selected by special education teachers due to	Reading comprehension	Ss were trained to use a story mapping strategy in order to build their schema and to improve reading comprehension. In addition to a concrete mapping structure, Ss were provided with precise teacher presentation in a model-lead test	Curriculum-based assessment was used to determine Ss' reading level for curriculum placement. These passages were	All Ss improved on most of the measures. Improved ability to answer comprehension questions was demonstrated by four Ss, whose performance was

(continued)

Author (year)	*N*	Selection criteria	Target domain(s)	Treatment(s)	Measures	Results
Idol & Croll (1987) (*cont.*)		serious reading comprehension problems during instruction in spite of adequate decoding skills. Four Ss were placed in resource programs; one was placed in a self-contained classroom.		format, feedback, and multiple practice opportunities. Graduate Ss with teaching experience provided intervention. Each received training in all features of the intervention prior to the study. Intervention occurred in a multiple BL A-B-A design. During BL, performance was monitored to obtain contrast data; only stories with structure were selected for this phase. Ss read orally for 10 min/day from a Ginn (1982) reader; errors were corrected as they occurred, except during a 100-word timed sample that was used to monitor reading accuracy and rate. Then the S retold the story and answered comprehension questions. Intervention conditions were the same with the exception of the teacher familiarizing the S with the story mapping procedures and providing feedback and opportunities for practice using the story map to retell the story. A second phase of BL conditions followed. Once a S stabilized at the criterion level of 80% correct responses, the story mapping procedures were stopped and BL procedures were followed to determine the degree of maintenance.	at least 100 words in length; measures were completed of comprehension, reading rate, and reading accuracy. Ten explicit and implicit comprehension questions were constructed. Additional measures were story retelling length, comparisons of story retelling responses to comprehension question answers, standardized reading tests, generalization probes, and listening comprehension measures.	also maintained following treatment and who increased in their use of story-mapping components in their story retelling. The fifth S only experienced marginal improvement on most measures, and his slow progress prevented implementation of a maintenance phase in his case. Finally, generalization results were mixed for the four Ss who did show improvement.

Jaben (1987)	50	Ss aged 11–12 yr old participated. Their WISC-R scores were in the normal range. Ss were chosen for this study if they could read at least at the 3rd grade level. Scores from the PIAT Reading Comprehension and Word Recognition showed that while all Ss could read at least at the 3rd grade level, they were underachieving by 2 yr.	Creative thinking	Ss met for 45 min, twice weekly for 14 wk. The treatment consisted of The Purdue Creative Thinking Program, a program designed to encourage divergent thought processes in the area of verbal and figural fluency, flexibility, and originality. The PCTP has 28 audiotapes and printed materials. Components have three parts each: (1) a 3–4 min lesson that teaches a principle related to creative thinking; (2) a 10–12 min story about a famous American pioneer; and (3) three or four exercises related to content of the story. Instructors were told to ignore errors in spelling, writing, and grammar. The control group received no treatment.	Torrance Tests of Creative Thinking, Written Verbal Subtests for Fluency, Flexibility, and Originality	Posttest group means were significantly greater than the control group's means on the verbal subtests of the Torrance Tests of Creative Thinking.
Jenkins, Heliotis, Stein, & Haynes (1987)	32	Ss were elementary LD Ss enrolled in suburban schools ($N = 24$) or a self-contained class in the University of Washington's Experimental Education Unit. They were selected from 3rd to 6th grade rooms. All had significant comprehension and decoding deficits, at least 1 yr below grade expectancies, and were identified LD as defined by state's criteria, including significant discrepancy between achievement and ability, plus demonstrated processing deficits.	Comprehension monitoring Reading	The strategy consisted of writing brief restatements of important ideas from text. The intervention employed scripted lessons designed to help Ss state the most important ideas from narrative text. Training was presented in three phases. 80% correct for the group was the criterion selected for proceeding to the next phase. Phases typically lasted 3 to 5 days. The entire program was typically completed in 10–15 days, and lessons lasted about 20 min each. All instruction occurred during regular reading period. Ss in the control condition worked on seatwork assignments. *First Phase:* Teachers used modeling, practice, and corrective feedback to identify the most	Four stories developed by Brown and Smiley (1977) were adapted by Jenkins et al. (1986); each consisted of about 400 words and represented around 3rd–4th grade reading level (Fry, 1968). Pausal unit analyses were performed on these stories, and these units were then rated according to structural importance, resulting in four categories, ranging from 1 (least	Analyses of variance were performed for Importance Levels (4) × Tests (pre- and posttests) and Group (experimental or control) with repeated levels on the first two factors. *Training Test:* More level 3 or level 4 stories were recalled. A significant Group × Test interaction was observed due to superior recall by the experimental group. However, trained Ss were not more selective than

(*continued*)

Author (year)	*N*	Selection criteria	Target domain(s)	Treatment(s)	Measures	Results
Jenkins, Heliotis, Stein, & Haynes (1987) (*cont.*)				important persons and/or major events in paragraphs. *Second Phase:* Instruction emphasized use of the fewest possible words to convey the gist of text; lined spaces were inserted between each paragraph used for written restatements. *Third Phase:* Ss were given regular narrative text without writing space, then shown how to write restatements on separate sheets of paper.	important) to 4 (most important). Short-answer comprehension questions were developed for each story requiring recall of information from pausal unit levels 3 and 4. Ss were tested under three separate conditions in which they silently read text, then answered questions. *Training Test:* Ss were explicitly to use the restatement while reading, including writing a summary of each paragraph. *Near Transfer Test:* The story was presented in normal format; an extra sheet of paper provided, but no explicit directions were given for use. *Remote Transfer Test:* The story was presented in normal format; no writing materials or explicit strategy directions were provided.	controls to the relative importance of passage ideas. *Near Transfer Test:* Trained Ss correctly answered significantly more questions than controls. Thirteen of 16 trained Ss used spontaneous strategy, and 1 control S adopted the strategy. Eleven of 16 control Ss wrote some type of notes, although their work lacked organization. *Remote Transfer Test:* Importance level and the Group × Importance Level Interaction were significant, although performance patterns across the two groups did not vary systematically. A significant effect was observed for the Group × Text I interaction, which was attributed to improved recall by the experimental group between the pre- and posttests.

Johnson, Gersten, & Carnine (1987)	25	High school Ss with LDs who scored at least 3 yr below grade level on the Reading subtests of the Woodcock–Johnson (Woodcock & Johnson, 1977). A 50-item pretest was administered to all Ss, who were then matched by pretest scores and randomly assigned to one of two treatments.	Vocabulary	The intervention used CAI to vary the amount of words taught and the cumulative review of vocabulary words. Instruction was provided 20 min/day, 4 days/wk. *Large Teaching Set:* The program presented words in two sets of 25 words each; mastery was defined as 84% correct on 2 consecutive days. After this criterion was attained, Ss completed a review, and played an arcade game for any time remaining. A sentence completion activity followed mastery. Small Teaching Set: Vocabulary words were also presented via computer (1) individualized lessons which provided teaching and practice with words unknown by the Ss, (2) in sets no larger than seven, (3) with mastery defined as correct response on two trials, and (4) cumulative review to ensure retention.	Reading subtests of the Woodcock–Johnson (Woodcock & Johnson, 1977). The Advanced 1 Level Reading subtest of the Metropolitan Achievement Test (Prescott, Balow, Hogen, & Farr, 1978). A multiple choice, 50-item vocabulary test developed for this study was used for pretest, posttest, and maintenance test. All Ss took a 10-item, open-ended oral test designed to measure recall of word definitions; an attitude survey was developed to measure response to CAI.	Time to mastery differed significantly for the two groups. Performance on posttest and maintenance test did not reveal a main effect for type of instruction, i.e., the amounts learned and retained were about equal. Performance dropped slightly for both groups between posttest and maintenance test. Differences between results obtained from an open-ended oral test were not significant. Ss generally responded positively to CAI, but Ss in the Small Teaching Set condition enjoyed using the computer more. LD Ss performed similarly to non-LD Ss in a comparison group on the 50-item multiple choice posttest.
Jones, Torgesen, & Sexton (1987)	30	Ss were 20 school-identified LD Ss who participated in the two treatment groups. The control group consisted of 10 regular classroom Ss. The LD Ss' mean age was 10.8 yr. Ss	Word recognition Oral reading	A new computer program designed to increase decoding fluency in reading was evaluated. Ss practiced 15 min daily for 10 wk. Three groups were included in this study: Group 1, *Computer* Ss, practiced with computer and speech	Word recognition: speed and accuracy	Ss in the experimental group showed substantial improvements not only on words directly practiced by the program, but also on generalization words that

(continued)

Author (year)	*N*	Selection criteria	Target domain(s)	Treatment(s)	Measures	Results
Jones, Torgesen, & Sexton (1987) (*cont.*)		mean IQ score (WISC-R) was 99.25, and the PIAT Reading mean score was 3.1. Ss were slow readers.		digitizer. Ss practiced the first level of *Hint & Hunt* for 15 min. The vowel sounds (medial and combinations) were practiced with the "Hint" portion. When Ss were able to perform on 10 consecutive trials, they were moved to the "Hunt" game. They began at the slowest speed and moved to faster speeds. Four days were spent practicing a given level, then Ss progressed to the next level. On levels 2–10, Ss practiced the "Hint" portion until they were able to perform without error on 10 trials. After completion of 10 levels, five posttests were given. *Group 2, Computer Experience Control* Ss, practiced on the computer with the spelling program for 15 min/ day. They were matched with a S in Group 1 and took posttests at the same time. *Group 3, Non-LD Control* Ss, received no treatment.		were never practiced during the training.
Larson & Gerber (1987)	68	LD and low-achieving incarcerated youth aged 16–19 yr participated. Ss were drawn from a population of institutionalized high school Ss eligible for reading intervention based on reading achievement at or below 6th	Impulse control	This study investigated the efficacy of social metacognitive training focused on impulse control, metacognitive awareness, and metacognitive control for improving the overt social adjustment of incarcerated delinquents. LD and NLD Ss were assigned to either social metacognitive training, or to attention	*Cognitive variables:* Meta-awareness Ss were asked to identify knowledge about themselves and others that would be needed for solving social problems. An	Compared to control Ss, those who received metacognitive training experienced significant improvement in (1) quantity of negative behavior reports, (2) staff rating of rehabilitation

grade level (Tests of Adult Basic Education, 1976). Ss were identified as either LD or NLD low achievers based on California state guidelines, i.e., normal or above normal IQ, significant discrepancy between achievement and aptitude, and a determination by a school planning team that the S is not able to effectively learn in a regular school program. Decision rules for LD classification included total reading grade level at or below 4.7 and PPVT standard score at or below 62; total reading grade level more than 2 yr less than PPVT grade level score; or spelling below 5th grade level and a rating by teachers on average of 3 or less on a teacher questionnaire. All low achieving delinquents participating in remedial classes and ineligible for parole for at least 6 mo were eligible to volunteer. Ss had felony offense histories. LD delinquents were randomly assigned to one of three conditions.

control or test-only control groups. Treatment and attention control Ss received twenty-two 90-min training sessions over a 7-wk period. Two trainers worked with both treatment and attention control Ss; one was assigned to LD and one to NLD Ss. There were three treatment components. Verbal self-instruction lessons (3) taught Ss to covertly cue themselves to stop and think prior to responding in social risk situations; they were also taught to consider whether ignoring provocative stimuli or engaging in systematic problem solving would be more adaptive. *Metacognitive awareness* lessons (9) taught identification of salient problem-solving variables during interpersonal situations and evaluation of the usefulness of information about these variables in assessing problem difficulty and determining response requirements. *Metacognitive control skill* lessons (10) taught a seven-step, general problem-solving strategy for effectively using social metacognitive awareness information. Ss read aloud and followed lesson plans; each lesson was organized around cartoonlike posters. Ss practiced applying problem-solving skills daily following presentation of social problem scenarios or episodes. Activities followed

independent rater used a protocol to score answers. The final score consisted of the number of specific variables identified as important for social problem solving. *Metacontrol knowledge:* Ss were asked which problem-solving steps they would recommend to a younger peer. Blind interviewers and independent raters were used. The scores on this measure consisted of the quantity of specific problem-solving steps recommended.

Behavioral variables: Overt problem-solving behavior was analyzed by multiple dependent measures prior to and following training, including quantity of institutional behavior reports; attainment of phase level promotion

achievement, and (3) institutional living unit phase level promotion. Although both LD and NLD Ss who received cognitively training improved their behavior significantly, a greater proportion of the LD Ss improved on every variable. Parallel increases in metacognitive skill and significant correlations between social metacognitive scores and indices of metacognition and effective behavior suggest that social metacognition was the mediating variable.

(*continued*)

Author (year)	*N*	Selection criteria	Target domain(s)	Treatment(s)	Measures	Results
Larson & Gerber (1987) (*cont.*)				a general sequence; training for generalization followed principles described by Meichenbaum (1980). Attention control Ss were taught daily living skills to solve employment, money management, law, and driver's education problems. Activities were similar to treatment lessons except content was not focused on interpersonal problem solving.	from pre- to posttest; quantity of good days credit; and routine staff ratings of progress toward institutionally defined social rehabilitation goals.	
Lenkowsky, Barowsky, Dayboch, Puccio, & Lenkowsky (1987)	96	LD, emotionally handicapped Ss between 12 and 14 yr old attending a special education only school; WISC-R Full Scale IQs between 92 and 114. Ss were divided into four equal groups. Groups were initially equivalent based on distribution of Full Scale IQ scores, CTBS reading levels, age, and sex.	Self-concept	*Group 1* read and reported about general interest books that contained no specific references to adolescent stresses. *Group 2* read the same books as Group 1, but also participated in a group rap session each week. *Group 3* participated in three bibliotherapy sessions/wk which employed literature focused on problems frequently experienced by the Ss; this group was not involved in discussion related to therapeutic topics. *Group 4* read the same literature as Group 3, but also participated in one discussion group/wk oriented toward problem topics explored through the literature.	The WISC-R (Weschler, 1974) and the Comprehensive Test of Basic Skills were administered prior to the intervention. The Piers–Harris Children's Self-Concept Scale (Piers & Harris, 1969) was used before and after the intervention to assess self-concept.	A one-way ANOVA revealed significant differences between groups following treatment. Scheffe comparisons indicated that the two bibliotherapy groups had significantly higher self-concept scores following treatment than Ss who participated in rap sessions after reading general interest literature or only read those types of books without discussion afterward.

Moore, Carnine, Stepnoski, & Woodward (1987)	27	Ss were middle school Ss with LD. No information was available regarding IQ and achievement.	Math computation	Only Experiment 1 is reported here. The efficacy of Teacher Net, an inexpensive computer networking system, was examined to see if it effectively reduced teacher grading time and if it had any effects on Ss' acquisition of facts. As Ss completed a problem on their worksheets, they typed in the problem number and corresponding answer on their keyboards. Control Ss completed worksheets with paper and pencil.	Math facts and computation Amount of teacher time spent correcting worksheets	The results suggest Teacher Net can save the teacher tremendous time by assuming the tasks of providing immediate feedback to Ss, correcting and summarizing S performance, and administering and scoring S tests. The experimental condition provided savings in teacher time of over 14 hrs. The teachers in the control condition spent 15.10 hrs correcting worksheets. A two-tailed *t*-test revealed no significant differences between the Teacher Net and control groups on either facts or computational problems.
Prior, Frye, & Fletcher (1987)	27	Ss were referred to the experimenters by the special education unit at a local technical (secondary) school on the basis of their long history of reading problems. None was receiving any systematic individual remediation. Ss' mean age was 13.5, ranging from	Spelling Word recognition	The experiment consisted of six 30-min sessions over successive school days for the Bradley SOS remedial procedure. Ss were divided into two groups: Phoenician (most able to use phonological decoding for lexical access) and Chinese (showed deficiencies in phonological decoding). Three word types were used: R = Regular, N = Nonsense, and E = Exception. During	Schonell Word Recognition Test Baron Word List Spelling	Significantly more regular than exception words were spelled correctly after training and more words were spelled correctly in the posttest than at follow-up. There was no difference in levels of performance between the groups, and there was no interaction.

(continued)

Author (year)	*N*	Selection criteria	Target domain(s)	Treatment(s)	Measures	Results
Prior, Frye, & Fletcher (1987) (*cont.*)		13–14.6. Ss' mean PPVT scores were: Chinese, 12.7; Phoenician, 13.4; and Mixed, 13.1. Ss' mean scores on the Schonell Word Recognition Test were: Chinese, 62.3; Phoenician, 70.2, and Mixed, 75.6.		Session 1, 10 randomly ordered words were presented to the child. Instructional steps included: (1) The word was written correctly by the experimenter with plastic script letters; (2) The child named the word; (3) The child wrote the word, saying each letter of the word; (4) The child named the word again, and checked if it was written correctly; (5) Steps 2 and 4 were repeated twice for each word. The stimulus word was covered or disregarded when the child felt confident and could manage without it. During Sessions 2 through 6, a similar procedure was used except the 1st step was omitted. The S, rather than the experimenter, was then given the task of constructing the word with plastic script letters, which the S was encouraged to manipulate until the word "looked right." All errors were corrected by the experimenter. The S was to construct the word correctly and write it three times. All sessions were tape-recorded and phonetically transcribed. The no-treatment control group was mixed, with half Phoenician and half Chinese Ss.		

Swanson, Kozleski, & Stegink (1987)	2	The Ss were 15 yr old. Their IQ scores were 92 and 101, and their percentile scores on the reading section of the Woodcock–Johnson Psycho-Educational Battery were 5% and 9%.	Reading	A multiple BL design was implemented across two Ss. During BL, Ss were individually instructed to listen to taped prose passages (3 min in length). Ss could make notes on main ideas (MI), and were told how many idea units were in the passage. A practice session with *Old Mother Hubbard* was used where the S and teacher together wrote MIs while listening to the tape. After, Ss turned over their papers and recalled what they had heard. There was no time limit. Responses were taped and played back later. During playback, for each MI remembered, Ss were asked "how" they remembered. Cognitive Training was then provided using procedures similar to those used during BL. Ss were also given a "mapping organizer" to enhance their remembering, instead of a plain piece of paper. This strategy training taught Ss to map MIs on paper with supporting ideas. Ss used this while listening to the taped passages. Then they turned the paper over and were asked to recall idea units, word for word. Verbal responses were coded along with strategies used, including lip movements, and verbalizations. *Reading Comprehension* treatment occurred after each BL and training session. Ss silently read one 50-word passage from the Barnell–Loft Skill Builders Series, Level F (3rd grade). Ss answered 10 literal comprehension questions on idea units.	Prose recall performance was measured on three dependent measures: percentage of idea units recalled, percentage of strategy verbalizations per idea unit recalled, and percentage of facts correctly recalled on the transfer (comprehension) task.	A qualitative shift in verbal strategy reports occurred across training sessions. The introduction of cognitive training (visual and verbal mapping of idea units) increased the recall of prose compared to the BL conditions, although concurrent effects on reading comprehension tasks were minimal. It was assumed that unstable cognitive processes during prose recall, as well as nonequivalent mental processes between the two tasks, accounted for the poor transfer of training effects.

(continued)

Author (year)	*N*	Selection criteria	Target domain(s)	Treatment(s)	Measures	Results
Vanden Meiracker (1986) Dissertation	9	Ss were 2nd through 5th graders with a mean age of 9.99 yr (range, 8.25–13 yr). IQ (WISC-R or Stanford–Binet) was 85 or greater. On the WRMT, Ss scored at least 1 yr below grade level.	Reading comprehension	The study used an alternating treatment design where treatments were altered each day. The treatment condition was CAI. The control condition was teacher instruction. In both treatments, the S read a short story twice and answered a series of multiple choice questions. Levels of time on task were collected daily. *CAI:* Ss read a story two times silently. The computer controlled the speed. If the S answered the multiple choice questions incorrectly, the computer program brought the S back to the appropriate paragraph and the correct answer was highlighted. If the S correctly answered 80% of the questions correctly, she/he was presented with colorful graphics and the S was praised. If the S scored less than 80%, the S was prompted to read more carefully the next time. *Teacher Instruction:* The same process was used except that there was no computer assistance. The teacher went over the answers to the test and discussed the incorrect answers. If the S received 80% or better, the Ss were told they had done well. If the S scored less than 80%, the S was encouraged to do better the next time.	On-task behavior Multiple choice questions generated from short stories	Comprehension performance under teacher-based conditions was the same for the two subgroups. However, reading comprehension performance under computer-based conditions was a function of subtype membership. LD Ss with maladaptive patterns of classroom behavior showed lower performance levels under the computer-based condition than under the teacher-based condition, while LD Ss with normal patterns of classroom behavior performed equally well under both conditions. All Ss showed high levels of time on task under both conditions. No clear pattern in time-on-task data could be detected between conditions or between subgroups. LD Ss with maladaptive patterns of classroom behavior, however, spent 25–50%

						more time completing the teacher-based sessions than the computer-based sessions, which might be a possible explanation for higher performance levels under teacher-based conditions for this subgroup.
Wade & Kass (1987)	76	LD Ss from 3rd to 5th grade attending a public school. Ss were randomly divided into two groups.	Reading fluency Decoding skills	Both groups received 9 wk of remediation. One group received 3 wk of component deficit remediation based on the developmental theory of deviance and 6 wk of academic deficit intervention based on the Stanford Diagnostic Reading Test (SDRT; Karlsen, Madden, & Gardner, 1976a). The second group received academic intervention for the entire 9 wk. *Component Deficit Remediation:* The goal was to develop deficient psychological processes through specific remediation techniques. Four tasks were designed which were implemented in 1-hr sequential time segments. A highly descriptive one-paragraph story was used for the first three tasks of each lesson. Task 1 focused on haptic discrimination. Task 2 was oriented toward visualization. Task 3 targeted	Stanford Diagnostic Reading Test (SDRT; Karlsen, Madden, & Gardner, 1976a), Forms A and B. Form A was administered as a pretest and to plan remediation; Form B was given at posttest.	The posttest SDRT scores of Ss receiving both types of remediation were higher than those of Ss receiving the academic remediation alone when effect size analyses were used. In addition, effect size analyses for each SDRT subtest indicated significant improvement after component deficit remediation.

(*continued*)

Author (year)	*N*	Selection criteria	Target domain(s)	Treatment(s)	Measures	Results
Wade & Kass (1987) (*cont.*)				figure–ground perception. Task 4 was homework designed to reinforce all three types of processing. *Academic Deficit Remediation:* This intervention was individualized for each S based on SDRT results. The diagnostic procedures described by the test's authors were analyzed to determine instructional priorities, then specific objectives were developed. These objectives were written on each S's IEP. The researchers prescribed methods and materials.		
Borkowski, Weyhing, & Carr (1988)	75	School-identified RD disabled Ss, ages 10–14; 26 girls, 49 boys were assigned randomly to one of four conditions.	Reading strategies Metacognition Motivation	The intervention consisted of a Pretest, Training (two phases, five sessions total), and a Posttest (two sessions). One group received strategy training combined with attributional training during both training phases. The second experimental group received attributional training during training Phase 2 only. Controls either received strategy training alone or were presented tasks without training.	Stanford Diagnostic Reading Test (Reading Comprehension subtest); Antecedent Attributions questionnaire; paragraph summaries; teacher ratings of impulsive behavior (Conners) and reading levels.	Reading skills improved in the two attributional conditions following training, although long-term beliefs regarding reasons for success and failure proved more resistant to change.

Bulgren, Schumaker, & Deshler (1988)	64	Ss were part of 475 Ss in 23 classes who participated in the study. Of those Ss, 32 were LD. A subset of the remaining 443 experimental Ss was randomly selected to serve as experimental comparison Ss. For each LD S, a NLD S was randomly selected who was enrolled in the same course, and was the same gender, age, and grade as the LD S. LD Ss' mean age was 16.6 yr, ranging from 15.5 to 17.7. Ss were enrolled in grades 9–12, with a mean of 9.8. Ss' mean IQ score was 90.7, with a range of 74–133 (no instrument was named). On reading achievement, Ss' mean score was 87.9, with a range of 67–119 (no instrument was named).	Concept acquisition	This study consisted of a multiple BL across-groups-of-Ss design used to evaluate the effectiveness of *Concept Diagrams* and a related *Concept Teaching Routine* when used by regular class teachers to present concepts to heterogeneous groupings of Ss, including LD pupils in regular classrooms. The study focused on both teachers and Ss. The teachers' ability to prepare *Concept Diagrams* and to implement a *Concept Teaching Routine* in the classroom was measured. Ss were evaluated relative to performance on tests of concept acquisition, regular classroom tests, and notetaking before and after implementation of the *Concept Teaching Routine*. Teachers were trained in a 4-hr workshop to identify, prepare, and present concepts, including a description of and rationale for the steps to be followed, demonstrated by the trainer, with an opportunity to practice and to receive feedback. During BL, teachers analyzed two concepts using one textbook chapter from a social studies text and one chapter from a science text. Teachers were asked to describe in writing how they would present the major concept in the selected chapters and were given materials with which to work. They then implemented the	Concept acquisition tests Regularly scheduled tests Note taking	Teachers were able to select concepts from content material, prepare Concept Diagrams from those concepts, and present concepts to their classes. Both Ss with and without LD showed gains in their performance on tests of concept acquisition and in notetaking when the Concept Teaching Routine was used in the classroom. Gains in performance on regular tests were associated with the Concept Teaching Routine combined with a review procedure.

(continued)

Author (year)	*N*	Selection criteria	Target domain(s)	Treatment(s)	Measures	Results
Bulgren, Schumaker, & Deshler (1988) (*cont.*)				*Concept Teaching Routine* in their classroom. Teachers were observed and S progress was analyzed via concept acquisition tests and used as pretests. Finally, fine tuning of the teacher presentation was done by the trainers. During the *Concept Training Condition*, a concept was trained in each unit of study. Ss took notes and handed them in at the end of class. *Concept Instruction Steps* included (1) The teacher chose a concept; (2) The teacher constructed a list of key words; (3) Characteristics were described via symbols; (4) The teacher made a *Concept Diagram;* and (5) The teacher used the *Concept Teaching Routine* (i.e., advanced organizer, list of key words from chapter, symbols reviewed on diagram, concept was named, concept was defined, characteristics were discussed, one example of the concept was discussed, one nonexample was discussed, each example was linked to characteristics, each nonexample was linked to characteristics, Ss determined if the example and nonexample were members of the concept class, and teacher provided a postorganizer). In the Review condition, Ss were asked questions and were then told to fill out a blank *Concept Diagram* from memory.		

Collins & Carnine (1988)	26	All of the Ss were in 9th, 10th, or 11th grade, aged 14 to 17, and currently receiving help in a resource room. Nineteen of the Ss were LD according to local school district criteria which included having an IQ within 1 SD of the mean on the WISC-R and a score 30% or more below grade level on the Woodcock–Johnson. The other seven Ss were considered to be remedial. Ss were randomly assigned to treatment.	Reasoning skills	Experimental Ss received intervention via Revised CAI. Control Ss were engaged in CAI activities. The intervention took place in the resource room during regular instruction over 12 sessions. The revised CAI program involved methods to more clearly teach Ss to evaluate evidence in an argument. The original CAI program (Reasoning Skills Program; Engelmann, Carnine, & Collins, 1983), taught Ss about overlapping, inclusive and exclusive classes, and the words associated with the relationships among classes. Using this information, Ss could draw conclusions based on evidence. Ss were also taught to identify unsound arguments and to specify one of three reasons why an argument was unsound. Similarities between the original and revised CAI programs include: 10 lessons, 32 questions, comparable amount of text, each error is followed by a correction tailored to the error, missed items reappeared, and explicit strategies are modeled. Guidance was systematically faded until Ss were working independently. The differences included four major changes: (1) introduction of invalid evidence earlier; (2) delay of drawing-conclusions tasks; (3) focus on evidence when critiquing arguments; and (4) deletion of nonessential vocabulary	The Reasoning Skills Test (Collins, 1986): time to completion and error rates	Scores significantly favored Ss in the revision group who made fewer errors per lesson, took less time to complete the lessons, and had higher posttest scores on the criterion-referenced test.

(continued)

Author (year)	*N*	Selection criteria	Target domain(s)	Treatment(s)	Measures	Results
Lovett, Ransby, & Barron (1988)	112	Children referred to the LD Research Program at the Hospital for Sick Children in Toronto. Referrals for remedial reading treatment originated from multiple sources, e.g., medical and psychology staff, parents, and Metropolitan Toronto area boards of education. Children between 8 and 13 yr old were screened for inclusion when reading underachievement coexisted with at least low average ability. Exclusionary criteria included brain damage, hyperactivity, hearing impairment, chronic conditions, serious emotional disturbance, and primary language other than English. *Accuracy-Disabled* (66): Scores at least 1.5 yr below age expectancies on at least four different measures of word recognition. *Rate-Disabled* (46): Scores ranging from near to above grade level on at least four word recognition measures	Oral language Word recognition	Matching was used to obtain initial equivalence between the two groups according to chronological age, WISC-R Verbal IQ and WISC-R Performance IQ. The two samples differed on several measures of oral language development. The accuracy-disabled group was inferior on all three language measures, suggesting a multifaceted language and reading disability for Ss in this group. The rate-disabled Ss displayed relative language integrity, possibly indicating language processing deficits specific to orthographic input. Ss were randomly assigned to one of three treatments, i.e., word recognition and decoding skills training (DS), oral and written language instruction (OWLS), or training in classroom survival skills (CSS), an alternative treatment control that offered no direct instruction to remediate deficient skills. Forty treatments total were conducted for each program. Intervention was implemented in special laboratory classrooms at a pediatric teaching hospital. Special education teachers administered the treatments, with each teacher implementing each treatment with exactly one-third of his/her assigned Ss from each category, i.e., rate- or accuracy-disabled.	Durrell Analysis of Reading Difficulty (Durrell, 1955, Oral Reading, Word Recognition, and Word Analysis subtests; Gates–McKillop Reading Diagnostic Tests (Gates & McKillop, 1962), Words Flashed, Words Untimed, and Phrases Flashed subtests; Gilmore Oral Reading Test (Gilmore & Gilmore, 1968); Peabody Individual Achievement Test (Dunn & Markwardt, 1970), Reading Recognition subtest; Slosson Oral Reading Test (Slosson, 1963); Test of Rapid Reading Responses (Doehring, 1976), WDR and WMD subtests; Biemiller Test of Reading	The experimental treatments affected significantly higher word recognition performance, but improvements in contextual reading and oral language skills were not obtained. There was a posttest advantage for both disability subgroups associated with DS training. Accuracy-disabled readers made treatment-specific gains for both regular and irregular words. Gains for rate-disabled readers were limited to irregular words, but their gains were associated with both DS and OWLS training. The rate-disabled children achieved significant growth regardless of experimental treatment, but DS training produced greater gains.

		combined with scores at least 1.5 yr or more below grade level on four of five reading speed measures.			Processes (Biemiller, 1981); Wide Range Achievement Test-Revised (Jastak & Wilkinson, 1984).	
Rivera & Smith (1988)	8	Middle school Ss with LD attending cross-categorical classes for at least 3 hrs daily who were mainstreamed in regular classes for the rest of the day were participants. Selection criteria included arithmetic achievement at least 1 yr below grade level, ability to accurately compute addition and subtraction problems, and some ability with the multiplication process. Ss were randomly assigned to one of two instructors. Assessment involved two steps. First, Ss were assessed to determine their level of computation skill ranging from addition to division; Ss completed three worksheets for addition, subtraction, multiplication, and division that contained problems representing the instructional sequence for	Mathematics (long division)	The influence of a modeling technique involving demonstration, imitation, and key guide words on acquisition of long division was examined. Worksheets from the Computational Arithmetic Program (CAP; Smith & Lovitt, 1982) were modified for this study to control for equal representation on S worksheets of different division problem types. Four different worksheets were used over a 4-day instructional week; a fact table for multiplication/division was available to Ss to reduce the possibility of fact errors during solution of the division problems. A multiple BL crossover design was used across four pairs of Ss; they were randomly assigned to staggered BL conditions ranging from 3 to 6 days in length. During BL, Ss completed division worksheets without instruction or feedback. During intervention, Ss were shown graphs of their daily progress. The demonstration strategy followed, including: (1) the teacher solved a sample problem while verbalizing key words for the solution	Each S's percentage of correct responses on the worksheets was computed and graphed daily. When the criterion of 2 out of 3 days at 100% correct was reached on the skill initially targeted for instruction, Ss began instruction on the next long division skill.	Although initial scores on division problems were 0%, Ss mastered each long division skill in minimal time with the application of this intervention.

(*continued*)

Author (year)	*N*	Selection criteria	Target domain(s)	Treatment(s)	Measures	Results
Rivera & Smith (1988) (*cont.*)		each operation. For inclusion in the study Ss were required to demonstrate 90% average accuracy in addition and subtraction, and ability to multiply without regrouping. Second, Ss were assessed on a task-analyzed sequence of long division skills; a score of 0% in a division skill was the basis for instructional placement.		steps; (2) the S imitated the demonstrated process by completing a sample problem while repeating the key words; (3) the demonstrated problem remained visible while the S completed the worksheet. The intervention was individually administered daily prior to the Ss' independent worksheet completion. Instruction averaged 10 min during 45-min class periods. If Ss completed the sample problem correctly, they proceeded to complete their division worksheet; incorrect completion of the sample problem was followed by instructor repetition of the strategy with new problems. Ss received feedback on computation errors during independent seatwork; they were told to check errors, and they were asked specific questions when having difficulty or when they asked for help.		
Salend & Nowak (1988)	3	Ss assigned to a resource room program receiving supplemental instruction in reading, math, spelling, and writing.	Oral reading	Target Ss were paired with a peer according to ability and age, with older and more proficient Ss serving as peer previewers. Peer previewers read randomly assigned passages aloud while targeted Ss listened and followed along using a passage photocopy. After peer previewer read orally, the targeted S	Oral reading errors were recorded on passage photocopies; teacher circled words read incorrectly; errors included mispronunciations, omissions,	Peer previewing was associated with marked decreases in the Ss' oral reading errors, with collateral improvement noted in the targeted Ss' correct and incorrect reading rates.

				read the same passage to the teacher who recorded reading errors on a photocopy of the text. Sessions lasted about 5 min each; intervention duration was 15 days for all Ss.	substitutions, and unknown words, with the exception of suffix errors, i.e., -ing, -ed, and -s; hesitations of more than 5 sec were coded as errors, self-corrections were not recorded as errors.	
Somerville & Leach (1988)	40	Ss had reading problems at school. Their mean reading age was 8.10 on the Schonell Word Recognition Test. Each S had average to above average general abilities (IQ 90+).	Reading	Three intervention programs were conducted over twelve 1-hr weekly sessions. *Psycho-Motor* Ss participated in a wide variety of exercises, including patterning and trampoline work. Ss were given supervised homework exercises of approximately 15 min/day. *Self-Esteem* activities were designed to establish trust and confidence among group members and to encourage positive feelings about self, school, achievement, parents, and teachers. Ss were to gain insight into personal strengths and weaknesses and order their priorities. Ss were given 15 min/day of homework. Direct Instruction Ss were taught with the *Corrective Reading Programme* (Engelmann, Hanner, & Haddox, 1980). Instruction included a task-analyzed reading program for decoding. Staff taught parents how to deliver the lessons to the Ss. Ss received 15 min/day of homework. *The Wait-List Control Group* received no treatment.	Reading (Schonell, 1961) Psycho-motor skills (Newton & Thompson, 1976) Self-esteem (Lawrence, 1982)	The direct instruction program resulted in gains in reading performance significantly greater than the other two programs and the control group.

(*continued*)

Author (year)	*N*	Selection criteria	Target domain(s)	Treatment(s)	Measures	Results
Bos, Anders, Filip, & Jaffe (1989)	50	Ss with LD attending a middle-class high school in a large metropolitan district in the Southwest; reading 3 to 7 yr below grade level, with Verbal, Performance, or Full Scale IQ scores between 85 and 115 on individualized IQ measures; attending intact LD social studies and English classes. Ss were randomly assigned to experimental or contrast conditions.	Reading comprehension Content area learning	Instructional materials included experimental and practice passages, a relationship chart, and instructional guidelines for the experimental condition and a vocabulary list and instructional guidelines for the contrast condition. The relationship charts consisted of matrices on which the important passage ideas were listed across the top and related vocabulary words were listed down the side. *Semantic Feature Analysis:* Discussions of content along with completion of relationship charts in order to activate and instantiate prior knowledge and to predict relationships between old and new knowledge as represented by the concepts and vocabulary presented in the relationship charts. Ss received copies of the chart, which was also presented on the board or overhead. The name of the chart and each important idea were introduced. Definitions were either generated by the Ss or provided by the teacher. Ss were encouraged to share their prior knowledge, and vocabulary items were introduced using the same procedures. Once a definition was generated, the Ss	Prior Knowledge Assessment: a 20-item, multiple choice test of Ss' knowledge of the major concepts in the experimental reading passage about the Fourth Amendment. This measure was developed according to Langer's Prereading Plan (PReP; Langer, 1981), a strategy designed to assess topic knowledge prior to instruction. Comprehension Test: One test of comprehension was developed for each passage, with the test for the experimental passage used as the dependent measure. This consisted of a 20-item multiple choice test consisting of 10 vocabulary and 10 conceptual items.	Comprehension was measured immediately after instruction and again 6 mo following instruction. Prior knowledge for passage content served as a covariate. Results indicated that Ss in the SFA instructional condition demonstrated significantly greater comprehension than contrast Ss immediately following and 6 mo after instruction.

				predicted the relation between the vocabulary words and each important concept. Then Ss read the passage to confirm predictions and to clarify unknown relations between concepts and vocabulary. After reading, the chart was discussed and reviewed. *Dictionary Method Condition:* The teacher introduced and led a short discussion on the reading passage topic, then wrote the vocabulary list on the board and read the words while Ss repeated them. The Ss then used the dictionary to find and write a definition and sentence for each word related to the concept. Then the Ss read the passage to verify and/or clarify the word meanings. After reading, Ss modified their definitions if necessary according to information obtained during reading.	Vocabulary items measured selected vocabulary instructed in the two conditions; conceptual items required Ss to apply concepts presented in passages to real-life situations. Each item had five options, with the final item option being "all of the above" or "none of the above." Topic Interest Assessment: Three items required Ss to rate their agreement on a 5-point Likert scale ranging from "strongly agree" to "strongly disagree."	
Ellis, Deshler, & Schumaker (1989)	13	Ss were 10th to 12th graders enrolled in a special education resource room program volunteered to participate in this study. Mean age was 17.3, with a range of 15.2–19.5. Ss had been classified LD based on a	Problem solving	A multiple BL across-Ss design was used for this study. The BL condition consisted of individualized training in the substrategies. BL lasted from 2.5 wk to 6.5 wk. The treatment condition also lasted from 2.5 to 6.5 wk. Ss received the intervention in the resource room daily for 20 to 40 min. The goal of the	Metacognitive knowledge measure Near-generalization measure Far-generalization measure	Dramatic increases were observed in the Ss' verbal expression of metacognitive knowledge and ability to generate task-specific strategies. Ss' regular class grades increased. For those Ss who did not

(continued)

Author (year)	*N*	Selection criteria	Target domain(s)	Treatment(s)	Measures	Results
Ellis, Deshler, & Schumaker (1989) (*cont.*)		standard score regression formula with a 15-point discrepancy between ability and achievement. Mean WISC-R score was 92.6, with a range of 82 –109. Scores from the Woodcock–Johnson Psycho-educational Battery were: mean Reading, 5.75 (range = 2.8 to 8.0); mean Math, 6.61 (range = 5.3 to 9.4); and mean Written Language, 5.72 (range = 2.8 to 12.5)		Executive Strategy Procedures focused on a problematic situation. Ss were to identify and analyze the critical features of the problem, then generate a series of problem-solving steps and monitor the effectiveness of the self-generated strategy and make necessary modifications. The strategy included three substrategies (Ellis, 1985): (1) Zero-in-IDEA—This was used to conduct assessments with problem situations, and of the S's relevant strengths and weaknesses. The result was the identification of specific weaknesses for which a strategy could be constructed. (2) TASC—This was used to generate a strategy. Ss identified any single step that was crucial to solving previously identified weakness. The S was to use the Before and After Rule. The result was a set of sequenced steps for solving the problem. (3) ECHO—This enabled Ss to test the new strategy by trying to use it, monitoring its effectiveness, and modifying it to meet situational demands. S reported ECHO until the strategy was refined. A superordinate strategy—SUCCESS (Ellis, 1985)—combined all three of the above. Training steps included: Ss were taught		spontaneously generalize use of the strategy to problems encountered in these classes, providing instruction to target-specific classes resulted in improved grades.

				each of the substrategies individually (BL); Ss were then given instruction in the SUCCESS strategy and asked to apply the strategy to problems in their regular classes; Ss who appeared not to be achieving were given extra training to facilitate generalization by targeting a specific class for strategy application.		
Graham & Harris (1989)	33	LD Ss identified according to school district criteria; IQ scores between 85 and 115 on an individually administered intelligence test; achievement at least 2 yr below grade level in one or more academic areas; significant composition problems. Normally achieving Ss identified by scores between the 29th and the 81st percentile on the Cognitive Abilities Test (Thorndike & Hagen, 1978); above the 29th percentile on the reading vocabulary, reading comprehension, language mechanics, and language expression subtests of the California Achievement Tests; normally achieving, competent writers served as contrasts.	Metacognition Self-efficacy Writing	Undergraduate special education majors followed scripted lesson plans to instruct cognitive strategies. Instructors met with small groups of three or four Ss for about 45 min, 2 to 3 days/wk, for 2 to 3 wk. A criterion-based approach was adopted, with number of sessions and time spent varied according to mastery learning requirements. Two self-instructional strategy training groups of LD Ss were included. Both received story grammar strategy instruction, including emphasis on significance of the strategy. One group also received direct instruction in explicit self-regulation.	Story grammar elements: The schematic structure of written stories was assessed with a scale developed for this study. For each of eight story elements (i.e., main character, locale, time, starter event, goal, action, ending, and reaction), a score from 0 to 2 is assigned, where 0 = absence of the feature, 1 = inclusion, and 2 = highly developed. When two or more goals were included in a story, a score of 3 was given; scores of 3 or 4 were assigned when story actions/events followed a logi-	Self-instructional strategy training was associated with meaningful and lasting improvements in Ss' story writing skills, as well as with significantly improved sense of self-efficacy as a story writer. Explicit self-regulation procedures did not significantly enhance instructional effects for either writing performance or self-efficacy. After instruction, composition performance among LD Ss did not differ meaningfully from that of normally achieving Ss in terms of story grammar elements. Normally achieving Ss' compositions were longer and received significantly

(*continued*)

Author (year)	N	Selection criteria	Target domain(s)	Treatment(s)	Measures	Results
Graham & Harris (1989) *(cont.)*					cal sequence or when more than 1 well-defined episode was presented. The maximum points possible for this scale = 19. Holistic Rating Scale: Story quality was measured on a 7-point scale, with 1 representing the lowest writing quality, and 7 the highest. Examiners read each story to obtain general impressions first, then used representative samples of low, medium, and high quality compositions to guide scoring. Self-efficacy measure: An individually administered self-efficacy scale for creative writing was developed for this study. Scores ranged from 10 to 100 in 10-unit intervals, with higher values indicating higher perceptions of creative writing self-efficacy.	higher quality ratings than those of LD Ss', however. Treatment validation and confirmation of mediating responses was obtained. The educational validity of self-directed cognitive strategy training was also supported.

Writing stimuli: Four different black-and-white pictures were used to stimulate writing samples. Four measures were obtained, i.e., pretest, posttest, generalization, and main. Pictures were presented in the same order to all Ss.

The use of story grammar elements was analyzed before and after instruction. To determine whether improvements in story quality were related to changes in schematic structure, overall quality was analyzed pre-and postintervention. To assess intervention effects on narrative structure, changes in story grammar elements were examined. The treatment was validated by analyzing the use of story grammar strategies during instruction and independently. Data related to LD Ss self-efficacy as creative writers were also collected before and after intervention.

(continued)

Author (year)	N	Selection criteria	Target domain(s)	Treatment(s)	Measures	Results
Guyer & Sabatino (1989)	30	Ss were LD college Ss attending university summer school. Ss ranged in age from 17 to 24, with a mean age of 20.3. Ss mean WAIS-R score was 105.7, with a range of 94 to 135.	Reading	College Ss were studied to determine whether they would make more progress in a summer program if taught by an adaptation of the Orton–Gillingham (O–G) approach. Progress of those exposed to this approach was compared to progress of those exposed to a nonphonetic approach or a no-treatment control group. Group 1 Control group: Ss received no intervention. Group 2 Multisensory Orton–Gillingham (1960) Phonetic Approach: Multisensory techniques were used, including letter or letter combinations unknown to the S were taught and included consonants, vowels, blends, dipthongs, prefix, suffix, etc. The six syllable division types were also taught using the acronym "CLOVER": closed syllable, consonant -le, open syllable, vowel, silent e, r-influenced vowel. Group 3 Nonphonetic Approach: No attention was given to word attack skills. Ss were provided with information on understanding the main idea and supporting ideas and how details are arranged. Ss learned new words when reading in context and how to recognize synonyms and antonyms, prefixes. Critical and practical reading (following written directions, reading charts, illustrations, and more) was also taught.	Wide Range Achievement Test—Revised Woodcock Reading Mastery Test	The group who received the Orton–Gillingham phonics approach was found to achieve statistically significant improvement in reading when compared to the group using the nonphonetic approach or no educational activity. No statistically significant difference was noted between the latter two groups. This study indicated that a modified O–G approach was useful in the teaching of reading to college Ss who are LD.

Lovett, Ransby, Hardwick, Johns, & Donaldson (1989)	178	Children referred to the LD Research Program at the Hospital for Sick Children in Toronto; referrals for remedial reading treatment originated from multiple sources, e.g., medical and psychology staff, parents, and Metropolitan Toronto area boards of education. Children between 8 and 13 yr old screened for inclusion when reading underachievement coexisted with at least low average ability. Exclusionary criteria included brain damage, hyperactivity, hearing impairment, chronic medical conditions, serious emotional disturbance, and primary language other than English. *Accuracy-Disabled:* Scores at least 1.5 yr below age expectancies on at least four different measures of word recognition. *Rate-Disabled:* Scores ranging from near to above grade level on at least four word recognition measures combined with scores at least 1.5 yr or more below grade	Word recognition	*Decoding Skills (DS):* Word recognition and spelling skills were targeted. Word sets were divided into orthographically regular and orthographically irregular. Regular words were taught in word families with emphasis on phonic and visual rules. Exception words were introduced and practiced individually using whole word methods. Regular words were taught according to the difficulty of the grapheme–morpheme correspondence rule for the word family. The order for exception words was determined by actual frequency of use. Consolidation and automatization lessons were included for both word types. Phonetic analysis and word blending, rapid word recognition, morphological analysis, and written spelling were emphasized. No training was provided to improve reading or listening comprehension, or for sentence structure appreciation. Oral and Written Language Stimulation (OWLS): Attempted to simultaneously remediate several levels of language system deficits. Instruction focused on improving semantic and syntactic linguistic function. Intensive stimulation of oral language comprehension, reading and reading comprehension, and written composition was integrated into lessons	Experimenter generated exception words: reading and spelling lists Regular words: reading and spelling lists	Both experimental treatments resulted in significantly greater improvements compared to the results associated with the control condition. DS instruction produced posttest advantages in recognition of both regular and exception words as well as reliable improvements on measures of two out of three word identification tests. Spelling skill improvements associated with DS treatment were also obtained, and the same Ss made reliable gains in knowledge of representing speech sounds in print, in spelling accuracy, and in spelling performance on experimental spelling dictation measures although transfer to lexical spelling achievement measures was not obtained. OWLS instruction produced significant posttest advantages in terms of contextual reading

(continued)

Author (year)	*N*	Selection criteria	Target domain(s)	Treatment(s)	Measures	Results
Lovett, Ransby, Hardwick, Johns, & Donaldson (1989) (*cont.*)		level on four of five reading speed measures. Disabled readers were randomly assigned to one of three treatments designed to remediate deficits in specific literacy skills through some form of cognitive or language rehabilitation. Special education teachers administered all treatments; each teacher implemented instruction for each treatment program with about one-third of his or her assigned class.		sequenced over a series of 4-day cycles. Instruction was organized around weekly themes varied according to S interests and ages. Each 3-day cycle of silent and oral reading culminated on the 4th day with teacher-assisted writing. Parallel instruction in oral and written language concentrated on developing vocabulary, grammar and structural analysis, and discourse comprehension. *Classroom Survival Skills* (CSS): This was an alternative treatment control program in which Ss received the same amount of clinic time and professional attention available to the experimental Ss. Instead of remedial academic activities, control Ss received instruction in social skills, classroom etiquette organizational strategies, life skills, self-help techniques, and academic problem solving. No direct instruction in academics and no print exposure were provided. Forty treatment sessions were conducted for pairs of Ss who were seen in lab classrooms at a hospital. Treatment sessions were 50–60 min, 4 times/wk over 10 wk.		skills, oral vocabulary, and general semantic/syntactic skills. Significant treatment-specific effects related to language skills targeted by the OWLS program were also obtained and generalized improvements on measures of basic literacy skill components were obtained as well.

Newby, Caldwell, & Recht (1989)	5	Children with dysphonetic (two) or dyseidetic (three) dyslexia aged 8 to 10 yr participated. Ss applied for tutoring services at a college-based, professionally staffed reading clinic. Three Ss were receiving LD services in the schools. All were diagnosed using Boder and Jarrico's (1982) dysphonetic, dyseidetic, and mixed criteria based upon specific patterns of reading and spelling. Additional criteria included: (1) at least average intelligence as measured by any of the global scales of the K-ABC (Kaufman & Kaufman, 1983); (2) scored at least 1 yr below current grade level in reading comprehension for grades 1 to 3 or at least 2 yr below grade levels for grades 4 and above on an informal reading inventory (Johns, 1985) and on school-administered standardized achievement batteries; (3) evidence confirming dysphonetic or dyseidetic miscues qualitatively judged using an	Reading comprehension	Ss received intervention using a story grammar strategy wherein instruction was differentially designed to match the processing strengths of each dyslexia subtype. A multiple BL design across Ss was used; each S was randomly assigned to begin with a BL of two, four, or six BL sessions of traditional remedial tutoring, followed by story grammar strategy instruction matched to each Ss' dyslexia subtype. Ss were given two 70-min, one-to-one tutoring sessions each week for 7 wk total. Five vocabulary words were selected and taught that were believed to be conceptually important for understanding the story content. The story grammar strategy involved the teacher dividing a piece of paper into four squares. The vocabulary word was written in the first square, discussed, and related to a real-life context. The S then generated an example and a nonexample that were written in the second and third squares, respectively; the S wrote a definition in his/her own words in the fourth square. These vocabulary words were displayed and periodically reviewed. Next, a narrative story written at each S's instructional level was presented. During BL, standard instructional procedures were followed, including the teacher setting	Outcome measures followed the word recognition skills component of the lesson, using the passage read during that session, including: (1) number of words read orally in one minute excluding miscues; (2) percentage of words taught during word recognition training that were correctly read in list format; and (3) number of idea units recalled from each passage. Quantitative and qualitative methods were used to analyze the idea units data.	Treatment involving instruction of a metacognitive reading strategy was associated with significant improvements in the proportion of qualitatively important story elements Ss recalled. Although qualitative improvements were observed in the reading of Ss representing both subtypes of reading disorder, a smaller proportion of those with the dysphonetic pattern than those with the dyseidetic pattern demonstrated increases in the ideas recalled during treatment.

(*continued*)

Author (year)	*N*	Selection criteria	Target domain(s)	Treatment(s)	Measures	Results
Newby, Caldwell, & Recht (1989) (*cont.*)		informal reading inventory administered by reading specialists; and (4) a mental processing score indicating average ability in the area of presumed strength.		the purpose for reading and oral reading by the S. During the experimental phase, the story grammar strategy was taught along with setting the purpose for reading and oral reading; Ss were also taught story parts, and that using these parts would help them to better remember the story. Instruction for dysphonetic Ss sought to capitalize on their simultaneous processing strengths through the use of pictographs; dyseidetic Ss were given sequentially based instruction using prepared outlines to achievement instructional goals.		
Rosenberg (1989)	6 4	Elementary Ss participated who were diagnosed as LD according to state criteria, including: (1) a Full Scale IQ of 80 or above on the WISC-R or Stanford–Binet administered by a school psychologist; (2) learning problems not primarily due to hearing, vision, or emotional problems; and (3) a severe discrepancy between ability and achievement, with overall achievement at least 1.5 *SD* below expectancies. In the	Multiplication facts Spelling	Two studies investigated the impact of supplemental homework assignments on basic skill acquisition. A teacher was trained to teach scripted lessons and to collect the data for both guided and independent practice in the experimental procedures. These studies took place in a university-based laboratory school; a quiet corner was used for instruction and practice. Before the first study began, pretesting identified which basic multiplication facts were unknown by all Ss and a common remediation unit of 40 facts was developed. Ten were assigned to each of the experimental conditions,	*Math Performance* (*Study 1*): 20 DI and 20 DI & HW facts randomly ordered on eight forms of a daily testing sheet. Ss were told to complete as many facts as possible, placing an X over problems they could not do. The teacher enforced a 5-min time limit using unobtrusive timing procedures. The number of facts correct per	*Study 1:* Although the impact of the treatment varied across Ss, three factors appeared to maximize the effectiveness of homework assignments, i.e., homework completion rate, percentage correct of homework assignments, and acquisition rate of the presented content. *Study 2:* Results confirmed the effectiveness of direct instruction combined with supplemental homework

first study, the IEP for each S indicated need to acquire or develop fluency in basic multiplication facts. In the second study, a conference with the resource teacher resulted in targeting spelling skills for intervention.		direct instruction alone (DI) and direct instruction with supplemental homework (DI + HW); stratified randomization was used to assign these facts to experimental condition. An adapted alternating treatments designed was used to evaluate differences between the two treatments. Equal numbers of facts from each of the two experimental conditions were presented during regularly schedule math periods according to a prearranged presentation and practice schedule. For 30 min, direct instruction was provided; each lesson consisted of six activities: introduction and group rule review, daily performance checks, review of previous work and assigned homework, demonstration of and controlled practice, independent seatwork, and homework assignment. With the exception of homework assignment, all components were balanced to ensure coverage of both fact types. Homework consisted of math fact worksheets similar to the daily seatwork assignments; Ss were given daily homework sheets and reminders about the importance of homework. In the second study, individualized spelling lists were taught using the same instructional and homework procedures.	condition was counted; testing forms changed daily *Spelling Performance* (*Study 2*): 10 spelling words were tested daily (5 DI and 5 DI + HW). Frequency counts of words mastered were the dependent measure; mastery was defined as correct spelling for a word on 2 consecutive days. As words were mastered, new words were added to the instructional and daily testing word list. *Homework Completion Rate* (*both studies*): During daily reviews, the teacher recorded whether or not homework was returned. To be considered complete, 90% or more of the assigned problems had to have either a number or an X in the answer space.	assignments on acquisition of basic skills taught using the same instructional and homework procedures.

(*continued*)

Author (year)	N	Selection criteria	Target domain(s)	Treatment(s)	Measures	Results
Rosenberg (1989) (*cont.*)					Homework completion rate was calculated by dividing the number of assignments meeting completion criterion by the total number of homework. *Percentage Correct on Homework Assignments* (*both studies*): Assignments were graded and scores recorded. A percentage was calculated by dividing the number of facts or words correctly completed by the number assigned. An average rate correct on homework assignments was obtained by computing the mean of the daily scores.	
Scruggs & Mastropieri (1989)	20	Ss were 7th and 8th graders with LD attending three history classes participated. All were classified as LD based on initial teacher referral, evaluation by school psychologist, special education personnel, and a multidisciplinary team	Social studies	Ss were taught U.S. history content over an 8-wk period; mnemonic and nonmnemonic materials were alternated in a within-Ss design. For the mnemonic instructional condition, materials were adapted from the regular curriculum; an outline was developed for each chapter. Transparencies were made of outlines and illustrtaions; scripts were developed	Chapter content was assessed at the end of each 2-wk chapter by a 20–30-item multiple choice test. In addition, teachers were asked to report grades at the end of the study that Ss	Ss obtained an average of 62.4% correct under mnemonic instruction compared to 46.8% correct under traditional instruction. Average grades of "B" were earned during mnemonic instruction compared to average grades

		meeting. Ss met state and federal guidelines for identification as LD, i.e., a significant discrepancy between ability and achievement not explained by sensory, emotional, environmental, or intellectual factors; enrolled in special education programs, spending at least five periods/day in special education classes; described by teachers as deficient in study skills		which detailed the information in each mnemonic picture and described the chapter outlines, informaiiton to be learned, strategy usage information, and review-and-practice pages. S booklets were also developed to accompany the chapters. Instructional materials were developed for the traditional instruction condition which closely paralleled those used in the mnemonic condition, with the exception that mnemonic pictures and strategy usage information were not included. Teachers were asked to use the model of effective instruction described by Mastropieri and Scruggs (1987a), including: (1) daily review, (2) statement of instructional objective, (3) presentation of new material by teacher, (4) guided practice, (5) independent practice, and (6) formative evaluation. The four chapters were taught over an 8-wk period; each class met for 50 min/day. Mnemonic and traditional instruction was alternated.	received under traditional and mnemonic instruction; these grades reflected S performance on tests, quizzes, worksheets, and class participation. Teachers were also asked to complete a Behavioral Intervention Rating Scale (BIRS, Von Brock & Elliott, 1987) for each S with respect to academic behavior under each condition.	of "D+" during traditional instruction; the difference between these grades was statistically significant. According to teacher reports on the FIRS, mnemonic materials were viewed as significantly more appropriate for content area instruction of LD Ss. Teachers also reported that Ss enjoyed using mnemonic materials, were more motivated under mnemonic instructional conditions, and engaged in substantially more class instruction during this type of instruction.
Smith (1989) Dissertation	34	Elementary Ss who ranged in age from 8 to 12 yr old were included. All Ss had 85+ IQ and tested at or below the 25 percentile on the WRMT.	Reading Phonetic analysis	The experimental group received mnemonic instruction in a direct instruction format. Ss met twice weekly for 25 min for a total of eight sessions. The treatment involved the use of key phrases paired with interactive pictorial prompts. Sample decoding exercises were incorporated into lessons. Children	Correct scores on other sounds Correct scores on letter clusters	An analysis of variance showed significant results in favor of the mnemonic method. The success could also be attributable to an interaction of the direct instruction approach and the mnemonic method.

(continued)

Author (year)	*N*	Selection criteria	Target domain(s)	Treatment(s)	Measures	Results
Smith (1989) (*cont.*)				learned the 10 mnemonic cards and associated phrases over five trials. Next, there were one to five recall trials, as needed. Missed items were reviewed. Ten target letter clusters were used based on high frequency use: ai, au, ay, oa, oi, oo, oy, ph, wh, wr. All words were represented by mnemonic pictures and letter combinations were matched with mnemonic pictures. Three cue questions were used with the letter combination and mnemonic cards: What does "oi" usually say? What do you think of when you see "oi"? Why will you think of *boiling soil* (mnemonic picture) when you see "oi"? The S then repeated the question without the mnemonic card and answered the question. The S also repeated the question without the letter cluster card and answered the question. Both real words and nonwords were used. The control Ss received no instruction. However, all control Ss were receiving some type of additional remedial instruction in reading, but unrelated to the experimental group.		

Snider (1989)	26	Junior high Ss at three different sites identified LD according to guidelines and receiving services in a resource room. Exhibited a significant discrepancy between ability and achievement not primarily the result of a physical handicap, mental retardation, social, and/or emotional factors. Potential Ss were excluded if WISC-R scores were below 85, included if decoding skills were adequate to easily read the passages presented in the study an a lack of information and vocabulary concepts as defined for this study. No attempts were made to randomly assign Ss to treatment conditions, although experimental Ss were drawn from one site, with Ss at the other schools serving as controls.	Reading comprehension	Experimental Ss received instruction that emphasized thetechniques and content of two direct instruction programs: *Comprehension B* of the *Corrective Reading Program* (Engelman et al., 1978) and *Reading Mastery* (Engleman & Hanner, 1983). Materials and worksheets were adapted from *Reading Mastery* III and IV. Lessons taught factual information and/or vocabulary about topics assessed in the reading passages. Each lesson consisted of three parts: (1) a structured oral presentation of lesson content, (2) application of the information by Ss, and (3) independently completed written exercises. Review was provided in game format after every 8 lessons were completed. There were 24 lessons total.	Decoding was assessed by the Reading Mastery IV (Engleman & Hanner, 1983) to determine skill levels. Prior knowledge was measured by an instrument designed by the experimenter for this study. The 24 tasks included were open-ended questions about topics that were covered in the experiment. Curriculum-based tests were constructed to correspond with topics instructed in each of the 24 experiment lessons. There were 24 sets, three passages each, with one focal topic per set.	Evidence was obtained from a split-plot factorial ANOVA for the utility of increasing background knowledge to improve reading comprehension performance. Comparisons of the marginal means revealed that experimental Ss were able to accurately answer more of the comprehension questions. Main effects for type of passage were also obtained, suggesting that degree of difficulty of a comprehension question is influenced by the quantity of information provided in the text. Post hoc analyses indicated that the differences between explicit and implicit questions accounted for much of the variance. Viewed overall, the results of this study suggest that many interrelated factors affect reading comprehension, and that some of these factors are hierarchical, implying that the emphasis of instruction should be varied accordingly.

(continued)

Author (year)	*N*	Selection criteria	Target domain(s)	Treatment(s)	Measures	Results
Trapani & Gettinger (1989)	20	Ss were boys in the 4th, 5th, and 6th grades attending public schools; diagnosed LD according to school district criteria, with placement in LD resource room for 50% of the school day. All Ss in this study were identified by specialists with LD certification as exhibiting problems with social skills according to ratings on the Walker Problem Behavior Identification Checklist. Ss were randomly assigned to participate in the experimental, the comparison, or the control group.	Social skills Spelling	The intervention involved two components: social skills training and cross-age tutoring. Experimental Ss received both types of treatment. Comparison Ss received only the social skills training. *Social Skills Training:* During this phase, children in the experimental and the comparison groups received direct instruction in five social communication skills. The control group remained in their LD resource room and completed typical activities. This phase lasted seven consecutive school days following completion of the pretest. The trainer was blind to the Ss' group assignments. These sessions lasted about 30 min/day. Each skill was instructed separately according to a standardized procedure using a scripted lesson. There were five phases total including pretesting and posttesting. *Cross-age Tutoring:* After the social skills training phase, experimental Ss tutored NLD 2nd grade boys in spelling. These sessions were about 20 min/wk over 4 consecutive school wk. Tutors and tutees met in rooms separate from their classrooms. The LD Ss were instructed	Three performance scores were collected for each child. Spelling achievement was pretested and posttested with the Test of Written Spelling (TWS; Larsen & Hammill, 1976). Children's classroom behavior was rated by teachers pre- and postteatment using the Walker Problem Behavior Identification Checklist (WPBIC; Walker, 1983). Observations of the frequency/appropriateness of each target behavior were made in the LD resource room during unstructured activities at three different points in the study: prior to social skills training, between the social skills training	Experimental Ss obtained significantly higher TWS scores than Ss in the control or the comparison groups. No meaningful differences were observed for the WPBIC. Experimental Ss showed higher rates of appropriate greeting and question response.

				to provide dictated practice with corrective feedback to children identified by their teachers as benefiting from extra practice. This phase was designed to ensure practice of the five social behaviors targeted by the initial phase of the study. The comparison Ss remained in the LD resource rooms and worked for an equivalent time period with an LD partner who was not a study participant.	and the cross-age tutoring, and after the cross-age tutoring was completed.	
Wallace & Bott (1989)	4	Ss were 8th graders with LD who were receiving resource room support services participated. All were identified as LD according to Kentucky state guidelines, and were nominated by special education teachers as having an IEP objective in the area of written expression. Although all Ss achieved overall scores within 1 *SD* below the mean on the TOWL (Hammill & Larsen, 1978), CBM data and BL measures collected for this study indicated these Ss had not mastered the specific skill of writing expository paragraphs.	Expository paragraph writing	The effects of teaching a metacognitive text structure strategy, called Statement Pie (Hanau, 1974) upon paragraph writing skills was examined. This strategy teaches Ss to understand the relation between supporting details and the main idea. Ss were taught to use an outline as a paragraph-planning guide, which was then used to transform the information into expository paragraphs. All BL probes and instructional sessions were completed in a one-to-one format in an LD resource room; generalization writing samples were completed in other resource rooms and mainstream classes in the same middle school. A certified LD teacher taught the strategy in a multiple probe design across three instructional phases and across four Ss for 8 wk; a series of consecutive probe	Data on writing performance were collected continuously throughout this study. During BL phases, data were collected on all three tasks: generating Pies, outlining, and writing paragraphs. A scoring guide was used to evaluate each paragraph, with points assigned according to the following criteria: (1) topic sentence present, 2 points; (2) related details fit topic, 1 point each, 3 points maximum; (3)	All Ss reached the criterion for instructional outcomes on writing compare/contrast and sequence paragraphs. In addition, Ss generalized their paragraph writing skills to other teachers and to different classrooms 1 wk after reaching mastery in the special education classroom. These results suggest that adolescents with LD to improve their paragraph writing skills when provided with intensive instruction in a text structure strategy.

(*continued*)

Author (year)	*N*	Selection criteria	Target domain(s)	Treatment(s)	Measures	Results
Wallace & Bott (1989) (*cont.*)				sessions were conducted between instructional phases. Instruction occurred daily, consisting of three phases of scripted lessons related to the three target behaviors; length of these sessions varied according to phase, averaging 23 min across sessions and Ss. Ss only received instruction if BL performance was below the mastery criterion of 80% correct for 3 days consecutively. Each phase consisted of the same general activity sequence: (1) instructional objective stated, (2) target behavior modeled, (3) examples and nonexamples provided, (4) guided practice, (5) independent practice with feedback, and (6) daily probes. Both compare/contrast and sequence text structures were instructed on a counterbalanced schedule of phases, including: (1) generating statement pies (*p*roofs, *i*nformation, and *e*xamples) according to a specific outline; (2) outlining statement and pie ideas from expository paragraphs; and (3) writing paragraphs. Generalization samples were obtained 1 wk following the final BL phase.	information logically or sequentially presented, 1 point; (4) transitional statements or text structure signal words present, 1 point; and (5) no intrusive or irrelevant material, 1 point. A percentage score for paragraph writing was obtained by dividing the points earned on two paragraphs (1 for each type of paragraph) by the total points possible.	

Wilson (1989) Dissertation	62	Ss in this study were between 9.7 and 10.2 yr old (mean ages) and were currently in a resource room or self-contained special education class. The mean IQ scores ranged from 89.5 to 96.7, and the mean reading scores ranged from 2.0 to 3.1 in grade equivalent.	Math	There were three groups in this study. A pool of 304 word problems were used in the pre-, post-, and follow-up tests and training materials were from 1st and 2nd grade math texts and workbooks. 4 problem types were used: (1) simple action, (2) classification, (3) complex action, and (4) comparison problems. Treatments 1 and 2 consisted of the direct instruction method (Silbert et al., 1981) and Treatment 3 (Control) used the school's basal text, *Math Today* (1985, No author given). *Treatment 1, Strategy Plus Sequence:* The teacher presented and the Ss practice sets of problems from one of the four problem types per session. Training for each problem type lasted for 3 consecutive days for a total of 12 lessons. *Treatment 2, Strategy Only Sequence:* Ss were presented with and practiced a balanced combination of the four problem types per session. Ss were taught to use the strategy, but the practice problems were presented without regard for the problem type. In both Treatments 1 and 2,the format for introducing word problems included three parts: (1) discrimination skill for problem type, (2) a structured board presentation, and (3) worksheet for individual practice	Experimenter generated mathematics test	Ss in the strategy plus sequence and strategy only groups scored significantly higher at posttest than those in the sequence only group 2 wk later, Ss in the strategy plus sequence group scored significantly higher than Ss in the other two groups. In sum, direct instruction to use a strategy was superior to the other approaches.

(continued)

Author (year)	*N*	Selection criteria	Target domain(s)	Treatment(s)	Measures	Results
Wilson (1989) (*cont.*)				*Treatment 3 Sequence Only* (control): No direct instruction was involved in this condition. Instructions were taught from the basal math series, *Math Today*. Teacher engaged Ss in discussion about the word problems, and included four steps in the lessons: (1) Ss wrote the numbers from the problems; (2) Ss identified the operation; (3) Ss wrote the equation; and (4) Ss wrote the answer. Ss were given problem types in the same manner as in Treatment a: training for each problem type lasted for 3 consecutive days.		
Ault, Wolery, Gast, Doyle, & Martin (1990)	5	The study included three experiments. The Ss for all three experiments were the same. One S moved after the first experiment. Ss ranged in age from 8.9 to 10.10 and were enrolled in both regular and special education classes in 3rd and 4th grades. Mean WISC-R IQ was 102.5, with range 90–118. Range on the word recognition subtest of the Brigance Diagnostic Inventory of Basic Skills (BDIBS) was 1.5–2.0.	Word recognition	*Experiment 1*: A progressive time-delay procedure was used to teach word reading in a small group. The effects of a single-trial, predictable sequence were compared to a single-trial, unpredictable sequence. *BL* 1:1 sessions to assess performance on all words in the study, daily for a minimum of 3 days or until stable performance was evident. 55 trials were recorded in 3-sec intervals. Ss received one trial on each S's target words, one trial on each of the other S's target words, and one trial on each of five known words. *Intervention* Each day Ss took part in a small group session. All	*Experiment 1:* Percent of correct responses with word recognition	The progressive time-delay procedure was reliably implemented and was effective in establishing criterion-level responding by all group members. Ss also learned words taught to other Ss through observation. In Experiment 1, the two trial sequences did not differ substantially, and in Experiment 3, two Ss initially produced higher levels of correct responding in the multiple-trial,

Ss were taught target words specifically for them at the second grade level. Ss responded individually rather than chorally. Each S received 15 trials/session; Ss received 34 sessions total.		predictable sequence. However, no substantial differences were found in observational learning. Across all investigations, no consistent effects of the trial presentation methods were noted.
Experiment 2: A progressive time-delay procedure was used in a small group to teach abbreviation identification. The effects of a multiple-trial, predictable sequence were compared to a multiple-trial, unpredictable sequence. BL Prior to instruction, all 32 abbreviations plus 5 known words or abbreviations were presented in 37 trial sessions. These sessions were conducted for a minimum of 3 days or until stable. Procedures were identical to Experiment 1. Intervention Each S was taught 8 abbreviations, 4 in each condition. Ss received one small group instructional session each school day. Abbreviations were taught using the progressive time-delay procedure. Each session included four trials on each of their four abbreviations. The intervention included two instructional conditions alternated across days (multiple trial and single trial).	*Experiment 2:* Percent of correct responses with abbreviations	
Experiment 3: A model-test procedure was used to teach a small group. The effects of the multiple-trial, predictable sequence were compared to the single-trial, unpredictable sequence. An	*Experiment 3:* Percent of correct responses—predictable and unpredictable sequence condition	

(*continued*)

Author (year)	*N*	Selection criteria	Target domain(s)	Treatment(s)	Measures	Results
Ault, Wolery, Gast, Doyle, & Martin (1990) (*cont.*)				adapted alternating-treatments design was used in all experiments. *BL* Prior to instruction, all 40 words plus 5 known words were presented in 45 trial sessions. Three BL sessions were conducted prior to a 1-wk school district vacation, with one session after the Ss' return. *Intervention* A small group instructional session was conducted each school day. Each of the other Ss read their list aloud. Two conditions were alternated across day (multiple and single trial); 5 words w ere taught per condition. Ss received 15 trials per group member in each session. In all three experiments, other children learned the words or abbreviations of the other children by watching.		
Bakker, Bouma, & Gardien (1990)	98	Ss classified as dyslexic. Mean age was 10.0 yr; IQ was equal to or greater than 80, and reading mean was 7.5.	Reading	Treatment was based on the assumption that L- and P-type dyslexia result from deviations in the development of hemispheric subservience. In this study, L-dyslexic Ss received HSS (hemisphere-specific stimulation) of the right hemisphere by the presentation of words to the fingers of the left hand. P-dyslexic Ss received HSS of the left hemisphere by the presentation of words to the fingers of the right hand. Ss met twice weekly for 20- to 25-min sessions. In	Number of substantive and fragmentation errors during oral reading	HSS-treated L-dyslexics, relative to controls, tended to show larger improvement in accuracy of text reading. HSS-treated P-dyslexics, relative to controls, showed larger improvement in fluency of word reading.

				both groups, treatment began with single letters and progressed to words and sentences. Special exercises followed. L-dyslexic Ss were given three words visually and then asked which matched the word on the planning board. P-dyslexics had to find a word that rhymed with a word that was traced by touch. Control Ss (L- and P-dyslexics) were treated according to the discretion of the remedial teacher with the stipulation that no experimental treatment be given.		
Bos & Anders (1990)	61	Ss were recruited from middle- and lower-middle-class junior high schools. Mean age was 13.80; mean IQ was 91.97. Woodcock–Johnson reading test mean was 81.30.	Reading comprehension Vocabulary	This study compared the effects of three interactive vocabulary strategies derived from the knowledge hypothesis with definition instruction derived from the access and instrumental hypotheses. The first intervention day varied by treatment. *Semantic Mapping* (SM) *Day 1:* The researcher and S constructed hierarchical relationships from a vocabulary list. *Semantic Feature Analysis* (SFA) *Day 1:* The researcher and Ss predicted the relationships among concepts using the relationship matrix. *Semantic Syntactic Feature Analysis* (SSFA) *Day 1:* Same as SFA with the addition of predicted answers for the cloze-type sentences using their matrix as a guide. _*Day 2 for all three groups:* The researcher and Ss set purposes for	Vocabulary, Comprehension, Relevant Vocabulary, Relevant Conceptual Units, Quality of Scriptal Knowledge, and Holistic Reading	Results from the multiple choice items suggested that Ss participating in the interactive strategies demonstrated greater comprehension and vocabulary learning than Ss receiving definition instruction. Results of the written recalls indicated qualitatively and quantitatively greater recalls at long term for Ss in the SFA and SSFA conditions compared with the DI condition.

(*continued*)

Author (year)	*N*	Selection criteria	Target domain(s)	Treatment(s)	Measures	Results
Bos & Anders (1990) (*cont.*)				reading according to their intervention and then read the passage. After reading, Ss received a postreading activity and again discussed the matrix and maps, or practiced and reviewed the vocabulary and definitions. *Day 3 for all three groups:* Ss were given 10 min with an aide to study for the posttest using the definitions, map, matrix, or matrix and sentences. The control group received *Definition Instruction.* This included direct instruction teaching of definitions of vocabulary terms. Oral recitation, correct and automatic pronunciation of each vocabulary word or phrase, and memorization of concise context-related definitions.		
Brown & Felton (1990)	42	Ss were drawn from a larger sample of public school children screened during spring of their kindergarten yr for risk of reading disability using teacher ratings and the Otis–Lennon Mental Abilities Test (Otis & Lennon, 1968). Excluded children were either teacher-rated as above average to superior in potential for reading success,	Beginning reading skills	General procedures for this study were adapted in order to allow evaluation of instruction effects within the regular classroom and avoidance of negative labeling. A project teacher worked with the teacher assigned to each classroom; the project teacher provided support services in the area of reading to the at-risk Ss in this study. Ss were randomly assigned to one of two instructional conditions throughout grades 1 and 2. The methods of reading instruction	Each child was administered measures of reading and spelling achievement at the end of 1st and 2nd grade, including the Woodcock Reading Mastery Test, Form A (WRM; Woodcock, 1973), the Test of Written Spelling—2	Ss in the code-emphasis group earned uniformly higher scores at the end of 1st and 2nd on all measures. At the end of 1st grade, insignificant differences were found between groups on spelling of phonetically regular words and on nonword reading. At the end of 2nd grade, significant.

		or those who had IQs below 80 on the Otis–Lennon. The remaining children were individually tested for phonological awareness, naming, and auditory short-term memory. To be included in this study, scores on at least three of the research measures of 1 or more *SD* below the group mean or in the bottom 16th percentile were required. Also excluded were children retained in kindergarten. Six groups of eight at-risk children were placed in regular 1st grade classrooms at five different schools; six Ss moved before the study was complete.		included a structured phonics code-emphasis approach or a context-emphasis approach. Criteria for selection of reading programs included (1) designed for instruction within the regular classroom; (2) structured to include emphasis on both word identification and comprehension; and (3) contained well-developed teacher manuals, as well as basal readers and work books for each child. The Houghton Mifflin program (1986) was chosen as the context-emphasis approach, and the Lippincott Basic Reading program (1981) as the code-emphasis approach.	(TWS; Larsen & Hammill, 1986), the Decoding Skills Test (DST; Richardson & DiBenedetto, 1985), and the Metropolitan Achievement Tests—Primary 1, Form L (MAT; Prescott, Balow, Hogan, & Farr, 1985).	differences occurred in decoding of monosyllabic and polysyllabic nonsense words and in reading of polysyllabic real words. The authors concluded that reading instruction exerts significant impact on early reading skill acquisition, and that structured, systematic phonics instructions has more powerful influence than context-emphasis approaches on reading acquisition
Chan, Cole, & Morris (1990)	78	*RD:* Intelligence within normal limits, but reading skills 2 or more yr below age expectancies, and deficiencies not primarily due to physical and/or emotional disabilities or environmental influences. The LD sample consisted of 39 upper elementary Ss. *Average Readers:* Younger Ss whose word recognition	Reading comprehension	Training was conducted with groups of 4 to 5 at Ss home schools; intervention occurred in one of three groups. *Visualization Only* Ss were trained to generate images. *Visualization Instruction with Pictorial Display* Ss were instructed to generate images plus they were shown a pictorial display that illustrated the story events sequentially. The *Read–Reread* control Ss were instructed to read without instructions to visualize.	St. Lucia Graded Word Reading Test (Andrews, 1973) Comprehension tests were constructed for passages used in this study in a multiple choice format. Individual interviews were employed to assess strategy use.	This study confirmed the benefits of strategy instruction for LD Ss. Comprehension was optimized by visualization instruction along with pictorial display. The benefits depended on training method and amount of help provided. Although comprehension

(*continued*)

Author (year)	N	Selection criteria	Target domain(s)	Treatment(s)	Measures	Results
Chan, Cole, & Morris (1990) (*cont.*)		scores were used to match them to LD Ss. Thirty-nine normal achievers served as reading level matches for this study. Ss were randomly assigned to one of three treatments.		Experimental Ss received strategy instruction prior to the first reading, were asked to use strategy while listening to a prerecorded tape of the story, and then were directed to use the strategy without audiotape or display. Controls read the story three times.		was enhanced, negative effects on generalization were also observed.
DiVeta & Speece (1990)	2	1st graders attending a public school that served only children with handicaps who were diagnosed as LD. IQ score for S1 was 100, and for S2 was 113, and the PPVT-R score was 85+ for both. Mean age was 7.1, with a range of 6.8 to 7.4.	Reading Spelling	An alternating treatment design was used in this study. Each training type was not repeated for more than two consecutive sessions. The sessions were 25 min. Ss were given three trials to correctly blend or spell the list of 12 words. The experimenter gave correction. After three incorrect trials, the experimenter gave the correct blending or spelling, next said the word, then had the child repeat it. Each session began with an explanation of the difference between real words and nonwords. The experimental condition was *Blending*. The S was given three tiles and shown the CVC word. The child was taught to say the first phoneme as a unit and add the last phoneme. The control condition was referred to as *Spelling*. Ss were given nine tiles. The experimenter then said a word and the child repeated it. The S selected letter tiles and pronounced the sound of each letter.	Percentage of words read correctly Phonemic segmentation task	Although neither intervention proved superior, the Ss met the learning criterion for both interventions and demonstrated both maintenance and generalization of their skills. They also improved their phonemic skills, even though independent training in this area was not provided. It appeared that the equivalence of the interventions might have been due to the intensive instructional setting and use of systematic error analysis procedures.

Ellis & Graves (1990)	47	LD with accurate decoding, but poor comprehension skills. Minimum Full Scale IQ of 85 on the WISC-R, plus 2 or more yr below grade level on the PIAT reading comprehension subtest with a minimum 15-point discrepancy between ability and achievement. Ss were screened to select those who could read 3rd grade level material at 100 wpm with 97% accuracy, and who scored 60% or less on comprehension tasks from *Reading for Concepts, Level C.*	Reading comprehension	Ss were trained to use specific procedures for deriving main ideas. Common features of training included (1) Ss taught the technique could increase comprehension; (2) Instruction included modeling, prompted practice, and corrective feedback; (3) Ss allowed 12 min/selection to read and apply the strategy; (4) Reading selections randomly assigned; (5) Ss required to select main ideas from multiple choices during the first 4 days of training, then generate main ideas during the second 4 days; (6) During the first 2 days of training, only one practice story was given, then two stories were provided per day; (7) Items for the first 4 training days were similar to those used on the screening measure, selections from the *Health Science Book* for 5th grade used thereafter. Four training conditions were used. *Control:* Following a brief definition of main idea, Ss read stories and answered multiple choice questions about main idea. *Repeated reading:* A brief definition of main ideas was provided, and the RR technique was modeled; Ss were instructed to read the story repeatedly within the allotted time to find main ideas. *Paraphrasing strategy instruction:* Ss were taught a task-specific paraphrasing strategy and told to	Ten-item multiple choice tests wer e constructed to accompany a pool of stories selected from *Reading for Concepts, Book C.* Ten stories were randomly chosen for use as a pretest, six were selected for training, and ten for evaluation of treatment effects.	Paraphrasing instruction was superior to the repeated reading method. Pairing both strategies was not more effective than only teaching the paraphrasing strategy.

(*continued*)

Author (year)	*N*	Selection criteria	Target domain(s)	Treatment(s)	Measures	Results
Ellis & Graves (1990) (*cont.*)				repeat this procedure for each paragraph read. Instruction initially included definition of main ideas and description of the strategy, followed by modeling, guided and independent practice, and corrective feedback. *Paraphrasing strategy instruction plus repeated reading.* PSI modified to include repeated reading.		
Fletcher & Prior (1990)	40	2nd and 3rd graders with a mean age of 9.8. Mean IQ was 96.6; mean reading age in word knowledge was 6.7 for the 2nd graders and 4.9 for the 4th graders. Reading age comprehension stanine scores were 6.2 for 2nd graders and 3.3 for the 4th graders.	Reading Phonics	Only Study 2 is reported here. The performance of RD and non-RD Ss was compared. Both groups received the same treatment. Ss met for three 15-min sessions in 1 week. Each S was presented with a set of 54 pseudoword cards and told that on each card was an unfamiliar word. The S was asked to read the first pseudoword. Immediate feedback was given. If the S was incorrect, she/he was encouraged to "Try again." If the S could not correctly say the word, the examiner gave the correct response. After Set 1 (abstraction condition), the S was given appropriate vowel rule instruction of a general phonic type (Hornsby & Shear, 1976), and asked to	Short vowels: number of errors Vowel digraphs: number of errors Rule of e: number of errors	The RD children performed less accurately than the NLD control Ss when they had to abstract rules, although this was restricted to the most difficult rule of e.

				read Set 2. Again, feedback and verbal encouragement was given. Ss were given more phonics instruction regarding vowels, then Set 3. Each session included the presentation of three sets of cards of one rule type and instruction.		
Graham (1990)	3	4th and 6th graders; mean IQ (WISC-R or Slosson) for the 4th graders was 93.4 and for the 6th graders was 92.8. Achievement scores, as tested by the Woodcock–Johnson (1978) or the PIAT (1970) showed that Ss were at least 1 yr below grade level (4th graders) and at least 2 yr below grade level (6th graders) in one or more academic areas.	Writing	There were three conditions in this study, and each S received all three. Each S wrote three compositions, each one on a different opinion essay topic. Ss were prompted to continue with more information or to extend their ideas in Conditions 2 and 3. Ss met once/wk for a total of three times. Each session was a different condition. *Writing Condition* (Control): Ss were told to write as much as they could on the assigned topic. If there were any words the experimenter could not read, the S was asked to read them at the end of the session. *Normal Dictation Condition:* The directions were identical to the first condition except that Ss were asked to speak their composition into a tape recorder and were told that the examiner would later type their composition from the tape. *Slow Dictation Condition:* Ss were asked to tell their composition to the examiner who wrote it down for them. All other conditions were the same as in Condition 2.	Frequency of words Quality of writing	LD Ss' writing problems appeared due, in part, to difficulties with mechanics and problems in sustaining production during writing.

(*continued*)

Author (year)	*N*	Selection criteria	Target domain(s)	Treatment(s)	Measures	Results
Hine, Goldman, & Cosden (1990)	11	Ss were participants in a summer school program for learning handicapped Ss. Mean age was 10.26, range 8.33–13.25. Mean Verbal IQ was 86, and mean Performance IQ was 98 (no instrument was named). The WRAT reading scores indicated that all Ss were functioning at least 2 yr below grade level.	Story writing	The study took place during 4 wk of a summer school program in a computer lab on a university campus. Ss generated text at computers both alone (control) and as members of dyads (treatment). During the first two sessions, Ss used a tutorial to practice the MacWrite Program. Ss repeated a 3-day sequence for each story, basing each on a different 3- or 4-frame picture set. The first day involved prewriting discussion of the picture set with the experimenter. On the first writing trial, Ss generated stories on the computer. On the second day, the Ss engaged in the second writing trial and continued generating the story. The third day involved editing at the computer with teacher prompting. Ss were encouraged to make their stories longer. Ss mostly worked in groups of three, one at the computer, with feedback from the other two. Ss rotated throughout the study, thus participating in both the experimental and control conditions.	Mean error rate Subject-identified errors Subject-corrected errors	Transcripts of the social interactions revealed differential degrees of cooperative behavior and involvement in the writing task among the LD Ss. The evidence supported the use of collaboration on computer writing activities to elicit editing and monitoring behaviors. Six of the 11 Ss had lower error rates when working in dyads compared to working alone. The 5 who did not show this pattern all had low error rates (below 10%) in both the single and dyad conditions.

Hurford (1990)	48	2nd and 3rd graders were selected from LD and RD classes; all Ss were white, middle-class children with no observable handicaps or emotional problems. *RD:* Reading scores below the 35th percentile; average intelligence; Full Scale IQs above 90; 1 SD below mean performance on a phonemic segmentation measure. *Nondisabled:* Regular classroom placement; cognitive academic scores were not reported.	Phonemic segmentation	The phonemic segmentation skills of LD and NLD Ss were compared in this study. *Phonemic Discrimination Training* Ss received instruction prior to training to increase understanding of the training procedure. Instructional tasks consisted of visual representations of the nature of the phonemic discrimination task. Training occurred around 1 wk after assessment. Trials began with computer presentation of tasks, followed by presentation of a comparison pair. The task required the subject to discriminate whether word pairs were the same or different, then to respond by pressing a key on the keyboard to indicate their choice. Intervention consisted of three training phases, each corresponding to a different syllable class. Each phase occurred on a different day. Training took place for 30–45 min/day for about 3 to 4 days. Ss were posttested on the phonemic segmentation task with a new word list.	Metropolitan Reading Test WISC-R (RD Ss only) Phonemic segmentation tasks: two lists of 12 words and 12 nonwords developed for this study. Words were selected based on their recognizability by 2nd and 3rd graders. Nonwords were constructed to follow orthographic rules	Significant performance differences were not observed for word versus nonword tasks. There were no significant differences related to deletion of initial versus ending phoneme. A main effect for time of testing was obtained. A Training Group × Time of Testing interaction occurred in which LD Ss who received training outperformed those who didn't. LD controls did not improve their performance significantly from pre- to posttest. The same main effect and interaction were observed at both grade levels. Although trained 2nd graders with RDs improved, their performance remained significantly inferior compared to Ss without LDs. In contrast, trained 3rd graders with LDs did not differ significantly from the NLD children.

(continued)

Author (year)	*N*	Selection criteria	Target domain(s)	Treatment(s)	Measures	Results
Hurford & Sanders (1990)	52	*Experiments 1 and 2:* Both experiments included 2nd and 4th grade LD Ss and NLD Ss. Ss in Experiment 2 were RD Ss drawn from Experiment 1 who scored less than 84% on the assessment. The RD Ss were selected from LD classrooms. The mean WISC-R scores for 2nd and 4th grade LD Ss were 97.7 and 96.9, respectively. Reading scores for the LD Ss were taken from the Woodcock–Johnson Psycho-Educational Battery or the CTBS. Mean scores for the 2nd and 4th grade Ss were 7.27 and 7.88, respectively.	Reading	*Experiment 1* examined 2nd and 4th grade RD and NRD Ss' ability to discriminate between combinations of two-syllable phoneme pairs with varying intersyllable intervals. Ss were shown a series of consonant–vowel (CV) cards. The S was asked to distinguish between two CV syllable combinations, whether they were the same or different. Next, assessment trials began with the computer presentation of a standard pair, consisting of one of the CV syllable combinations, followed by a comparison pair. The speed increased from 1000 ms to 320 ms, shorter interstimulus intervals (ISIs). The control Ss were the NDRs. They received the same treatment as the treatment Ss.	Percentage of correct responses on the 400 ms and 320 ms trials The number of trials to criterion for grade, reader group, and ISI	*Experiment 1:* 2nd grade disabled readers performed significantly worse than nondisabled grade-mates and the 4th grade disabled and nondisabled readers, all of whom performed similarly. 2nd grade nondisabled and 4th grade disabled readers matched on r eading level performed almost identically, suggest-ing a developmental lag in phonemic processing.
	32			*Experiment 2* involved training disabled readers on phonemic stimuli that became increasingly complex. The purpose of the experiment was to investigate if the RD Ss from Experiment 1 could be trained to overcome their processing deficit. Disabled readers who underwent phonemic training were given trials in which the stimuli became increasingly more complex and the ISIs shorter.		*Experiment 2:* The training significantly improved their performance up to the level of the nondisabled readers in Experiment 1. Control training with nonspeech, steady-state stimuli did not improve phonemic discrimination. Overall, the results suggest that disabled

				Three categories of stimuli were presented in the phonemic training segment of this experiment: vowels, CV syllables with initial liquid and nasal consonants, and two CV syllables with initial voiced plosives that each participant received in the assessment phase. The syllables were created with the same recording and digitization procedures as in Experiment 1. The control Ss were trained nonphonetically. They were given an assessment task that was the same as in Experiment 1. Ss made decisions regarding two different tones instead of vowels, liquid consonant and plosive syllables. ISIs were the same as for Experiment 1.		readers do experience a phonemic processing deficit, but that it can be remedied with appropriate training.
Kershner, Cummings, Clark, Hadfield, & Kershner (1990)	26	Participants were children 8 to 14 yr old diagnosed LD according to guidelines from Ontario Ministry of Education. Criteria included (1) no evidence of neurological disorders, emotional disturbance, sensory losses, or inadequate environmental or instructional opportunities; (2) not hyperactive or taking stimulant mediation; (3) English as the primary language; (4) individually diagnosed by a registered	Auditory processing	During the first yr of this study, children with LD were randomly assigned to one of two groups. The Tomatis Listening Training Program (LTP) was combined with regular remedial programming for experimental Ss. The LTP treatment consisted of graduated stages of auditory training using an audio vocal conditioning device called the Electronic Ear. To control for the effects of attention, the second group received simulated experimental treatment along with the regular remedial program. The regular remedial program provided to both groups of Ss was based on the	Testing was administered blindly by the Ontario Institute for Studies in Education. Measures at pretest, posttest, and follow-up included WISC-R (Weschler, 1974); WRAT Reading, Arithmetic, and Spelling (Jastak & Jastak, 1978); TOWL (Hammill & Larsen, 1983); Verbal Fluency	Irrespective of group assignment, LD children in this research showed gains from pretest to follow-up in WRAT arithmetic, TOWL, Verbal Fluency, Auditory Closure, Seashore Rhythm, and Coopersmith SEI. The placebo group demonstrated superior performance compared to the LTP group on the Seashore Rhythm Test at follow-up. There were no

(continued)

Author (year)	N	Selection criteria	Target domain(s)	Treatment(s)	Measures	Results
Kershner, Cummings, Clark, Hadfield, & Kershner (1990) (*cont.*)		psychologist based on a psychoeducational assessment battery including (a) WISC-R (Weschler, 1974) IQ > 80, (b) writing < 30th percentile on the Test of Written Language (TOWL; Hammill & Larsen, 1983), and (c) at least a 2-yr discrepancy between CA and both reading comprehension and word recognition measured by the Monroe Sherman Diagnostic Reading and Aptitude Tests (Monroe & Sherman, 1966).		Orton–Gillingham multisensory approach to teaching (Cox, 1984; Gillingham & Stillman, 1956), including remedial instruction directed toward the development of language skills within the context wherein tasks are to be learned and applied. The present study was a 2-yr follow-up comparing Ss in the LTP intervention with those who received simulated auditory training (i.e., a placebo).	(Reitan, 1983); Auditory Closure or Phoneme Blending (Kass, 1964); Seashore Rhythm (Reitan & Davidson, 1974); and Coopersmith Self-Esteem Inventory (SEI; Coopersmith, 1981).	other significant effects associated with these treatments.
Lalli & Shapiro (1990)	8	All Ss selected for participation in this study were enrolled in an independent, licensed, nonprofit school for the LD. Criteria for placement in the school followed federal and state standards requiring a severe discrepancy between achievement and intellectual ability in one or more basic learning skills.	Word recognition	The study investigated the effects of two treatments on sight word acquisition. *Self-monitoring:* A three-step training procedure was followed. First, the experimenter provided instructions on how to self-monitor while demonstrating the procedure. Next, Ss were required to imitate the self-monitoring procedure and corrective feedback and descriptive praise was provided. Finally, there was a trial session wherein independent performance was monitored by the experimenter. *Self-monitoring plus continent reward:* All procedures were the same as the self-monitoring condition with the addition of predetermined rewards at the end of each session contingent on reaching a set criterion.	Experimenter generated word lists	Both treatments were found to increase sight word vocabulary. However, results indicated that the introduction of contingent reward did not enhance the reactivity of self-monitoring for the majority of Ss.

Leong, Simmons, & Izatt-Gambell (1990)	30	*Experiment 1:* 5th graders with a mean age of 10.78. Mean score on the British Ability Scale, Matrix E subscale, was 8.9 yr. Ss were 14 less skilled readers and 16 skilled readers.	Reading	*Experiment 1:* Compared different levels of word knowledge training: *Enriched* (E), *Partial* (P), and *Minimal* (Control). The 30 Ss were placed into one of the three groups. All lessons were on a 5-day cycle that included thirty 25-min sessions over 6 wk. Stimulus words were taught on days 1 through 4 with overall revision and evaluation on day 5. On the average, 8 words were taught/wk. Prior to the teaching of each target word, the children in the subgroups were shown (without vocalization) the word and were asked to answer four simple questions as a further check on their lack or level of question. *Enriched* training emphasized multiple exposure of the target words in different sentential contexts with emphasis on word meaning, words of similar and opposite meanings, and words in prose passage integration to bring out particular aspects of meanings. *Partial* training focused on the dictionary definition of the lexical items with little attempt at multiple exposure and/or prose passage integration. *Minimal* training required Ss to read short passages embedding the target words, but there was little explanation of the different shades of meaning of the lexical items.	*Experiment 1:* Word meaning: pretests and posttests	The results of the two interrelated exploratory training studies suggest that systematic, sustained in situ training helped the poor readers, although both the training approaches and stimulus materials would need refinement.

(*continued*)

Author (year)	*N*	Selection criteria	Target domain(s)	Treatment(s)	Measures	Results
Leong, Simmons, & Izatt-Gambell (1990) (*cont.*)	41	*Experiment 2:* Ss were a mean of 12.72 yr old, enrolled in 7th grade. The Ss were poor readers who scored below the 25 percentile for 7th grade on the aggregate Vocabulary and Reading Comprehension subtest scores of the Canadian Test of Basic Skills.		*Experiment 2:* This study took place over 4 wk in 30-min daily sessions and consisted of three conditions: *Full Elaboration Training* (FE), *Partial Elaboration Training* (PE), and *Minimal Elaboration Training* (ME, Control). The poor readers and the average readers were each placed in one of the three groups. The *Elaboration Training* was based on the model of Anderson (1980) with these traits: (1) information processing, (2) response–demand events, (3) student responding, (4) response judging and feedback, and (5) heuristics on the next step. Also included were teacher modeling, describing and interacting with Ss, and direct, systematic instruction. Ss helped to develop their comprehension monitoring with self-questions. *Full elaboration:* Introduction of motivation set with discussions of the purposes of reading, skimming, and getting main ideas. Verbal praise was provided as was a general procedure with teacher modeling of self-questioning summarizing. Use of extended or enriched procedure with teacher emphasizing main ideas, drawing out inferences with feedback on both comprehension and its monitoring.	*Experiment 2* Self-questioning Metacognitive awareness Comprehension	

				Partial elaboration: The above procedure was not used in this group, and no specific instruction for summarizing and paraphrasing the passages was given. *Minimal elaboration:* Ss were asked to answer the general questions rather than to generate specific and inferential questions.		
Lovett, Warren-Chaplin, Ransby, & Borden (1990)	54	Children were referred to the LD Research Program at the Hospital For Sick Children in Toronto. Referrals for remedial reading treatment originated from multiple sources, e.g., medical and psychology staff, parents, and Metropolitan Toronto area boards of education. Children between 7 and 13 yr old were included when reading underachievement coexisted with at least low average ability. Exclusionary criteria included brain damage, hyperactivity, hearing impairment, chronic medical conditions, serious emotional disturbance, and/or primary language other than English. *RD:* Scores below the 25th percentile on measures of oral	Word recognition	Each program consisted of 35 sessions total; lessons lasted 60 min each and were conducted 4 days/wk. Instruction was presented to pairs of Ss in special laboratory classrooms at a pediatric teaching hospital. Special education teachers implemented each program with about one-third of his or her assigned caseload. Intensive, systematic instruction in word recognition was used for both experimental word-training programs. Instructional format was varied. *Grapheme–Phoneme Rehearsal:* For one group, training of regular words emphasized grapheme–phoneme correspondence. Whole word methods were employed for exception words. Both regular and exception words were taught and rehearsed by whole word methods alone. The amount of practice time allocated to both regular and exception words was equated across both conditions. Spelling instruction for the	Word lists for reading and spelling	Significant gains in word recognition accuracy and speed, and in spelling, were achieved by Ss in both experimental groups. Training effects were transferred to uninstructed spelling words, but not to uninstructed vocabulary. Efficacy of word training programs was equivalent for instructed content, but the whole word method demonstrated superiority at posttest on some transfer measures. Support was obtained for usage of word training methods with disabled readers, although differential effects for the two methods employed in this study were not observed.

(*continued*)

Author (year)	*N*	Selection criteria	Target domain(s)	Treatment(s)	Measures	Results
Lovett, Warren-Chaplin, Ransby, & Borden (1990) (*cont.*)		reading performance; results replicated on four of five measures; underachievement in written language evident on multiple standardized instruments; children whose reading problems were potentially secondary to attentional deficits were excluded. Disabled readers were randomly assigned to one of two word recognition and spelling interventions or to a problem-solving and study skills training control group.		first group emphasized word segmentation, with focus on phonological coding and sequence. *Letter Rehearsal* The second group rehearsed letter sequences orally and in writing, with emphasis on letter name sequences. The *Classroom Survival Skills Program* (CSS) was presented to control Ss who received the same amount of clinic time and teacher attention as experimental Ss. This condition consisted of instruction related to classroom etiquette, life skills, organizational strategies, self-help skills, and academic problem solving. No direct instruction or print exposure was presented in this condition.		
MacArthur, Haynes, Malouf, Harris, & Owings (1990)	44	5th and 6th graders in self-contained classrooms in a suburban school district in a major metropolitan area. LD classification was determined according to the following criteria: normal intelligence demonstrated by WISC-R or K-ABC scores between 85 and 115; functioning at least 1.5 yr below grade level expectancies in math or reading as documented by	Spelling	Ss received 4 wk of paper and pencil (PPI) or computer-assisted (CAI) spelling intervention that replaced regular spelling instruction and conformed to typical classroom routines. Both programs required only occasional teacher support, with practice occurring throughout the day during normal seatwork time. Weekly spelling tests were given as regularly scheduled. Both programs had identical content and similar activities. Response opportunities were about equal. Ten new words were	*Spelling:* Paper-and-pencil spelling tests wer e given weekly on Friday; a retention test composed of five randomly selected words from each of four wkly lists was given 1 wk following the 4th wk of instruction. *Social skills:* Engagement rate and	Achievement and engagement were strongly correlated, with scores for CAI significantly greater. A priori hypotheses regarding the nature of the group effects on achievement were supported by the relationship patterns observed in path analyses, although conclusions regarding the mechanisms underlying these

	recent scores on an individually administered, standardized achievement test; no significant behavior disorders, lack or educational opportunity, or primary language other than English. Ss were matched by classroom, gender, and Morrison–McCall scores, then randomly assigned to experimental or control groups.	presented weekly, including discussion of word meanings and usage. Independent seatwork was assigned for 20 min/day. Monday and Tuesday practice focused on a 5-word subset each day, and consisted of word copying, practice from memory, and sentence completion. An entertaining activity was provided after each subset was presented. Practice for the remaining days included multiple choice, sentence completion, riddles, scrambled words, and a short-term memory task. No homework was assigned. All Ss received the same word lists comprised of words familiar to 75% of 4th grade Ss. Prior to the experiment, Ss were pretested on 60 words divided into three lists presented over 3 days. No student knew how to spell more than 15% of the words selected for this experiment. *CAI* Ss worked independently at a computer, with immediate corrective feedback provided responses, with correct response required before continuing. Incorrect words were presented for practice later in the same day. The CAI program completely controlled activity sequence, and even regulated pacing to some extent. Practice time was regulated by a timing device within the computer program. *PPI* Ss worked alone in a learning center in a separate area. They each had a folder with pockets containing corrected work	Ss' interactions with teachers and peers were evaluated through systematic observations using and instrument designed for this study. *Response frequency and accuracy:* Response frequency and accuracy were analyzed based on responses made during four practice sessions, including the proportion of responses correct. *Attitudes toward spelling and computers:* Attitudes were analyzed according to responses on two rating scales administered 2 wk prior to instruction and again 1 wk after instruction was complete.	observations were noted as preliminary since this study was not designed explicitly to analyze the influences mediating between the two variables.

(*continued*)

Author (year)	*N*	Selection criteria	Target domain(s)	Treatment(s)	Measures	Results
MacArthur, Haynes, Malouf, Harris, & Owings (1990) (*cont.*)				from the previous day. Study time was regulated by an electronic time; feedback was provided by self-checking and delayed teacher feedback. Self-checking was not forced. Ss were taught study strategies.		
McCurdy, Cundari, & Lentz (1990)	2	Both Ss were classified as seriously emotionally disturbed and attended a private laboratory school for Ss with behavior disorders including aggression and noncompliance to directions. S1 was 8 yr old and functioned within the borderline classification of IQ (WISC-R). He was reading at 1st grade level and had difficulty recalling material previously learned. S2 was 9 yr old and also had reading difficulties and was reading at the 1st grade level. His WISC-R scores fell within the low average range.	Word recognition	A multiple BL design was used to compare two strategies, *Time-Delay* and *Trial and Error.* During BL Ss were assessed each day on 40 words and results were recorded. During treatment, 5 words were directly instructed to each S using the Trial and Error strategy for the first paired data series. During the second series, 5 words were directly instructed to each S using the time-delay strategy. While one S received instruction, the other S observed instruction. *Time-Delay Strategy* Ss were instructed that if they did not know the word, to wait until the instructor said the word first. The teacher said the correct response simultaneously with the S. Ss then received two pennies for correctly naming each before the prompt and one penny for correctly naming each word after the prompt. *Trial and Error Strategy* Ss were told to say the word if they knew it. Ss received two pennies for correctly naming each word. In both conditions, each S received three trials for each instructed word per day.	The number of correct words read from a list of 40 two-syllable words was the dependent measure.	Both direct instruction and the opportunity to observe instruction were effective procedures, with the progressive time-delay strategy somewhat more effective than trial and error.

Ruhl, Hughes, & Gajar (1990)	30	Ss were LD and NLD college Ss. LD Ss had been diagnosed based on a severe discrepancy between achievement and ability (at least 40 percentile points) in reading, mathematics, written language, foreign language, and/or general knowledge. Ss mean age was 22.64 yr. Their mean WAIS-R score was 109.2.	Memory	The study focused on a pause procedure that involved three 2-min pauses spaced at logical breaks during videotaped lectures. A four-group, three-phase experiment was conducted which included six 1-hr sessions. Group B was the control condition; Groups A and B were mixed. During Phase 1, both groups received a lecture without pauses. During Phase 2, Group A received a lecture with pauses while group B received the same lecture without pauses. During Phase 3, both groups received a lecture with pauses. After each of the three phases, recall and objective test measures were administered.	Immediate free recall of facts Long-term free recall of facts Objective test measure	The pause procedure was effective for enhancing student performance on immediate free-recall and objective test measures.
Simmonds (1990)	60	4th to 6th graders between the ages of 9 and 12; classified LD by a local committee on special education. IQ scores ranged between 85 and 115.	Use of questioning strategies	The study investigated the relative effectiveness of two methods of teaching an efficient questioning strategy to LD Ss. The methods compared were *Cognitive Modeling Alone* in the use of constraint-seeking questions and *Cognitive Modeling and Verbalization* in the use of constraint-seeking questions involving explicit and consistent instruction feedback. The Ss met for four weekly, 20-min sessions. Both groups used the 20-question game *The Flowers Problem* (McKinney, 1972) that included 48 cards varied in size, color, and number. The examiner consistently asked four	Number of questions required	Both groups showed significant reductions from pretreatment to posttreatment in the number of questions required. The two methods of instruction did not differ significantly in effectiveness.

(*continued*)

Author (year)	*N*	Selection criteria	Target domain(s)	Treatment(s)	Measures	Results
Simmonds (1990) (*cont.*)				constraint-seeking questions with and without verbalization to eliminate half of the cards and at least two hypothesis-seeking questions to zero in on the correct response. This guaranteed solution in a maximum of six questions. *Cognitive Modeling with Verbalization:* Ss were given explicit and consistent instructions in the use of the constraint-seeking questioning strategy. Ss were taught to arrange and order the items and cards, and ask questions about the sets in order. The instructor and S took turns and feedback was given after each question. *Cognitive Modeling Alone* (Control): The 20-questions game was played alternately by the model and the S after instructions were given. Ss first observed the model who used the constraint-seeking question strategy in finding the correct answer with and without verbalizing the procedure. Ss then played the 20-question game without assistance or corrective feedback.		
Tenney & Osguthorpe (1990)	32	Ss attending a special education resource program. Each student was referred by a teacher or a parent and was identified LD (22) or BD (10) according to state special education criteria.	Keyboarding skills	The intervention took place in a resource room and was implemented with Apple IIe computers and tutorial software. Two research assistants, adult volunteer tutors, and a teacher supervisor were involved. Nine hours of instruction were presented over a 27-day	*Reading:* The Woodcock–Johnson (Woodcock & Johnson, 1977) reading section of the standard battery was employed to determine	Every student made some improvement on speed and accuracy following treatment. An analysis of the four speed and accuracy tests showed that self-trected Ss typed at about

	Ss were randomly assigned to one of two groups: self-directed or tutor-assisted. The Woodcock–Johnson Reading subtest was used to verify initial equivalence of the two groups in terms of reading level.	span, with daily sessions provided at 30 min/day. Prior to the intervention, tutors were trained to assist special education Ss with basic reading and math skills. The tutors began working with Ss in reading, math, spelling, and study skills after initial training, after which each tutor received an individual introduction to the software, with modeling of correct keyboarding skills provided. *Self-directed:* Ss were told to follow the instructions given by the computer. Tutoring prompts were limited to those included in the software. Ss kept track of their own progress on a management sheet. Other than controlling off-task behavior and responding to specific questions about the software, the tutors were directed to allow the Ss to work independently. *Tutor-assisted:* Volunteers sat beside the Ss at least 80% of the time helping them to find the place to begin and to remain on task, modeling correct techniques, maintaining records, and giving continuous verbal feedback to supplement the computer feedback.	each student's reading level; the composite mastery score was obtained to analyze the relation between reading level and keyboarding aptitude. *Speed and accuracy tests:* One-min timed writings designed to increase in difficulty as keyboarding skill improved. Scores were obtained by counting the letters and spa ces correct, then subtracting errors, producing a letters/min score. The scores for each testing date were collected and analyzed. *Keyboarding technique:* Ss were rated on a scale from 1 to 5, wher e 1 indicated "never" and 5 meant "always," on how ofte n they exhibited six keyboarding skills. *Testing schedule:* Besides the reading	the same speed as the tutor-assisted Ss after 9 hrs of intervention. In terms of keyboarding technique, tutor-assisted Ss had better scores at posttest than the self-directed Ss. Results also indicated a linear relationship between grade level and typing speed. Finally, a strong relationship between the Woodcock–Johnson Reading Cluster scores and the speed and accuracy scores was observed.

(*continued*)

Author (year)	N	Selection criteria	Target domain(s)	Treatment(s)	Measures	Results
Tenney & Osguthorpe (1990) (*cont.*)					and keyboarding tests, initial assessment included a pretest average of speed and accuracy derived from three 1-min timed samples. Once/wk, a timed keyboarding skills test was given following the same procedure. A posttest was administered on the last day of the study.	
van Daal & Reitsma (1990)	31	Ss were enrolled in special education schools. Mean age was 9.58; IQ scores were 90+ (no instrument named). Ss scored a mean of 20.9 words/min on the Standard Dutch Reading Achievement Test, Form B.	Reading	This study investigated the use of speech feedback during independent word reading and its effects on the remediation of reading deficits. All stimuli and feedback were presented by a computer equipped with headphones. The task was to read words from the computer screen. The study included 10-min sessions presented daily for 10 to 16 days. Three different independent practice conditions were employed. *Segmented Word*: S was presented with the word on the computer screen. If help was needed, she/he could click the speech feedback button and the word	Easy and difficult words: proportion of requests for speech feedback; mean latency of first help calls; mean practice time for words Practiced and nonpracticed words: words read within 10 sec at posttest; reading fluency Segmented and whole words: reading backwardness; proportion of help calls	It was concluded that whenever the goal of reading instruction was to memorize particular words, whole word sound as well as segmented word sound could be used. However, when more productive skills were aimed at, the most promising way of giving support was to present segmented word sound, although only a nonsignificant tendency for transfer was found in the present study.

				was sounded out. *Whole-Word:* The same as the above condition except that the S was told the word without it being sounded out. *Control:* Ss were given no opportunity for speech feedback. The word was visually displayed only.		
Bell, Young, Salzberg, & West (1991)	1	Only one subject in this study was LD. He was 16 yr old and was identified as LD based on a discrepancy between his expected performance (WISC-R IQ was 83) and his actual performance on achievement tests. His high school GPA was below 1.6 on a 4.0 scale.	Driving skills	A multiple BL design was used in this study to evaluate the effects of peer tutoring on driving skill. BL included 8–14 sessions, and the treatment lasted three to six 10-min sessions. During BL, the S left driver's education class for 5 min each day and was asked to write as much of each maneuver as he could in 1 min. During treatment, *peer tutoring* was provided for 10 min at the end of the driver's education class. Direct instruction was used as the peer tutor modeled; tested, retested, acknowledged correct responses, used the correction procedure of interrupt, model, test, and timed. The maneuvers included both narrative and diagram sections. The S was taught to say complete narrative, and then to write it. He also drew the maneuvers and was timed for 1-min responses. Corrective feedback was given. *Maintenance* consisted of daily, 1-min timed responses about items on which he had already reached criterion.	Training responses Classroom performance	The S passed the written tests in the driver education classroom, obtained a driver's license, and produced similar or better driving records than Ss who did not require assistance.

(*continued*)

Author (year)	*N*	Selection criteria	Target domain(s)	Treatment(s)	Measures	Results
Berninger, Lester, Sohlberg, & Mateer (1991)	14	*Experiment 1:* 1st, 2nd, and 3rd graders with dyslexia ranging in age from 6.8 to 8.11; WISC-R IQ scores ranged from 89 to 126, and Woodcock Reading Mastery scores ranged from K.8 to 2.8. (A second experiment was conducted with one S, but is not included here.)	Decoding skills Sight word vocabulary	This study investigated the effects of two alternated treatments on the dyslexic Ss reading skills. Ss met for 10 sessions and were divided into two groups. *Written Reproduction / Selective Reminding:* The written reproduction component consisted of computer presentation of single words letter by letter in a left-to-right sequence. In each learning trial, the same 10 words were presented in a different random order. The task was to write the word from *memory* after the display disappeared, using pencil and paper. If the S was correct, the examiner pronounced the word. If incorrect, no feedback was given. The selective reminding component consisted of presenting 3 × 5 cards on which single words were typed. On testing and teaching trials, all 10 words were presented and the child was to pronounce them. On the initial teaching trial, all 10 words were presented. On subsequent teaching trials, only the missed words were presented and named by the examiner. *Selective Reminding / Written Reproduction* (Control): Ss experienced selective reminding first. They were then presented with the	Words correct	The analyses indicated the relative superiority of selective reminding over written reproduction. Selective reminding may have an advantage because it facilitates the process of rapid, automatic retrieval of a name code. Written reproduction may have been relatively ineffective because some RD children are also writing disabled.

				written reproduction task using the same procedures as the experimental group, with the exception that words were typed and presented on 3 × 5 cards instead of computer. The S was to *copy* the word rather than write it from memory.		
Boyer (1991) Dissertation	3	Ss were between 12 and 13 yr old, with a mean age of 12.33. WISC-4 IQ scores were 83, 126, and 91. Ss had difficulty with writing assignments Paragraph writing	The effectiveness of	a directly taught expository writing strategy which paralleled the first three steps identified as crucial in the writing process were evaluated using a multiple probe design across three learning phases and replicated across three 6th grade Ss who were labeled mildly LD. Probe Conditions 1, 2, and 3 were completed in one session each, lasting 90 min. Probe Condition 4 and the three Instructional Conditions consisted of one to three sessions each. Probe 1 measured BL performance for all skills taught in the three instructional phases for each S. The remaining probes measured performance for skills taught during instructional phases. Instruction sheets were identical for probe and instructional sessions. *Instructional Conditions* consisted of modeling, interactive guided practice, independent practice, instructional probes, prompts, and prompts during group and Accuracy in use of organizing	sheet/template The intervention was effective in teaching	correct use of the sheets/temp lates in a minimum number of sessions. Ss maintained criterion or above criterion level scores after instruction in each learning phase. Social validity question-naires revealed high levels of parent and student satisfaction with the procedure.

(*continued*)

Author (year)	*N*	Selection criteria	Target domain(s)	Treatment(s)	Measures	Results
Boyer (1991) (*cont.*)				individual computer instruction. Task completion was reinforced by verbal praise and a token economy system paired with backup reinforcement. The focus was not on spelling, capitalization, or grammar, but on ideas. If the S did not reach criterion over three sessions, that S would receive additional instruction/remediation before the next instructional session. *Writing Process* instructional steps included: (1) Correctly fill in a planning, organizing, or paragraph drafting sheet/template, *Target the Topic;* (2) Determine the audience, purpose, and what is already known about the topic; (3) Write a draft, check it, revise it; and (4) Write the final copy. *Phase Sequences* included: (1) Probe Condition 1 on all three instructional skills; (2) Group strategy instruction on Phase 1, *Use of planning sheet/template;* (3) Probe 2 on all three instructional skills; (4) Group strategy instruction on Phase 2, *Use of the organizing sheet/template;* (5) Probe 3 on all three instructional skills; (6) Group strategy instruction on Phase 3, *Drafting Expository Paragraphs;* and (7) Probe Condition 4 on all three instructional skills		

Campbell, Brady, & Lineham (1991)	2	Ss attending a part-time, self-contained classroom of 14 Ss with mild handicaps. Selection criteria included regular attendance, willingness to participate in a study that required actively teaching their classmates, positive social behavior, and compliance with adult instruction.	Written capitalization skills	A multiple BL design across peer partners was utilized. Peer-mediated instruction combined with student letter-writing activities. Peer partner (1) reviewed the capitalization rules, (2) quizzed the student on the rules, (3) provided correct examples of each rule, and (4) asked the student for other examples.	Identification of words that should be capitalized—permanent product recording	Both Ss demonstrated acquisition of capitalization rules after participating in the teaching sessions with one or two peer partners. Across peer generalization was also demonstrated in a letter writing procedure that included multiple peers.
Chan (1991)	60	*Disabled Readers:* 5th and 6th graders receiving resource services; IQ not subnormal; no primary physical, sensory, or emotional disabilities; reading 2 or more yr below expectancies for chronological age. *Average Readers:* NLD Ss attending same school as LD Ss; reading level matches selected from 3rd grade by word recognition ability comparable to LD; chronological matches chosen from 5th and 6th grade classes. Ss were randomly assigned to either a standard instruction condition or a generalization induction condition.	Metacognitive strategies Reading comprehension	Instruction was delivered to groups of five or six similar-age Ss in a resource room by the same teacher. *Standard Instruction* consisted of demonstrating the use of text to answer a standard set of questions, followed by independent practice. *Generalization Induction* involved teacher explanation of self-questioning during reading, followed by explication of five stages of guidance in strategy use, i.e., cognitive modeling, overt external guidance, overt self-guidance, faded self-guidance, and covert self-guidance. Posttesting Ss' regular class teachers to assess transfer across settings. During the week after training, two additional posttests were administered under cued conditions.	St. Lucia Graded Word Reading Test (Andrews, 1973); GAP Reading Comprehension Test (McLeod, 1977); three main ideas tests constructed for this study (pretest, cued and uncued posttests)	The generalization induction procedure was more effective than the standard instruction method for improving Ss' identification of main ideas regardless of group assignment. Generalization of self-questioning was more likely for LD Ss in the generalization induction condition. Strategy instruction improved LD Ss' identification of main ideas regardless of instructional method.

(continued)

Author (year)	*N*	Selection criteria	Target domain(s)	Treatment(s)	Measures	Results
DiGangi, Maag, & Rutherford (1991)	2	Ss with LD attending a resource room 5 hr/wk for remedial math instruction; identified as LD based on IQ scores between 85 and 115 on the WISC-R (Wechsler, 1974) and achievement scores on the WRAT-R at least 2 yr below grade or age expectancies in one or more academic areas. Ss were also nominated by their resource teacher as having significant problems in attention and academic performance.	Self-monitoring of on-task behavior and academic performance	This study evaluated the differential effects of self-graphing, self-evaluation, and self-reinforcement on improving the reactivity of self-monitoring on-task behavior upon on-task behavior and academic productivity and accuracy. Treatment and observation occurred in a regular classroom during independent seatwork. Subjects were given 20 min to complete a math practice worksheet consisting of 40 addition and subtraction problems provided by their resource teacher. Accuracy was monitored daily by the regular classroom teacher who provided assistance, correction, or praise as needed. Data on academic performance and on-task behavior were collected throughout the study; self-monitoring was only implemented for on-task behavior, defined as any time a subject's eyes were focused on assigned materials or self-monitoring card or she was writing answers, checking problems, or receiving help from the teacher. In addition, the subject had to be seated and not talking unless asking a question directly related to the assignment; other behaviors were recorded as either motor or verbal off-task. A multitreatment design was employed for a total of six	*On-task behavior:* Observations of on-task behavior were made four times/wk using time sampling at intervals of 10 sec for 10-min recording session. Observations of on-task behavior were made by special education student teachers; percentage of on-task behavior was calculated by dividing the number of on-task intervals by the total number of on- and off-task intervals and multiplying by 100. *Academic performance:* Measures of academic performance were obtained by monitoring the number of problems correctly answered and the number of problems completed.	On-task behavior and academic performance (productivity and accuracy) improved for both Ss during self-monitoring, with additional increases observed with self-graphing. However, improvements in on-task behavior and academic productivity were minimal when self-reinforcement and self-evaluation were introduced, although academic accuracy improved slightly for both Ss.

				phases. During BL, on-task, off-task, and math performance was recorded during independent seatwork; Ss were told to complete as many problems as possible on practice worksheets, and to skip any problems they could not solve. During the first treatment phase, Ss self-monitored on-task behavior on index cards in response to audiotaped tones. During the second treatment phase, Ss self-graphed their on-task behavior at the end of sessions in addition to the self-monitoring during their seatwork. During the third treatment phase, self-reinforcement was added, and self-evaluation was added during the fourth treatment phase. The last phase involved fading to determine the extent of maintenance.	The observer recorded totals for these behaviors at the end of each work session. Prior to treatment, both Ss were administered the computation survey of the Multi-Level Academic Skills Inventory (MASI; Howell, Zucker, & Morehead, 1982) to develop instructional objectives.	
Englert & Mariage (1991)	28	Ss were enrolled in grades 4 through 6, and were drawn from five classrooms. Two of the classes participated in the experimental group and three in the control group. Ss were identified as LD and had a mean IQ of 95.4 and a reading achievement mean of 3.2. No instruments were named.	Reading comprehension	The study investigated a comprehension procedure that made visible to the Ss their prior knowledge about a topic and the structures in expository text. The procedure used reciprocal-like teaching formats for the design of group interactions during instruction, as well as semantic mapping to make text structures apparent to Ss. (Reciprocal teaching refers to the process in which Ss take turns leading the teacher discussion about short sections of the text by using four reading strategies: questioning,	Written free recall (holistic) Strategy knowledge Total number of ideas Total number of main ideas	Strategy instruction using this procedure significantly affected recall of expository ideas and knowledge of comprehension strategies among Ss with learning disabilities. The extent to which teachers were able to transfer control of reading strategies to Ss that appeared to affect Ss' developing strategy knowledge was impressive.

(continued)

Author (year)	*N*	Selection criteria	Target domain(s)	Treatment(s)	Measures	Results
Englert & Mariage (1991) (*cont.*)				summarizing, clarifying, and predicting text information.) The intervention took place over 2 mo. The strategy used was POSSE: *Predict:* Background knowledge was activated through various cues (title, headings, and pictures); *Organize:* Ss organized their brainstormed ideas into a semantic map; *Search/Summarize:* Ss searched for the author's text structure as they began reading the passage (The main ideas were searched throughout the paragraphs and were transferred to a semantic map corresponding to a given category); and *Evaluate.* Three reading strategies were used to further guide the group: *Compare:* The semantic maps were compared with current information and new information added; *Clarify:* Ss were asked questions about unfamiliar vocabulary and unclear referents; and *Predict:* Ss confirmed their predictions. Predict and Organize were prereading strategies presented by the teacher. The Search, Summarize, and Evaluate steps took place during reading strategies and were led by the student leaders.		

Englert, Raphael, Anderson, Anthony, & Stevens (1991)	174	4th and 5th graders from 12 schools participated, including learning disabled (LD), low achievers (LA), and high achievers (HA). IQ scores were average to above average. On the SAT, HA Ss scored 56+ percentile; LA Ss scored 39 or lower percentile. The LD Ss scored a mean GE of 2.8.	Story writing	The study examined the effects of an intervention that attempted to improve Ss' expository writing abilities through an instructional emphasis on teacher and student dialogues about expository writing strategies, text structure processes, and self-regulated learning. Instruction in CSIW (Cognitive Strategy in Writing) occurred in four phases for each text structure taught. *Text Analysis* Ss were introduced to the types of questions that different text structures address, the text structure signals that authors use to help their readers locate information, ways of formulating introductions that catch the reader's attention, and the types of questions the audience has about the topic. Writing samples and nonexamples of the target text structure were presented with teacher think-aloud discussion on the variables within a good writing sample. Teachers also did a think-aloud procedure with their own comprehension problems related to the text and solved problems with the Ss about the type of information that would answer readers' questions. Finally, using four student passages, Ss were invited to participate in the text analysis and carry on the dialogue themselves about text structure questions, signal words,	Two direct measures of writing performance; the measures produced Holistic, Primary Trait, Productivity, and Reader Sensitivity scores	The findings suggested that the dialogic instruction was effective in promoting Ss' expository writing abilities on two text structures taught during the intervention (explanation and comparison/contrast) and in leading to improved abilities on a near transfer activity, in which Ss wrote using a text structure not taught during the intervention. The results support the importance of instruction that makes the writing processes and strategies visible to Ss through teacher–student and student–student dialogues.

(*continued*)

Author (year)	N	Selection criteria	Target domain(s)	Treatment(s)	Measures	Results
Englert, Raphael, Anderson, Anthony, & Stevens (1991) (*cont.*)				readers' questions, and more. *Modeling* was provided for each writing process structure being taught. Ss used a planning think-sheet as an aid to record their plans and thinking for later reference. *Dialog* (guided practice) was carried on about the writing process as Ss constructed a class paper on a topic related to the text structure they were learning. Ss used self-questioning and planning strategies along with the planning think-sheet. *Independence* in writing was developed. The total set of strategies was referred to by the acronym POWER: *P*lan, *O*rganize, *W*rite, *E*dit, and *R*evise. Ss received think-sheets for each element in the acronym. Each of the other think-sheets were introduced in a similar manner: (1) Teachers introduced think-sheets by modeling and thinking aloud; (2) teachers and Ss jointly applied the strategies and dialogue to a class paper; (3) teachers provided guided practice as Ss applied the strategies to writing papers on topics of their own choosing; and (4) Ss were encouraged to share ideas and strategies during peer conferences. In the control condition, teachers and Ss engaged in their regular writing activities and routines. They used writing lessons related to a district process writing program.		

Griffin, Simmons, & Kemeenui (1991)	28	Ss were classified LD according to state and federal criteria, and were integrated with NLD peers during P.E., art, music, recess, and lunch. They received academic instruction from special education teachers. Ss were randomly assigned to either a *graphic organizer* condition or a *no graphic organizer* conditioner and taught identical content from the same basal science text for 4 days.	Science	Two experimenters served as trainers. Sessions were counterbalanced between trainers to ensure equal distribution of trainer effects across groups. All sessions were 45 min long and occurred in the special education classroom. *Graphic Organizer Condition* (GO): Four graphic organizers were constructed that emphasized the important facts and concepts in each passage. Content and visual–spatial organization were varied. Information quantity was minimized through use of single words and phrases to highlight the most salient ideas in each passage. Lessons for this condition began with prior knowledge activation and development of each day's content. This was followed by vocabulary development activities and presentation of the graphic organizer. *No Graphic Organizer:* Ss in this condition read and studied the same material in the same order as the GO group. The words and phrases used for the GO Ss were presented to this group in vertical lists without an organizing structure. Other features of the lessons were the same as those used for the GO group. The main thing differentiating the two groups was the presence or absence of the visual–spatial display.	*Pretest:* a 13-item, short-answer test of prior knowledge to ensure initial equivalence of the groups; Ss with extensive knowledge were excluded from this study. *Posttests:* The effects of instruction on Ss' recall and comprehension of science content was measured by oral free-retells, a short-answer essay test, and a multiple choice response test. Posttests were administered immediately following instruction and again 2 wk following training.	Significant differences between the two groups were not obtained, although Ss did not make gains be tween pre- and posttesting.

(*continued*)

Author (year)	*N*	Selection criteria	Target domain(s)	Treatment(s)	Measures	Results
Hughes & Schumaker (1991)	6	7th and 8th graders enrolled in a resource room program for one or two periods. WISC-R scores ranged from 80 to 101, with a mean of 88; reading grade level scores from the Metropolitan Achievement Test ranged from 4.0 to 7.1, with a mean of 5.2. Ss had been classified LD, were enrolled in a mainstream science or social studies class, were capable of reading at or above the 4th grade level, and were receiving below-average or failing test scores in at least one science or one social studies course.	Study skills Test-taking strategies	Ss met daily for 20-min sessions over 18 days. The study was a multiple-probe across-subjects design. During BL, Ss took probe tests and were simply told to do their best. Treatment consisted of instruction designed to promote strategy acquisition and generalization. There were seven strategy components organized according to the acronym PIRATES: *P*repare to succeed; *I*nspect the instructions; *R*ead, remember, reduce; *A*nswer or abandon; *T*urn back; *E*stimate; and *S*urvey. Instructional steps included: *Describe* Introduce the purpose of test-taking strategy and strategies, e.g., underline key words; *Model* Experimenter modeled how to complete each strategy step; *Verbal Rehearsal* Rapid-fire exercise in verbally rehearsing the steps of PIRATES; and *Initial Practice* and *Advanced Practice* activities.	Percent of strategic responses performed	Increases in the use of the strategy corresponded to participation in instruction. Follow-up probes indicated that the Ss maintained their use of the strategy for up to 11 wk after instruction was terminated. Permanent-product evidence indicated that all six Ss applied the strategy while taking tests in selected mainstream classes, and their test grades in those classes were higher after test-taking strategy instruction than before the instruction. This study demonstrated that LD Ss can learn to apply a comprehensive test-taking strategy in a generative way to contrived tests and mainstream class tests.
Lenz, Ehren, & Smiley (1991)	6	7th to 9th grade LD Ss ranging in age from 12 to 14. They were enrolled in summer school and attending three separate LD classes for 3 hr, 4 days/wk. Mean WISC-	Goal attainment Task completion	The study explored the impact of a goal-attainment intervention related to the completion of project-type assignments. A multiple BL across-subjects design was employed and replicated once. Ss were enrolled in summer school and attended	Completion of projectlike assignments	Training the goal-attainment procedures was effective in increasing the number of projects successfully completed and the quality of goal setting

		R score was 95.7; mean reading percentile (WRAT or PIAT) score was 14.6, with a range of 3.0 to 5.7.		three separate LD classes for 3 hr/day, 4 days/wk. During BL, the Student Management Guide (SMG) form was given with no instructions. The intervention included two phases. During *Phase 1,* Ss were trained in goal setting as it related to selecting and evaluating various aspects of project-related goals. During *Phase 2,* Ss were trained in goal actualization as it related to identifying steps and strategies to create a plan that would facilitate project completion and monitoring step implementation. The SMG was a two-sided form used as a concrete organizational aid, for memory and cueing related to goal setting and goal actualization. It included seven steps: (1) task evaluation; (2) options generation; (3) goal specification; (4) plan identification; (5) plan expansion; (6) demands consideration; and (7) self-monitoring		and goal actualization responses. All Ss had significant difficulty generating alternatives when given choices. Performance patterns indicated that some Ss readjusted the way they attacked the goal-setting process as they learned what they could actually plan for and accomplish during the goal-actualization phase.
Losh (1991) Dissertation	64	Mean age was 13.98, ranging from 12.5 to 16.4. IQ was average (no instrument was named), and mean reading score on the CAT was 5.3. Ss' reading scores were 1.3 SDs below their IQ.	Word recognition Language achievement	The intervention used in this study was the Strategies Intervention Model (SIM; Deshler & Schumaker, 1986). The SIM differed from the resource room in that Ss were taught how to learn instead of mastering specific content. SIM instruction included several components.	California Achievement Test	Experimental Ss performed slightly poorer than their control group counterparts on six of the seven pretest CAT measures. After SIM instruction, the experimental group

(*continued*)

Author (year)	N	Selection criteria	Target domain(s)	Treatment(s)	Measures	Results
Losh (1991) (*cont.*)				*Word Identification:* Ss were taught a problem-solving strategy for use in identifying unfamiliar words in content-area materials. Ss learned the use of contextual cues and how to apply common principles of structural analysis through a series of systematic steps. *Paraphrasing:* This was used to improve the recall of main ideas and specific facts. Ss read short passages and rephrased the content, focusing on the main idea and supporting facts. *Sentence Writing:* Ss learned a set of skills to assist them in constructing correctly punctuated, simple, compound, complex, and compound-complex sentences. Control Ss received no treatment.		performed higher on all seven of the posttest measures. The differences were not all statistically significant but several might be of practical significance. The 1st-yr SIM curriculum used with 7th through 9th grade LD Ss had a positive and statistically significant impact on language achievement, as measured by the CAT.
MacArthur, Schwartz, & Graham (1991)	29	4th, 5th, and 6th grade Ss from four self-contained classes for LD Ss. Ss were drawn from the population in a large, suburban district. Identified LD based on the following criteria: intelligence scores between 85 and 115 on an individualized test; reading and writing achievement at least 1.5 yr below grade level	Writing	The process approach to writing instruction was implemented for one semester prior to intervention. Writing workshops occurred weekly in each class for 30–45 min. Writing mainly consisted of personal narratives related to self-selected topics. Minilessons were provided several times weekly, and individual teacher–student conferences occurred frequently. Peer group readings of writing occurred	The WISC-R (Weschler, 1974) or the K-ABC (Kaufman & Kaufman, 1983) and an individual achievement test, e.g., the Woodcock Reading Mastery Test, the Woodcock–Johnson Tests of Achievement,	Treatment affected acquisition of the strategy and demonstrated the utility of its use to improve the quality of student writing. Experimental Ss made more revisions and their changes were of higher quality than those produced by control Ss. Strategy usage was also

expectancies as documented by a recent individual achievement test; absence of English proficiency limitations or other handicapping conditions.	regularly. Five or six computers, two printers, and desktop publishing software were available in each classroom. Classes were randomly assigned midyear to either control or strategy conditions. *Strategy Group:* Training was provided for 6 to 8 wk within the writing workshop context. Two Ss meetings were conducted each wk. One focused on substantive revision in a reciprocal teaching format wherein a peer listened and read along as the author read, summarized the meaning, and told which part he/she liked best, reread the paper making notations about revision questions, and discussed suggestions with the author. The second meeting emphasized mechanical error correction using an error checklist. These meetings were followed by independent revision at a computer. The two experimental group teachers taught this strategy to their entire classes, then provided guidance. Strategy instruction involved (1) modeling, (2) relating strategy to previous knowledge, (3) highlighting importance of revision, and (4) emphasis on motivation via peer reinforcement and feedback.	or the Kaufman Tests of Achievement administered to determine special education eligibility. *Writing Samples:* Prompted writing samples were collected before and after instruction. Prompts were designed to facilitate production of personal narratives, to be interesting, and to be unbiased in terms of race, gender, or economic status. Prompt order was counterbalanced. *Metacognitive Interview:* Designed to draw on student's knowledge of writing processes and the criteria for good writing. This measure was administered before and after instruction to a random sample of 20 Ss.	associated with significant reductions in mechanical errors. The effects on quality were particularly noteworthy, with an effect size of 1.33 observed for Ss in the peer editing condition. Transcripts of peer interactions suggest that improvements were mediated by strategy usage. Results from the metacognitive interview indicated that Ss learned the specific evaluation criteria taught in the strategy and were more conscious of the benefits associated with peer review of one's writing. Contrary to expectations, the interview did not support group differences resulting from training when Ss were asked to evaluate and make revision suggestions for their own writing or the writing of others besides their peer editing partners. Thus, limited transfer effects were associated with strategy implementation as defined for this study.

(continued)

Author (year)	N	Selection criteria	Target domain(s)	Treatment(s)	Measures	Results
McIntyre, Test, Cooke, & Beattie (1991)	1	A 10-yr-old, black, 4th grade student with LD; nominated by the special education teacher as a student needing extra multiplication fact instruction; parental permission to participate. The subject met the North Carolina definition of LD, including: (1) achievement in standard score units of 15 or more points below intellectual/cognitive functioning; (2) not primarily the result of other handicapping conditions and/or environmental, cultural, and/or economic influences.	Multiplication facts fluency	A teacher with experience teaching LD Ss taught the subject a count-by technique that involved learning to translate a multiplication problem into a count-by problem (e.g., 3 × 4 translates into count by 3 four times—3, 6, 9, 12). The subject learned to count by numbers not generally taught (e.g., 4s, 7s, and 8s) as a way to quickly derive answers for difficult-to-master facts. Oral and written count-bys were practiced prior to daily probes of multiplication facts; a multiple-probe design across multiplication tables was employed. Count-by instruction began once a stable BL was established on the first fact set; instruction continued on the fact set until a criterion of 80 correct DPM was reached. A stable BL was verified by probing for the remaining facts to be taught; instruction on the next set was then initiated and the steps were repeated until the subject reached criterion on that fact set.	Correctly written digits/min (DPM) in response to single-digit multiplication fact worksheets were charted. Each session, the subject was presented with one of five equivalent probes generated for each fact set; the subject was given 1 min to answer as many facts as he could. Probes were assigned randomly on a daily basis in blocks of five; each pro be was used once/wk. Besides daily probes, measures used to assess stimulus generalization included (1) a test that included all single-digit facts presented randomly was used as a pretest and posttest; and (2) a 1-min timed test using a mixed probe of randomly	Substantial increases were observed in the subject's correct rate per minute. In addition, rates were maintained and generalized to other situations when the study ended.

					ordered facts from the three fact sets identified for intervention was given after pre- and posttesting and when the subject reached mastery on each fact set.	
Morgan (1991) Dissertation	81	Mean age was 11.9 yr; mean WISC-R score was 86.93. No information was available regarding achievement scores.	Language Impulsivity	This study investigated the integration of an attribution retraining program and a cognitive self-instruction procedure as a means of improving the academic performance and component attentional skills and modifying the cognitive–behavioral beliefs and behaviors of elementary-age children served in self-contained learning disabilities (SCLD) programs. The intervention took place over 10 wk. Ss met daily for 30-min sessions. There were two treatment groups. Control Ss received no treatment. *Group 1, Cool Cats are Stars:* "Cats" = Can do-Ability–Try hard–Strategy–Success. "Stars" = Stop–Think–Act–Review–Success. Ss in this group were given attributional retraining, and cognitive self-instructional methods. Ss engaged in a group-processing session every Friday instead of receiving instruction. Three sequential phases included controlled	Woodcock–Johnson: Reading, Mathematics, Written Language Probe Sheets: Reading, Mathematics, Written Language Burks' Behavior Rating Scales: Poor attention, poor academics, poor impulse control, poor ego strength, excessive dependency Nowicki–Strickland Internal–External Control Scale Matching Familiar Figures Test: Latency, Errors Visual–Aural Digit Span Test	Analysis of covariance and post hoc least squares means analysis revealed significant primary treatment growth in cognitive–behavioral outcomes (poor attention, poor ego strength, and excessive dependency) and probe sheet mathematics. Significant primary treatment growth versus either secondary treatment or control conditions was noted in cognitive–behavioral areas (poor academics and poor impulse control) and standardized reading. No significant differences were noted in mathematics or written language on the standardized instrument,

(continued)

Author (year)	*N*	Selection criteria	Target domain(s)	Treatment(s)	Measures	Results
Morgan (1991) (*cont.*)				instruction, transition, and direct instruction. Ss were regularly assessed in strategy conceptualization, recall and application. *Group 2, Stars:* Ss received cognitive self-instruction only.		reading or written language on probe sheets, trends toward internality, general attention/memory, and latency (near significance) or error rate.
Prater, Joy, Chilman, Temple, & Miller (1991)	5	Junior high and high school Ss with LD; identified by multidisciplinary teams using local district criteria that conformed to the state definition of LD. Criteria included (1) demonstrated interference with learning that may be the result of weaknesses in learning processes, including attention and concentration; (2) impact of the LD must be reflected by the student's degree of academic deficiency in at least one of the seven areas identified in PL 94-142; and (3) discrepancy between academic achievement and grade placement. Teachers described Ss as easily distracted and/or noncompliant; additional characteristics included	On-task behavior	Five single-case studies evaluated whether self-monitoring procedures implemented in special and regular education settings are effective for improving the on-task behavior of adolescents with LD. Treatment was provided by graduate Ss assigned to either a junior or senior high school where they spent 15 hr/wk assisting a special educator; each designed a self-monitoring procedure based on individual needs of the Ss and teachers involved. Settings ranged from regular mainstream classrooms to a self-contained special education class; three studies occurred in resource rooms. Each graduate student operationalized "on-task" with assistance from their cooperating teacher; definitions all included eyes on teacher or materials and sitting in seat. All interventions incorporated self-monitoring using auditory tones and visual prompts; all studies involved training the subject to	*On-task behavior:* Momentary time sampling was used by the graduate student observers in all cases, with variations in interval (15–60 sec) and observation periods (15–30 min); observers looked at the subject at the end of each interval, noting on a recording sheet whether she/he was on- or off-task. Percentages of on-task behavior were calculated as the total number of on-task intervals divided by the total intervals observed multiplied by 100. *Comparative classroom data:* Data were collected in some settings	Adolescen ts with LD successfully implemented self-monitoring procedures in both special and regular education settings, with corresponding improvements noted in their on-task behavior. These improvements were obtained regardless of whether comparison Ss in the Ss' classes demonstrated on-task behavior that was either as high or as low as the Ss' on-task behavior. In some cases, it was necessary to combine self-monitoring with reinforcers to affect improvements, although fading and withdrawal of both were affected without decreasing on-task behavior. However, self-monitoring

academic problems, poor concentration, daydreaming, poor social skills, and inappropriate talking-out.		use self-monitoring procedures (including self-recording sheets), implementing self-monitoring, and fading. Variation occurred in terms of specific treatment and data collection procedures and research design. In Study 1, an AB with fading design was used in the subject's resource math class. In Study 2, treatment was implemented in an ABC with fading design in a special day class; in addition to BL (A) and self-monitoring (B), it was necessary to include a self-monitoring with reinforcement condition (C). Study 3 involved an ABAD with fading design with a reinforcement program delivered in a resource room. Study 4 was a multiple BL across-settings study with fading design, with treatment in the subject's regular education study hall and social studies class. Study 5 involved a multiple BL across-settings (resource government and resource English) with fading design. Comparative data with classroom peers was obtained in studies 3, 4, and 5.	on Ss attending the same class as the subject. Due to variations in teacher structure and expectations, comparisons were made between the subject's behavior and that of his/her classmates. Comparative classroom data were obtained by randomly selecting the order in which the Ss' classmates were observed along with the targeted subject. *Self-monitoring recording:* Researchers discussed on-task definitions and provided Ss with a written copy or a visual prompt representing targeted behaviors. Then, Ss were presented with a self-recording record form and received instructions in recording procedures; Ss were directed to record a "+" if on-task and a "0" if off-task in response to audiotaped tones presented via personal or desk-type cassette players.	was more effective during independent seatwork than du ring instruction and class interaction. In sum, it was demonstrated that self-monitoring is an adaptable, generalizable, and effective intervention for adolescent Ss with LD.

(continued)

Author (year)	*N*	Selection criteria	Target domain(s)	Treatment(s)	Measures	Results
Reilly (1991) Dissertation	39	The elementary LD Ss had a mean age of 11.8 with an average IQ.	Reading comprehension Locus of control	This study evaluated the effectiveness of a cognitive–behavioral approach to reading comprehension instruction. An important component of the intervention was a training course for teachers designed to communicate a conceptual framework for understanding the comprehension deficits of LD children. The treatment group received a five-step verbalizing strategy known as Self-Instruction. They were given a four-step process in which to look for clues as they read: Summarize, Clarify, Question the content, Predict. The treatment took place over 5 wk. Ss met for 50-min sessions on a daily basis. Control Ss received no treatment.	Gates–MacGinitie Reading Comprehension Subtest Locus of control	Ss in the cognitive–behavioral treatment showed significant improvement in reading comprehension when compared to control group Ss who were exposed to their normal routine of reading instruction. The treatment did not affect locus of control.
Ross & Braden (1991)	94	Ss classified as LD in math based on a 1 *SD* discrepancy between ability and math achievement, along with evidence of a psychological processing deficiency. IQ was measured by either the WISC-R (Weschler, 1974) or the K-ABC (Kaufman & Kaufman, 1983). Cognitive processes were assessed by measures of perceptual–motor	Math skills Cognitive strategies	Two treatments and one treatment control were used in this study. Intervention was provided for nineteen 60-min sessions spanning 4 wk. One experimental group was trained to use cognitive behavior modification to remediate deficient math skills. Token reinforcement was used for the second experimental group. The third group continued to receive direct instruction in math.	The computation portion of the Stanford Diagnostic Mathematics Test (STMT; Beatty, Madden, Gardner, & Karlsen, 1986) was administered at the pretest and posttest. Estimates of typical classroom math performance were	All three techniques were effective, although none appeared superior to the others. However, standardized math achievement only improved among the Ss in the cognitive behavior modification and the token reinforcement conditions.

		skills, short-term memory, and receptive language. Nine teachers (and their Ss) were randomly assigned to one of three treatment groups.			obtained from rates of problems correct, or timings of basic addition and subtraction problems.	
Schulte, Osborne, & McKinney (1991)	67	Ss were attending 1st through 4th grades and were receiving LD resource room services. Ss scored in the average range of intelligence (IQ > 85) and evidenced at least 1 SD discrepancy between IQ and achievement in the area of reading or written language.	General academic achievement	Ss in this study met for 30 min three times weekly over 26 wk, for approximately 78 sessions. The experimental group was divided into two groups as was the control group. *Experimental Groups: Group 1, Consultive Services and Direct Instruction* (CD): The consulting teacher collaborated with the classroom teachers to identify instructional and behavioral objectives for the Ss. The consulting teacher then worked with the classroom teacher to develop weekly lesson plans for the Ss. The consulting teacher then focused on modifying classroom behavior, enhancing motivation, and teaching organizational strategies. *Group 2, Indirect, Consultive Services* (CI), In addition to identifying objectives, the consulting teacher also provided direct instruction in the classroom based on modifications of the classroom teacher's lesson plans for the rest of the class. Included were task analysis, monitoring student understanding, using manipulatives and concrete examples, and self-instruction.	Woodcock–Johnson Tests of Achievement, Reading, Written Language, Mathematics Essential skills assessment in reading/study skills	Ss receiving a combination of consultation and direct services showed small but significantly greater overall gain s in achievement than did Ss placed in the resource room.

(continued)

Author (year)	*N*	Selection criteria	Target domain(s)	Treatment(s)	Measures	Results
Schulte, Osborne, & McKinney (1991) (*cont.*)				*Control Groups: Group 1,* Resource Room for one period/day. *Group 2,* Resource Room for two periods/day. Ss received no treatment, only normal resource room activity.		
Wilson & Sindelar (1991)	62	2nd to 5th graders with LD from nine elementary schools. Ss were labeled LD by the district criteria, attended a special education math program, scored at 80% or better on a test of basic addition and subtraction skills, read on at least a 1.5 grade level, and were identified by their LD teacher as needing instruction in word problem solving. Ss had average IQ and scored a mean of 2.0–3.1 in reading, and 2.4– 3.6 in math on the Woodcock–Johnson.	Math word problems	The effect of strategy on word problem-solving performance was analyzed in this study. There were three groups: *Strategy Plus Sequence* (SPS), *Strategy Only* (SO), and *Sequence Only* (Seq O). Ss met daily for 30 min for a total of 14 sessions. *SPS and SO:* Ss responded in unison to questions. During the first 2 days, Ss were given instruction on the fact-family concept. Steps included: Teach the rule; Demonstrate on the board; Teach the rule to use when the big number is not given; Provide boardwork then seatwork practice. On the third day, Ss were taught how to apply the rule to word problems. The groups differed in the practice problems given. SPS Ss completed 3 days of action problems, 3 days of classification problems, 3 days of complex action problems, and 3 days of comparison problems. SO Ss completed a balanced combination of problems each day.	Experimenter generated math problem-solving tests	Ss in the SPS group and in the SO group scored significantly higher than Ss in the Seq O group. Findings indicated that strategy teaching was the more effective of the two instructional components.

				SEQ O (Control): This group used the *Mathematics Today* (1985) basal math series. During the first 2 days, Ss were given computation. Word problems were given on day 3. The questioning technique was used to prompt completion of board problems, followed by seatwork problems. Ss received 3 days each of action problems, classification problems, complex action problems, and comparison problems.		
Bay, Staver, Bryan, & Hale (1992)	68	4th to 6th graders from three elementary schools. All were LD and BD Ss who normally received science instruction in the general education setting and who were granted parental permission to participate. Ss had low average or higher IQ.	Science	The study took place over five 40–60 min sessions. Two groups were included in the study; both conditions used the same content. The purpose of the lessons was to learn the process called controlled experimentation. By using rafts and focusing on factors related to the amount of weight a raft can support in water, the concept of controlled experimentation was presented. The purpose of the *Discovery-Based* treatment was for the Ss to have meaningful interaction with their environment. Ss constructed concepts and ideas about their world. Activities were used that encouraged Ss to engage in identifying important questions, gathering data to respond to those questions, brainstorming solutions to problems, manipulating materials, and observing consequences. During Session 1, Ss explored displacement and	Experimenter-generated science concepts test	Ss in both groups learned equally well as measured by an immediate posttest. However, Ss in the discovery teaching condition outperformed their direct instruction counterparts on a retention test administered 2 wk after the posttest. Finally, LD Ss in the discovery condition performed better than their direct-instruction counterparts on a performance-based measure designed to assess generalization.

(*continued*)

Author (year)	*N*	Selection criteria	Target domain(s)	Treatment(s)	Measures	Results
Bay, Staver, Bryan, & Hale (1992) (*cont.*)				why objects float or sink, using SAVI/SELPH materials. During Session 2, Ss used materials to discuss relationships among such concepts as displacement, balancing weights on a raft, and thickness of a raft. During Session 3, Ss used thick and thin rafts to conduct experiments on the amount of weight each could hold. During Session 4, Ss made and tested predictions as to the amount of weight that a medium-sized raft could hold. During Session 5, the posttest was given. Retention and generalization tests were given 2 wk later. The *Direct Instruction* approach was the control condition. Steps included: Teacher presents/demonstrates the model; Ss ask questions; Ss practice what they have learned; teacher gives feedback; and teacher gives frequent evaluation. Content of the lessons followed the same order as the treatment group. Advance organizers that gave the purpose of the lesson and reviewed previous lessons were used along with presentation of content. Demonstration/modeling of content using the SAVI/SELPH material was part of the study, as was guided practice including worksheets for reinforcement and immediate feedback. Independent practice also included immediate feedback.		

Bos & Anders (1992)	73	Bilingual elementary and English-speaking junior high school Ss were participants. Ss were identified as LD according to school district criteria including a discrepancy between intellectual functioning and academic achievement with low achievement in reading. IQ was 85+.	Recall of content-area concepts	This study included three phases. During Phase 1, the effectiveness of the interactive teaching strategies was investigated with researchers as the teachers. During Phase 2, an interactive staff development component was used and the effectiveness of the interactive teaching strategies when teachers provided the instructional intervention was tested. During Phase 3, the focus was on interactive learning strategies that combine teaching of strategic and content knowledge. The study investigated whether interactive learning strategies could be used in cooperative learning groups. Phase 3 included three sessions: (1) Ss participated in prereading activities using specified instructional materials and procedures; (2) The researcher/teacher and Ss reviewed their instructional materials and read a chapter to confirm their predictions and learning, then Ss reviewed their instructional materials and offered changes; and (3) Ss reviewed materials and completed a multiple choice test. Three interactive teaching strategies were used. *Semantic Mapping* (Pearson & Johnson, 1978); Scanlon, Duran, Reyes, & Gallego, 1992). A relationship map or web was used. The concepts were listed and then arranged.	Experimenter-generated multiple choice test	Overall, the interactive strategies of semantic feature analysis and semantic mapping were found to be more effective than instruction that emphasized definitions for Ss striving to learn content-area concepts.

(continued)

Author (year)	*N*	Selection criteria	Target domain(s)	Treatment(s)	Measures	Results
Bos & Anders (1992) (*cont.*)				*Semantic Feature Analysis* (Anders & Bos, 1986; Johnson & Pearson, 1984): A relationship chart or matrix was used. Coordinate and subordinate concepts were charted and used to make predictions and confirmations. *Definition Instruction* (Control): The teacher taught content-related definitions using instructional techniques that emphasized high S engagement through oral, recitation, correct and automatic pronunciation of each concept and its definition, and teacher monitoring and feedback (Engelmann & Carnine, 1982; Pany, Jenkins, & Schreck, 1982)		
Brigham, Scruggs, & Mastropieri (1992)	16	Junior high school LD Ss with a mean age of 14.3, ranging from 12.9 to 15.4. The mean WISC-R or Stanford–Binet IQ score was 84.81. Standard scores obtained from either the WJPB or the WRAT in reading yielded a mean reading score of 71.73 and a mean mathematics score of 74.87. Ss attended special education classes an average of 3.71 hr/day and had been	Science On-task behavior	This study evaluated the effects of teacher enthusiasm on the academic and behavioral performance of Ss with LD. Two classes were involved in a crossover design. *Class A* received *Enthusiastic Teacher* treatment for the first unit, and received *Unenthusiastic Teacher* treatment for the second unit. *Class B* received the same treatment in the opposite order. Both instructional units were on "weather." Each class received a 30-min lecture and had 20-min guided and independent practice activities.	Student involvement: int erest in the lesson, degree to which Ss appeared to be learning Unit test: experimenter generated Off-task behavior	More enthusiastic presentations resulted in significantly higher academic achievement as well as lower levels of off-task behavior. In addition, Ss were rated by preservice teachers as more interested in instruction and more likely to be learning during enthusiastic instruction.

		in special education classes a mean of 4.35 yr. Ss were reported as having chronic academic failure.		*Enthusiastic Teacher:* Components included rapid, uplifting vocal delivery; dancing wide-open eyes; frequent and demonstrative gestures; varied and dramatic body movements; varied, emotive facial expression; selection of varied words; ready, animated acceptance of ideas and feelings; exuberant overall energy level; moving briskly around the room; and frequent eye contact		
Case, Harris, & Graham (1992)	4	5th and 6th graders identified as LD and receiving self-contained classroom services. Mean age was 11.4, ranging from 11.1 to 11.8; mean WISC-R score was 79.25, ranging from 77 to 82. Scores on the Woodcock–Johnson math and reading tests were 2 yr below grade level. Math scores ranged 2.0–3.2. Reading scores ranged 2.1–2.8.	Math problem solving	The study focused on four LD Ss whose main difficulty in solving simple word problems involved performing the wrong operation. They were taught a strategy for comprehending the problem and devising an appropriate solution. Ss learned to apply the strategy first to addition word problems, then to subtraction word problems. During BL, Ss were given instructions in using cues. Pretreatment measurements were taken. The intervention was called Problem-Solving Strategy and used the self-regulated development procedures (Harris & Graham, 1985). Interactional scaffolding and Socratic dialogue were included. Ss were taught strategies for word problems using cue words. Ss were taught self-instruction (five steps) and rehearsed the steps until	Addition and subtraction: number of equations and answers correct	Upon completion of instruction, Ss overall performance on mixed sets of addition and subtraction word problems improved, and they were much less likely to perform the wrong operation. The effects of instruction generalized to a different setting; however, maintenance of strategy effects was mixed.

(continued)

Author (year)	*N*	Selection criteria	Target domain(s)	Treatment(s)	Measures	Results
Case, Harris, & Graham (1992) (*cont.*)				they were memorized. Problem-solving steps included: (1) Ss read the problem aloud; (2) Ss look for important words and circle them: (3) Ss draw pictures to tell what is happening; (4) Ss write the math sentence; and (5) Ss write the answer. A teacher–student conference was provided at the beginning of each new phase of instruction. BL included 3–12 sessions and treatment duration was ten to sixteen 35-min sessions. Ss met two to three times weekly over 5 wk.		
Commeyras (1992) Dissertation	14	7th graders ranging in age from 11 to 13 yr. WISC-R IQ scores ranged from 90 to 110. Reading	Critical thinking The study	investigated the effects of reading instruction that emphasizes critical thinking on LD Ss reading and thinking skills. Ss met twice weekly for 40 min for 20 sessions total. The treatment group received 10 dialogical thinking-reading lessons. The goal of each dialogical thinking-reading lesson was to engage the Ss in reasoning and reflective thinking in order to decide what to believe about a central issue related to a story. Ss were asked to consider the evidence for two hypothesized explanatory conclusions regarding an important question. Each lesson had two phases: (1) Reading Teacher and Ss read	Illinois Goal Assessment Program in Reading: Rummage Test, Arnie Test, and Cartoon Critical Test	Differences were found between the two groups on the post dialogical-thinking reading lessons. The instructional group was better at arriving at sound defensible evaluations of the reasons they had generated to support the two hypothesized conclusions. They also gave better final conclusions regarding the central issue than did the comparison group. There was no evidence of improvement

				each page silently, one page at a time, and shared an understanding of what had been read; and (2) Discussion Teacher and Ss discussed the two explanatory conclusions which were written on the chalkboard. Ss had four rules: One at a time, Listen carefully, Do your best, and Be kind. Lessons 8, 9, and 10 were rewritten as plays to heighten the Ss' interest in reading texts they perceived were too long to read independently. Control Ss received no treatment.		on the paper and pencil tests of reading comprehension and critical thinking for either group. Comparing the Ss' performance in discussion settings revealed significantly differing views of competency.
Dowis & Schloss (1992)	4	Ss in two general education classrooms classified as LD by public school district according to Missouri state eligibility criteria, including (1) achievement not commensurate with ability; (2) severe discrepancy between ability and achievement in one or more academic areas; and (3) learning difficulties not the result of another handicapping condition. All four Ss (two girls, two boys) were identified as having written language problems according to the diagnostic summary in their IEPs.	Written language	Analysis of the LD student's pretreatment writing samples resulted in the identification of adverbial phrases and possessives as instructional objectives. The Ss in both classrooms were divided into two groups with one LD subject in each group. In each classroom, minilessons on adverbial phrases were given to one group while the other group received minilessons about possessives; each group received instruction while the other completed work independently, then the groups were switched. Ss wrote daily. Lessons consisted of about 10 min of teaching, with presentation on the chalkboard or overhead projector. Then, the group was given a topic and allowed 40 min to write. A replicated multiple BL across-behaviors design, with counterbalanced treatment order, was used to analyze treatment effects on written expression.	Following each writing session, Ss completed two probes used to measure the number of adverbial phrases and possessives correctly used. The adverbial phrase probe contained 14 sentences with the potential of correctly using adverbials with 18 verbs. The possessive probe contained 20 sentences with the potential for correct usage of 20 possessives.	Treatment averages compared to BL averages revealed skill improvement by all four Ss from BL to treatment. In addition, maintenance scores indicated six of the eight average were higher than the Ss' criterion levels. Three of the four Ss increased their use of adverbial phrases from BL to treatment or generalization. In addition, three of the four Ss also increased their use of possessives across these intervention phases. Finally, two out of the four Ss increased their use of possessives in the maintenance phase.

(*continued*)

Author (year)	N	Selection criteria	Target domain(s)	Treatment(s)	Measures	Results
Duvall, Delquadri, Elliott, & Hall (1992)	3	Three of four children chosen for the study qualified for the local school's LD program and were, despite adequate intelligence, experiencing reading difficulties (below grade level).	Reading	A combination of a multiple BL and a reversal design were used to test effects of an intervention that involved parents as reading tutors. The intervention was carried out at home during the summer. Parents initiated tutoring procedures for 10 sessions. After making a starting point in the book and setting a timer for 10 min, they instructed the children to begin reading the passage orally and intervened when the child made the following errors: word substitution, word omission, word addition, hesitated more than 4 sec during reading. Error-correction procedures were used: pointing to location of error, correctly stating the error word(s), having the child pronounce the modeled words, and directing the child to reread the sentence correctly.	Woodcock–Johnson Psycho-Educational Battery, Reading Words read accurately/min (on untutored passages)	Increases in correct rates of reading were noted across settings. Parent tutoring with school basal texts during summer produced marked increases in reading rates that generalized at home to different academic tasks and at school to different and similar tasks.
Englert, Raphael, & Anderson (1992)	63	Ss were randomly selected from a pool of 500 4th and 5th grade Ss involved in a study of expository writing and reading. Thirty-two Ss had participated in a yr-long cognitive strategy instruction program, and 32 had not. Within each group, about half were LD and the remaining half were not. All LD Ss met	Metacognitive knowledge about writing	Pretesting of the control Ss occurred in the spring. The Cognitive Strategy Instruction in Writing (CSIW) program was conducted from October to April of the following school yr followed by postintervention interviews in May. Ss wrote an explanation and a compare/contrast paper to document between-group comparability prior to intervention. Then CSIW instruction was provided at least two to three	A metacognitive knowledge interview about writing was developed for this study which consists of three vignettes, each describing a hypothetical student with writing problems. Ss in this study were asked to help the Ss identified	A MANOVA of student responses to the metacognitive questionnaire revealed significant main effects for treatment and ability, with no significant interaction observed between these factors, suggesting that Ss' talk about the writing process differed as a function of ability and treatment in

	state and local guidelines for special education placement, including average to above average intellectual ability; significant discrepancies between achievement and age expectancies; no evidence of emotional disturbance, mental retardation, or cultural disadvantage; and receptive or expressive language abilities below mental age expectancies. For every LD student, a grade level peer was randomly selected from a pool of normally achieving Ss in the same school district.	times/wk for 6 mo. This process consisted of four recurring phases: text analysis, writing process modeling, guided writing, and providing opportunities for independent practice. Classroom observations were conducted once/wk to analyze the fidelity of intervention across classrooms. Though some variations were observed, all teachers met the minimum requirements for implementation.	in the vignettes by identifying their writing difficulty and making suggestions for improvement. Two composition measures assessed Ss' ability to employ the explanation and the compare/contrast text structures. Recall of expository text was analyzed by presenting information about two topics in the explanation and compare/contrast text structures followed by Ss written of production of facts from this reading. A series of "think sheets" was developed that emphasized relevant writing strategies and text structures to use during the writing activities, guide teacher modeling, build a common language related to writing, and serve as written records to stimulate discussion throughout the writing process.	stable ways. Ss' ability to describe the steps in the writing process made one of the largest contributions to the main effect for treatment. Control Ss tended to focus on the superficial aspects of writing, expressing incorrect or limited assumptions. Many described a simple "write and look-it-over" approach. For LD Ss, there was a focus on procedural and mechanical aspects of writing. Ss' awareness of when a paper was complete, i.e., met task requirements, also made a significant contribution to the treatment main effects with differential effects observed according to group assignment and treatment. In sum, support was obtained for the utility of a socially mediated approach to writing instruction.

(*continued*)

Author (year)	N	Selection criteria	Target domain(s)	Treatment(s)	Measures	Results
Farmer, Klein, & Bryson (1992)	14	Ss with reading disabilities from a special school volunteered to take part in the experiment. All were reading at least 2 yr below expected grade level and their average reading level was Grade 4.65 (Slosson Oral Reading Test). IQ scores were in the average or above average range (WISC FSIQ 81–121)	Word recognition Reading comprehension	Computer speech feedback of correct pronunciation of words was provided on one-half of the words that could be tagged as unknown by the student reader. In the tagged, DECtalk on condition, the computer provided feedback, in the tagged DECtalk off condition, the computer would not prounounce the tagged words. The remaining two conditions were the untagged, DECtalk on condition and the untagged, DECtalk off condition.	Percentage of comprehension questions answered correctly Accuracy of word recognition of tagged and untagged words from stories	Use of the reading tutor system with DECtalk speech feedback made no significant difference to word recognition ability. There was no difference in the mean percentage of comprehension questions answered correctly when DECtalk was on. The main reading time per story in the two conditions was virtually identical.
Gajria & Salvia (1992)	30	6th through 9th graders classified as LD were participants. Ss were adequate decoders, but poor comprehenders. They had 4th grade decoding skills at 90% accuracy level, with comprehension scores at least 2 yr below grade level, but not below grade 4. Their scores on measures of main idea reproduction were below 40%, and their scores were below 40% on two criterion texts of comprehension. Thirty LD Ss were stratified	Comprehension	Ss in the experimental group were taught five summarization rules developed by Brown and Day (1988). The method used was direct instruction (e.g., Pearson, 1984) in a mastery learning structure (Bloom, 1976). Control Ss continued their regular resource reading program. Training sessions were about 35–40 min/day, with three to four Ss/group. All training was provided in the resource room. Total time ranged from 6.5 to 11 hr.	Pretest, posttest, and delayed posttest data were collected from six expository passages similar to training materials. Ten multiple choice questions were constructed for each passage. The Gates–MacGinitie Reading Test was administered before training to all Ss with LDs. The experimental group	The experimental groups' performance was significantly greater then either the control or the normal comparison groups' on condensation questions immediately after treatment. The experimental group obtained significantly higher scores than the control group, but performed equivalently to the comparison group, on factual questions. Further, maintenance of

		by reading levels on the Gates–MacGinitie, then randomly assigned to either experimental or control conditions; 15 age-matched, normal readers from the same grades provided normative comparisons.			was given an alternative form of the same test after the intervention was complete.	summarization skills was observed and this affected maintenance of experimental effects on comprehension performance.
Graham, MacArthur, Schwartz, & Page-Voth (1992)	4	5th graders, age ranging from 11 to 13, with LDs receiving resource room services. Ss met the following criteria: identified as LD by the school district, IQ scores between 85 and 115 on the WISC-R or Slosson, achievement at least 2 yr below age or grade level in one or more academic areas as measured by the Woodcock–Johnson Psycho-Educational Battery, absence of any other disability, and interviews with teachers indicating that significant composition problems were evident. The Vocabulary and Thematic Maturity subtests from the Test of Written Language (TOWL) were also administered to each subject. On the Vocabulary subtest, Ss' scores ranged from 3 to 8,	Writing compositions	This study used a multiple-probe design across subjects with four phases. Preteaching Ss received instruction in using the word processor and on the components of a good essay and story. BL Established pretreatment response rates on writing essays. Treatment Instruction was started for the first participant after a stable BL in terms of total number of functional essay elements was established. Instruction continued until the S demonstrated independent mastery of the strategy and was able to write essays that contained all the basic parts. Instruction was not started for the next participant until S1's posttreatment essay performance reached a criterion level of at least one and a half times the mean number of elements produced during BL. The treatment included the following elements in the 40-min sessions: (1) After BL, S and instructor discussed S's performance; (2) Ss learned the	Written composition: total number of story elements	Strategy instruction had a positive effect on Ss' essay writing performance and knowledge of the writing process, and effects were maintained over time.

(*continued*)

Author (year)	*N*	Selection criteria	Target domain(s)	Treatment(s)	Measures	Results
Graham, MacArthur, Schwartz, & Page-Voth (1992) (*cont.*)		and on Thematic Maturity, Ss' score ranged from 5 to 9.		composition strategy Do PLANS (*P*ick goals, *L*ist ways to meet goals, *A*nd make *N*otes, *S*equence notes); (3) Write and say more; and (4) Test goals. The teacher modeled the strategy while "thinking aloud." Ss learned problem definition, planning, self-evaluation, and self-reinforcement. Ss recorded on small charts their own self-instructions for using the strategy. Ss kept goal charts. They rehearsed the steps of the strategy until it was memorized. The instructor and S jointly composed an essay using the strategy and self-instructional statements. The S independently composed two to three essays using the strategy and self-instructional statements. Generalization and Maintenance were assessed in the final session. The S and the instructor discussed how the strategy could be used with other classroom assignments.		
Humphries, Wright, Snider, & McDougall (1992)	103	Children with LD and sensory motor integration impairment referred by family doctors to the Child Development Clinic and Rehabilitation Services of the Hospital for Sick Children in Toronto; referred for motor coordination problems negatively impacting school	Sensorimotor integration	Ss were assigned to one of two treatments. Sensory Integration (SI) Therapy Intervention was provided to encourage development of a foundation for motor skills, attention, social emotional response, and other functions. SI activities included the use of equipment to provide tactile and vestibular	*Sensorimotor instruments:* the Southern California Sensory Integration Test (Ayres, 1980); the Southern California Postrotary Nystagmus Test (Ayres, 1975); the long form of the Bruinicks–Oseretsky	Perceptual–motor training resulted in significantly higher motor performance gains among the PM Ss compared to the other two groups. SI therapy resulted in a motor planning advantage for SI Ss. Reliable group differences were not observed in visual

performance and social interactions. Verbal, Performance, or Full Scale scores on the WISC-R or the WPPSI of 85 or above; a significant discrepancy (more than 1 SD) between their highest IQ score and their standard score for reading, spelling, or math on the WRAT. If there was no significant discrepancy between their Verbal and Performance IQs, the Full Scale IQ was used to determine a discrepancy between IQ and achievement. Exclusionary criteria included primary sensory impairment or physical handicap, emotional disturbance, cultural difference, bilinguals or English as a second language. Evidence of sensory integrative dysfunction was based on (1) a deviant score on the Southern California Sensory Integration Test, (2) deviant score clustering, (3) clinical observations consistent with standardized testing results, and (4) reliability of positive clusters evaluated by therapists. Ss were randomly assigned to one of three groups.	experiences and proprioceptive input requiring adaptive responses. The SI treatment group received 72 hr of sensory integration training during three, 1-hr sessions/wk for 24 wk. Perceptual–Motor Therapy (PM) Intervention consisted of motor training to remediate weakness in specific motor skills. In contrast to SI therapy, no attempts were made to control and refine the amounts and types of sensory input. Ss in the PM group received seventy-two 1-hr sessions of therapy for a total of 3 hr/wk. This study also included a control group who did not receive treatment.	Test of Motor Proficiency (Bruinicks, 1978); the Test of Visual Motor Integration (Beery, 1982) *Psychoeducational tests:* the WISC-R (Weschler, 1974); the WPPSI (Weschler, 1967); the Test of Visual Perceptual Skills (TVPS; Gardner, 1982); the Gestalt Closure and Number Recall subtests from the K-ABC (Kaufman & Kaufman, 1983); the WRAT Reading and Spelling subtests (Jastak & Jastak, 1978); the Zaner–Bloser Printing Evaluation Scale (Zaner-Bloser & Staff, 1975); a 10-point rating of print readiness from the Basic School Skills Inventory (Hamill, 1975) *Language measures:* the Grammatic Closure subtest from the ITPA (Kirk, McCarthy, and Kirk, 1968); the Sentence Repetition	ability, perception, copying, handwriting readiness, cognitive, academic, language, and attentional skills or in self-concept.

(*continued*)

Author (year)	*N*	Selection criteria	Target domain(s)	Treatment(s)	Measures	Results
Humphries, Wright, Snider, & McDougall (1992) (*cont.*)					subtest from the Clinical Evaluation of Language Functions (CELF; Semel-Mintz & Wiig, 1982); the Listening Comprehension subtest from the Durrell Analysis of Reading Difficulty (DARD; Durrell & Catterson, 1980); the short form of the Rosner Test of Auditory Analysis (Rosner, 1975) *Attention:* the 10-item short form of the Conners Parent and Teacher Questionnaire (Conners, 1973); an informal continuous performance task requiring detection of identical pairs of letter strings; the Matching Familiar Figures Test (MFFT; Kagan, Rosman, & Day, 1964); informal parents' and teachers' ratings of the child's organizational skills. *Self-concept:* the New York Self-Concept Scale (New York School Board, 1980).	

Hutchinson, Freeman, Downey, & Kilbreath (1992)	16	9th and 10th grade Ss identified as having a LD. Ss had average IQ and were registered in basic-level and general classes.	Career awareness and maturity	The study investigated the effects of a counseling program designed to promote career maturity among youth with LD and other youth at risk of dropping out of school. Activities focused on self-awareness and an exploration of career options. Discussion, teacher modeling, and cognitive processing/thinking aloud were utilized in the treatment. The treatment was divided into three parts. Part 1 (7 sessions) Activities that focused on self-awareness, including teacher modeling of activities, student completion of activities with a partner, class discussion, emphasis on cognitive processes, and thinking aloud. Part 2 (2 sessions) Ss explored a range of career options using a card-sorting exercise focused on job field educational level required. Part 3 (3 sessions) Activities focused on matching people with jobs. All sessions of Part 1 were audiotaped and later transcribed for analysis. There were a total of twelve 40-min sessions. Control Ss received no treatment.	Employability Maturity Interview (EMI)	The Ss in the intervention group improved significantly from pretest to posttest on a measure of career maturity. Ss in the control group did not show similar improvement. Most of the improvement in intervention Ss' scores were attributed to an improved understanding of career options.
Kim (1992) Dissertation	8	High school Ss with LD. Ss had a mean WISC-R score of 95.5.	General academic achievement	This study investigated the relationship between a test-taking strategy intervention and academic improvement of high school Ss with LD. Ss in the treatment group met for thirty-two 30-min sessions over 4 wk. Ss were taught a	Classroom assessments Letter grades	High school Ss with LDs were positively affected by test-taking strategy instruction. They were able to utilize at least one subskill from the test-taking

(continued)

Author (year)	*N*	Selection criteria	Target domain(s)	Treatment(s)	Measures	Results
Kim (1992) (*cont.*)				first letter mnemonic strategy and a paired associates strategy, and were also taught to use checkmarks and numbers on their tests to monitor test completion. The sessions included eight steps: (1) Pretest; (2) Test-taking strategy instruction (examples of how and where they could use the strategy, advantages of using the strategy, results they could expect, and goal setting for learning the strategy); (3) Teacher modeling; (4) Self-instruction and verbal rehearsal; (5) Controlled practice with teacher feedback; (6) Strategy practice on grade-appropriate tests; (7) Posttest; and (8) Ss were encouraged to use the strategy in a variety of settings (across subject areas). Generalization steps included Orientation, Activation, and Maintenance Control Ss received no treatment.		strategy for any academic classroom assessments. The posttest scores increased significantly (.0001) for the experimental sample as demonstrated by an analysis of variance.
King-Sears, Mercer, & Sindelar (1992)	37	Ss in this study were in the 6th, 7th, and 8th grades, and included 30 with LDs and 7 with emotional or behavioral disorders. Mean IQ scores were 85+; mean achievement scores were significantly lower (no instruments were named).	Science vocabulary	Ss were separated into three groups: Systematic Teaching (Control), Imposed Keyword Mnemonic, and Induced Keyword Mnemonic. In all conditions, the teachers used immediate and corrective feedback, positive reinforcement, prompts, and elicitation of active student involvement. Teachers	Written definitions at the 2nd and 3rd wk Written definitions and matching definitions at the 4th wk	Favorable results were obtained for both the imposed and induced keyword methods.

				were cued by audio tape when to begin, when they had just 1 min left, and when the time was ended. The Ss met 12–15 min, three times wkly, for 4 wk. Imposed Keyword Two cards were used, 5 × 8 and 8.5 × 11. The smaller card had a vocabulary word on one side and the keyword on the other. The larger card had the keyword, vocabulary word, its definition and an interactive illustration of the keyword and its term. Induced Keyword The same instruction and identical materials were used as in the first condition during the first of the 4 wk. During the second week, a strategy was taught to help Ss make up their own keywords. A poster prompt was displayed. Systematic Teaching (Control) The 8.5 × 11 cards contained words, their definitions, and illustrations of the definitions displayed on them. The card for each term was used for presentation and rehearsal of the term and definition.		
Malone & Mastropieri (1992)	45	LD Ss grades 6, 7 and 8 who met the federal, state, and local guidelines for classification; minimal decoding skills, weak comprehension skills; teacher recommendation based on serious problems in reading	Reading comprehension Cognitive strategies	All Ss received 2 days of training followed by 1 day of posttesting. Treatment was delivered in a tutorial format in a quiet room near the Ss' regular classrooms. Teachers read from standardized scripts. All Ss were interviewed prior to the investigation regarding their use of strategies to	Training and testing passages: 19 stories were randomly selected from *Reading for Concepts, Level D* (Liddle, 1977). All passages were about 200 words long with	ANOVAs were used to analyze the results of the posttest, near-transfer, and far-transfer tests. *Test of training:* There was a significant main effect for treatment condition favoring the two

(continued)

Author (year)	*N*	Selection criteria	Target domain(s)	Treatment(s)	Measures	Results
Malone & Mastropieri (1992) (*cont.*)		comprehension. Specific criteria included (1) decoding scores of at least 2.0 grade equivalent; (2) comprehension GEs of at least 2.5 on a standardized reading test; (3) a reading rate of at least 70 words/min. Ss were stratified by sex and grade, then assigned randomly to one of three treatment groups.		facilitate comprehension and recall. The content to be remembered/understood and tutorial format were held constant across conditions, with instruction varied. All Ss received instruction followed by practice tests and condition-specific feedback on the first day. Condition-specific review, practice with another passage, and another practice test followed on the second day. Ss in all conditions read new passages and completed posttests on the third day. *Summarization Training* Ss were taught to identify important information in text, to monitor their own comprehension, and to summarize after reading each paragraph. *Summarization Training with Monitoring* consisted of the same strategy instruction provided for the above condition with the addition of training to use a self-monitoring checklist on a card to check use of the summarization strategy. *Traditional Instruction* Ss read stories and answered questions. Instruction included preview and word practice.	readability estimated at level 3.2 (Spache, 1974). Two passages were used for training, two for posttesting, and the rest were available for extra reading when Ss finished the required tasks before the time limits expired during individual sessions. Strategy questionnaires: An item instrument developed and administered prior to training and again after posttesting was completed. Questions related to Ss' techniques for remembering important information. A think-aloud measure was developed and administered which required Ss to describe	experimental groups. A significant Treatment Condition × Question Type interaction was obtained indicating the summarization Ss performed better on nonsummary items, the monitoring group performed comparably on both summary and nonsummary items, and the control group displayed higher performance on summary-related items. *Near transfer:* Significant main effects for treatment condition and question type favored experimental Ss, but a significant interaction between Treatment Condition and Question Type did not occur. *Far transfer:* Significant main effects for Treatment Condition and Question Type occurred, but there were no significant

what they were doing while reading. A third measure assessed Ss' satisfaction with the strategies. Recall measures: 12 short-answer questions were developed to accompany training and testing materials. Half of the items pertained to summary information in each paragraph, with the other half focused on nonsummary information. Examiner scripts: Length of time for instruction each day was held constant. Ss received strategy interviews and instruction on the first day, review and the "think-aloud" protocol on the second day, followed by posttesting and strategy measures on the third day. Scripts only varied for condition-specific aspects of the intervention.	interactions. Ss trained to summarize and to monitor their own understanding performed at the highest levels, followed by the summarization group Ss. The traditional condition produced the poorest. *Strategy data:* Self-reported use of strategies increased significantly from pre- to postintervention interview for Ss in the summarization conditions. Control Ss' responses remained at equivalent levels throughout the study. However, no significant differences were noted in analyses of the think-aloud protocols or the retrospective strategy probes. Experimental Ss responded positively overall to questions related to satisfaction with the instructed strategies.

(continued)

Author (year)	*N*	Selection criteria	Target domain(s)	Treatment(s)	Measures	Results
Montague (1992)	6	Middle school Ss who met school district criteria for placement in the LD program. Mean age was 13.6; mean WISC-R score was 98; mean Woodcock–Johnson mean grade equivalent in Broad Math was 5.8 and in Calculation was 6.6.	Math problem solving	The study investigated the effects of cognitive and metacognitive strategy instruction on mathematical problem solving. A multiple BL, across-subjects design was used. One 6th, one 7th, and one 8th grade subject were assigned randomly to one of two groups. The experimental phases included BL, two levels of treatment, setting generalization, near and far temporal generalization, and retraining. The study investigated the effects of cognitive and metacognitive strategy instruction on the mathematical problem solving of the six Ss. The treatments included strategy acquisition training, strategy application practice for CMSI (Cognitive, Metacognitive Strategy Instruction) only, and testing sessions. BL included data collection on test scores and time required for test completion. Ss were told that word pronunciations and definitions would be provided upon request. *Treatment 1:* Direct Instruction in Cognitive *Strategies* (CSI) and Meta-cognitive Strategy Instruction Strategy (MSI) Acquisition training included demonstration, guided practice, and	Math problem-solving test: number and percent of correct responses Test session length: number of minutes	Ss generally improved their mathematical problem solving as measured by performance on one-, two-, and three-step word problems.

testing. For CSI, Ss learned the names of the processes and their descriptions: read, paraphrase, visualize, hypothesize, estimate, compute, check. Ss were told to use the initial letters RPV-HECC (for remembering). For MSI, Ss were taught: Say, Ask, Check. Strategy acquisition training included: (1) Discussion of current performance; (2) Description of the cognitive processes or metacognitive activities; (3) Verbal rehearsal of the process or activities; (4) Teacher modeling of strategy application; (5) Student–teacher role exchange during demonstration exercises; (6) Corrective and positive feedback during guided practice; (7) Mastery check for the CSI Ss of recitation of the cognitive processes from memory (100% mastery required); and (8) Testing Sessions.

Treatment 2 focused on strategy instruction in cognitive processes for the MSI condition and metacognitive strategy for the CSI condition. There was no instruction package. Ss received the same strategy acquisition training as in Treatment 1. Ss practiced strategy application. Ss received testing sessions.

(*continued*)

Author (year)	*N*	Selection criteria	Target domain(s)	Treatment(s)	Measures	Results
Olofsson (1992)	33	2nd to 7th graders with RD attending regular classes but receiving special education support weekly.	Decoding skills Only	Experiment 2 is reported. Computer-aided reading was used in special education classes for about 10 wk. On the average, Ss participated in 25 computer sessions, and read between 16 and 30 texts of very different length and content. Ss were tested, instructed, and observed by their special education teachers. During instruction, the teacher was sitting by the pupil and giving information about when to request help and how to monitor the reading. Gradually, the S was engaged in more independent reading. Control Ss had the same amount of training and were taught by the same teachers as the experimental group. They did not receive training via the computer.	Word decoding: word reading, pseudoword reading, and the word chain test Reading comprehension: sentence reading, passage reading	Older children, from grade 4 and up, benefited more from the computer-aided reading than did younger ones. However, both experimental and control groups showed gains in several aspects of reading. Some children did not seem to have metacognitive skills enough to benefit from the computer-aided system. These children may initially need more extensive training in how to use the system and how to monitor their own reading.
Olson & Wise (1992)	35 149	3rd through 6th graders referred by teachers based on poor classroom performance in reading and on various standardized tests of reading given in the schools. IQ of at least 90 on the WISC, without obvious sensory or neurological deficits such as seizures. Ss had normal school attendance and English as a first language.	Word recognition Decoding	Two phases of treatment were conducted. The difference between Phase 1 and Phase 2 was that the first group was trained during the 1988 spring semester over 10 hr, while Phase 2 Ss were trained in the fall semester of 1988 and received five sessions/wk for 30 min each over an 18-wk semester. There were three conditions, *Whole word*, *Syllable*, and *Onset-rime*. Training consisted of computer remediation with a large number of short stories and book.	Word recognition Nonword reading	Both whole word and segmented feedback resulted in almost twice the gains in standardized word recognition scores compared to control groups that spent an equal time in their normal remedial reading program. The computer-trained groups improved their phonological decoding of

		Stories were presented daily by computer. Ss were trained to request synthetic-speech feedback (DEC Talk) for difficult words. Multiple choice comprehension questions were inserted into the text, every 5–10 pages. Comprehension monitoring and targeted word review was also included. Each new word from the stories was coded into a dictionary. When feedback for a word was requested, the word (whole word) or its segments (syllable) were initially highlighted without speech and the subject was encouraged to attempt decoding the word. After a brief delay (onset-rime training) the word or its orthographic segments were sequentially highlighted by reverse video in synchrony with the speech segments. The segments were highlighted for an interval based on time × number of letters in segment, and 300 ms where time = 300 ms for whole word and 400 ms for segmented conditions. Control Ss received no training on the computer, but did receive normal reading instruction in class.	nonwords at about four times the rate of the control group. There was a significant interaction between level of deficit severity and optimal feedback condition. The most severely disabled readers showed the largest phonological decoding gains from syllable feedback, while the largest gains for the less severely disabled readers were from onset-rime feedback. The disabled readers' level of phonological awareness at pretest was the strongest predictor for gains in word recognition and phonological decoding.

(continued)

Author (year)	*N*	Selection criteria	Target domain(s)	Treatment(s)	Measures	Results
Salend, Reeder, Katz, & Russell (1992)	9	Ss ranging in age from 11 to 13 and identified as needing special education by the school multidisciplinary team in accordance with New York State guidelines. WISC-R scores ranged from 75 to 105. Ss were given the Stanford Diagnostic Math Test, Level H, and scored a mean of 16, with a range of 3 to 43.	Inappropriate verbalizations	The study incorporated a reversal design with two BLs consisting of 11 sessions, and two treatments with seventeen 42-min daily sessions. *BL 1 and 2:* Inappropriate verbalizations were recorded using event recording. Tokens and verbal praise were awarded for appropriate behavior, effort, work completion, and accuracy. Inappropriate verbalizations received a teacher reprimand. *Treatment 1 and 2:* At the beginning of each intervention session, the teacher distributed two evaluation forms to each member of the group. Each S was to rate the group's behavior on a 5-point Likert scale. The system was implemented twice during each session at 15-min intervals. The teacher also rated the group and was compared with one of the S's evaluations. Tokens were given for the teacher/student match for positive behavior.	Inappropriate verbalizations frequency	A dependent group evaluation system was effective in decreasing the group's inappropriate verbalizations. Student satisfaction data revealed that group members had positive reactions to the system.
Sawyer, Graham, & Harris (1992)	56	*Learning Disabled:* Thirty-three 5th and 6th grade Ss with LD were randomly assigned to one of three experimental groups. Each LD student was receiving resource room services in one	Composition skills Cognitive strategies	Four preservice teachers with extensive experience delivered instruction to experimental Ss. Training and practice in the implementation of instructional approaches was provided until error-free role-playing was attained. Instructors worked with small groups of two or three Ss in a quiet area at each school.	Story grammar scale: This scale is used to evaluate the schematic structure of stories as defined by the inclusion and quality of eight common story elements.	No significant between-group differences were apparent prior to intervention. Ss in the normally achieving group and those in the explicit self-regulation instruction group received higher story gram-

of four suburban elementary schools. Ten additional LD Ss participated in a nonrandomized practice-control condition. All of the LD Ss met the following stepwise criteria: identified by their local district as LD; IQ scores between 80 and 120 on a norm-referenced intelligence test; at least 2 yr below grade level in one or more academic areas; absence of other handicapping conditions; and resource teacher report of significant composition deficits. *Normally Achieving:* Thirteen randomly selected Ss attending the same schools as the LD Ss assigned to one of the three experimental conditions. These Ss were not receiving special education or remedial services, and were capable writers according to classroom teacher report.	There were four instruction groups in each condition. Instructors met with each group of Ss for three sessions/wk for about 3 wk, with session length ranging from 20 to 56 min. *Self-Regulated Strategy Instruction:* (SRSD): The instructional procedure used for SRSD typically involves learning an effective strategy through a self-instructional format, as well as explicit individual self-regulation techniques, including goal-setting and self-monitoring of strategy usage. For this study, the amount of support provided was varied to create three experimental conditions.	Self-efficacy measure: An individually administered measure for assessing self-efficacy related to story writing. This instrument includes 10 items for probing the self-perceived capacity to create a "made-up" story. Strategy usage: The notes and writing samples produced by experimental Ss were analyzed to obtain direct evidence that the strategies instructed were actually used. Writing stimuli: Black-and-white pictures (5) were used to stimulate writing in response to writing probes (5). This medium was selected because teachers at the schools involved typically used pictures for this purpose. These pictures were selected	mar scores. The schematic structure of the stories written by LD Ss in the three experimental groups did not significantly differ from the stories written by Ss in the normative comparison group. While no significant differences were documented between LD Ss in the practice-control group and instructional groups at the start of intervention, Ss in the full SRSD and SRSD without specific strategy instruction groups received significantly higher schematic structure scores than were obtained by Ss in the practice-control group. The only significant difference at posttest was the significantly higher quality scores received by the normally achieving Ss in the practice-control condition. No significant differences were observed among the three strategy intervention conditions on either the 2- or 4-wk maintenance probes.

(*continued*)

Author (year)	*N*	Selection criteria	Target domain(s)	Treatment(s)	Measures	Results
Sawyer, Graham, & Harris (1992) (*cont.*)					because content was previously identified as interesting to 5th and 6th grade Ss, they were easy to write about, and they were similar in nature. Picture assignment was counterbalanced to ensure that each student responded to a different picture after each writing prompt, and an equivalent number of Ss in each condition responded to each of the pictures.	
Schunk & Rice (1992)	33	Elementary school Ss regularly receiving remedial reading comprehension instruction after being placed in remedial classes. Their scores were at or below the 30th percentile on the reading subtest of the SRA Survey of Basic Skills.	Learning strategies Reading comprehension	*Experiment 1:* Some Ss received strategy instruction, while others were informed of the link between strategy usage and improved performance. Pretesting included a self-efficacy test and a measure of reading comprehension. Children were randomly assigned within sex and grade level to one of three experimental groups: strategy instruction, strategy-value feedback, and instructional control. Ss received 35 min of instruction/day for 15 consecutive	Ss were pretested to determine initial equivalence in terms of self-efficacy and comprehension skills. The self-efficacy test measured perceived capacity for accurately answering comprehension questions that focused on main ideas. This scale ranged in 10-	*Experiment 1:* Improved self-efficacy was experienced by Ss in the strategy-value feedback condition. Comprehension skill increases were obtained by Ss in the two experimental conditions. A MANCOVA of the self-efficacy and skills scores with the corresponding pretest scores as covariates

school days, during which they completed packets of materials. Five to six Ss assigned to the same treatment met in groups with a teacher from outside their school. These groups met in a classroom, with only one group present during each session. The instructional materials consisted of reading passages followed by comprehension questions in a multiple choice format. Ss worked on these packets during each session. Comprehension instruction in their regular classroom was suspended during this experiment. Experimental Ss received either (1) strategy instruction without specific feedback regarding the value of strategic comprehension efforts, or (2) the same strategy instruction plus feedback about the benefits associated with strategic reading behaviors. Control Ss received the same amount of instruction except it did not include the reading comprehension strategy. *Experiment 2:* 33 Ss were drawn from one elementary school; all Ss were 4th and 5th graders enrolled in remedial reading classes. Ss' characteristics and selection procedures were similar to those employed in Experiment 1 with some modifications. Ss were assigned within sex and grade level to one of three conditions: strategy instruction,	unit increments from "not sure" (10) to "really sure" (100). Reading materials were passages drawn from *Scoring High in Reading* books (Cohen & Foreman, 1978), with number of sentences varied between 4 and 8. Passages were followed by 1 to 4 questions, for a total of 20 questions. A maintenance test was given 6 wk after the posttest.	revealed significantly higher judgments of self-efficacy as a result of the strategy-value condition. Experimental Ss verbalized more steps than control Ss. Strategy-value feedback Ss verbalized more than strategy instruction Ss. *Experiment 2:* Ss in the strategy modification condition made significant improvements in self-efficacy, skill, and self-reported strategy use. Strategy instruction Ss demonstrated gains in self-reported strategy use. A MANCOVA of the posttest self-efficacy scores showed significant between-conditions differences. Strategy modification Ss obtained higher self-efficacy scores than control Ss, and they also demonstrated higher skill than Ss in the other two conditions. Experimental Ss reported more usage of the strategy than was claimed by controls.

(continued)

Author (year)	*N*	Selection criteria	Target domain(s)	Treatment(s)	Measures	Results
Schunk & Rice (1992) (*cont.*)				strategy modification, and instructional control. Ten instructional sessions on finding main ideas were conducted, followed by 10 sessions on locating details. Format was similar for these sessions to the first experiment with the addition of methods for adapting the strategy for finding details in the strategy modification group. Ss in the strategy instruction and the instructional control conditions received instruction on locating details, but they were not taught the modified strategy.		Maintenance was significantly higher for strategy modification Ss than for those in the other two groups. Overall, it appears that teaching remedial readers to use strategies enhances their comprehension self-efficacy, skill, strategy use, and achievement
Scruggs & Mastropieri (1992)	20	Middle school Ss attending two self-contained special education classes. The sample included thirteen 6th graders, three 7th graders, and four 8th graders who had a mean chronological age of 13.8 yr. The Ss had an average WISC-R IQ score of 80.1, an average reading percentile of 6.9, and an average math percentile score of 5.4 from the Basic Achievement Skills Individual Screener.	Science concepts	This study involved a crossover design in which each of two classrooms received both mnemonic and traditional instruction for life science, with units counterbalanced across classrooms for 2 wk. For both conditions, each instructional unit was taught for 1 wk with a unit test on Friday. A review before the test was given on the 4th day, Thursday. During the generalization preparation phase, the third unit was taught to both classes. Feedback was given on mnemonic strategies used by the Ss. Ss were encouraged to make their own mnemonics.	Unit tests of science concept acquisition	Mnemonic instruction resulted in substantial increases in initial content acquisition, and substantially higher delayed-recall scores over more traditional instructional procedures. Further, it was found that trained Ss were able to successfully generate and apply their own mnemonic strategies to novel content. Ss overwhelmingly preferred mnemonic instruction over traditional instructional methods.

The Ss were asked to learn the fourth unit during the 4th wk for the generalization phase.

Mnemonic: The mnemonic strategy treatment included using pictures that were developed to represent all important content information, according to the model of reconstructive elaborations (Mastropieri & Scruggs, 1989). When information was considered to be concrete and familiar to mildly handicapped learners, mimetic reconstructions were developed in which target stimulus and response information was depicted interacting pictorially. For abstract information, symbolic reconstructions were employed in which pictorial representations were shown pictorially interacting with relevant target information. When information was considered to be unfamiliar to learners, acoustic reconstructions were employed in which target information was linked with acoustically similar keywords. Mnemonic pictures were developed for three of the four chapters. In addition, mnemonic transparencies and teacher scripts, student workbooks and worksheets were provided.

Traditional: No explicit strategy or retrieval information was provided to learners. Ss were told to work hard and to try their best.

(*continued*)

Author (year)	*N*	Selection criteria	Target domain(s)	Treatment(s)	Measures	Results
Simmonds (1992)	447	1st through 9th graders classified as LD by local committees on special education in accordance with New York State guidelines. Stepwise selection criteria included average or above IQ, 50% discrepancy between ability and achievement, and absence of a primary physical, sensory, or emotional disorders. Ss were enrolled in grades 1 through 9 in regular classes and received supplementary instruction in resource room programs.	Reading comprehension	The experimental and control groups met for a total of four sessions, for 45 min, over the period of 3 wk. The question-answer-response (QAR) strategy was used (Raphael, 1982) by the experimental group. The control group used traditional methods for recalling factual information and main ideas, for locating supporting details, and for drawing conclusions. The control condition is referred to below as *Skill.* *Session 1:* Included four phases *Phase 1:* Charts defining QAR or the skill (Control) were displayed. *Phase 2:* Ss were given four sentences from a familiar story or topic. Questions were discussed and teachers discussed the type of QAR or skill that each question represented. *Phase 3:* Passages with questions and answers were given and Ss were required to identify the QARs or skills for each as a group. *Phase 4:* Ss were given passages with questions and required to give the appropriate QAR or skill and the answers. Feedback was given and dicussion on the differences between the text-based and knowledge-based answers.	Reading comprehension and maze tasks	Teachers were able to effectively acquire and implement both QARs and skills with explicit training and supportive feedback. QARs accommodated to content-area reading material readily; and QARs significantly elevated the question-recognition and location performance of LD Ss.

				Session 2: Teachers reviewed and modeled quided practice using a short, familiar story. Teachers then gave two passages with six questions that required different answer types. Ss first worked in groups, then individually. *Session 3:* A passage was divided into four sections with two questions for each of the three types (QARs or skills) for each section. Review, clarification, and feedback were part of the session. *Session 4:* Classroom materials on social studies and science were used. Ss read a unit of 300–500 words with three questions. Ss were to identify each type of question and answer. All charts were removed for posttesting.		
Simpsons, Swanson, & Kunkel (1992)	63	13- to 18-yr-old inmates selected from two detention facilities. One facility provided residential care for 60 wards of the court with an average length of stay of 92 days. The other facility provided residential care for 120 wards of the court and a day school program for another 60. The average length of stay was 37 days for the residential program and	Word recognition	The Ss met for 90-min daily sessions for an average of 45 sessions. Ss in the experimental group received remedial reading instruction with the Orton–Gillingham Approach, a multisensory, highly structured phonics approach that integrates reading, writing, and spelling through primary modes of hearing, vision, and kinesthesia. Control Ss received reading instruction in their regular classroom.	Woodcock Test of Reading Mastery Rate of recidivism Average number of arrests Frequency of arrests	Ss who received less than 23 hr of remedial instruction would have zero to negative growth. Most Ss who made large gains in reading had extensive remediation: 80% of the Ss who made a yr or more growth in reading had more than 50 hr of remedial reading instruction. Results clearly indicated that the

(*continued*)

Author (year)	*N*	Selection criteria	Target domain(s)	Treatment(s)	Measures	Results
Simpsons, Swanson, & Kunkel (1992) (*cont.*)		162 days for the day school program. Ss were selected for this project on the basis of full English proficiency, hearing and vision within normal limits, verbal or performance IQ at or above 80, discrepancy between reading and verbal or performance IQ of 15 points or more, and a history or adequate elementary school attendance.				Orton–Gillingham Approach could produce significant results in reading growth.
Swanson & Trahan (1992)	120	4th, 5th, and 6th graders were randomly selected from 12 elementary and middle schools (40 Ss/grade level). LD Ss were randomly selected from those served in resource rooms. LD identification was based on verbal intelligence within normal limits (85–115) on the WISC-R (Weschler, 1974), but achievement at or below the 25th percentile for reading total on the Comprehensive Test of Basic Skills.	Reading comprehension	Comprehension passages were selected from *Steps to Comprehension* (Adams & Adams, 1984), a computer program hierarchically arranged according to level of difficulty (1st through 11th grade). Two different types of comprehension skill practice are provided: (1) a "Regular Step" presents a story followed by three literal and three inferential questions: (2) the "Cloze Step" begins at the 2nd to 3rd grade level and requires the student to fill in a missing word. The experiment occurred over a 3-wk span, with one 60–90 min session presented/wk. In the experimental groups, Ss were required to (1) read the instructions, (2) read and study a passage, (3) answer questions	Metacognition/attribution: An adaptation of a questionnaire by Paris, Cross, and Lipson (1984) was presented in a multiple choice format for this study. It had 20 items covering basic comprehension activities, as well as items related to person, task, and strategy variables. The Nelson Reading Skills Test (Hanna, Schell, & Schriener, 1977) was given to	*Between-group analyses: Comprehension:* Average readers obtained significantly higher scores than LD Ss. All other effects were nonsignificant. When verbal ability was controlled, interactions related to passage difficulty disappeared. *Cloze Passages:* Skilled readers outperformed disabled readers across all levels of passage difficulty. *Time:* Disabled readers took longer than average readers in the computer reread condition, while no

about the passage, and (4) proceed to the next passage. Each subject read 12 passages ordered by reading difficulty, then responded to 6 multiple choice and 16–20 cloze format, textually implicit comprehension questions. Control Ss were given the same pretest and posttest assessment, but received no direct comprehension intervention related to the passages. Their classroom program continued as usual. Method of presenting the passages and the question were varied, with the same text presented to all Ss. The researcher or an assistant used a stopwatch to record each student's start and stop time. *Paper (Offline):* LD and average readers received both traditional and cloze comprehension passages in printed form. Passages were presented in fixed order and Ss were not allowed to reread. Six comprehension questions followed each passage; cloze items were completed as the passage was read. *Computer Presentation–No Optional Rereading:* LD and average readers read the traditional and cloze passages once before answering the comprehension questions. The test was computer-mediated. Ss were not allowed to reread prior to task completion. Ss were provided with an alphabetical list of	both reading ability groups to measure (1) *reading comprehension:* questions of simple recall, inference, and cause and effect follow questions related to the humanities, science and social studies curricula; (2) *word meaning :* identification of stimulus word meanings when words are presented in isolation in a phrase, and in a pragraph; and (3) *reading rate:* a 1-min sample of the proprtion f words read from a 600-word passage. Working memory span test (Swanson, Cochran, & Ewars, 1989): A children's adaptation of the Reading Span Test developed for adults by Daneman & Carpenter (1980).	significant group effects were obtained for the computer no reread and paper conditions. Average readers required less time than LD readers to finish passages at the low and medium levels of difficulty, but did not at the high levels. There was an overall advantage for average readers compared to LD readers in terms of passage difficulty. *Posttest Scores:* *Reading Comprehension:* Significant differences between the LD and average reading ability groups were observed. *Word Meaning:* Average readers consistently scored higher than LD readers, although this advantage was only significant for Ss in the treatment conditions. Average readers performed best in the comprehension no reread condition while LD Ss favored the paper (off-line) condition. *Reading Rate:* No significant main

(*continued*)

Author (year)	*N*	Selection criteria	Target domain(s)	Treatment(s)	Measures	Results
Swanson & Trahan (1992) (*cont.*)				all words possible for the cloze tasks. *Computer–Rereading:* LD and average readers were directed to reread all or part of the passages before answering comprehension questions or completing cloze items. The text was computer-mediated for this group as well .	This version consists of eight sets of sentences. The number of sentences in each set rages from two to five. After listening to each set, Ss are asked to write the last word in each sentence according to the order in which they were presented. Prior to writing these words, the Ss are required to answer a question about one of the sentences	effects were observed. *Total Reading:* Average readers scored significantly higher. *Working Memory:* Average Ss scored higher than LD Ss on computer reread conditions. The two groups performed similarly on all other conditions. Significant differences occurred between treatment conditions within ability group. For average readers, treatment was independent of instructional manipulation. Performance for LD Ss was more depressed in the computer reread condition. *Metacognitive Questionnaire:* Average readers obtained significantly higher score than LD readers. *Attributions:* A chi-square analysis produced no significant effects related to treatment or pretest–posttest performance, either between or within ability.

Van Daal & van der Leij (1992)	28	In the Dutch school system, pupils with different kinds of handicaps attend sepearate schools for special education. Five percent of all children in elementary schools are referred to special education. Placement decisions for schools for Ss with primary LD (2% of all Ss) are positive if medical and psychological assessments show that the student does not have gross emotional, sensory, neurological, or intellectual handicaps. IQ must fall within the normal range, between 90 and 110 on the Dutch version of the WISC-R. Ss in this study were of the above description. Their mean age was 9.7. In reading, Ss were 2 yr below age level.	Reading Spelling	To examine the effects of computer-based reading and spelling practice on the development of reading and spelling skills, a pretest–training–posttest experiment was conducted. Ss practiced hard-to-read words under three conditions. For all words, whole word sound was available on call during practice. To assess learning effects, both a dictation and and read-aloud task were administered in which nonpracticed control words were also presented. During training, the computer kept record of several aspects of the pupils' learning behavior. During the pretest, Ss took part in computer-assisted reading. They were given 42 hard-to-read words that were used in a dictation test the next day. The experimenter pronounced the words and the S wrote them down. For the next 15 days, Ss were given 10-min practice sessions of repeated practice with sets of 24 hard-to-read words and 6 easy-to-read words. The remaining selected words were not practiced, but were used as control words in the posttest. *Reading from the computer screen:* Ss could request speech feedback from the computer, but speech feedback requests were limited to 10/words.	Number of speech feedback requests, speed feedback tests during typing, practice time, errors	Copying words from the screen resulted in significantly fewer spelling errors on the posttest than writing words from memory, and that both forms of spelling practice let to fewer spelling errors than only reading words during practice. All three forms of practice improved to the same degree both the accuracy and fluency of reading the practiced words aloud.

(*continued*)

Author (year)	*N*	Selection criteria	Target domain(s)	Treatment(s)	Measures	Results
Van Daal & van der Leij (1992) (*cont.*)				*Write from memory:* A written word was presented, and the subject was to indicate that she/he was ready for typing, after which the word was erased and the S given 2 min to type the word *Copying from the screen:* The target word remained on the screen during typing. In both typing conditions, the word sounds could be requested up to five times *before* typing, and up to five times *during* typing. When the S spelled the word correctly, the computer said "Well done." The computer also alerted the S to errors. *Control:* Ss were presented 16 hard-to-read words and 16 easy-to-read words from the pretest which were not used in the intervention. There was no repeated practice.		
Weinstein & Cooke (1992)	3	Four Ss were selected for this study who were certified as LD according to North Carolina state guidelines. (One student had an IQ of 74, and was therefore not included in this meta-analysis.) Ss had been assessed on intellectual and	Reading	Prior to the initial reading each intervention session, Ss were given an opportunity to listen to an audiotaped model of the passage. After listening to the model. Ss were instructed to read the passage as quickly and as well as they could. No errors were corrected during or after the reading. Each student was given two opportunities to reread each	Correct words read/min on a reading passage	All Ss made gains in their mean correct words read/min with the repeated reading technique, regardless of the type of criterion. The difference between fluency means for the improvements phases and

		achievement measures and had attained age standard-score units 15 or more points below their intellectual/cognitive functioning.		day until they met the specified criterion. In the *Fixed-Rate Intervention Phase,* Ss continued to reread a story passage until they reached a criterion of 90 correct words/min. In the *Improvement Phase,* Ss continued to reread a story passage until they achieved three successive improvements on correct words/min.		was 10.4 CWPM, with the difference favoring the fixed-rate criterion; however, this difference was interpreted by the authors as small.
Welch (1992)	18	6th grade Ss with specific LDs from a suburban area of the intermountain west. Seven of the Ss were enrolled in classes taught by two teachers who had taken a summer workshop on learning strategies. Eleven Ss from another school in the same district served as a control group. Ss were not aware of their group assignment.	Metacognition Learning strategies	The experimental Ss were taught a mnemonic strategy (PLEASE) in the resource room three times a week during 30-min lessons for about 20 wk. Comparison Ss received language arts instruction during 20-min lessons for 20 wk. *PLEASE:* This strategy involves the use of a first letter mnemonic that cues Ss on how to finish a writing task independently. To facilitate metacognitive problem solving, the student is provided with a list of behavior to be performed. "p" represents "pick," which reminds Ss to pick a topic, and audience, and the appropriate format. "L" refers to "list," which prompts the generation of information to be used. "E" reminds Ss to "evaluate" their list and then plan the best way to organize the information to generate supporting sentences. "A" stands for "activate," which instructs the writer to	Ss completed a brief survey designed to measure their knowledge of metacognitive processes associated with prewriting, planning, writing, and proofing/revising. In addition, actual writing samples were examined to determine whether or not the strategy was actually implemented. The teacher individually administered an attitudinal measure. This consisted of showing the Ss 33 index cards containing positive statements	Although analyses of pretest date supported initial equivalence of the two groups, the posttest scores of the experimental group were significantly higher than those of comparison Ss.

(*continued*)

Author (year)	N	Selection criteria	Target domain(s)	Treatment(s)	Measures	Results
Welch (1992) (*cont.*)				generate a short and simple declarative sentence to activate the written idea for the reader. "s" refers to take information from the list to "supply supporting sentences." "E" prompts the writer to "end" with a concluding sentence and to "evaluate."	about writing paragraphs. These cards were flashed to the student who indicated if the statement reflected his or her own attitudes.	
Barbetta & Heward (1993)	3	Two boys and one girl, ages 10 to 11, enrolled in a primary, self-contained class for children with LD. Each was mainstreamed for geography class, and they were selected based on their need to learn state and country capitals.	Geography facts	Students were pretested to identify a set of 14 unknown capitals during each of week of the study. An alternating treatments design was used to evaluate the extent to which active student response (ASR) and no response (NR) affected differential effects on student learning of the names of state and country capitals. ASR error correction consisted of the experimenter stating the correct capital, then having the student repeat it. Praised followed each correct repetition. NR error correction consisted of the experimenter stating the capital and the subject looking at the card. Each week seven capitals were taught using ASR error correction and seven capitals were taught using NR error correction. Presentation order of the two error correction feedback strategies was randomly determined and frequently chances by shuffling the whole set of	The amounts of correct responses by each subject during both types of instruction were counted. Data included initially correct practice trial responses plus active responses made during error correction. Because no active student responses were made during NR error correction, NR active response data includes only initially correct practice trial responses plus records of inadvertent student responses made during NR error correction episodes.	During instruction, each subject correctly stated more capitals following ASR than NR error correction. Results of same-day and next-day testing showed that all three subjects learned more capitals with ASR than with NR error correction. These subjects also correctly stated more ASR capitals on 1-wk maintenance tests. In sum, these subjects learned and maintained more capitals taught with ASR than with NR error correction, lending further support to research demonstrating that active student responding is a powerful instructional variable.

				geography cards (seven ASR and seven NR) following each practice and testing session. One-to-one sessions occurred 4 days each wk; a new set of facts was introduced wkly, with each session lasting 12–15 min and consisting of a next-day test, instruction with ASR and NR error correction, and a same-day test (given right after instruction). Maintenance tests followed same-day tests. The geography cards were shuffled, then presented during a practice trial one card at a time; the subject read aloud the name of the state or country printed on the card and tried to name the capital. Praise followed correct statements; either the ASR or NR error correction procedure followed incorrect responses.		
Cole (1993) Dissertation	12	3rd through 5th graders with WISC-R/WPPSI mean IQ scores of 85, with a range of 71 to 103.	Writing	The study investigated the effectiveness of an instructional intervention that was designed to teach students with LD to write a sequential expository paragraph (i.e., a set of directions) through strategy instruction and the use of a set of structured writing frameworks. BL conditions required the Ss to write a paragraph on a "how to" topic. No further instructions or discussion was given. BL lasted for 6 days. During the 12 treatment sessions, each S received a packet of writing framework sheets at the beginning of each session. The instructional procedure	Writing Fluency: number of words/session	The three groups of Ss attained criterion performance levels on the writing measure, and increased fluency over BL levels. Maintenance of performance and generalization to another setting were also demonstrated.

(*continued*)

Author (year)	*N*	Selection criteria	Target domain(s)	Treatment(s)	Measures	Results
Cole (1993) (*cont.*)				involved model-lead-test methodology. Generalization was programmed by the teachers frequently asking the Ss whether they could think of another time or place when using a particular part of the framework would be helpful. *Treatment:* Each session included: (1) Introduction of the topic, during which the instructor modeled and demonstrated a self-questioning technique; (2) Ss were then led through the self-questioning technique; (3) Ss and teacher discussed which materials were necessary and Ss made a list of them; (4) Ss wrote and verbalized the steps to the process; (5) Ss looked at the steps again and asked themselves whether a younger child could follow the steps and do the task without instruction; (6) Ss made a final format of the instructions; (7) Ss learned how to write a topic sentence, then the paragraph using signal words (sentence starters) for the above instructions, ending with a summary sentence; (8) Ss made a final draft; and (9) After each session, Ss were tested with a "how to" topic and asked to do the above steps without help or modeling *Maintenance:* After five consecutive test sessions without training, Ss were given a topic and the blank writing packets, but no instruction. *Generalization:* Ss were asked to write paragraphs in different settings within the school.		

Danoff, Harris, & Graham (1993)	6	Four 5th graders and two 4th graders. Two of the 5th grade Ss and one of the 4th grade Ss had been identified as having a LD disability by the school district. Mean WISC-R IQ score was 97.33, ranging from 89 to 105. WRMT showed a reading mean of 80.66, with a range of 76–88. The LD and NLD Ss were paired.	Story writing	The study examined the efficacy of embedding strategy instruction in the context of a process approach to writing in inclusive classrooms. During BL, Ss' preinstructional response rates on writing stories were established. *Intervention:* Ss were fully mainstreamed. The special education teacher and the regular classroom teacher worked together in teaching the series of extended minilessons in writing strategies. The special education teacher was a consultant and a coteacher in some classes. Sometimes, she was the developer and teacher of lessons, and the regular teacher provided backup. Writing took place throughout the day. However, there was a specific class period, Writer's Workshop, where this intervention took place. Ss chose their own topics and genre, content and purpose, selected pieces for completion and publication, and consulted with peers when planning and revising work. The Self-Regulated Strategy Development Model (SRSD) was used (Graham et al., 1987, 1992). Seven instructional phases were included: (1) *Initial conference:* Discussed purpose of instruction and common parts of a story; (2) *Preskill development:* Defining, identifying, and generating common story parts by discussion, then by	Story-grammar scale Number of words written Holistic rating scale Strategy usage Self-efficacy measure Social validity interviews	The strategy instruction procedures had a positive effect on the participating Ss' writing. The schematic structure of their stories improved substantially following instruction and remained improved over time and with a different teacher. The quality of what was written also improved for four of the six Ss following instruction. Overall, improvements in story quality were maintained and generalized by all of the Ss, except for the younger 4th graders and one 5th grade S who failed to maintain quality gains on a generalization probe. In addition, one of the Ss who had not evidenced quality gains immediately following instruction wrote qualitatively better stories on the generalization and maintenance probes. Finally, data collected during instruction demonstrated that the best results were obtained when all stages and components of instruction were enacted.

(continued)

Author (year)	*N*	Selection criteria	Target domain(s)	Treatment(s)	Measures	Results
Danoff, Harris, & Graham (1993) (*cont.*)				recognizing examples in literature, and how to graph the story parts; (3) *Composition strategy discussion:* A five-step writing strategy and a mnemonic for remembering seven questions about the basic parts of the story; (4) *Modeling:* The teacher modeled thinking aloud about her story to further develop it and also modeled five types of self-instruction (problem defining, planning, self-evaluation, self-reinforcement, and coping); (5) *Strategy and mnemonic memorization*; (6) *Collaborative practice:* The goal was for the teacher to help by fading support and for the Ss to become more independent with the strategies they had been given; (7) *Independent performance:* Ss independently planned and wrote two stories using the five-step strategy and accompanying self-regulation procedures (goal-setting, self-monitoring).		
DuPaul & Henningson (1993)	1	S was a 7-yr-old boy who was referred by his classroom teacher to an outpatient psychiatry clinic due to problems with attention span, impulse control, and activity	Math computation On-task behavior	The study focused on classwide peer tutoring (CWPT) involving instructional procedures (provision of frequent, immediate feedback) that are known to be successful for children with attention-deficit/hyperactivity disorder (ADHD).	Math computation: digits written correctly on curriculum-based measurement probes	The implementation of peer tutoring with the student with ADHD showed results indicating significant improvements in attention to instruction,

	level. The S was underachieving academically, and was diagnosed as having ADHD.	An ABAB reversal design was used to evaluate the effects of peer tutoring on the S's classroom performance. *BL 1 and 2:* Mathematics instruction was provided by teacher-directed lessons to the whole class with sample questions being done at the board by selected students. The S then worked on seatwork independently using worksheets. The S received corrective feedback. *Treatment 1 and 2: Classwide Peer Tutoring* (Greenwood et al., 1998): The S was randomly paired with another student for math instruction. The tutor was given a script of math problems and dictated the problems to the tutee one at a time. The tutee then responded orally, using a black piece of paper to solve the problem, if needed. Rewards and reinforcers for correct answering were awarded. Corrective feedback was provided for incorrect responding. The tutee then practiced the correct answer. The items were presented as many times as possible for 10 min after which Ss switched roles.	On-task behaviors: interval recording of on-task and fidgeting behaviors.	task-irrelevant activity level, and acquisition of mathematics skills.

(*continued*)

Author (year)	*N*	Selection criteria	Target domain(s)	Treatment(s)	Measures	Results
Fawcett, Nicolson, & Morris (1993)	12	Ss were10 to 12 yr old, with a mean age of 11.4, and diagnosed as dyslexic. Diagnosis based on standard exclusionary criteria (i.e., an 18-mo or more deficit in reading age over chronological age, together with normal or above normal IQ, and no primary emotional or neurological problems). Mean IQ scores were 112.3, with a range of 105 to 128. On the Schonell Test, mean reading score was 8.4 and mean spelling score was 6.6.	Spelling	Ss met for three, 20-min sessions for each set of words. During the pretest, each parent identified 20 words which were of particular significance and difficulty for their child. They dictated the words and timed the child's performance. Next, the parents discussed the words with the child and asked him/her to rank them in order of difficulty. The lists were given to the experimenters and were used to make two sets of words. The words were then compared with the Schonell Spelling List. *Self-Spell:* Experimental Ss received treatment in four phases: (1) Pretest; (2) The experimenter created a passage using the selected words from the pretest and typed it into the computer with mistakes; (3) The child read through the passage with the teacher's help, identifying all of the mistakes (bugs) and made up a rule to remember the correct spelling; (4) The child read through the passage without help and fixed all of the errors. *Spellmaster* (control): A word list was typed into the computer and each word was presented until it was understood and learned. Immediate feedback was provided.	Spelling: percent correct spellings out of 10 possible words	The rule-based approach resulted in significant improvement of spelling. However, use of a mastery learning technique for learning spellings was just as effective as the rule-based approach. These findings were interpreted in the light of Frith's influential framework for the development of reading and spelling ability. It was suggested that the multimedia presentation approach provides a uniquely effective method for helping dyslexic children to acquire the "alphabetic" stage of linguistic processing.

Hollingsworth & Woodward (1993)	37	Secondary students from the Pacific Northwest or Canada. All Ss were identified as LD per individualized educational plans (IEPs), with reading at least 2 yr below grade expectancies. Following a 3-day preliminary orientation to a computerized health curriculum, students were matched on reading and randomly assigned to either an experimental or a comparison group.	Problem solving Health facts and concepts Cognitive strategies	A writing curriculum was used to teach basic health facts and concepts. A computer simulation was implemented to affect student involvement in complex problem solving. The content of the curriculum covered secondary health information with readability controlled at between 4th and 5th grade level. The goal of the simulation is improving longevity through behavioral change. All Ss participated daily in a 50-min health class for 14 days. The first 25 min of each class consisted of health instruction. One teacher delivered a 20-min lesson to the entire group of students participating in this study. Concepts and vocabulary presented in the orientation were covered in depth at this time. For the last 5 min of this section, the students were separated into two groups. In the *Explicit Strategy* group, the teacher explained the use of a pictorial presentation of a decision tree, including the use of each step, as well as the advantage of using the tree to solve health-related problems as presented in a computer simulation. *Comparison* Ss reviewed supplemental materials from the health curriculum. For the remaining 25 min of each class, Ss completed two to four simulation activities, with the teacher circulating to facilitate problem solving. Experimental Ss were reminded	To assess the effects of intervention, three different measures were administered. A 30-item, fill-in-the-blank measure, the Nutrition and Disease Test, was used as a pretest and as a posttest to measure Ss' retention of health facts and concepts. The Health Diagnosis Test was given immediately following the intervention. This instrument consists of three written health profiles which must be evaluated to identify and prioritize health problems, to prescribe needed behavioral changes, and to identify lifestyle changes needed for stress reduction. The Video Diagnostic Test was another posttest measure that assessed the ability to generalize knowledge of health problems to another medium.	*Nutrition and Disease Test:* A 2 × 2 (Treatment x Time of Test) ANOVA with repeated measures on the Time factor revealed no significant between group effects. *Transfer Measures:* Significant between-group effects were observed in an ANCOVA performed on the results of the Health Diagnosis Test using the Nutrition and Disease posttest as a covariate. Ss in the explicit strategy group displayed significantly greater prioritization skills related to the identification of needed changes in health-related behaviors according to between-group comparisons of the three major factors of the Health Diagnosis Test. The ability to transfer health problem solving skills to new situations was also assessed by the Video Diagnostic Test. Using the Nutrition and Disease posttest as the covariate

(*continued*)

Author (year)	*N*	Selection criteria	Target domain(s)	Treatment(s)	Measures	Results
Hollingsworth & Woodward (1993) (*cont.*)				of the relevant steps in the decision tree; comparison Ss were encouraged or given succinct answers, supportive feedback, or general responses. Teacher assignment to treatment was counterbalanced; the two teachers switched places after the first wk of intervention. again, significant between-group		differences were identified. The evidence indicated that explicit strategy instruction affected more effective solutions to computer generated health problems.
Hutchinson (1993)	20	8th through 10th graders with LD attending small-group learning assistance classes in mathematics at two junior high schools. Ss were between the ages of 12.5 and 15.83 yr, with a mean age of 14.45 yr. WISC-R IQ scores between 85 and 115; Ss had been identified as having a specific learning deficit and a discrepancy of more than 3 yr on a standard achievement test in mathematics.	Algebra problem solving	The study included single-subject and group data. The treatment lasted from 3 to 7 days. *BL:* Ss met in BL conditions twice for 2 days each. During BL, Ss completed two sets of 10 problems of one mathematical structure containing two problems of each story line. *Treatment:* Ss met individually with the instructor for one 40-min session on alternate days for 4 mo. Ten procedures were followed by the instructor during treatment in a teach/test cycle: (1) Ss were reminded of that day's purpose and graph results were discussed; (2) Ss were given a task sheet of five problems and a prompt card for self-questioning; (3) Ss were asked to read self-questions; (4) Ss read the first problem silently; (5) Strategy use was modeled by thinking aloud for the first and second problems; (6) Prompts were provided with	Relational problems: percentage correct representation, solution, and answers Proportional problems: percentage correct representation, solution, and answers	Two variable, two equation problems: percentage correct representation, solution, and answers Visual analysis of the single-subject data showed the strategy to be an effective intervention for this sample of Ss with deficits in algebra problem solving, but with criterial knowledge of basic operations and one-step problems. Statistical analyses of the two-group data showed that the instructed Ss had significantly higher posttest scores than the comparison group. Overall, the instructed Ss demonstrated

encouragement and corrective feedback while the S utilized the think aloud procedure for the third and fourth problems; (7) Corrective feedback was provided after the fifth problem was complete; (8) Fade out prompts, encouragement, and gradual feedback were provided; (9) Ss were tested with an assessment task sheet to be completed independently; and (10) Ss were shown the graph of progress and informed about the purpose of the next session. Six phases were included in the treatment: Representation and solution for relational, proportional, two-variable, and two-equation problems. *Transfer:* A test of 5 near-transfer problems in the session following post-testing for each problem type mastered by each subject. *Maintenance:* Six weeks subsequent to transfer testing, the posttest was readministered, consisting of five problems of each instructional type under the same conditions as the two previous administrations. In addition, 28 think-aloud protocols about following instructions depicted Ss thinking through steps in the problem cued by the worksheet and monitoring their attempts.	improved performance on algebra word problems. Maintenance and transfer of the strategy were evident.

(*continued*)

Author (year)	*N*	Selection criteria	Target domain(s)	Treatment(s)	Measures	Results
Kennedy & Backman (1993)	20	LD students between 11 and 17 yr old enrolled in a nonprofit residential school. Most students at this school are publicly funded and must qualify for services based on stringent criteria, including at least average cognitive ability, a severe ability and academic achievement discrepancy, and failure to make adequate school progress in spite of several yr of intensive remediation efforts. Ss were randomly selected for this study based on speech and language results from the Lindamood Auditory Conceptualization Test (LAC; Lindamood & Lindamood, 1979). Controls were matched to experimental Ss based on WISC-R scores, chronological age, Slosson Oral Reading Test scores (SORT; Slosson, 1963), and the Stanford Achievement Test, Spelling List Scores.	Phonological skills Phonetic reading and spelling skills	The curriculum at this school typically emphasizes remediation of weaknesses and reinforcement of strengths. Programming is individualized and instruction is delivered through tutorial and small group formats. Experimental Ss received the Lindamood program, Auditory Discrimination in Depth (ADD), in addition to the typical intervention program. Control Ss received the individualized program without the Lindamood component. *Teaching Programs:* The individualized tutorial program emphasizes a skills-based, bottom-up approach to language arts instruction. Discrete skills are taught and reinforced through multisensory activities. The Lindamood program involves the identification and classification of speech sounds, followed by sound–symbol association activities. Students are taught to use auditory, visual and articulatory feedback to classify and label consonant and vowel sounds. Tracking and representation of sounds is encouraged through multisensory activities. After these discrete skills are mastered, students are encouraged to integrate their auditory tracking skills with	Sound–symbol WISC-R scores were obtained from students' preadmission records. The Gray Oral Reading Test (GORT; Gray, 1955) was given as a pre- and posttest. Six additional measures were administered at the beginning of the school year, at midyear, and at the end of the year. *LAC:* The student must identify sounds and sound sequences in spoken nonsense words and by pointing to colored blocks which represent the sounds. This test is administered individually. *SORT:* An individually administered reading test that requires word pronunciation at	Both groups made significant gains across the study period as measured by a repeated-measures MANOVA of SORT and SAT-S; scores using age as a covariate. A significant Group × Time of Testing interaction did not occur, indicating that the experimental Ss did not make significantly more progress than controls. All Ss made gains in GORT performance across the year, i.e., there were no significant between-group differences at the end of the year when age and pretest scores were considered. A significant main effect for testing time was obtained in analyses of LAC scores, indicating that both groups improved in terms of phonological skills during this study. A significant Group × Time of Testing interaction indicated significantly greater gains

associations. Instruction culminates with reading, i.e., the decoding of syllable pattern sequences. Experimental Ss received the Lindamood program for three 50-min class periods daily for 6 wk (75 hr). The regular reading and spelling program was initiated after this period, and was continued for the remainder of the school year. Lindamood strategies were reviewed throughout the school year, with encouragement for transfer provided to enhance students' generalization and development of automaticity. Control Ss received the regular reading and spelling program. Class size for both groups was maintained at between four and six students except for tutorial periods (50 min/day). Overall time allocated for instruction was the same for both groups.	different levels of difficulty. *SAT-Sp:* This test involves standard administration of spelling items to small groups of students. First the word to be spelled is dictated by the teacher, then the word is used in a sentence, after which the word is repeated again. *GORT:* A measure of oral reading proficiency that is individually administered. *Phonetic Reading—Nonwords:* An individually administered diagnostic sound–symbol battery completed at the beginning of the school year to assist in planning individual programs. Subtests using mainly one- and two-syllable, phonetically	by the experimental Ss than the controls in terms of growth in phonological skills. Although both groups improved their phonetic accuracy, the degree of improvement varied according to treatment. All Ss in this study made significant gains on reading and spelling measures during this intervention, including tests of word recognition, paragraph reading, and spelling. However, there was only limited evidence to support the efficacy of providing the Lindamood program in addition to a comprehensive remedial program such as the one provided by the private school where this study was conducted.

(*continued*)

Author (year)	*N*	Selection criteria	Target domain(s)	Treatment(s)	Measures	Results
Kennedy & Backman (1993) (*cont.*)					based nonwords were also administered to Ss in January and May to evaluate the use of phonetic principles in reading. *Phonetic Spelling—Stanford:* Misspelling analysis was employed to determine if experimental Ss had greater improvements in their use of phonetic spelling compared to control Ss. *Phonetic Spelling—Nonwords:* 75, one-syllable words and 12 two- and three-syllable words were selected from the school's auditory and tutorial testing battery.	

Lundberg & Olofsson (1993)	33	Ss were RD, divided into two age groups. The *beginners* (10 experimental and 8 controls) were in grades 2–3. The *readers* (8 experimental and 7 controls) were in grades 4, 6, and 7. The treatment Ss were attending regular classes but were referred to special education (reading remediation) for some hours a wk.	Reading comprehension	The authors assumed that one major obstacle for successful reading comprehension among poor readers was related to problems with decoding of individual words encountered in the text. A computer-based system for dealing with this obstacle was designed using the IBM-PC/AT and a Scandinavian multilingual text-to-speech unit. The reader of a text file could easily request immediate pronunciation of a problem word encountered. The child read the text on the screen and when a difficult word was encountered, the computer provided speech support. The child could target the word with the mouse. The word was highlighted and the immediate speech feedback was provided. All actions were logged onto a special file for each S. Ss met for about 25 sessions over 10 wk. Control Ss received traditional reading tasks and materials.	Word decoding Reading comprehension	Older Ss gained more from the computer-aided reading than did younger ones. One reason for this differential effect might be related to the metacognitive demands implied by the request option.
Maag, Reid, & DiGangi (1993)	6	All Ss in this study were classified as LD according to their school district's criteria, which were similar to those of the federal government. Ss were currently enrolled in 4th and 6th grades, with mean ages of 9.3 and 11.5. According to their WISC-R	Math computation Problem solving	A multiple BL design was used in this study. The study included the following: BL, Self-Monitoring, Choice, Fade, and Follow-up. *BL* consisted of 5–10 sessions. Tape-recorded tones were introduced. The tape began at different intervals. Ss worked on math practice sheets; however, no instructions were provided.	Attention: self-monitoring	Differential results were obtained across age groups. Fourth graders' mathematics performance improved most when self-monitoring productivity, whereas 6th graders' performance improved most when self-monitoring accuracy.

(continued)

Author (year)	*N*	Selection criteria	Target domain(s)	Treatment(s)	Measures	Results
Maag, Reid, & DiGangi (1993) (*cont.*)		IQ scores, Ss' mean scores were 92; one S scored 81. Ss' mean WRAT-R scores were 69.83.		Ss verbalized class rules. For *Self-Monitoring*, Ss received training in three types of self-monitoring. *Self-Monitoring Attention* Ss were instructed to self-record on their recording sheets if they were on- or off-task when cued by a taped tone. *Self-Monitoring Productivity* When cued by a taped tone, Ss marked the problems on which they were working and counted the number of completed problems and then recorded on the sheet. No emphasis was placed on accuracy. *Self-Monitoring Accuracy* Ss recorded how many problems they had completed accurately between tones on a tally card. *Choice* Ss chose which of the three self-monitoring techniques they preferred to use.		
Maron (1993) Dissertation	13	Ss in this study had a mean age of 10.7, ranging from 10.2 to 11.0. WISC-R/K-ABC mean IQ score was 98.86. Achievement scores from the PPVT showed a 2 *SD* difference from the IQ scores.	Word recognition	Ss met twice/wk for 30 min for a total of eight sessions. Two groups were compared, *Explicit Training* and *Implicit Training*. Both groups received intervention in test-taking skills in the same content area, *Reading Vocabulary*, with the same format, i.e., multiple choice worksheets. Skills for both groups included: (1) careful reading of test questions and answer choices; and (2) choosing the answer from dissimilar answer choices, visually similar foils,	Gates–MacGinitie Reading Tests (Pre and Post) Probe tests Percent of foil errors on probe tests (visually similar foils, miscue foils, and shared semantic features foils)	Performance on the training worksheets, which increased in vocabulary level difficulty, suggested that foil avoidance learning might have occurred for some subjects. Four Ss from each training group appeared to learn to avoid visually similar foils. All of the Explicit Group Ss and half of the Implicit Group

				foils with potential miscues, and foils with a shared semantic feature. Feedback was different for each of the two groups. *Explicit Training* Worksheets that were modeled after *Vocabulary Structured Practice Lessons* from *Super Score* (Scruggs & Williams, 1985) were used in conjunction with instruction designed to make particular test-taking strategies explicit or more salient. Associated scripts adapted from *Super Score* were also used. Four worksheets were used during each section. Feedback was given for the correctness of answers and direct instruction was given for how to avoid future errors. *Implicit Training* Worksheets were used to provide test-taking practice. The script was selected from *Super Score*. Feedback was only given for the correctness of answers.		Ss appeared to learn to avoid shared semantic features foils. Worksheet performance improvements would appear to be the result of training, but may be due to chance. Examination of individual subject characteristics revealed a common significant positive correlation for both groups between miscue pretest probes and posttest Gates–MacGinitie performance. IQ and Gates–MacGinitie negative correlation was large but not significant.
Mathes & Fuchs (1993)	67	4th through 6th grade students identified as LD who were receiving support for reading in special education resource rooms. Criteria for inclusion included an identified LD, receiving resource support, an IEP with reading objectives, an instructional reading level at least at the primer level and at	Reading	A basal reading series that was novel to both groups of Ss was used. Pretesting was completed to determine the instructional and independent reading level of each subject. Manipulation of type of peer-mediated instruction and level of difficulty resulted in a two-factor, multiple-treatment, pretest and posttest design. Classwide peer-mediated reading instruction occurred in the students' resource classrooms three times/wk for 10	Reading achievement was tested using the comprehensive Reading Assessment Battery (CRAB; Fuchs, Fuchs, & Hamlett, 1989). Individual testing was completed before and after the 10-wk intervention, with	Initial differences were noted based on a MANOVA of the CRAB pretest that indicated a main effect for treatment, although neither a main effect for text level nor a Group × Text difficulty interaction was observed. Due to this nonequivalence, a two-way

(continued)

Author (year)	N	Selection criteria	Target domain(s)	Treatment(s)	Measures	Results
Mathes & Fuchs (1993) *(cont.)*		least one grade below age expectancies. LD identification was based on a discrepancy of more than 1 SD between ability and achievement. Inclusion in this study required that a discrepancy be apparent in terms of reading achievement. Treatment assignment for students was determined by their teacher's random assignment to either an experimental or a control condition. Ss were randomly assigned within classrooms to read either independent or instructional reading materials.		wk total during regularly scheduled intervention periods. Two peer-mediated conditions were designed according to the classwide peer tutoring structure. All students in each of 12 resource teachers' participating classrooms were involved in peer-mediated instruction in one of two conditions. Teachers were randomly assigned to incorporate either a sustained reading condition or a repeated reading condition. Ss in the sustained reading group read orally continuously from a basal reading text for 9 min. Students worked in pairs, with each peer tutor monitoring word recognition errors as his or her partner read. The roles of tutor and peer student were switched after 9 min, and the process was repeated with new text. Ss assigned to the second experimental condition, repeated-reading, read three different passages three times for 1 min during each reading session, for a total of 9 min/session, with the goal of reading further in the text each time with fewer errors recorded across sessions. Control Ss continued with typical resource room activities. Total overall time for reading intervention in control and experimental classrooms was approximately equivalent. Oral reading time	Reading Instructional Time Use (RITU; Mathes & Fuchs, 1991), and the Teacher Effectiveness Rating Scale (TERS; Simmons, Fuchs, & Fuchs, 1989). Experimental teachers and their students also responded to questionnaires evaluating their satisfactions with the peer-mediated techniques.econd experimental condition, repeated-reading, read three different passages three times for 1 min during each reading session, for a total of 9 min/session, with the goal of reading further in the text each time with fewer errors recorded across sessions. Control Ss continued with typical resource room activities. Total overall time for	multivariate ANCOVA was used to analyze posttest scores with pretest scores employed as covariates. This analysis revealed a significant main effect for treatment groups, but again did not suggest either a main effect for text difficulty or an interaction between these factors. Reliable differences were found among groups for word reading accuracy, but not for questions correct. Analyses of the tutoring fidelity measure did not suggest reliable differences between the two experimental groups in terms of implementation. Data from the two observation instruments, i.e., the RITU and the TERS, were analyzed by one-way ANOVAs. Results from the RITU suggest groups did not differ according to time allocated to reading, student focus on

was the same for both experimental groups.	reading intervention in control and experimental classrooms was approximately equivalent. Oral reading time was the same for both experimental groups.	instruction, oral reading practice, silent reading practice and noninstructional waiting or off-task time. However, a significant difference occurred in terms of the proportion of students doing independent seatwork, with the sustained-reading group spending more time on this type of activity. In terms of teacher satisfaction, no differences were found between treatments, with both groups responding favorably to the treatment. Students' responses to the satisfaction surveys, however, did reveal important differences, with repeated-reading Ss reporting that they liked their peer-mediated activities more than the sustained-reading group liked theirs.

(continued)

Author (year)	*N*	Selection criteria	Target domain(s)	Treatment(s)	Measures	Results
Miller & Mercer (1993)	9	Of the nine Ss in this study, five were already classified as LD, three were classified as at risk for an LD program, and one was classified as educable mentally handicapped, although he received instruction with students who were identified as LD. The six LD Ss were receiving math instruction in a resource room, and the other three were receiving math instruction in general education classes. Mean age was 9.4, ranging from 7.7 to 11.2. IQ scores were as follows: one S = 85 (WISC-R), five Ss = 63–80 (KABC), and no scores were available for three Ss. Math achievement scores were reported as follows: MAT GE scores (three Ss) ranged from K.7 to K.9; CAT GE scores (three Ss) ranged from 3.4 to 3.8; KTEA GE scores (three Ss) ranged from pre-K to pre-1.	Math	Systematic math instruction using the concrete–semiconcrete–abstract teaching sequence was provided to nine Ss who were identified as having math disabilities. Data were collected via a 1-min probe at the end of each lesson. *Phase 1:* BL data were collected daily using 1-min abstract-level probes without teacher feedback. Rate of correct and incorrect responses/min were recorded a minimum of 3 days. *Phase 2, Treatment:* Instruction was implemented, with lessons and instruction limited to 20-min scripted sessions. Each lesson involved four instructional steps that included self-instruction. The teacher began instruction with an advanced organizer that illustrated benefits of the skill, rationale for the skill, description of the skill being taught, and skill instruction. Three problems were demonstrated, then Ss modeled the skill. The teacher verbalized the process while modeling, then asked Ss questions while working another problem. Guided practice was provided, which consisted of giving Ss several problems while the teacher provided prompts and cues and assistance if needed. Finally, Ss were given independent practice with 10	Skills: accuracy of response Division: accuracy of response	The concrete–semiconcrete–abstract sequence was an effective intervention for the Ss in this investigation. Moreover, through simple classroom data collection, it was determined that the Ss needed between three and seven lessons using manipulative devices and pictures before they were able to transfer this learning to abstract-level problems presented on a probe sheet after the lesson was completed.

				problems and no feedback. This treatment phase began with *concrete-level* instruction, which included three-dimensional objects to solve math problems. Different objects were used during each lesson. Next, *semiconcrete* instruction was used which entailed drawings begin used to solve math problems. Ss learned how to keep tallies. Finally, in the *abstract-level* lessons, Ss were asked to solve the problem without using objects or drawings. During all three levels, there were three lessons taught by the division teacher, and five lessons by the coin sums and addition teacher. *Phase 3, Posttreatment:* One week after completion of all lessons, a 1-min probe was administered.		
Montague, Applegate, & Marquard (1993)	96	LD Ss were divided into three treatment groups.	Math problem solving	This study investigated the effects of cognitive strategy instruction on math problem-solving performance. Three treatment conditions and two cycles of treatment were implemented. Treatment was not given to the fourth group. Treatments included: *Cognitive Strategy Instruction, Metacognitive Instruction*, and *Cognitive Metacognitive Instruction Combined.* The first treatment cycle consisted of 7 instructional days for each condition. The second treatment cycle consisted of 5 instructional days in the complementary component of the instructional program for the *Cognitive* and	Word problem tests: 6- and 10-problem tests	Ss improved in math problem-solving performance on two different measures of one-, two-, and three-step word problems. In addition, their performance compared well with that of a normally achieving peer group.

(*continued*)

Author (year)	*N*	Selection criteria	Target domain(s)	Treatment(s)	Measures	Results
Montague, Applegate, & Marquard (1993) (*cont.*)				*Metacognitive* groups and a continuation of the combined treatments for the third group. Both treatment cycles included strategy acquisition training (scripted) and strategy application practice sessions. *Group 1, Cognitive:* Through direct instruction, Ss learned only the names and description of the processes. Ss were required to recall the seven processes. The teacher modeled the problem-solving strategy, but did not explain how to apply the strategy. Ss practiced with corrective feedback. Verbalization of the strategy processes was required at a criterion of 100%. *Group 2, Metacognitive:* Only the metacognitive activities associated with each cognitive process were taught. Ss paraphrased rather than memorized the metacognitive activities. The teacher modeled using word problems. Ss practiced individually and were given corrective feedback. *Group 3, Combined:* Ss were required to memorize the seven processes and paraphrase the metacognitive activities associated with strategy implementation. Verbalization of the cognitive processes from memory was required at a criterion of 100% prior to administration of the first posttest. The teacher modeled strategy recitation and application. Ss received corrective and positive feedback.		

Reid & Harris (1993)	28	LD Ss were selected from a pool of students in ungraded, self-contained classrooms. Mean age was 11 yr, with a range from 9 to 13. Mean scores on the WISC-R/KABC or Stanford–Binet were 87.54–88.67. Woodcock–Johnson Reading Cluster means were 78.39–72.68; Math Cluster means were 77.62–79.40. On the Test of Written Spelling, the means were 73.54 and 70.40.	Spelling On-task behavior	The study compared the effects of two types of self-monitoring on attention and academic performance. A factorial design with two groups was utilized in which each group received the same treatment, but in reversed order. LD Ss were taught a spelling study procedure (SSP), followed by instruction in self-monitoring of performance (SMP) and self-monitoring of attention (SMA). *Group 1* Ss received the interventions in the following order: SSP, SMP, and SMA. *Group 2* Ss received the same interventions, but in the reverse order. Ss spent 1 wk in each intervention. *SSP Phase* (first wk): Ss used the spelling study procedure, but they did not receive training in self-monitoring procedures. *SMA or SMP* (second and fourth weeks) *No Treatment* (third wk). The experimenter was not present. Ss participated in regular classroom activities. *SSP* included five steps: (1) Look at the word; (2) Say the Word; (3) Cover the Word; (4) Write the word three times; and (5) Check spelling accuracy. *SMP* components included: Discussion about the importance of spelling practice; (2) Instruction to count up and graph the number of correct spelling practices after each session; (3) Mastery demonstrated by correctly and	On-task behavior: percentage of observed behaviors Spelling: number of correctly practiced words; percent correct on wkly spelling tests and maintenance spelling test	On-task behavior was significantly higher in both the SMA and SMP conditions than in the SSP condition. Number of correct practices was significantly higher in SMP than in SSP. Spelling achievement was significantly lower in SMA than in SSP, and spelling maintenance was significantly lower in SMA than in SSP and SMA. Subject interviews indicated that SMA was experienced as intrusive. The type of self-monitoring used may have direct, significant effects on academic outcomes; there does not appear to be a "best" method of self-monitoring for all students on all tasks.

(*continued*)

Author (year)	*N*	Selection criteria	Target domain(s)	Treatment(s)	Measures	Results
Reid & Harris (1993) (*cont.*)				independently performing and verbalizing all steps; and (4) No feedback was given on self-recording accuracy. *SMA* procedures included: (1) Ss discussed the importance of paying attention; (2) Ss discussed what determines attention in spelling tasks; (3) Ss were instructed to ask themselves, "Was I paying attention?" when cued by a taped tone, and to self-record results on a tally sheet; and (4) Ss graphed results daily.		
Van Daal & Reitsma (1993)	46	Three groups were included in this study. Group 1 consisted of normal beginning readers with a mean age of 7.3 attending the 3rd and 4th grades. Ss in Groups 2 and 3 were RD with a similar reading level as the normally progressing beginners. Group 2 Ss' mean age was 8.86 yr, and Group 3 Ss' mean age was 9.15 yr. IQ for both groups was greater than 90 (no instrument was listed). The mean score for Group 2 on the Dutch Reading Achievement Test was 19.8.	Reading fluency	Disabled readers and normal beginning readers were compared on requesting help in the form of *speech feedback* during computer-based word reading. This study examined whether it was best to give feedback on all words or to allow the disabled readers to choose. Normal beginning readers and reading-age matched pupils with reading problems engaged in reading practice with speech feedback on call for both difficult and easy words. A set of both difficult and easy sums was completed as a control task. Another group of RD pupils who were also matched on reading level practiced the reading of words with	Speech feedback: number of requests Practiced/nonpracticed words: reading accuracy, mean reading time Reading speed	Both disabled readers and beginners were very sensitive to sum difficulty but not to word difficulty, though in the present study the Ss were more selective than in a previous study. The inclusion of more easy words might account for this finding. The beginners requested help only during the first sessions of reading practice, whereas the disabled readers remained dependent on the speech feedback. The RD pupils

They were 18 mo below grade level. Group 3 Ss' mean age was 9.15 yr, with a mean reading score of 19.1, which was 2 yr below grade level.	unsolicited speech feedback. *Group 1* (Control): Normal, beginning readers received speech feedback on call. *Group 2:* LD Ss received speech feedback on call. *Group 3:* LD Ss received unsolicited speech feedback. Groups 1 and 2 were run first to compute the mean practice time/word. Ss were instructed how to use the mouse, and how to obtain speech feedback. Groups 1 and 2 were also administered the arithmetic task, a list of 20 sums presented based on ability. The Ss were asked to examine each sum, but not to solve it yet. The Ss were then asked to indicate which sums they could solve alone and on which they needed the experimenter's help. A week later, on the second occasion, Ss were asked to solve all problems without help. Group 3 practiced 25 difficult and 5 easy words selected during pretesting. Practice time gradually was decreased from 10 sec to 3 sec/word. Ss would attempted reading the word on their own, speech feedback followed, and then time was allowed for Ss to evaluate attempts.	did not learn less when the computer delivered the spoken form of all words without request than when they were allowed to choose.

(*continued*)

Author (year)	*N*	Selection criteria	Target domain(s)	Treatment(s)	Measures	Results
Vaughn, Schumm, & Gordon (1993)	48	Twenty-four LD and 24 non-LD students were drawn from 10 classes located at three middle-class schools in the same district. Criteria for inclusion as an LD subject included a significant discrepancy between ability and achievement; evidence of a processing deficit; learning difficulties that were not primarily attributable to other handicaps or cultural/social conditions; and identification by classroom teacher and achievement tests of significantly below average spelling performance.	Spelling	Instructional procedures were held constant across treatments. Elements included the development of an individual word list for each student; limiting instructional set size to three words/session; teaching to mastery; providing time for students to self-check for accuracy; providing corrective feedback and modeling error analysis; and reducing information in the targeted spelling words until the student could spell the word without a model. Each subject received 11 days of spelling intervention. On the first day, a 50-word paper-and-pencil pretest was administered to each student to develop a core list of 30 spelling words that each student could not spell correctly, with selection for instruction limited to words that students had not learned through general classroom instruction. Spelling words were randomly assigned to one of three treatment conditions (10 words/condition): writing, tracing, and the computer. One word from each treatment condition was taught each day for a total of three words/day. Spelling training occurred from Day 2 to Day 11, with students taught individually in 20-min sessions. Each session consisted of	On the 6th and 11th days, Ss were individually assessed on their ability to correctly spell the 15 words learned during that segment of the intervention. A researcher read each word, used it in a sentence, and then repeated the word. Presentation order was varied from the instructional order for these assessments, with words repeated at student request. One month following completion of this study, each S was again tested individually tested on retention of all 30 words. Ss were also interviewed individually following intervention to determine their preferred method and opinion regarding the method that affected the best results.	Results from a repeated measures ANOVA indicated significant Group and Time effects, but there were no significant interactions. In terms of spelling accuracy, reliable between-group differences occurred favoring the NLD Ss. Both groups experienced significant declines on the retention measure, with the proportion of words retained about equal across groups. Neither LD nor NLD Ss performed differentially as a result of varying treatment. Furthermore, the effects of treatment did not vary as a function of time. Analyses of the proportion of bigrams correctly spelled produced similar results, with significant between-group differences observed at posttest and follow-up. Again, main effects for group and time were not

				learning one word from each treatment condition, with method of motoric practice varied, i.e., one word was written, one word was traced, and one word was practiced on a computer. A standard, 10-step procedure was employed for instructing all words.		reliably different, and there were no significant interactions. The method of choice for both LD and NLD Ss was the computer. However, when questioned about the most efficient method, i.e., the technique which affected the best results, both LD and NLD Ss chose writing, followed by tracing, with the computer chosen the least amount of times.
Wood, Rosenberg, & Carran (1993)	1	Nine Ss took part in this study; only S3 is reported here. S3 was 8 yr old, had a mean IQ of 96, and scored at 3rd grade beginning level on the WRAT-R math subtest. Overall achievement on the CAT was 2.4.	Math computation	The effects of tape-recorded cues on the mathematics performance of a student with RDs was investigated in a multiple probe design. *BL:* Ss worked on worksheets with no taped self-instructions. Treatment conditions included: (1) Self-instruction training (SIT) 30- to 40-min sessions in which the Ss were paired with another S who served as an observer; (2) Ss served as observers of Ss in the SIT condition; and (3) a no-treatment control condition. Ss were introduced to the procedure, after which the experimenter modeled the 10 instructions for solving the math problem. A tape recorder was used to record the experimenter, which was later	Self-instruction steps: percentage completed Math problems: percentage attempted and correctly completed	Time elapsed: time for task performance Without access to taped cues, experimental and observer Ss did not successfully utilize the SIT after the first self-instructional training. However, when experimental Ss were trained to use taped cues, they demonstrated the ability to accurately solve their problems. Ss were able to successfully use SIT procedures when the taped cues were faded.

(*continued*)

Author (year)	*N*	Selection criteria	Target domain(s)	Treatment(s)	Measures	Results
Wood, Rosenberg, & Carran (1993) (*cont.*)				used as a prompt to finish the other problems on the worksheet. Each SIT S then composed instructions, wrote them down, and recorded them. The observer student observed. The experimental S was next given a worksheet and was asked to solve the problems with the aid of her/his recorded instructions. Ss were praised for correct answers. Incorrect answers were modeled and rehearsed with the S. *SI Generalization 1:* The three groups of Ss were asked to do a worksheet with the use of the tape-recorded instructions. *SI Generalization 2:* This was the same as the previous generalization condition except that the group of Ss no longer had use of the tape and were expected to remember and whisper the instructions. There were three Ss in the no-treatment control condition.		
Daly & Martens (1994)	4	Ss had LDs in reading and were receiving 1 hr/day of special education instruction. The Ss' mean age was 10.8, with a range from 8.83 to 11.92. Ss' mean WISC-R score was 93.5, with a range from 89 to 98. On the KABC, Ss' reading achievement mean was 71, with a range of 61 to 80.	Oral reading fluency	The study used the instructional hierarchy to compare the effects of three instructional interventions (listening passage preview, subject passage preview, and taped words) on Ss' oral reading performance on word lists and passages. Ss received 1 hr/day of instruction in a 3-day instructional sequence for 21 days under three conditions. *Subject Passage Preview*	Four dependent measures were used to assess the effects of treatment conditions on reading performance. These instruments measured accuracy and fluency on the passages and the word lists.	The listening passage preview intervention (which contained modeling, drill, and generalization components) produced the largest performance gains.

				(SPP): Emphasized development of accuracy and fluency. Ss read a passage orally without help, read a corresponding word list, then read the same passage again. Taped Words (TW) Ss read word list with audiotape and then read the word list and passage. *Listening Passage Preview* (LPP): Ss listened to an audiotape while following along in the passage with a finger. Ss then read the word list and passage.		
Fuchs, Fuchs, Hamlett, Phillips, & Bentz (1994)	120	Teachers delivered treatment in their math classes to all of the Ss in the class. However, some Ss were identified within the class as LD. Ss' mean age was 9.5. The range of grade levels was 2 to 5. The mean IQ score was 93.5. Using Curriculum-Based Measurement (CBM), the mean math measurement for LD Ss was 2.8.	Mathematics	The study examined the effectiveness of innovative curriculum-based measurement (CBM) on classwide decision-making structures within general education mathematics instruction, with and without recommendations for how to incorporate CBM feedback into instructional planning. There were two intervention, *CBM-IN* (feedback with instructional recommendations) and *CBM-NO IN* (feedback without instructional recommendations). Teachers implemented treatments with all Ss in their math classes. Teachers identified three Ss for whom treatment effects would be evaluated: (1) *LD*, a S who was chronically low achieving in math, and classified as LD; (2) *Low Achieving* (LA), a S chronically low achieving in math, and never assessed for LD; and (3)	Math operations test Curriculum-based measurement	Only the CBM teachers who received instructional recommendations designed better instructional programs and effected greater achievement for their students.

(continued)

Author (year)	*N*	Selection criteria	Target domain(s)	Treatment(s)	Measures	Results
Fuchs, Fuchs, Hamlett, Phillips, & Bentz (1994) (*cont.*)				*Average Achieving* (AA), a S whose math performance was near the middle of the class. Group 1 Teachers (CBM-IN) taught their students using the classwide peer tutoring method (CWPT) in four 30-min sessions. Every S in the class was paired to work on a math skill. Pairings were based on the CBM data to determine who needed remediation on which skills. Each CWPT session was divided into 5–8 min of coaching, and 3–5 min of practice. During coaching, Ss worked through 12 examples of the target math skill. The coach used a question sheet to prompt the tutee to complete each step of the first problem correctly. Also used was a digit-by-digit correction procedure. In a 6-wk interval, each student would have the opportunity to be a tutor for at least 2 wk. Ss in the control condition received no CBM, but rather continued with regular math instruction. Control Ss did not participate in CWPT.		

Harris, Graham, Reid, McElroy, & Hamby (1994)	4	*Experiment 1:* 4th and 5th graders in a self-contained class for children with LD. Ranging in age from 9.6 to 11.8. WISC-R scores ranged from 86 to 104. On the Test of Written Spelling, Ss scored 1 SD below the mean. *Experiment 2:* The Ss ranged in age from 10.4 to 12.2. Ss' WISC-R scores were between 85 and 115. Their TOWL scores were 1 SD below the mean.	*Experiment 1:* Spelling *Experiment 2:* Story writing	The effectiveness of two self-monitoring interventions on the attentional and academic performance of Ss with RDs was compared in two separate experiments. *Experiment 1:* The investigation was designed to study whether attention and performance monitoring had differential effects on the spelling study behaviors of four students. The intervention included on-task behavior and performance with spelling. For 15 min, Ss studied spelling words according to Fitzgerald's method, which was taught before the intervention began. The intervention included self-monitoring and attention. During an individual conference, teacher and student discussed the importance and meaning of paying attention. The Ss were instructed to ask themselves the question, "Was I paying attention?" upon hearing a taped tone at random intervals of 10 to 90 sec during spelling practice sessions. Ss were also instructed to self-record if on task. The Ss graphed the number of times they marked yes. During the self-monitoring of performance, Ss discussed the meaning and importance of practicing spelling words. The Ss were asked to count the number of times spelling words were	*Experiment 1:* On-task behavior: percentage of time on task Academic performance *Experiment 2:* On-task behavior: percentage of time on task Academic quality	In both interventions, positive effects were observed for on-task behavior as well as the number of times Ss correctly practiced spelling words. Two of the Ss were more productive when using self-monitoring of performance and all of the Ss preferred this self-monitoring procedure. Both self-monitoring interventions had a positive effect on the length and quality of Ss' stories as well as their on-task behavior during writing. Neither of the self-monitoring interventions was clearly or consistently superior to the other.

(*continued*)

Author (year)	*N*	Selection criteria	Target domain(s)	Treatment(s)	Measures	Results
Harris, Graham, Reid, McElroy, & Hamby (1994) (*cont.*)				correctly practiced and to then record that number on a graph. *Experiment 2:* The same design and procedures, but the self-monitoring interventions were applied to story writing. The intervention included on-task behavior and performance as in Experiment 1, and quality of performance.		
Kerstholt, Van Bon, & Schreuder, (1994)	48 49	Ss were drawn from schools for children with LDs, and were selected because of their difficulties with reading and writing. The Ss were screened for their knowledge of grapheme–phoneme correspondences and their phonemic segmentation skill. Ss' mean age in Experiment 1 was 8.4 yr, and in Experiment 2 was 8.7 yr. For both experiments, the Raven's Coloured Progressive Matrices indicated average IQ for the Ss.	Decoding skills Spelling	Two experimental studies examined the effects of different types of phonemic segmentation training on phonemic segmentation, reading, and spelling. Ss who were weak in phonemic segmentation were trained with the use of diagrams and alphabet letters, alphabet letters only, or with no visual support at all. The study incorporated CAI. During each of the three treatment groups, the child and experimenter sat at the computer. The experimenter stated the word to be segmented. The S then segmented the word. *Experiment 1: Structure:* After the experimenter said the word to be segmented, the S named the first sound of the word and then clicked on the first square. The pattern followed for each sound until the total grapheme was displayed and the S could "see" it. No	Phonemic segmentation Reading Spelling Mean proportion errors Deletion, Substitution, Contraction, Reverse Order, and Addition Mean proportion correct in five word structures CCVC, CVCC, CCVCC, CCCVC, CVCCC	*Experiment 1:* In each training program, the Ss improved their phonemic segmentation skill. However, no significant differences were found among the three training groups. The results may have been influenced by the different types of feedback that were provided in the three training programs. *Experiment 2:* The differences in feedback were eliminated and all of the Ss were trained with the same three programs. The results of the experiment were the same as those of the first

				corrective feedback was given. *Memory:* The S said the word and clicked on the square in the middle of the screen, after which the matching grapheme appeared in the middle of the screen. When the S thought that she/he had spoken all segments, the child clicked the arrow on the screen. If an incorrect number of segments had been spoken, an auditory warning signal sounded after the arrow click. *Standard Treatment* (Control): The same square and arrow as in the Memory Treatment was shown in the middle of the screen. The same procedure as the Memory Treatment was used, although no graphemes were presented on the screen. Errors were corrected orally by the experimenter after the S segmented the word *Experiment 2:* The only difference from Experiment 1 was that Explicit Immediate Oral Feedback was added and provided to Ss in all three treatment conditions.	experiment. The finding that visual support had no beneficial effects could therefore not be attributed to differences in explicit feedback. It was concluded that with Ss of this age group, in contrast to preschoolers, phonemic segmentation training using visual support did not have any advantage over auditory training alone.	
Lovett, Borden, DeLuca, Lacerenza, Benson, & Brackstone (1994)	6	Ss were screened for oral reading performance on a screening battery which included the Goldman–Fristoe–Woodcock (GFW) Sound–Symbol Tests, Reading Symbols subtest, the	Decoding skills	This study compared two forms of word identification training to promote transfer of learning by children with dyslexia. Ss met four times weekly for 60-min sessions for a total of 35 sessions.	Transfer to real words: Tests of Transfer, Challenge, Regular, and Exception words	Evidence of transfer was obtained after treatment of the Ss' core reading deficits. Both training approaches were associated with large positive effects, transfer on several

(*continued*)

Author (year)	*N*	Selection criteria	Target domain(s)	Treatment(s)	Measures	Results
Lovett, Borden, DeLuca, Lacerenza, Benson, & Brackstone (1994) (*cont.*)		PIAT Reading Recognition subtest, the WRAT-R Reading subtest, and the WRMT-R Word Attack and Word Identification subtests. Ss who were selected scored below the 25th percentile with this result was replicable on four of the five different measures. The chosen Ss had RDs. Their mean age was 9.6 yr, with a range of 7 to 13 yr. The mean WISC-R score was 100.9. WRAT-R mean scores in percentiles were: Reading = 2.5, Spelling = 3.4, and Arithmetic = 13.0. WRMT-R mean percentile scores were WI = 3.7 and WA = 3.2.		*Word Identification Strategy Training (WIST):* Ss were trained in the acquisition, use, and monitoring of effective word identification strategies. A metacognitive phonics program was used (Gaskins et al., 1988). Four strategies were incorporated into the study: Word identification by analogy; Seeking the part of the word that the S knows; Attempting variable vowel pronunciations; and "Peeling off" prefixes and suffixes in multisyllable words. A metacognitive mnemonic was also used: SAME (select, apply, monitor, evaluate). *Direct Instruction, Phonological Analysis and Blending (PHAB):* Ss received printed presentations. Letter–sound and letter cluster–sound correspondences were taught via direct instruction. A corrective reading program was used (Engelmann, 1978, 1988). The treatment also included word segmentation, sound blending, and cumulative, systematic review. *Classroom Survival Skills (CSS):* Ss received training in the areas of classroom etiquette, life skills, organizational strategies, academic problem solving, and self-help techniques. No instruction was provided in the area of reading.	Transfer to nonwords: GFW and WRMT-R nonword reading Word attack strategies: Select strategies, Apply strategies, Monitor success, and Word identification success Word identification: WRAT-R and WRMT-R Spelling: WRAT-R, PIAT-R, and GFW Phonological processing skills: GFW Sound Analysis, Sound Blending, and Sound–Symbol Association Additional measures: WRMT-R Passage, WRAT-R Arithmetic, and the Piers–Harris Self-Concept Scale	measures, and generalized achievement gains. The phonological program resulted in greater generalized gains in the phonological domain and the strategy program in broader-based transfer to real words.

Montague & Leavell (1994)	8	Junior high students identified LD by the school district and also met subject selection criteria for participation in the study. Criteria included: at least 50 words in response to the picture stimulus on the Test of Written Language (TOWL); a minimum score of 4 on the Thematic Maturity subtest of the TOWL; a Full Scale score of 90+ on the WISC-R; a minimum reading stanine of 3 on the district-administered Stanford Achievement Test; and poor composition skills as determined by each child's special education language arts teacher. The WISC-R range in scores was 91 to 133; mean age was 13.6.	Writing	This study investigated the effects of procedural and substantive facilitation to affect character development. A multiple BL design across triads was used to determine the effects of treatment. The study lasted for 2 mo. *BL:* Ss were given a story-ender on a 5 × 8 card and were asked to write a story. Mechanical errors were not counted against the student. The teacher met individually with the S. *Treatment 1,* Procedural Facilitation: Ss were given a story-ender, the story grammar cue card, and instructions to check off story parts as they included them in their stories. Three stories over 2 wk were written. The teacher met individually with the S. *Treatment 2,* Substantive Facilitation: Ss received 3 days of small group instruction. Steps included review of story grammar elements, lessons on internal responses and plans of characters, reading and writing stories as a group, and evaluating stories. Two stories were written over 2 wk. Two weeks later, Ss wrote a final story with only a story-ender and the story grammar cue card to determine maintenance and generalization.	Quality ratings: coherence, organization, and episodic structure	Over a period of 2 mo, Ss generally made substantial increases in the amount they wrote and mild to moderate increases in the quality of the stories produced.

(continued)

Author (year)	*N*	Selection criteria	Target domain(s)	Treatment(s)	Measures	Results
Seabaugh & Schumaker (1994)	11	9th through 12th graders classified as LD by a validation team composed of two certified school psychologists and two certified secondary teachers of the LD. Three NLD Ss also participated in the study. Ss' mean age was 16.0. Their mean WISC-R IQ scores were 102 for LD Ss and 106 for NLD Ss. Mean WJPB scores for LD Ss were: Reading, 42nd percentile, Math, 22nd percentile, and Writing, 21st percentile. Mean WJPB scores for NLD Ss were: Reading, 60th percentile, Math, 41st percentile, and Writing, 44th percentile. All Ss were attending a small, private alternative school for grades 9 to 12. All Ss had a prior history of school failure and low lesson completion rates. This school was their "last chance." It had two large classrooms. Ss enrolled in this class at the beginning of the semester and in addition were	Rate of lesson completion General academic achievement	A multiple BL design across the three academic areas of reading, writing, and math was combined with a reversal design for each of the Ss. During BL, the number of lessons completed by a S in each of the three skill areas was monitored without intervention. Ss met in the BL condition for 5–10 sessions. The intervention took place over 80–85 sessions. Self-instruction was taught in reading, writing, and math, and the number of lessons completed each day was recorded. Lessons increased in difficulty and Ss graded the assignments using an answer key. The teacher also graded the paper. Each S then picked up the assignment and filed it in her/his notebook. At the end of each school day, the number of completed assignments placed in each S's notebook was counted. Four skills were taught with instructional procedures: (1) self-recording of behavior; (2) self-evaluation; (3) self-reinforcement; and (4) self-contracting. The instructional procedures included: Teacher described the skill and provided a rationale for using it; Teacher demonstrated; Ss practiced,; and Teacher provided positive and corrective feedback.	Lessons completed: reading, writing, and math	All participants substantially increased their rate of lesson completion after the intervention. These increases occurred in the academic areas targeted by the Ss for the application of the self-regulation skills.

		required to attend one large-group activity each Friday which included therapeutic activities, field trips, and guest speakers.		Achievement scores were reviewed with the S and it was explained how certain deficits in achievement might hinder the S's success. Also demonstrated was how to write a goal for each academic area, including: (1) how to write a goal; (2) reasons for the goal; (3) a task analysis; (4) descriptions of contingencies for completing the goal; and (5) Ss were taught how to record their progress on a graph.		
Van Reusen & Bos (1994)	21	The Ss were 9th graders labeled LD according to district criteria, including a significant discrepancy between ability and achievement. The mean WISC-R score was 86.4 and the mean scores on the WJPB were 5.4 for Reading and 5.1 for Written Language. Ss' mean age was 16.3.	Active participation of students with LD in IEP meetings	This study investigated the effectiveness of strategy instruction designed to foster Ss' active participation in IEP conferences. High school students with RDs and their parents participated in either strategy instruction or an orientation lecture/discussion (control group). *IEP Participation Strategy* (IPARS, Van Reusen et al., 1989): Ss received instruction in the use of the IEP participation strategy (IPARS) and participated in an informational discussion on the purpose and procedures of the IEP conference. After intervention, Ss and their parents participated in the Ss' annual IEP conferences. The strategy involved helping Ss at the secondary level to realize that they have the communication skills and	Student verbal contributions: identifies learning strengths and weaknesses; identifies goals and choices for learning; clarifies test performance; statements/questions about IEP, and about school Student performance: rating of student performance (by parents, teacher, student) Types of information: parent and teacher perceptions	Srategy-instructed Ss identified more goals and communicated more effectively during their conferences than did the contrast Ss.

(continued)

Author (year)	*N*	Selection criteria	Target domain(s)	Treatment(s)	Measures	Results
Van Reusen & Bos (1994) (*cont.*)				motivation to take an active role in planning their own educational programs (Strategies Intervention Model; Ellis et al., 1991). The IPARS included five steps with substeps. These procedures included: (1) *I*nventory Step Identify S's learning strengths, weaknesses to improve, goals and interests, and preferences for classroom learning and studying (Van Reusen & Bos, 1990); (2) *P*rovide inventory information during the IEP conference; (3) *A*sk questions; (4) *R*espond to questions; and (5) *S*ummarize the IEP goals. Communication skills that were developed included active listening, eye communication, pleasant tone of voice, and open body posture. Steps for teaching the strategy (Learning Strategies Model; Ellis et al., 1991) included orientation, description, model and prepare, verbal rehearsal, strategy practice and feedback, generalization. Three types of sessions took place, i.e., student, partner (parent and student), and generalization. The sessions were held on 3 consecutive days for 50 min, and included groups of three to five Ss at one time. *Control:* Ss participated in an informational lecture/discussion on the		

				purpose and procedures of an IEP conference, parent's legal rights, review of assessment results and implications, identification of a S's learning problems, and IEP goals development. These sessions were also 2 hr long and included two to four Ss and their parents. A generalization session followed wherein information was reviewed and questions asked.		
Williams, Brown, Silverstein & deCani (1994)	69	Criteria established by the experimenter for inclusion in the study included a Full Scale IQ of 85 or higher, achievement level at least 1.5 grade levels below expectation, and no gross behavioral problems as assessed by psychological evaluations by school psychologists.	Reading comprehension	Treatment consisted of nine lessons were organized around a single story and consisting of five parts: (1) prereading discussion of the purpose of the lesson and the topic of the story to be read; (2) reading of the story; (3) discussion of the important story information using organizing (schema) questions as guides; (4) identification of a theme for the story and generalization of it so it is relevant to a variety of situations, and (5) application of the generalized theme to real-life experience. Control Ss continued to receive their regular program.	Experimenter-generated test measured concepts of theme and perseverance, story details, story components, theme identification, and theme application	Instructed students outperformed noninstructed students. Instructed students were significantly better than noninstructed students in their knowledge of what is meant by "theme." They also had a better understanding of the concept of perseverance.

(continued)

Author (year)	*N*	Selection criteria	Target domain(s)	Treatment(s)	Measures	Results
Wong, Butler, & Ficzere, Kuperis, Corden, & Zelmer (1994)	31	8th and 9th graders whose WISC-R scores were in the average range, while their Gates–MacGinitie Reading Test scores revealed significant underachievement, despite adequate intelligence. No scores were available.	Writing	Ss met three times/wk for 50 min. The study included two treatment groups and a control group. *Group 1,* Dyadic Student– Student Interactive Dialog: During Phase 1, Ss were given keyboard training skills for 2 mo. Phase 2 consisted of training to plan while writing. This phase lasted for 1 wk during which Ss were involved with group discussion. The importance of planning for a rock concert was the topc that led into a group discussion on planning to write essays. Ss were taught to: Be clear about the topic, Stick with the goal, and Have a sense of direction. The researcher then modeled a three-step planning strategy which included: (1) Memory access, (2) Reliving the event visually and auditorially in their imagination, and (3) Reactivating emotions associated with the event. Ss planned their essays aloud using the previous steps and then typed plans on the computer. Phase 3 activities focused on writing and revising. Ss wrote drafts, revised their papers with the teacher's help, and were taught to be specific and to not make the reader "guess" what they are saying. Ss were also told to be "clear" about the theme and title. During Phase 4, Ss read and critiqued each other's essays. *Group 2,* Individual S–Researcher with Interactive Dialog: The only difference between Group 1 and Group 2 was that Group 2 did not include Phase 4. Control: Ss received a modified course in English in the resource room.	Clarity and thematic salience were compared between the pre-, post-, and maintenance tests for the individual and dyad conditions. Attitudes, self-efficacy, and metacognition were compared between individual and dyad conditions.	Results from multivariate analyses of variance and effect sizes clearly indicated both intervention conditions were equally effective in promoting clarity and thematic salience in trainees' reportive essays. Trainees also maintained their learned skills. Moreover, Ss in both interventions surpassed those in the control condition in writing performance.

Bulgren, Hock, Schumaker, & Deshler (1995)	12	The Ss were all 9th through 12th graders receiving at least 50 min of special education services/day and had been classified as LD. Mean age was 16.9, ranging from 15 to 18.7 yr; mean WISC-R score was 95.82. The Ss' overall achievement mean was 8.83; their reading mean percentile was 9.17, with a range of 1 to 53.	Memory-mnemonics	This study evaluated the effects of instructing Ss to use a mnemonic strategy to identify and remember pairs or small groups of information. A multiple BL across-Ss design was used. *BL:* Pretests were administered. *Intervention:* Ss were to identify pairs or small groups of information they needed to recall. They selected the best of four mnemonic techniques to help them recall. The Ss then created an appropriate mnemonic device and used a self-testing technique to master the information. The steps of the LISTS strategy included: *L*ook for clues; *I*nvestigate the items; *S*elect and design a mnemonic device; *T*ransfer the information to a study card; and *S*elf-Test. The *S*elect component included the substrategy CRAM, which stood for *C*reate a mental image, *R*elate to something familiar, *A*rrange boxes around key syllables, and *M*ake a code. The intervention also included clarification of goals and procedures, modeling of a paired associates strategy and self-statements, demonstration of fluent knowledge of procedure by students, student rehearsal, and independent practice.	Controlled test: percentage of points earned Content test score: percentage of points earned Controlled study card score: percentage of points earned Content study card score: percentage of points earned	The Ss made substantial improvement with regard to the creation of study cards and test performance as a result of learning the strategy. Results further indicated that Ss had distinct preferences for different types of mnemonic devices, that they made changes in the strategy, and that they called on previous experience with other learning strategies as they adapted the strategy.

(*continued*)

Author (year)	*N*	Selection criteria	Target domain(s)	Treatment(s)	Measures	Results
Cuvo, Ashley, Marso, Zhang, & Fry (1995)	5	Male adolescents attending a self-contained high school class for students with BDs. Most were mainstreamed throughout the school day, with integration individually determined.	Spelling Sight vocabulary	An alternating treatments designed was used to assess the effects of three practice procedures on the number of spelling or sight vocabulary words learned. In the One Relevant Practice condition, error correction occurred after each incorrect response, including verbal feedback and modeling of the correct response. Error correction in the Five Relevant Practice condition was similar except the participant was required to correctly respond five times. In the Five Irrelevant Practice condition the subject was required to practice a no-training word five times following each error. There was also a no-treatment control condition wherein the 15 untrained words were tested at the end of the experiment. Training involved random presentation of the words from each experimental condition; praise was contingent on correct responses in all three conditions. Sessions of about 20 min occurred about 4 or 5 times/wk in the school library; Ss were individually screened, tested, and trained. Each session involved an initial test of the words to be taught that day, followed by three training trials, and concluded with a second test of the words trained that	The number of words correctly read or spelled during each condition was recorded. A maintenance check was completed at the end of the final session each wk, with presentation of all words previously learned to criterion.	Sufficient stimulus control was obtained with one-time relevant practice. The additional practice associated with the five-relevant practice condition was not necessary for learning. In addition, Ss learned just as well in the five-irrelevant practice situation than in the five-relevant practice condition.

				day. All sessions were audiotaped; interscorer agreement was calculated every fourth session. Ss were screened to construct individualized word lists for training; screening yielded a total of 60 words for training/student; 45 words were randomly selected for training, 15/condition, and the remaining 15 were used as no-training controls.		
Das, Mishra, & Pool (1995)	51	Ss demonstrating word-decoding problems were selected for remediation. They were between 8.9 and 11.11 yr of age and were selected from four schools. The basis for inclusion was their poor performance on the Word Identification and Word Attack subtests of the WRMT-R and selected tests from the Cognitive Assessment System. Ss were at least 12 mo behind their expected age levels on any portion of this test. Ss' mean on the Matrix Analogies Test was 88.	Decoding skills	Cognitive remediation of decoding deficit was attempted by following a theoretically based program. The theory identifies four major cognitive processes: Planning, Attention, Simultaneous, and Successive (PASS) processing. The *P*ASS *Re*medial *P*rogram (PREP) provided 10 structured tasks that were aimed at developing internalized strategies for mainly successive processes (six tasks) and simultaneous processes (four tasks); deficits in either of the two may lead to poor decoding. Through its "global process" training and curriculum-related "bridging" training, PREP facilitates application of internalized strategies arrived at inductively for learning word decoding and spelling. It does not provide direct teaching of rules or exercises. The Ss met for 15 sessions, one to three times/wk for 55 min. The Woodcock Reading Mastery Test	WRMT-R, Form G, Word Identification and Word Attack subtests Cognitive Assessment System (CAS Test)	The largest improvement in word decoding occurred for the PREP combined global and bridging treatment.

(*continued*)

Author (year)	*N*	Selection criteria	Target domain(s)	Treatment(s)	Measures	Results
Das, Mishra, & Pool (1995) (*cont.*)				study included two parts. *Part 1, PREP Training:* Ss were individually shown a series of shapes and told to put them in the same order by memory. If incorrect, Ss were given another choice and this time asked to name each shape and practice the order. Ss were asked to verbalize how they put the shape together, and were encouraged to look for patterns; these "puzzles" had three to six shapes. Then a bridging activity from puzzles to words was provided which included the same. Control Ss received no treatment. *Part 2:* Experimental Ss received no treatment. The control group was divided into two remediation groups that received either Global Training Sessions or Bridging Training Sessions.		
DeLaPaz (1995) Dissertation	42	5th, 6th, and 7th grade students with LD, between the ages of 9.11 and 14.3. Ss were identified according to stepwise criteria: (1) school district identification; (2) Verbal or Full Scale IQ score between 80 and 126 on the WISC-III (Weschler, 1991), WISC-R (Weschler, 1974), or the McCarthy Scales of Children's Abilities	Writing	Ss were randomly assigned to one of four groups: (1) an experimental group given instruction on making oral plans for composing essays followed by oral production of their essays; (2) an experimental group given instruction on making written plans for composing essays followed by written essay production; (3) a comparison group instructed in essay structure followed by oral production of essays; and (4) a comparison group instructed in essay	Outcomes variables included time for advanced planning, number of propositions in Ss plans, type and percentage of transformations, composing rate, type and number of essay components, coherence, quality, subordination index scores, and	Combination of dictation and planning instruction had the strongest effect on Ss' essay composition abilities. Ss who composed via dictation and received planning instruction created essays that contained more essay elements and were higher in quality compared to Ss in all other conditions.

(McCarthy, 1972); (3) achievement in one or more academic areas at least 1 *SD*, but not more than 3 *SD* below the mean on the Woodcock–Johnson Psycho-educational Battery, Tests of Achievement—Revised (Woodcock & Johnson, 1989), the Woodcock Reading Mastery Tests-Revised (Woodcock, 1987), the KeyMath-Revised (Connolly, 1988), the WIAT (Psychological Corp,., 1992), or the TOWL-2 (Hammill & Larsen, 1988); (4) writing performance at least 1 SD but not more than 3 SDs below the mean on the Spontaneous Writing Composite score from the TOWL-2, Written Expression subtest, or the Writing Composite score from the WIAT; (5) able to write at least three T-units (Hunt, 1970) in a row on the same topic; (6) absence of sensory, motor, or emotional handicaps; and (7) English as the primary language. Teachers identified Ss as having problems with writing, and written language goals were identified on each Ss IEP.	structure followed by written essay production. All Ss were taught basic essay structure and components of good essays, and all received instruction in the use of linking words and phrases to signal transitions. All Ss practiced essay composition throughout instruction, providing control for confounding factors, e.g., motivation, instruction time, in evaluating the effects of the planning strategy. Comparisons also included two production modes, i.e., dictation and writing.	essay length. Data were collected at pretest, posttest, maintenance, and 2 wk following intervention. Following a preinstruction session, Ss wrote a pretest essay. Pretesting was done individually; instructors worked with each subject while the other students read unrelated class material. Each S was told to remember to plan before composing; Ss in oral conditions were reminded to watch the examine write down their dictated compositions. Ss in the essay planning groups each completed a posttest following the same procedures used in the pretest; Ss in the comparison groups also completed a posted following the same procedures. Two weeks later, each subject was administered a maintenance	Their essays were also longer and judged to be more cohesive at posttest, while differential effects for cohesion occurred at maintenance for Ss who differed by initial levels at pretest. Planning instruction benefited those Ss who received it, although there were differential effects between good and poor writers. Dictation alone had a minimal effect on Ss' plans and essays. At posttest, Ss composed at faster rates when dictating, and at maintenance sentence cohesion was higher. Social validity data revealed that both Ss and teachers found dictation, planning instruction, and essay component instruction to be effective and meaningful.

(continued)

Author (year)	N	Selection criteria	Target domain(s)	Treatment(s)	Measures	Results
DeLaPaz (1995) (*cont.*)					writing probe. After completing the maintenance probe, the Ss and their classroom teachers were separately interviewed to assess perceived effectiveness of the interventions, recommendations, and other comments. Treatment effects were also examined by examining plans and transformation between plans and essays.	
Lucangeli, Galderisi, & Cornoldi (1995)	166	3rd through 5th graders with normal intelligence of 100+ as measured by the WISC-R. On the MT Reading Comprehension Tests or the M+ Mathematics Achievement Test, 121 of the Ss scored in the 18th percentile.	Reading comprehension Decoding skills Math computation Math problem solving Metamemory Metacognitive knowledge	Only Study 2 is reported here. Ss were placed into one of three groups. Reading Metacognitive Group (RMG; DeBeni & Pazzaglia, 1991): Ss were taught how to clarify reading goals and were also taught reading strategies. Training also focused on developing the Ss' ability to reflect on mental functioning and on establishing general ideas about cognition. Memory Cognitive Group (MMG; Cornoldi & Caponi, 1991): The goal of this treatment was also to develop Ss' ability to reflect on mental functioning and on establishing general ideas about cognition. Control: Ss received training devoted to improving all of their school abilities.	Reading: MT Reading Tests Mathematics: M+ Mathematics Achievement Tests Reading Metacognitive Knowledge: a measure by DeBeni and Pazzaglia Metacognitive Knowledge in Mathematics: a questionnaire designed for this study	Results suggested that improving children's ability to reflect on their cognitive processes might improve their specific and general academic performances as well as their general cognitive attitude.

MacArthur & Haynes (1995)	10	Students with LD in grades 9 and 10 at two high schools in a suburban area volunteered to participate. Ss were identified with LD by schools using state procedures and criteria: (1) achievement not commensurate with ability; and (2) a severe discrepancy between ability and achievement that is not due to sensory disability, emotional disturbance, or environmental disadvantage. Ability was measured by the WISC-R (Weschler, 1974); comprehension was measured by the WRMT, Passage Comprehension subtest (Woodcock, 1987). All Ss received resource room support from special education teachers in one or two subject areas and were mainstreamed for other subjects; all had reading comprehension IEP goals.	Reading	Hypermedia versions were prepared of the biology text materials currently used by the Ss. The Student Assistant for Learning from Text (SALT) software was used to prepare a basic computer version and an enhanced computer version of two passages selected from chapters that none of the Ss had previously read; readability of the two passages was comparable. The basic version included the components found in the printed textbook and a notebook; the enhanced version added speech synthesis, an on-line glossary, links between questions and text, main idea highlighting, and supplementary explanations summarizing important ideas. A repeated measures design was employed, wherein each Ss read one passage with the basic version and another passage with the enhanced version of the text; both versions were developed for each reading passage. Ss were randomly assigned to use either the basic or enhanced version of the first passage; the two versions were counterbalanced across passage and presentation order. Intervention included two training sessions and 2 wk of intervention sessions.	Paper-and-pencil measures of comprehension were constructed for each passage to assess knowledge of main ideas and key terms; these tests consisted of short answer and matching items. An interview was constructed to evaluate Ss' overall opinions about the SALT program, including their opinions about intervention features.	All Ss learned to use the SALT system within about 1 hr of training, and they enjoyed using the system and felt that it helped them to learn the science content. Significantly higher comprehension scores were obtained when Ss used the enhanced version. In addition, Ss preferred the enhanced version, reporting they thought it helped them to better learn the material.

(*continued*)

Author (year)	N	Selection criteria	Target domain(s)	Treatment(s)	Measures	Results
Martin & Manno (1995)	3	7th graders with a mean age of 13 yr who were receiving resource room services for 1 hr/day for learning problems associated with LDs or emotional disturbance. Three of the four Ss were LD. Mean IQ score was 87.67, ranging from 85 to 90; writing abilities were 1 *SD* below the expected level.	Writing	The study examined the effects of a self-management procedure designed to teach Ss with RDs to improve the completeness (inclusion of identified story elements) and quality (organization and coherence) of their story compositions. The procedure was based on two strategies: teaching the Ss to plan stories composed in a narrative style, and teaching them to monitor the inclusion of elements from the plan with a check-off system. A multiple BL design was used to assess the effectiveness of the procedure and a combination of holistic and atomistic ratings was used to assist the completeness and quality of the Ss' written work. Treatment sessions were provided for 20-min, three times/wk. *BL:* Ss were given a folder with two pictures and two pieces of paper, three times/wk. Ss chose one of the pictures and wrote a story about it for 15 min. *Intervention:* Each S received one training session. They were then given two pictures, paper, and a Story Planner Form with the story elements defined on the form. The teacher modeled how to use the form and the Ss were shown how to make notes on it. Story planning elements included: main character, other characters, setting, problem, plan (action), and ending. Ss were shown how to self-monitor the use of the story planning steps.	Atomistic/objective measures (based on Parker et al., 1991, and Tindal & Parker, 1989): writing quality, percentage of words/min, and writing fluency Holistic measures (adapted from the Story Quality Scale by Montague, cited in Graves & Montague, 1991): coherence, flow of ideas, and organization Number of story elements	Stories were more complete when Ss used a simple check-off system to plan and monitor their work. In addition, there was a moderate correlation between the atomistic and holistic measures used to assess stories, with the total number of words written correlating most strongly ($r = .49$) with the overall rating for story quality.

Van Strien, Stolk, & Zuiker (1995)	40	Ss were 8 to 12 yr of age and had IQ scores higher than 80 on the WISC-R. Using a standardized Dutch text-reading test (AVIA-A; van den Berg & Te Lintelo, 1977), Ss showed reading scores of at least 1.5 yr below expectancy level, based on yr of education. To classify Ss with P- and L-dyslexia, a text reading test with levels of difficulty of 5 to 7 mo above each S's current level was administered. The procedure resulted in a sufficient number of reading errors in each S to allow for such a classification. Ss classified with P-dyslexia were accurate but slow readers; Ss with L-dyslexia were inaccurate but fast readers.	Reading fluency	Ss with P-dyslexia and L-dyslexia were treated with visual hemisphere-specific stimulation employing the HEMSTIM computer program. Stimulation was produced by presenting words to the left (L-dyslexia) or to the right (P-dyslexia) visual field. Ss received the HEMSTIM computer program treatment with 99 anxiety-laden words (three to five letters long). All Ss received the HSS (hemisphere-specific stimulation) through HEMSTIM sessions. Single words were printed in the standard typeface (Roman) flashed for 240 ms to the left or right side of the computer screen. If the child responded correctly, the next word was shown. If the child responded incorrectly, the word was repeated. If the S responded incorrectly again, the word was presented in free vision. Flash times were reduced from 100 to 60 msec and word difficulty was increased. The two treatment groups were the L-dyslexic and the P-dyslexic Ss. The Ss in the control condition were also divided into two groups and Ss received 99 neutral words (three to five letters).	Reading: substantive errors, fragmentations, and reading time	After treatment, the Ss with L-dyslexia in the experimental group made fewer substantive errors and more fragmentations on a text-reading task than did the Ss with L-dyslexia in the control group. The results are explained as being the consequence of additional activation of the right hemisphere caused by the anxiety-laden words. It was concluded that children with L-dyslexia benefit from the use of such words in the HEMSTIM program.

(*continued*)

Author (year)	N	Selection criteria	Target domain(s)	Treatment(s)	Measures	Results
Zipprich (1995)	13	Participants were students ranging from 9 to 12 yr old. Ss were identified by school personnel as having LD as a primary disability; receiving resource room instruction for students exhibiting LD, communication disorders, and/or BDs; demonstrated significant writing deficits as measured by the TOWL (Hammill & Larsen, 1983), and their IEPs indicated the need for writing instruction.	Narrative writing	A multiple BL design across Ss instructed in three groups was used to determine if a functional relationship exists between instructional methods used in this study and the obtained results; the study was performed in the resource room during regularly scheduled sessions. All Ss began the BL phase together, and the data were examined to ensure that all Ss needed to improve in the behaviors targeted. Intervention was staggered for the groups, with Groups 2 and 3 receiving treatment after Group 1. Ss met prescribed performance criteria. During BL, Ss were shown a picture poster from the Peabody Language Development Kit. They were told to carefully look at the picture, then given 30 min to write their best story. Intervention consisted of three phases. *Phase 1:* The teacher showed the Ss a picture poster, then displayed an overhead of a prestructured web labeled with critical story elements and questions to aid clarification of these elements, then read and explained the terms and questions, guiding the Ss to generate ideas for a narrative story. A brainstorming activity followed, with the teacher writing ideas on the overhead as	Twelve target behaviors were evaluated; a scale was developed for each target behavior that enabled recording of all data points on each S's charts. Stories were analyzed and data recorded and charted daily. Measures included: planning time, the number of words and number of thought units (T-units), story quality, and sentence types. Data analysis included both visual–graphic and mean-to-mean comparisons across individuals and phases.	Ss showed improvement in the target behaviors of planning time and holistic story quality following web technique instruction, but showed inconsistent results for the remaining target behaviors, i.e., number of words, T-units, density factor, sentence types, and mechanics. Inconsistent gains were observed for the number of words and T-units produced; no pattern of gains was obtained for the density factory, sentence types, and writing mechanics.

				they were generated, then Ss were given 30 min to plan and write their own best story. *Phase 2:* Ss were shown a picture poster and an overhead transparency of a story web. Each subject received a copy of the web, and was told to study the picture and independently fill in the web with his or her own story ideas. Then Sswere told to use any individually- or group-generated ideas and given 30 min to write. *Phase 3:* Ss were shown a picture poster and given a copy of the prestructured story web, then were asked to use the poster to generate ideas and given 30 min to complete the web and write. Once data stability was observed during intervention, BL conditions were reinstated to assess maintenance.		
Klingner & Vaughn (1996)	26	7th and 8th grade ESL students with LD participated. Selection criteria included (1) a significant discrepancy between ability and achievement, with evidence that learning problems not due to other conditions; (2) Spanish spoken as primary language; (3) decoding skills in English at least at the 2nd grade level; and (4) comprehension at least 2 yr below grade level.	Reading comprehension	Modified reciprocal teaching sessions were provided for 27 days for 35–40 min/day. All 26 Ss participated in reciprocal teaching strategy instruction for 15 days, then Ss were randomly assigned to one of two groups for an additional 12 days. Ss in the *Cross-age tutoring* group tutored younger students in the use of the reciprocal teaching strategies. Ss in the *Cooperative learning* group implemented the strategies in groups of three to five students.	Measures of reading included the Gates–MacGinitie Reading Comprehension Test (MacGinitie & MacGinitie, 1989) and Passage Comprehension Tests (10 passages with comprehension questions, constructed by Palincsar & Brown, 1984). In addition, a strategy interview was	Ss in both groups made significant progress in reading comprehension; there were no significant differences between the two groups. Comparisons of more and less successful learners in both groups suggest several conclusions. First, initial reading ability and oral language proficiency appeared related to comprehension

(*continued*)

Author (year)	*N*	Selection criteria	Target domain(s)	Treatment(s)	Measures	Results
Klingner & Vaughn (1996) *(cont.)*					administered to evaluate acquisition of the reciprocal teaching strategies.	gains. Second, a broader range of Ss benefited from reciprocal reading strategy instruction than would be predicted based on previously research. Finally, improvements in comprehension continued when Ss in both groups received minimal adult support.
Marsh & Cooke (1996)	3	3rd grade students with a history of low achievement in math. Participants met North Carolina state criteria for LD in the areas of reading, writing expression, and mathematics. Ss were selected based on accurate basic computation skills with poor success in the area of word problem solving as measured by the Woodcock–Johnson Psycho-educational Battery Tests of Achievement (Woodcock & Johnson, 1977) and the KeyMath Revised (Connolly, 1988).	Math problem solving	An elementary school in a small mill town in North Carolina was the site for this study. The Ss and experimenter were assigned to a large multiage classroom where team teaching involving the special education teacher and three general education teachers occurred; treatment was delivered at a large table which served as the classroom math center. Ss participated daily in treatment sessions and math instruction in heterogeneous groups with other students in the class. No other word problem-solving instruction was given during the regular math session for the duration of this study; Cuisenaire rods were only available to the Ss for use	Probes were constructed with 10 word problems each. The experimenter developed individual problems prior to the research that were organized by operation into four numbered boxes. Problem type order was established randomly by the roll of a die. A different version was created from the pool of available items and	The use of manipulatives during word-problem solving instruction was associated with immediate and durable improvement for all three Ss on probes administered without manipulatives available.

				during the experimental treatment. A multiple BL design across subjects was used to evaluate the effects of using manipulatives to teach word problem solving processes; the goal was to determine if a functional relation exists between manipulative use and accurate selection of the operations needed to solve word problems. Intervention was introduced in a staggered manner, with each subject after the first receiving treatment when an ascending trend was observed for the preceding subject; data were simultaneously collected for all Ss. Word problem probes and worksheets were constructed; results were recorded and graphed by the Ss.	given each day to all Ss. Word problems were constructed to require only one operation for solution; readability was controlled at 3rd grade level. Recording sheets and progress charts were placed in student folders; results were recorded daily by each subject. Results were also graphed by the Ss every 2 days using a computer program.	
Scanlon, Deshler, & Schumaker (1996)	204	12 middle school teachers and their students participated in this study. Experimental Ss included 11 6th, 7th, and 8th graders with LD and 98 without LD; comparison Ss included 6 with LD and 89 without LD in the same grades. Ss with LD had been identified as LD according to Kansas Guidelines for Identifying Children and Youth with Specific RDs (Kansas State Dept. of Education, 1987).	Strategy knowledge and use	A multiple-probe design was used to examine the effects of inservice training on instructional practices in class; a comparison group design was used to examine the effects of strategy instruction on student performance. Experimental group teachers chose one social studies class with mainstreamed resource students in which to deliver strategy instruction; comparison group teachers learned and implemented an assignment-giving routine in the same type of class (Rademacher, 1993). Each experimental teacher taught the ORDER strategy to Ss in a regularly schedule	Strategy implementation: Checklists were created with sections organized according to instructional phase; five general strategic teaching behaviors common to all three sections were listed at the bottom of each. Percentages were calculated for each lesson by dividing the total number of teaching behaviors observed by	Teacher training was associated with increased use of strategy instruction by teachers in the experimental group, although these teachers also reported that competing instructional demands interfered with their use of strategy instruction as frequently as they would prefer. While posttesting revealed significantly higher performance of

(continued)

Author (year)	N	Selection criteria	Target domain(s)	Treatment(s)	Measures	Results
Scanlon, Deshler, & Schumaker (1996) (*cont.*)				class. Developed through collaboration between the teachers and researchers, this strategy consisted of the following steps: (1) Open your mind and take notes; (2) Recognize the structure; (3) Design an organizer; (4) Explain it; and (5) Recycle it. The third component consisted of a substrategy, FLOW, with four steps: (1) Find and list; (2) Look and check; (3) Organize the information; and (4) Work out an organizer. Ss were taught to employ the ORDER strategy with sequentially structured information; the mnemonic keywords ORDER and FLOW were developed to assist Ss in remembering the names of strategy steps and the behaviors associated with each in which they were to engage.	the total number of items listed. Strategy knowledge: Ss were asked to write what each letter in ORDER and FLOW represent. Percentages were obtained of steps correctly named by each subject and of the students who correctly wrote all steps. Student creation of organizers: The first page of the strategy Performance Test contained instructions, a stimulus paragraph, and an example graphic organizer. The second page contained a different stimulus paragraph and three questions requesting that the subject: (1) describe in his/her own words the stimulus paragraph organization; (2) name	experimental Ss without LD compared to control Ss without LD, significant differences did not occur between conditions for Ss with LD. However, some significant differences across times were observed, i.e., some Ss with LD benefited from strategy instruction and others did not.

the manner in which the information was organized; and (3) draw a diagram to illustrate the organization. Responses were scored using a point-by-point system; a holistic scoring system evaluated the overall conceptualization of each graphic organizer.

Consumer satisfaction: Ss and teachers rated their satisfaction with the strategy and the goals, procedures, and strategy instruction outcomes according to a 7-point Likert scale. For each item, the average rating was calculated by dividing the ratings for that item by the total respondents.

(continued)

Author (year)	N	Selection criteria	Target domain(s)	Treatment(s)	Measures	Results
Vellutino, Scanlon, Sipay, Small, Pratt, Cheven, & Denkla (1996)	183	The initial pool consisted of 1,407 kindergartners from 17 schools in six school districts in the Albany, New York, area. The 1st cohort (n = 708) began the study in fall, 1990, and the 2nd cohort (n = 699) entered in fall, 1991. Of these, 1,284 were initially evaluated in November of 1st grade, when classroom teachers rated each S's progress in reading, writing, spelling, and math on a 1- to 5-point Likert scale. Teachers were also asked to identify Ss who met any of the following exclusionary criteria: severe vision or hearing problems; frequent ear infections; severe emotional problems; limited intellectual ability; daily medication, English as a second language; or diagnosed and pervasive neurological disorder. About 15% of the children were considered as candidates for the intervention based on ratings of 1 in reading.	Reading	Two groups of kindergartners completed the kindergarten test battery in 2 consecutive yr. From the lowest achieving students in these groups, Ss were selected to receive remedial tutoring during 1st grade. To distinguish between reading problems caused by cognitive deficits and those related to experiential deficits, these Ss were retested midyear, and only those who did not respond to the tutoring were included as poor readers in this intervention; a group of normal readers was selected from the same classrooms. Poor readers were randomly divided into two groups, tutored and nontutored. Tutored Ss received 30 min/day, one-to-one tutoring for a minimum of 15 wk. Tutoring was individualized according to each subject's needs. Fifteen min of each session was allocated to reading connected text. Treatment goals included reading for meaning and fun; foster use of a variety of word identification strategies; sight vocabulary development; and development of phonemic awareness, the alphabetic principle, and phonetic decoding and writing skills. Fourteen tutors provided the treatment; all were certified teachers.	Pre- and posttest measures were administered during kindergarten and 1st grade. *Kindergarten Battery:* *Language and Language-Based Measures: Phoneme Segmentation; Rapid Automatized Naming* (Denckla & Rudel, 1976a, 1976b); *Rapid Articulation* (adapted from Stanovich, Nathan, & Zolman , 1988); *Syntactic Processing* (measured by the CELF-R Linguistic Concepts subtest; Semel, Wiig, & Secord, 1987); and *Semantic Processing,* (evaluated by the PPVT-R; Dunn & Dunn, 1981). *Memory Measures: Sentence Memory* (verbatim recall of orally presented sentences ranging in length from 4 to	After one semester of assistance, most of the original group of 1st grade poor readers were found to be within or above the average range. At this point, Ss who did not improve demonstrably performed below both those who were readily remediated and normal readers on kindergarten and 1st grade tests evaluating phonological skills, but not on tests evaluating visual, semantic, and syntactic skills. Following treatment, normal readers and tutored Ss were found to differ on some, though not all, measures of the cognitive abilities presumed to underlie reading ability. The authors conclude their results are consistent with previous research findings suggesting that some poor readers' deficits are attributable to phonological processing deficits.

Normal readers of the same sex were randomly selected from each classroom containing the poor readers. Children scoring below the 15th percentile on the WRMT-R Word Identification and Word Attack subtests (Woodcock, 1987) were eligible for inclusion in the poor reader sample; those scoring above the 40th percentile were qualified for the group of normal readers. Children who qualified based on the reading criteria were given the WISC-R (Wechsler, 1974); only those children scoring at or above 90 were qualified for inclusion. Altogether, 118 children qualified as poor readers, and 65 were included as normal readers.	Sessions were audiotaped; 1 of every 10 sessions was selected for review by one of the authors. Individual and biweekly meetings were held to ensure treatment fidelity. Untutored Ss received the remediation provided by their home school. Since these treatments varied across schools, only those Ss receiving small group instruction were included in this study. Ss in the normal reading control group only received the formal reading instruction provided by their classroom teacher.	12 words; *Word Memory* (randomly reordered words from the Sentence Memory Test; task requires recall of the words in the order of presentation); *Visual Memory* (task required reproduction of dot patterns); and *Paired-Associate Learning* (the first 57 items of the WRMT-R Auditory Learning subtest). *Cognitive Processing and General Knowledge Measures: WPPSI-R* Information and Block Design subtests (Wechsler, 1989); and Concrete *Operations* (Piaget, 1952; tasks of conservation, seriation, and class inclusion). *Attention and Organization Measures: Modified MFFT* (adapted from Kagan, 1965); *Target Search* (adapted from Rudel, Denckla, & Broman, 1978).

(*continued*)

Author (year)	*N*	Selection criteria	Target domain(s)	Treatment(s)	Measures	Results
Vellutino, Scanlon, Sipay, Small, Pratt, Cheven, & Denkla (1996) (*cont.*)					*Precursor / Rudimentary Reading Skills Measures: WRMT-R* Letter Identification, Word Identification, and Word Attack; *Print Awareness* (Huba & Kontos; 1985; assesses understanding of communication value of text; and *Print Conventions* (assesses understanding of common print conventions in written English). *Math Measures: WPPSI-R* Arithmetic (assesses understanding of terms referring to quantitative attributes, and comprehension of rudimentary number concepts); and *Experimental math measure* w (assesses the ability to count by rote to 40, skip count to 40, read 1-, 2-, and 3-digit numbers, and solve written number sentences.	

1st Grade Battery:

Intellectual Ability Measure: WISC-R

Reading Achievement Measures: WRMT-R Word Identification, Word Attack, and Basic Skills Cluster; and *Phoneme Segmentation* (the same measure administered in kindergarten).

Intervention Effects:

Reading Achievement Measures: WRMT-R Word Identification, and Word Attack; *Oral Reading Connected Text*; and *Silent Reading Comprehension* (from the Spache Diagnostic Scales; Spache, 1981).

Math Achievement Measures: Woodcock–Johnson Tests of Achievement-Revised Calculations and Applied Problems (Woodcock & Johnson, 1989)

Cognitive Tests:

Phonological Processing Measures: Phoneme

(*continued*)

Author (year)	N	Selection criteria	Target domain(s)	Treatment(s)	Measures	Results
Vellutino, Scanlon, Sipay, Small, Pratt, Cheven, & Denkla (1996) (*cont.*)					*Segmentation* (similar to kindergarten and mid-1st grade); *Phonological Memory* (free recall of auditorially presented items). *Syntactic Processing Measures: Token Test* (DiSimoni, 1978); *Test of Language Development-Primary 2* Grammatic Understanding (TOLD-P:2; Newcomer & Hammill, 1991); *Grammaticality Judgments*; and *Oral Cloze*. *Semantic Processing Measures: WISC-R* Vocabulary and Similarities subtests (Wechsler, 1974). *Naming and Fluency Measures: Rapid Automatized Naming* (similar to kindergarten measure); *Boston Naming Test* (Kaplan, Goodlass, & Weintraub, 1983); and *Verbal Fluency* CELF-R, Semantic Category	

Fluency, and the Controlled Word Association Test, Phonological Category Fluency subtests (Benton & Hamsher, 1989)

General Language Processing Measure: DRS, Listening Comprehension subtest.

Verbal Memory Measure: WISC-R, Digit Span; *TOLD-P 2* , Sentence Imitation; *Recall of Concrete and Abstract Words* (measures immediate and delayed recall); *Phonological Memory* (described above); and *Syntactic Word Order* (working memory task; requires unscrambling of scrambled words from sentences).

Visual Processing Skills Measures: Visuomotor and Visuospatial Ability WISC-R Performance IQ and Block Design; *Visual Memory* (described above).

(*continued*)

Author (year)	N	Selection criteria	Target domain(s)	Treatment(s)	Measures	Results
Wong, Butler, Ficzere, & Kuperis (1996)	38	Adolescents with LD and low achievers in grades 8 and 9 enrolled in modified English classes. LD was defined as (1) adequate intelligence as measured by the WISC (Wechsler, 1974); (2) significant academic delays despite adequate ability; (3) no emotional problems and no physical or sensory handicaps. Low achieving students in this study were those whose best grade was a C–, with a mixture of C–, D, and F grades. Teacher input and formal test performance indicated a need by all Ss for intervention in writing.	Writing (opinion essays) Two groups of	Ss participated in this study. In one group, Ss received explicitly and elaborately modeled training to plan, write, and revise opinion essays. These Ss were randomly divided into pairs, then taught to collaboratively use interactive dialogue to plan and revise their writing, although their essays were independently written. The other group severed as untrained control participants. Training was delivered in several phases. First, use of the planning strategy for writing opinion essays was explicitly and elaborately modeled. Then, Ss were randomly paired and given planning sheets and time for collaboratively planning their essays. Once their plans were judged satisfactory, they began writing independently on a computer. The last phase involved collaborative revision through interactive teacher and peer dialogues. Ss were allowed three periods of about 50 min each for composition of each essay.	Opinion essays were written as pretest, posttest, and maintenance measures. These essays were scored for clarity and cogency. Clarity was defined and scored in terms of the degree to which Ss' writing was free of ambiguity. Cogency was defined as the degree of persuasiveness revealed in Ss' written arguments. Both dimensions were scored on a scale of 1 to 5, with 5 representing the strongest writing.	MANOVAs and effect sizes revealed the clarity and cogency of opinion essays written by trained Ss improved significantly from pre- to posttest. In addition, maintenance of these gains was demonstrable. Further, the performance of trained Ss surpassed that of the untrained control participants.

Johnson, Graham, & Harris (1997)	59	*LD:* 4th and 5th graders (47) receiving services in special education classrooms in one of four suburban elementary schools in Washington, DC. LD Ss met the following stepwise criteria: identification by local school district, WISC-R scores between 80 and 120, Woodcock–Johnson reading scores 1 *SD* or more below the mean, classroom reading placement at a 2nd or 3rd grade level, and absence of other handicapping conditions. *Normally Achieving* (NA)*:* Normative comparison Ss (12) attending the same schools. These Ss were not provided with special education or remedial services, had no reported academic or behavioral problems, were average readers according to their teachers, and had reading scores within one-half an *SD* of the reading test mean. NA Ss were matched with LD Ss on race, sex, and grade. This group only served as a social validation group to assess instructional effectiveness.	Reading comprehension	All conditions in this investigation included features believed essential to the effective implementation the *Self-Regulated Strategy Development* model (SRSD; Graham & Harris, 1993; Harris & Graham, 1992a, 1992b). LD Ss were assigned to one of four instructional conditions: strategy instruction, strategy instruction plus goal setting, strategy instruction plus self-instruction, or strategy instruction plus both goal setting and self-instruction. Five graduate students with field experience serving students with LD were the instructors. Each instructor worked with no more than two groups in each of the experimental conditions. These instructors were trained to implement study procedures and document their provision of lesson steps. Instructors worked with groups of two to three Ss for about 45 min, 2 days/wk, for between 4 and 6 wk. In each condition, active collaboration by Ss was emphasized, with stress on interactive learning and responsibility for strategy selection and use gradually transferred from instructor to student. Interactional scaffolding and Socratic dialogue were used, tailored feedback was provided, strategies were explicitly modeled, and the goal/significance of strategy usage was made clear. Instruction was	Comprehension probes: Five stories, three of which were individually administered by the intervention providers, and two generalization probes administered by classroom teachers. Intervention probes employed a retelling format and were administered as pretest, posttest, and maintenance measures. Generalization probes consisted of a multiple choice format to assess comprehension and were administered just prior to instruction (generalization pretest) and immediately after instruction (generalization posttest). Assignment of both types of probes was counterbalanced. Selection was based on story interest as measured by normally achieving students. Readability was at up-	Reading strategy instruction was associated with significant and generalizable effects on Ss' story comprehension scores. Following instruction, the comprehension of Ss with LD was indistinguishable from that of social comparison Ss. However, explicit instruction in goal setting and self-instruction did not influence significant improvements in the comprehension of Ss with LD.

(*continued*)

Author (year)	N	Selection criteria	Target domain(s)	Treatment(s)	Measures	Results
Johnson, Graham, & Harris (1997) (*cont.*)				criterion-based. Ss in all four conditions received the same program, with the exception that self-regulation procedures were taught in the *strategy plus* conditions. Instructional steps included: (1) preskill development; (2) conferencing; (3) discussion about the learning strategy; (4) modeling; (5) strategy mastery; (6) collaborative practice; and (7) independent practice. Throughout treatment, Ss were encouraged to share their learning with parents and teachers.	per 2nd grade level; length ranged from 800 to 943 words. Retelling measure: Comprehension was operationalized as the amount of information recalled. After reading, Ss were asked to retell the story from memory, and their retellings were audiotaped. A checklist was provided listing main events and details to assist instructors in asking follow-up questions. Three scores were obtained: main ideas, proportion recalled; details recalled, total percent, and a rating for story grammar parts recalled. Strategy usage: Ss' behavior during pretest, posttest, and maintenance probes was observed to document evidence of overt strategy and self-regulation behaviors. Examiners were provided with recording forms to assist them in documenting overt evidence of self-regulation or strategy use.	

Lovett & Steinbach (1997)	122	RD Ss from 7 to 12 yr old; grouped into three developmental levels, i.e., grades 2/3, 4, and 5/6; referred to a clinical research unit for remediation of specific RD. Selection criteria included: substantial underachievement (<20th percentile), replicated on four of five standardized measures of reading (WRAT-3 Reading; WRMT-R Word Identification; WRMT-R Word Attack; PIAT-R Reading Recognition; GFW Sound–Symbol); English as the primary language; average intelligence on both verbal and nonverbal measures (WISC-R, WISC-III: mean VIQ = 91.8; mean PIQ = 99.6). Ss represent a severely impaired sample of RD students, with performance on multiple standardized measures of reading and spelling between 3rd and 4th percentile more than 2 SDs below age expectancies at referral, and half of these Ss were below the 1st percentile. Ss were randomly assigned to one of two word identification training conditions or to a study skills control condition.	Reading	Ss were randomly assigned to groups and teachers who taught all three programs; thirty-five 60-min sessions total were provided to groups of two to three Ss in each condition four times. Both remedial reading treatments consisted of intensive, systematic word identification training which taught procedures for identifying unknown words, with a focus on print training mainly at the words and subword levels. The Phonological Analysis and Blending/Direct Instruction Program (PHAB/DI) focused on remediating deficient phonological analysis and blending skills, with direct instruction of letter–sound mappings. PHAB/DI training was done at the oral level as well as in the context of print presentation and direct instruction of letter–sound and letter cluster–sound correspondences. A special orthography was used to highlight salient features of some letters; it also provided visual cues to facilitate initial learning. Content introduction was structured and gradually sequenced; multiple opportunities were provided for overlearning of content and skills. Cumulative review, massed practice, and teaching skills to mastery were also provided. The Word Identification Strategy Training Program (WIST) taught Ss to acquire, use, and monitor	Pretests and posttests included tests of trained content, transfer-of-learning measures, and a small set of standardized achievement and phonological processing measures. *Training measures:* Tests of instructed content included: (1) 120 *Key Words;* (2) 37 *Letter–Sounds* presented in isolation; and (3) 30 *Letter–Sound* Combinations. *Transfer-of-learning, real words:* The *Test of Transfer* included 371 words that systematically varied from the 120 key word spelling patterns. The *Regular and Exception Word Lists* was an inventory of 149 regular and 149 exception words was administered as a measure of distant transfer of word identification skill.	Both reading interventions were associated with significant improvement in the word identification and word attack skills of RD Ss, including sizable transfer effects. The PHAB/DI program resulted in greater skill transfer across the domain of phonological processing skills. The WIST program resulted in broader transfer from real word training to both regular and irregular words. All Ss experienced equivalent gains from remediation independent of grade level. Overall, the results from this research suggest that RD learners' phonological processing deficits can be remediated through focused and intensive remediation throughout the elementary yr.

(*continued*)

Author (year)	*N*	Selection criteria	Target domain(s)	Treatment(s)	Measures	Results
Lovett & Steinbach (1997) (*cont.*)				four metacognitive decoding strategies; each strategy was taught and practiced with a focus on using current knowledge to aid Ss in decoding unfamiliar words. A system of metacognitive mnemonics was taught to help Ss acquire general routines for implementing and evaluating strategy usage. The control condition involved training with the Classroom Survival Skills Program (CSS). Specific literacy training was not offered; Ss received training in organization strategies, academic problem solving, study, and self-help methods. Control Ss were involved in discussion and planned activities	*Transfer-of-learning, non-words:* Measures of non-word reading included the GFW Reading of Symbols (Goldman, Fristoe, & Woodcock, 1974) and the WRMT-R Word Attack (Woodcock, 1987). *Standardized measures:* Phonological measures included the Goldman–Fristoe–Woodcock Sound Analysis, Sound Blending, and Sound–Symbol Association subtests (Goldman, Fristoe, & Woodcock, 1974). Reading measures included the WRAT-R/WRAT-3 Reading (Jastak & Wilkinson, 1984, 1991) and the WRMT-R Word Identification subtests. Spelling measures included the WRAT-R/WRAT-3 Spelling, PIAT-R Spelling (Markwardt, 1989), and the GFW Spelling of Sounds subtests.	

McNaughton, Hughes, & Ofiesh (1997)	3	High school students with LD were selected according to the following criteria: (1) between the ages of 15 and 18; (2) identified LD as defined by the Commonwealth of Pennsylvania for placement in special education; (3) experienced in using Microsoft Word and able to demonstrate basic competency in using a spell checker; (4) identified as being functionally disabled in spelling as defined by a spelling error rate more than 2 *SD* below the performance of peers when a spell checker was used; (5) spelling scores 2 *SD* below academic peers on a standardized norreferenced test; and (6) referred by the resource teacher for proofreading skills instruction.	Proofreading performance	This study investigated the effect of training an integrated proofreading strategy, InSPECT, combining a computer-based spell checker and student strategies. Ss were taught to apply a five-step proofreading strategy using controlled and student written materials. Each set of controlled proofreading materials contained a passage with spelling errors typical of those made by students with LD and a list of words identified as problematic for secondary and college students. A multiple-probe across-subjects design was used; sessions occurred three times/wk, with maintenance data collected 1, 2 and 4 wk following treatment. During BL, data were obtained on preintervention spelling performance. Ss completed probe activities; they also participated in norm-referenced testing activities and two sets of generalization activities. During intervention, instruction was introduced for the first subject once stable a BL was achieved; the remaining Ss remained in BL conditions until the first subject's data revealed an upward trend, then treatment was introduced to the second subject. Introduction of treatment for the third subject followed the same procedures. Intervention continued until	Data were collected on strategy use, spelling error correction rate, and final error rate during probes across all three phases. In addition, generalization data were obtained using subject written and subject transcribed compositions collected during BL and maintenance.	The data revealed increased strategy use and improvements in spelling errors corrected on both controlled proofreading materials and on subject written compositions. Postintervention, all three Ss produced writing that contained final spelling error rates that fell within the performance range of their NLD peers.

(continued)

Author (year)	*N*	Selection criteria	Target domain(s)	Treatment(s)	Measures	Results
McNaughton, Hughes, & Ofiesh (1997) (*cont.*)				80% success for strategy use was observed on three successive probes. A six-step instructional sequence was followed: (1) Pretest and make commitments; (2) Describe strategy; (3) Model the strategy; (4) Verbal practice; (5) Practice with controlled and student-written materials; and (6) Provide generalization training. During the maintenance phase, proofreading probes with controlled materials were used. During generalization activities, Ss wrote on an assigned topic and transcribed a dictated passage. No comments were made by the investigator about using the proofreading strategy.		
Torgesen, Wagner, Rashotte, Alexander, & Conway (1997)	*Study 1:* 180 *Study 2:* 31	*Study 1:* Ss were not held back either in kindergarten or 1st grade, and selected based on scores from measures of letter name knowledge and phonological awareness. Children likely to be in the bottom 10% of readers by the end of 2nd grade were identified using logistic regression; those with verbal IQs below 75 on the Stanford–Binet Vocabulary subtest (Thorndike, Hagen, & Sattler, 1986) were eliminated.	Word reading Phonological awareness	Prevention and remediation of severe RD were examined in two studies. One focused on alternative approaches to prevention; the other examined the efficacy of remediation using similar methods. Two intervention programs containing relatively explicit phonics instruction were contrasted. *Phonological Awareness Plus Synthetic Phonics* (PASP), based on the Auditory Discrimination in Depth method (Lindamood & Lindamood, 1984), targets the stimulation of phonological awareness through articulatory position and movement exercises and explicit		

	Study 2: Children identified by the public school system as LD; nominated by the special education teachers as those having the greatest problems acquiring word level reading skill. Ss were screened to verify: (1) average standard scores on two measures of word level reading at least 1.5 SDs below average for age; (2) estimated verbal intelligence above 75; (3) phonological awareness below minimum levels for grade as measured by the Lindamood Auditory Conceptualization Test (LAC; Lindamood & Lindamood, 1979); and (4) no evidence of sensory impairment, neurological damage or disease, or English as a second language. Average Full Scale IQ for Ss in this study is 92. Ss were randomly assigned to one of two treatments.	instruction in letter–sound relations. *Embedded Phonics* (EP) consists of systematic, though less intensive, phonics instruction within the context of early and meaningful reading and writing experiences. The *Prevention* study provided supplemental reading instruction since kindergarten to Ss randomly assigned to one of four groups: (1) phonological awareness training plus synthetic phonics instruction (PASP); (2) implicit phonological awareness training plus phonics instruction embedded within classroom reading and spelling activities (EP); (3) individual instruction provided in a regular classroom group to support attainment of goals in the regular classroom reading program (RCS); and, (4) a no-treatment control group. Ss in each group received 80 min of one-on-one supplemental instruction/wk. In the *Remediation* study, Ss with LD received 2 intensive one-to-one instruction in PASP or EP for 80 min each week during a 2½-year period.

Note. LD = learning disabled, NLD = nonlearning disabled, CAT = California Achievement Test, Full Scale = Full Scale Intelligence score, *SD* = standard deviation, BD = behavior disordered, SLD = severe or specific learning disabled, WRAT = Wide Range Achievement Test, WISC = Wechsler Intelligence Test for Children, WISC-R = Wechsler Intelligence Test for Children—Revised. SORT = Slosson Oral Reading Test, Stanford–Binet = Stanford–Binet Intelligence Test, SIT = Slosson Intelligence Test, PPVT = Peabody Picture Vocabulary Test, PIAT = Peabody Individual Achievement Test, Bender–Gestalt = Bender Visual Motor Gestalt Test, KeyMath = KeyMath Diagnostic Arithmatic Test, WAIS = Wechsler Adult Intelligence Test, VIQ = Verbal Intelligence, PIQ = Performance Intelligence, GORT = Gray Oral Reading Test, WRMT = Woodcock Reading Mastery Test, ITPA = Illinois Test of Psycholinguistic Abilities, EFT = Embedded Figures Test, VMI = Visual Motor Integration Test, DTLA = Detroit Test of Learning Aptitude.

Index

Note. Tables and figures are indicted by "*t*" and "*f*," respectively. Notes are indicated by "*n*."

D

F

G

J

K

L

N

Q

R

S

U

V

W